M O N

Breast Pathology
Diagnosis by Needle Core Biopsy
THIRD EDITION

Breast Pathology
Diagnosis by Needle Core Biopsy
THIRD EDITION

■ PAUL PETER ROSEN, M.D.

Emeritus Professor of Pathology
Weill Medical College of
Cornell University
Formerly, Chief of Breast Pathology
New York Presbyterian Hospital
Cornell Center
New York, New York

■ SYED A. HODA, M.D.

Professor of Clinical Pathology
Weill Medical College of
Cornell University
Attending Pathologist
New York Presbyterian Hospital
Cornell Center
New York, New York

●. Wolters Kluwer | Lippincott Williams & Wilkins
Health
Philadelphia · Baltimore · New York · London
Buenos Aires · Hong Kong · Sydney · Tokyo

Senior Executive Editor: Jonathan W. Pine, Jr.
Product Manager: Marian Bellus
Vendor Manager: Bridgett Dougherty
Senior Manufacturing Manager: Benjamin Rivera
Senior Marketing Manager: Angela Panetta
Creative Director: Doug Smock
Production Service: MPS Limited, A Macmillan Company

Two Commerce Square
2001 Market Street
Philadelphia, PA 19103

© 2006, 1999 Lippincott Williams & Wilkins.

Printed in the People's Republic of China.

Cover images: Top Row: Myoepithelial hyperplasia in adenosis in fat; myoepithelial hyperplasia in adenosis in fat; myoepithelial cell nuclei are highlighted by the p63 immunostain; intraductal myoepithelial carcinoma; intraductal myoepithelial carcinoma with diffuse nuclear reactivity for p63. *Bottom Row:* Florid intraductal lobular carcinoma *in situ* composed of cells with cytoplasmic mucin; florid intraductal lobular carcinoma *in situ*; E-cadherin immunoreactivity is absent; granular cell tumor surrounding a duct; intraductal papillomas with histiocytes in fibrovascular stroma.

Library of Congress Cataloging-in-Publication Data

Rosen, Paul Peter.
Breast pathology: diagnosis by needle core biopsy/Paul Peter Rosen, Syed A. Hoda.—3rd ed.
      p. ; cm.
   Includes bibliographical references and index.
   ISBN 978-1-60831-670-0 (alk. paper)
   1. Breast—Needle biopsy. 2. Breast—Diseases—Diagnosis.
   3. Breast—Histopathology. I. Hoda, Syed A. II. Title.
   [DNLM: 1. Breast Neoplasms—pathology. 2. Biopsy, Needle.
   3. Breast—pathology. WP 870 R813b 2010]
   RG493.5.B56R67 2010
   616.99'44907—dc22
                                                          2010011834

                                   9 8 7 6 5 4 3 2

In memory of
Flora Caspari and Paul Caspari, M.D.
Rose Rosen and Morris Rosen
and for
Mary Sue Rosen
Deborah, Madelyn, John
Jon, Karen, Jordan, Mitch
Stacy, James, Paige, Denis

In memory of
Rabia Hoda and Qamar Hoda
and for
Rana Hoda and Raza Hoda

Contents

Preface to First Edition (Updated) vii
Preface to Third Edition ix
Acknowledgments x
Introduction xi

1 Anatomy and Physiologic Morphology 1

2 Inflammatory and Reactive Tumors 9

3 Specific Infections 23

4 Benign Papillary Tumors 27

5 Myoepithelial Neoplasms 52

6 Adenosis and Microglandular Adenosis 61

7 Fibroepithelial Neoplasms 77

8 Ductal Hyperplasia and Intraductal Carcinoma 97

9 Invasive Duct Carcinoma 144

10 Tubular Carcinoma 161

11 Papillary Carcinoma 171

12 Medullary Carcinoma 187

13 Carcinoma with Metaplasia 191

14 Squamous Carcinoma 202

15 Mucinous Carcinoma 205

16 Apocrine Carcinoma 213

17 Adenoid Cystic Carcinoma 223

18 Secretory Carcinoma 229

19 Cystic Hypersecretory Carcinoma 233

20 Other Special Types of Invasive Duct Carcinoma 237

21 Lobular Carcinoma In Situ and Atypical Lobular Hyperplasia 246

22 Invasive Lobular Carcinoma 263

23 Mesenchymal Neoplasms 274

24 Lymphoid and Hematopoietic Tumors 303

25 Metastases in the Breast from Nonmammary Malignant Neoplasms 313

26 Pathologic Effects of Therapy 319

27 Breast Lesions in Men and Children 329

28 Pathologic Changes Associated with Needling Procedures 340

29 Specimen Processing, Pathologic Examination, and Reporting 348

Index 360

Preface to First Edition (Updated)

Prior to the widespread implementation of breast conservation therapy, the role of the pathologist in breast cancer care was limited to making the diagnosis from tissue obtained by surgical biopsy and documenting the extent of the tumor after a mastectomy was performed. These two events typically centered around a single operative procedure in which the diagnosis made with a frozen section was followed by a mastectomy and axillary lymph node dissection. Presently, considerably more information is required to recommend breast cancer treatment that may employ more than one of the major existing therapeutic modalities: surgery, radiation, and chemotherapy. An important part of the data used for therapeutic decisions is generated by the pathologist using routine histopathologic procedures and immunohistochemistry.

The complex multifactorial description of breast pathology now considered to be standard practice has expanded the diagnostic report from a brief one- or two-line statement, such as "Infiltrating duct carcinoma, grade II; negative lymph nodes" to a catalogue of data one or more pages in length, often including many statements indicating the absence as well as the presence of features regarded as relevant to therapeutic decisions and to prognosis. A partial list of this information includes classification of the carcinoma, histologic grade, nuclear grade, tumor size, and statements about vascular invasion, the proportion of the in situ component in invasive lesions, subtype of in situ carcinoma, multifocality, and proximity of carcinoma to margins of excision. Immunohistochemistry is used to characterize distribution of estrogen and progesterone receptors, as well as other biomarkers and oncogene expression which are part of pathology reports. Proliferative activity may be estimated by the pathologist using immunohistochemistry.

Other advances have added to the complexity of the pathologist's role in breast cancer treatment. Primary among these is the widespread use of needle core biopsy procedures, especially for the diagnosis of nonpalpable mammographically detected lesions. Stereotactic needle core biopsy is an extremely valuable tool in planning breast conservation therapy because it can establish the diagnosis of nonpalpable lesions before operative surgical intervention. Needle core biopsy procedures often yield diagnostic samples, but in a significant number of cases the material obtained offers ambiguous findings that do not provide a specific diagnosis on which to base

therapy. This is a limitation of the procedure and not a failure on the part of the pathologist or radiologist. When this situation arises, it is necessary for physicians caring for the patient to consider the entire clinical situation. This process of reflection is often referred to as "clinical correlation."

Many mammographically detected nonpalpable lesions present the pathologist with challenging diagnostic problems when excised intact and viewed in context with surrounding tissues. The appearance of such lesions in the incomplete and often disrupted form of needle core biopsy samples can substantially increase the degree of difficulty. The major differential diagnostic problems encountered in these specimens include:

- reactive changes vs. recurrent carcinoma after lumpectomy
- benign sclerosing lesions (radial scar) vs. infiltrating carcinoma
- papilloma vs. papillary carcinoma
- fibroadenoma vs. cystosarcoma
- atypical duct hyperplasia vs. intraductal carcinoma (DCIS)
- DCIS vs. DCIS with (micro)invasion
- spindle cell tumors (metaplastic carcinoma vs. sarcoma)
- vascular lesions (angioma vs. angiosarcoma)

Although self-evident, it is important to understand that the diagnosis made with a needle core biopsy specimen can only be based on the samples available to the pathologist and that these samples are not always representative of all of the pathologic findings in a given case. Consequently, carcinoma may be found in up to 50% of surgical biopsies after a needle core biopsy diagnosis of atypical hyperplasia, and microinvasion may be present in about 20% of surgical excisions after a needle core diagnosis of intraductal carcinoma. Three principles offer guidance in the use of the needle core biopsy procedure for the diagnosis and treatment of breast lesions:

- Anything can turn up.
- What you see is what you have and it may not be all there is.
- What you have may be all there is.

The emergence of the needle core biopsy procedure as a major diagnostic tool epitomizes the growing complexity of the interaction of radiologists, surgeons, and pathologists in the diagnosis and management of mammary diseases, especially in the era of breast conservation therapy. Specialization in medicine has created circumstances in which the specialist physician is increasingly dependent on the assistance of colleagues who have acquired complementary expertise. This evolving situation has contributed to the team approach to disease management reflected in this volume. The intentional limited scope of this presentation, which focuses on diagnosis, does not permit inclusion of contributions from other important members of the team, including surgeons, radiotherapists, and medical oncologists who depend on these diagnoses to implement therapy.

Paul Peter Rosen, M.D.

Preface to Third Edition

This third edition of *Breast Pathology Diagnosis by Needle Core Biopsy* builds upon the two preceding volumes. A substantial number of images have been added, and a few images have been replaced. New and updated information is provided on laboratory procedures for processing needle core biopsy samples, the use of immunohistochemistry and molecular studies in the diagnosis of breast lesions, and differential diagnosis. The advantages and limitations of needle core biopsy sampling are emphasized throughout the text. New topics include basal-like and triple negative carcinoma.

As new information, references, and illustrations have been added, it has become necessary to omit selected references and text that appeared in the second edition to limit the book to a manageable size. As a consequence, we are no longer able to include chapters on the clinical aspects of imaging and needle core biopsy techniques that appeared in prior editions.

This edition has been thoroughly reviewed, rewritten, and subjected to rigorous scrutiny by the publisher's excellent staff at various stages in the production process. The choice of illustrations and references, the selection of data cited, and the conclusions expressed reflect the authors' experience and opinions.

Paul Peter Rosen, M.D.

Acknowledgments

The potential for the team approach to cancer treatment is epitomized in the management of patients with mammographically detected breast lesions, the most likely candidates for the needle core biopsy procedure. This effort draws upon the skills of mammographers, pathologists, and surgeons, as well as radiation therapists and medical oncologists. We are grateful to the hundreds of pathologists, surgeons, medical oncologists, and radiologists throughout the United States and abroad who contributed cases for pathology consultation that may be illustrated in this book, and to their patients.

The new illustrations in this book were taken from cases seen in consultation submitted from other institutions or diagnosed and treated at the New York-Presbyterian Hospital. Each specimen is vitally important to the individual from whom it was obtained, and we endeavor to provide a specific diagnosis that will contribute to the clinical care of that patient. This material is also a priceless resource for research and teaching. Thousands of adult women as well as many hundreds of men and children afflicted with breast diseases who cannot be recognized individually are acknowledged for their anonymous contributions to this and prior editions of *Breast Pathology, Diagnosis by Needle Core Biopsy*.

Knowledge gained in the course of providing this clinical service contributes to providing better care to patients with breast diseases. In this sense, each patient who has had a diagnosis made in the nearly 40 years of this consultation practice has participated in the academic undertaking and contributed to improving the diagnostic skill in breast pathology of hundreds of pathologists in training, to the benefit of still more individuals.

We also wish to recognize the superb support of the publisher for this project, most notably Marian Bellus, product manager, and Johnathan Pine as senior executive editor, from the earliest discussions of the concept for this third edition to the final publication.

We are indebted to Mary Sue Rosen for her loyal commitment, editorial assistance, and close attention to detail in preparing this manuscript. She is largely responsible for the timely completion of this edition.

All new photographic images in this edition were processed digitally by Ms. Patricia Kuharic in the Medical Arts Department of the Weill Cornell Medical College. We express our deep appreciation for her high professional standards that have made an essential contribution to this volume. We acknowledge with gratitude Daniel M. Knowles, M.D., the David D. Thompson, Professor of Pathology and Chairman of Pathology and Laboratory Medicine, for his continued support in establishing and fostering the growth of the Breast Pathology Consultation Service at the New York Presbyterian Hospital.

Introduction

Noninvasive techniques have been employed to study breast lesions since the beginning of the 20th century. The usefulness of this approach in the clinical setting has been dependent on technical advances that permitted the radiologist to detect lesions that were inapparent to the patient and physician, including clinically occult carcinomas. A consequence of this advance has been the need for a close working relationship between the practitioners of several medical specialties. The result is certainly one of the important examples of "team" management that requires the cooperative efforts of medical specialists to provide effective patient care.

Two methods of nonsurgical investigation of the breast were studied in the 1920s and early 1930s, namely, transillumination and radiography. As Cutler (1) reported, the idea for transillumination as a means of diagnosis "was first developed among the members of the laboratory staff of Memorial Hospital during the routine examination of breast specimens." Cutler also stated that "at the suggestion of Dr. Ewing, . . . Adair attempted to transilluminate breasts but encountered technical difficulties, chiefly due to the excessive heat developed by the transilluminating lamp." Although Cutler improved upon the light source, it is clear that transillumination offered little as a method of diagnosis except possibly as a way to distinguish between cystic and solid lesions. With widespread acceptance of needle aspiration of cysts, transillumination was abandoned and has now been replaced by ultrasonography.

The earliest radiologic studies of the breast reported in the United States in the 1930s by Fray and Warren, by Seabold, and by Lockwood were contemporaneous with similar investigations in Europe (2–7). When first employed clinically, it was apparent that roentgenography might prove helpful in the diagnosis of so-called early breast carcinoma. The definition of "early" has changed appreciably since this concept was introduced. This change is exemplified in a 1932 report by Fray and Warren (2) that described a 54-year-old woman who, on clinical examination, was thought to have chronic cystic mastitis. Roentgenologic examination revealed "a small area of dense tissue with irregular margins . . . in the left breast." The lesion proved on biopsy to be a carcinoma "the size of a walnut." It was concluded by the authors that the early status (of the tumor) was reflected not only by its small size but in the absence of macroscopic involvement of pectoral muscles. Today, the case described by Fray and Warren would be considered operable and potentially curable but not "early." Within a relatively short period, the term early has come to be used for lesions of microscopic dimensions, often detectable only by imaging techniques that include mammography, ultrasonography, and magnetic resonance imaging (MRI).

The initial mammography studies were met with skepticism. In 1931, Seabold (5) described the mammographic findings in a series of cases presented to the Philadelphia Academy of Surgery. The summary of the discussion that followed his report included the following comment:

> Dr. J. Stewart Rodman said that any attempt to make the diagnosis more exact is certainly praiseworthy. Being a surgeon, however, he is not sure but that sometimes x-ray men have somewhat vivid imaginations.... The clinical diagnosis of carcinoma of the breast and chronic cystic mastitis is not ordinarily difficult, and therefore until we have x-ray evidence of a more positive value we had best go a little slow in accepting evidence which is contrary to clinical findings.

Gunsett and Sichel (7) stated in 1934 that their x-ray images might be useful in some cases, but that radiologic distinctions between benign and malignant lesions were not precise enough to form a basis for surgical treatment. They concluded that mammography would not replace biopsy as a diagnostic procedure. The warning offered in these comments is applicable today. The clinician faced with a palpable abnormality in the breast should not depend only on mammography to decide whether biopsy is required. On the other hand, advances in clinical mammography and the development of stereotactic biopsy instruments have made it possible to detect and perform biopsies on nonpalpable lesions found by "x-ray men" who "have vivid imaginations" (5).

The need to relate radiologic findings to the histopathologic examination of breast tissue has been appreciated since the earliest x-ray images of the breast were obtained. In 1913 Albert Salomon (8), a surgeon at the University of Berlin, described a method for obtaining roentgenograms of serial sections of surgical breast specimens in order to correlate histologic observations with the specimen x-rays. The histologic appearance of calcification within a mammary carcinoma was described in his paper. Salomon may be credited with the first reported example of breast specimen radiography, and he deserves recognition for investigations that anticipated later developments in mammography and specimen radiography.

Detailed pathologic–radiologic correlations were carried out in the late 1920s by Dominguez (9–11) in Montevideo,

Uruguay. Dominguez was especially interested in studying the properties of calcifications in breast lesions. In addition to specimen radiography, he undertook biochemical analyses of the calcium content of breast tissue. Conway (12) described the clinical radiologic appearance of calcification in breast cysts and sarcomatous tumors, but failed to appreciate the potential usefulness of calcification as an x-ray marker for carcinoma. Lockwood (3) stressed the importance of correlating pathologic and radiologic findings, but did not obtain x-rays of specimens, and there was no mention of mammary calcification as an indicator of carcinoma in his report. Warren (6) described two cases thought roentgenologically to be carcinoma but reported to be benign on pathologic examination that "could not be studied because the specimens were thrown out before films could be made to locate the supposed small area of malignancy seen at the original examination."

The observations of Salomon, and later Dominguez, that calcium deposits in mammary carcinoma could be visualized radiologically remained largely unappreciated for nearly two decades. They were again brought to attention by Leborgne (13,14) in Montevideo who developed a technique for soft tissue roentgenography that made it possibly to identify small tumors and calcifications in clinical mammograms. He noted that "the roentgenographic study of the operative specimen also permitted the localization of the tiny calcifications for histopathologic study, and thus aided in finding a small cancer that would otherwise have been overlooked." As had Gershon-Cohen (15) some years earlier, Leborgne anticipated the role of mammography for detecting preclinical cancer:

> We firmly believe that the recognition and demonstration of this roentgenographic sign constitutes one of the easily observed aspects in which mammary cancer is presented, especially in its ductal form . . . and (is) therefore susceptible of detection in prophylactic examinations of women who do not yet present clinical tumor symptomology. With a systematic prophylactic roentgenographic examination of all women with antecedents of cancer in their family, we enter a new stage in the fight against mammary cancer.

The origin of modern needle core biopsy sampling of the breast to obtain a tissue specimen for histologic diagnosis is entwined with the history of needle aspiration biopsy and parallels the development of clinical mammography. Needles have been used to obtain samples for diagnosis from various anatomic sites since the middle of the 19th century (16). Needle aspiration sampling of the lung (17,18) and lymph nodes (19–21) was described by 1914. Many of the early biopsy attempts involved aspirating cells with a needle attached to a syringe. The aspirated blood and cellular material were expressed onto a slide and spread thinly to create a cytologic preparation.

The application of the needle aspiration biopsy technique to the diagnosis of neoplastic conditions attracted attention early in the 20th century. In 1921, Guthrie (22) reported that needle aspiration could be employed to evaluate the causes of lymph node enlargement. A method for aspirating cells from lymph nodes and the preparation of stained slides from this material was described in detail by Forkner (23) who also reported his experience using these samples for the diagnosis of cancer, including three women with adenocarcinoma in axillary lymph nodes (24).

The first concerted effort to employ the needle aspiration technique to the diagnosis of cancer was undertaken at Memorial Hospital in New York. In 1922, E.B. Ellis (25), a technician working under Dr. James Ewing, described cancer cells in cell block specimens of pleural fluid. Ellis concluded that "the diagnosis of cancer from direct smears is hazardous, but when one has made thin paraffin sections of suspected material and their evidence is fortified by some confirmatory clinical data, positive diagnosis may often be obtained." Four years later, Hayes Martin, a surgeon at Memorial Hospital, Fred Stewart, then the junior associate of Dr. Ewing, and Ellis began to use the aspiration biopsy technique in patients with head and neck cancer (26). In succeeding publications, they documented the applicability of the aspiration biopsy technique to a variety of tumors and defined the role of this procedure in the clinical management of cancer patients (27,28).

The Memorial Hospital technique proved to be the forerunner of what are now two largely separate methods of diagnosis: fine-needle aspiration (FNA) and needle core biopsy.

The specimens obtained by Martin and his clinical colleagues included disaggregated cells for cytologic examination, equivalent to FNA today, and fragments of tissue that they described as the clot, a counterpart of the modern needle core biopsy specimen. Ewing, Stewart, and their colleagues were not prepared to rely entirely on cytologic smears as evidenced by the importance they attached to the "clot," described in following commentary by Godwin (29):

> After the material is obtained in the syringe, the negative pressure is released to obviate splattering of the aspirate in the syringe. With the rake, the material is placed on several slides and gently smeared by approximating two slides and pulling them apart. The remaining material is placed on a small piece of blotting paper or fibrin foam and put in formalin for later paraffin section. This is designated as the clot.

The clot was "helpful in many instances where the smear is not diagnostic and in making a more definitive diagnosis as to the type of tumor" (29).

The system of aspirating tumors for diagnosis implemented at Memorial Hospital in the 1920s and 1930s evolved as a result of experience gained by the participants in this effort. In a later review, Godwin (30) observed:

> The interpretation of aspirates, as with other pathological material, is certainly not without pitfalls. It requires experience. It is necessary that a sufficient number of cases be available for both clinician and pathologist to maintain their efficiency. The pathologist must know the clinical setting, the normal cells of the region, and the nature of lesions to be anticipated in the area.

Technologic developments in imaging have played a major role in advancing the use of needles to obtain tissue samples from lesions in superficial and visceral locations. The impetus for improving needle biopsy techniques for breast lesions began with the increasing utilization of mammography in the 1960s and 1970s. The mammographic detection of nonpalpable lesions presented a diagnostic challenge to the radiologist, surgeon, and pathologist and led to the development of methods to localize nonpalpable lesions so that they could be found and excised by surgeons and sampled in the pathology laboratory. Various localizing procedures were introduced, employing needles, wires, dyes, and other markers placed in or near the lesion under mammographic or ultrasound guidance. After localization by the radiologist, the surgeon was guided by the marker. Radiographic examination of the specimen (specimen radiography) has been employed to confirm excision of a nonpalpable abnormality and to help the pathologist pinpoint the lesion for histologic examination (31–33). Specimen radiography has been particularly useful for lesions containing calcifications.

Under optimal conditions where a surgical biopsy was recommended for mammographic abnormalities with calcifications that were considered to be suspicious for carcinoma, 25% to 30% of the excised lesions proved to be carcinoma (32,33). Thus, for each patient with a biopsy sample that revealed carcinoma, three underwent surgical excision of a benign lesion. The surgical management of nonpalpable breast lesions without calcifications was more difficult because specimen radiography was not very reliable for confirming the adequacy of excision. The availability of the modern needle core biopsy procedure to sample nonpalpable mammographically detected lesions made it possible to avoid surgical biopsy in a substantial number of women. Friese et al. (34) analyzed Surveillance, Epidemiology, and End Results (SEER)-Medicare data for 45,542 patients with intraductal and invasive stage I–II breast carcinoma diagnosed between 1991 and 1999. The frequency of needle core biopsy as the first procedure increased from approximately 20% in 1991 to 30.9% in 1999 ($p < 0001$), and there was a concomitant decrease in initial surgical biopsy procedures. Women who had a needle core biopsy procedure initially tended to have fewer surgical procedures overall than those whose first biopsy specimen was obtained surgically.

The introduction of stereotaxic devices in the 1970s resulted in improved needle localization and made it possible to obtain needle biopsy samples from nonpalpable lesions more efficiently (35,36). One of the first papers described a "stereotaxic instrument" that facilitated "percutaneous needle biopsy of the breast for microscopic diagnosis" (37). The authors reported that "the sampling site can be located at a precision of ± 1 mm. The instrument can also be used for positioning of metal and dye indicators for guiding surgery and for post-operative identification of excised tumors." Linkage of this computer-guided localization system with the automated

biopsy gun introduced in the 1980s (38) led to the development of modern stereotaxic core biopsy instruments (39). Ultrasound-guided core biopsy has proven to be particularly effective for nonpalpable lesions without calcifications. Stereotaxic MRI and ultrasound-guided core biopsy procedures are now widely used for the diagnosis of breast diseases. These technologies provide efficient methods for sampling small areas rapidly, with less morbidity and expense than surgical excision (40–42). Multifocal lesions are also accessible with this approach (43).

Needle core biopsy procedures provide the pathologist with tissue specimens that are processed to produce histologic sections. While satisfying the preference of surgical pathologists for a tissue sample rather than a cytology specimen, needle core biopsy samples create new diagnostic problems and challenges. To some extent, these difficulties arise from the partial view of a lesion in the core biopsy specimen. This problem can be compounded by the heterogeneous nature of some tumors such as papillary and fibroepithelial lesions as well as carcinomas (44). The context of surrounding tissue afforded by sections of surgical biopsy specimens, important in some instances, is largely lacking in needle core biopsy samples. Nonpalpable lesions are frequently small abnormalities that can be difficult to interpret even in a complete excisional biopsy specimen, and they should not be submitted for frozen section examination except in extraordinary circumstances (45).

False negative results for needle core biopsy samples are lower when specimens are obtained by using techniques that produce larger samples such as 11-gauge and vacuum-assisted instruments (46,47). Failure to sample a carcinoma that is present is more likely to occur in cases where the target is solely microcalcifications than a mass lesion (48). Consequently, intraductal carcinoma, especially the noncomedo type, is more likely to be missed than is invasive carcinoma. False-negative needle core biopsy samples can usually be appreciated prospectively because of discordance between the imaging studies for which the procedure was performed and the pathology diagnosis (49).

The accuracy of needle core biopsy sampling is so precise that imaging evidence of the target may be lost after the procedure, and in some cases the lesion itself may be entirely extirpated (50, 51). When all imaging evidence of carcinoma has been removed, up to nearly 80% of patients have residual carcinoma in a subsequent excisional biopsy. Lee et al. (52) reported that the MRI targeted lesion was completely extirpated in 30% of carcinomas diagnosed by MRI guided vacuum-assisted needle core biopsy. Nonetheless, 64% of patients whose MRI-detected lesion had been removed had residual carcinoma. Liberman et al. (53) found that the mammographic target was entirely removed in 100 of 214 (47%) carcinomas and that carcinomas remained in 79% of cases after complete removal of the imaging abnormality.

To assist the surgeon and pathologist in finding the site of a prior needle core biopsy where part or all of the lesion may have been removed, a clip may be placed in the biopsy cavity at the conclusion of the procedure. Sometimes multiple clips are used to bracket a lesion or to mark more than one biopsy site. Clips of differing shapes are available and various types may be employed with mammographic, sonographic, or MRI-guided biopsy procedures (52,54,55). Migration of clips (56), extraction of the clip during a vacuum-assisted biopsy procedure (57), and loss of the clip during surgical excision (54) have been reported.

Relatively common diagnostic problems encountered in needle core biopsy specimens include the following: columnar cell lesions and atypical hyperplasia, radial sclerosing lesions and papillary tumors, lobular atypia, and lobular carcinoma in situ. Unusual tumors previously encountered only in surgical biopsy specimens such as pseudoangiomatous stromal hyperplasia, mucocele-like lesions, myofibroblastoma, metaplastic carcinoma, and hemangiomas are now the targets of stereotaxic needle core biopsy procedures (45,58). Today, virtually any lesion that occurs in the breast may appear on the pathologist's microscope in a needle core biopsy sample. The purpose of this book is to provide guidance in the interpretation of diagnosis of needle core specimens and the pathologic changes that occur in the breast as a result of these procedures.

REFERENCES

1. Cutler M. Transillumination as an aid in the diagnosis of breast lesions, with special reference to its value in cases of bleeding nipple. *Surg Gynecol Obstet.* 1929;48:721–729.
2. Fray WW, Warren SL. Stereoscopic roentgenography of breasts. An aid in establishing the diagnosis of mastitis and carcinoma. *Ann Surg.* 1932; 95:425–432.
3. Lockwood IH. Roentgen ray evaluation of breast symptoms. *Am J Roentgenol.* 1933;29:145–155.
4. Seabold PS. Roentgenographic diagnosis of diseases of the breast. *Surg Gynecol Obstet.* 1931;53:461–468.
5. Seabold PS. Diagnosis of breast disease by x-ray. *Ann Surg.* 1931;94:443.
6. Warren SL. Roentgenologic study of the breast. *Am J Roentgenol.* 1930; 24:113–124.
7. Gunsett A, Sichel G. Sur la valeur praticque de la radiographie du sein. J de radiol et d électrol. 1934;18:611–614.
8. Salomon A. Beiträge zur Pathologie und Klinik der Mammacarcinome. *Archiv für Klin Chirurgie.* 1913;101:573–668.
9. Dominguez CM. Estudio sistematizado del cancer del seno. *Boll Liga Uruguay contra el cancer genit gemen.* 1929;1:23.
10. Dominguez CM. Estudio radiologico de los descalcificadores. *Boll Soc Anatomia Patologica.* 1930;1:175.
11. Dominiguez CM, Lucas A. Investigacion radiografica y quimica sobre el calcio precipitado en tumores del aparato genital feminio. *Boll Soc Anatomia Patologica.* 1930;1:217.
12. Conway JH. Calcified breast tumors. *Am J Surg.* 1936;31:72–76.
13. Leborgne R. Diagnostico de los tumores de la mamma por la radiografia simple. *Boll Cir Uruguay.* 1949;20:407.
14. Leborgne R. Diagnosis of tumors of the breast by simple roentgenography. Calcifications in carcinomas. *Am J Roentgenol.* 1951;65:1–11.
15. Gershon-Cohen J, Colcher AE. An evaluation of the roentgen diagnosis of early carcinoma of the breast. *JAMA.* 1937;108:867–871.
16. Webb AJ. Through a glass darkly. (The development of needle aspiration biopsy). *Bristol Med Chir J.* 1974;89:59–68.
17. Horder TJ. Lung puncture: a new application of clinical pathology. *Lancet.* 1909;2:1345–1346;1539–1540.
18. Leyden OO. Ueber infectiöse Pneumonie. *Dtsch Med Wochenschr.* 1883; 9:52–54.
19. White WC, Pröscher F. Spirochaetes in acute lymphatic leukemia and in chronic benign lymphomatosis (Hodgkin's disease). *JAMA.* 1907;69:1115.
20. Grieg EDW, Gray ACH. Note on the lymphatic glands in sleeping sickness. *Lancet.* 1914;1:1570.
21. Chatard JA, Guthrie CG. Human trypanosomiasis: report of a case observed in Baltimore. *Am J Trop Dis Prev Med.* 1914;1:493–505.
22. Guthrie CG. Gland puncture as a diagnostic measure. *Bull Johns Hopkins Hosp.* 1921;32:266–269.
23. Forkner CE. Material from lymph nodes in man. I. Method to obtain material by puncture of lymph nodes for study with supravital and fixed stains. *Arch Intern Med.* 1927;40:532–537.
24. Forkner CE. Material from lymph nodes of man. Studies on living and fixed cells withdrawn from lymph nodes of man. *Arch Intern Med.* 1927;40: 647–660.
25. Ellis EB. Cancer cells in pleural fluid. *Bull Int Assoc Med Museums J Tech Methods.* 1922;8:126–127.
26. Martin HE, Ellis EB. Biopsy by needle puncture and aspiration. *Ann Surg.* 1930;92:169–181.
27. Martin HE, Ellis EB. Aspiration biopsy. *Surg Gynecol Obstet.* 1934;59:578–589.
28. Stewart FW. The diagnosis of tumors by aspiration. *Am J Pathol.* 1933;9:801–812.
29. Godwin JT. Aspiration biopsy: technique and application. *Ann NY Acad Sci.* 1956;63:1348–1373.
30. Godwin JT. Cytologic diagnosis of aspiration biopsies of solid and cystic tumors. *Acta Cytol.* 1964;8:206–215.
31. Rosen PP, Snyder PE, Foote Jr., FW, Wallace T. Detection of occult carcinoma in the apparently benign breast biopsy through specimen radiography. *Cancer.* 1970;26:944–953.
32. Rosen PP, Snyder RE, Urban J, Robbins G. Correlation of suspicious mammograms and x-rays of breast biopsies during surgery: results of 60 cases. *Cancer.* 1973;31:656–660.
33. Snyder R, Rosen PP. Radiography of breast specimens. *Cancer.* 1971;28: 1608–1611.
34. Friese CR, Neville BA, Edge SB, et al. Breast biopsy patterns and outcomes in Surveillance, Epidemiology, and End Results-Medicare data. *Cancer.* 2009;115:716–724.
35. Fox CH. Innovation in medical diagnosis: the Scandinavian curiosity. *Lancet.* 1979;1:1387–1388.
36. Nordenström B. New instruments for biopsy. *Radiology.* 1975;117:474–475.
37. Bolmgren J, Jacobson B, Nordenström B. Stereotaxic instrument for needle biopsy of the mamma. *Am J Roentgenol.* 1977;129:121–125.
38. Lindgren PG. Percutaneous needle biopsy: a new technique. *Acta Radiol Diagn.* 1982;23:653–656.
39. Burbank F. Stereotactic breast biopsy: its history, its present, and its future. *Am Surg.* 1996;2:128–150.
40. Nields MW. Cost-effectiveness of image-guided core needle biopsy versus surgery in diagnosing breast cancer. *Acad Radiol.* 1996;3:S138–S140.
41. Liberman L, Fahs MC, Dershaw DD, et al. Impact of stereotactic core biopsy on cost of diagnosis. *Radiology.* 1995;195:633–637.
42. Groenewoud JH, Pijnappel RM, vandenAkker-van Marle ME, et al. Cost-effectiveness of stereotactic large-core needle biopsy for nonpalpable breast lesions compared to open-breast biopsy. *Br J Cancer.* 2004;90:383–392.
43. Rosenblatt R, Fineberg SA, Sparano JA, Kaleya RN. Stereotactic core needle biopsy of multiple sites in the breast: efficacy and effect on patient care. *Radiology.* 1996;201:67–70.
44. Morris EA, Lieberman L, Trevisan SG, et al. Histological heterogeneity of masses at percutaneous breast biopsy. *Breast J.* 2002;8:187–191.
45. Association of Directors of Anatomic and Surgical Pathology. Immediate management of mammographically detected breast lesions. *Am J Surg Pathol.* 1993;12:850–851.
46. Hoorntje LE, Peeter PH, Mali WP, Borel-Rinkes IH. Vacuum-assisted breast biopsy: a critical review. *Eur J Cancer.* 2003;39:1676–6183.
47. Kettritz V, Rotter K, Schreer I, et al. Stereotactic vacuum-assisted breast biopsy in 2874 patients: a multicenter study. *Cancer.* 2004;100:245–251.
48. Liberman L, Dershaw DD, Glassman JR, et al. Analysis of cancers not diagnosed at stereotactic core breast biopsy. *Radiology.* 1997;203:151–157.
49. Schueller G, Jaromi S, Ponhold L, et al. US-guided 14-gauge core-needle breast biopsy: results of a validation study in 1352 cases. *Radiology.* 2008; 248:406–413.
50. Brenner RJ. Lesions entirely removed during stereotactic biopsy: pre-operative localization on the basis of mammographic landmarks and feasibility of free-hand technique-initial experience. *Radiology.* 2000;214:585–590.
51. March DE, Coughlin BF, Barham RB, et al. Breast masses: removal of all US evidence during biopsy using a hand held vacuum-assisted device-initial experience. *Radiology.* 2003;227:549–555.
52. Lee J-M, Kaplan JB, Murray MP, Liberman L. Complete excision of the MRI target lesion at MRI-guided vacuum-assisted biopsy of breast cancer. *AJR.* 2008;191:1198–1202.
53. Liberman L, Kaplan JB, Morris EA, et al. To excise or to sample the mammographic target: what is the goal of stereotactic 11-gauge vacuum-assisted breast biopsy? *AJR.* 2002;179:679–683.
54. Calhoun K. Giuliano A, Brenner RJ. Intraoperative loss of core biopsy clips: clinical implications. *AJR.* 2008;190:W196–W200.
55. Mercado CL, Guth AA, Toth HK, et al. Sonographically guided marker placement for confirmation of removal of mammographically occult lesions after localization. *AJR.* 2008;191:1216–1219.
56. Philpotts LE, Lee CH. Clip migration after 11-gauge vacuum assisted stereotactic biopsy: case report. *Radiology.* 2002;222:794–796.
57. Brenner RJ. Percutaneous removal of post biopsy marking clip in the breast using stereotactic technique. *AJR.* 2001;176:417–419.
58. Hoda SA, Rosen PP: Observation on the pathologic diagnosis of selected unusual lesions in needle core biopsies of breast. *Breast J.* 2004;6:522–527.

Pathology and the Origin of Specialization in Medicine

The development of modern medical specialism during the latter part of the nineteenth century and the early part of the present century . . . would hardly have taken place had not physicians accustomed themselves to the idea of distinct disease entities consisting of localized organic lesions connected with certain clinical pictures. . . . The development and application of a concept of localized pathology laid the groundwork for modern specialism by providing a number of foci of interest in the field of medicine. Each such focus of interest, that is, a disease or the diseases of an organ or region of the body, provided a nucleus around which could gather the results of clinical and pathological investigation.

On the technological side the influences represented in specialization manifest themselves in the multiplicity of technical skills, devices, and theories applied to the achievement of human aims in the field of medicine.

From *The Specialization of Medicine* by George Rosen, M.D., 1944

Anatomy and Physiologic Morphology

EMBRYOLOGY AND INFANTILE BREAST DEVELOPMENT

Mammary glands develop from mammary ridges or milk lines, thickenings of the epidermis that appear on the ventral surface of the 5-week fetus, extending from the axilla to the upper medial region of the thigh. In the human, much of the ridge does not grow further and disappears during fetal development. Persistence of segments of the milk line is the embryologic anlage for the development of ectopic mammary glandular tissue, which occurs most often at the extreme ends of the mammary ridge in the axilla or vulva. The development of the fetal breast is characterized by the differential expression of keratins 14, 18, and 19 and of actin in the breast ducts and lobular buds. Myoepithelial cells appear to arise from basal cells between weeks 23 and 28 of gestation (1). They contribute to the branching morphogenesis of the mammary gland by influencing the synthesis of basement membrane constitutents and growth factors (2). Endocrine and paracrine factors involved in fetal and neonatal mammary development were reviewed by Sternlicht (3).

In most girls, functional breast development does not begin until puberty. *Premature thelarche* is the unilateral or bilateral appearance of a discoid subareolar thickening before puberty. The incidence in white female infants and children up to 7 years old in the United States in 1980 was 20.8 per 100,000 (4). The nodular breast tissue formed in premature thelarche measuring 1.0 to 6.5 cm tends to regress slowly over the subsequent 6 months to 6 years (2). Excision of this tissue is inappropriate because of the resultant amastia after puberty. Premature thelarche has been associated with precocious puberty (5) but not with a predisposition to develop breast carcinoma (2).

Histologically, the breast tissue in premature thelarche resembles gynecomastia because it is characterized by epithelial hyperplasia in the duct system with a solid and micropapillary configuration. Growth and branching of the proliferating ducts results in an increased number of duct cross sections surrounded by moderately cellular stroma.

With the onset of cyclic estrogen and progesterone secretion at puberty, adolescent female breast development commences (Fig. 1.1). Growth of ducts and periductal stroma is estrogen dependent (6). Lobules are derived from solid masses of cells that form at the ends of terminal ducts. The greatest amount of breast glandular differentiation occurs during puberty, but the process may continue into the 20s and is enhanced by pregnancy (3). Most lobules in the mature breast are located in the fibrocollagenous stroma, but normal lobules may also be found in mammary adipose tissue (Fig. 1.2).

ANATOMY AND HISTOLOGY

The functional glandular and ductal elements are embedded in fibrofatty tissue that forms the bulk of the mammary gland. The relative proportions of fat and collagenous stroma vary greatly among individuals and with age. The combination of stromal and epithelial components is responsible for the radiographic appearance of breast structure in normal and pathologic states. Magnetic resonance imaging (MRI) provides a relatively precise method for discriminating between fatty and fibroglandular tissue in the breast. By comparing images obtained with mammography and MRI, Lee et al. (7) found a mean fat content of 42.5% (SD $\pm$ 30.3%) in mammograms and 66.5% (SD $\pm$ 18%) in MRI images. The ranges of fat content obtained by mammography and MRI imaging were 7.5% to 90% and 17% to 89%, respectively. The correlation coefficient for estimates of fat content obtained by both methods was 0.63, with the strongest correlation ($r = 0.81$) in postmenopausal women.

Each of the major lactiferous ducts terminates in and exits from the breast at the nipple via a secretory pore forming the lactiferous duct orifice. The squamocolumnar

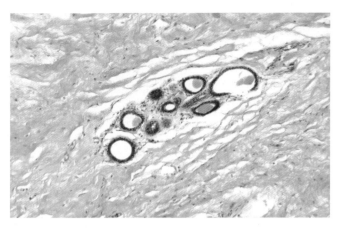

Figure 1.1 **Immature breast.** Breast tissue at the onset of puberty in an 11-year-old girl showing early lobular differentiation with glandular secretion and intralobular stroma.

junction, where the squamous epithelium joins the glandular duct epithelium, is normally distal to a dilated segment of the lactiferous duct, the lactiferous sinus, located just beneath the nipple surface. Extension of squamous epithelium into or below the lactiferous sinus is a pathologic condition termed *squamous metaplasia.* This may result in obstruction of the affected duct system.

Lactiferous ducts in the nipple are surrounded by circular and longitudinal arrays of smooth muscle fibers embedded in fibrocollagenous stroma. The lactiferous ducts extend distally from the nipple through a series of branches diminishing in caliber from the nipple to the terminal ductal–lobular units that are embedded in specialized, hormonally responsive stroma. Extralobular ducts are lined by cuboidal or columnar epithelium that is supported by myoepithelial cells, a basement membrane, and surrounding elastic fibers. In the nonlactating breast, the major ducts cut in cross section have contours marked by numerous folds or indentations that create a foliate or serrate border. The epithelium in the baylike pouches of the duct lumen can give rise to ductular branches. Fully formed lobules can originate directly from these pouches in lactiferous ducts

in the nipple and in more distal segments of the mammary duct system (8).

The majority of the cells that form the duct epithelium are columnar or cuboidal cells lining the lumen. Their cytoplasm is endowed with abundant organelles involved in secretion. Myoepithelial cells lie between the epithelial layer and the basal lamina. The cytoplasm of the myoepithelial cells, distributed in a network of slender processes that invest the overlying epithelial cells, is rich in myofibrils. The histologic appearance and immunoreactivity of myoepithelial cells is variable, especially in pathologic conditions, and depends on the degree to which the myoid or epithelial phenotype is accentuated in a particular situation. Myoepithelial cells display nuclear reactivity for p63 that is the most useful marker for detecting these cells in normal and lesional tissue. However, epithelioid myoepithelial cells can have absent or reduced p63 reactivity.

The normal periductal stroma contains fibroblasts, elastic fibers, a sparse scattering of lymphocytes, plasma cells, mast cells, and histiocytes. Ochrocytes are periductal histiocytes with a cytoplasmic accumulation of lipofuscin pigment. These pigmented cells become more numerous in the postmenopausal breast and in association with inflammatory or proliferative conditions (9).

Mammary secretion originates in the lobules. These structures are composed of alveolar glands encompassed by specialized vascularized stroma. The alveoli are connected by intralobular ductules that combine to form a single terminal lobular duct that drains into the extralobular duct system. The resting lobular gland is lined by a single layer of cuboidal epithelial cells supported by loosely connected myoepithelial cells. The normal microscopic anatomy of the lobules is not constant because the structure and histologic appearance of the lobule in the mature breast are subject to changes associated with the menstrual cycle, pregnancy, lactation, exogenous hormone administration, aging, and the menopause. Furthermore, there is variation in the functional state of individual lobules regardless of physiologic circumstances, an observation

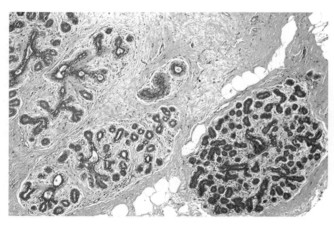

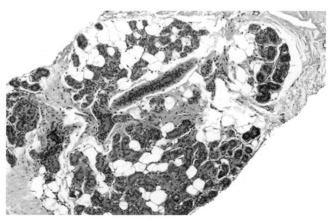

A **B**

Figure 1.2 **Normal lobules. A:** A lobule in fibrocollagenous stroma. **B:** A lobule in mammary adipose tissue.

that suggests that individual lobules or regions of the breast have intrinsic differences in response to hormonal and other stimuli. This is reflected in the substantial variability in labeling indices, indicating different proliferative rates among lobules in a given individual (10). Immunoreactivity for hormone receptors is also variably expressed in lobules.

PHYSIOLOGIC MORPHOLOGY

Histologic cellular and structural alterations occur in the normal breast during the *menstrual cycle* (11). According to some authors, the *proliferative phase*, days 3 through 7, features the highest rate of epithelial mitoses and of apoptosis (12,13). Other investigators who defined this phase as days 0 to 5 reported that "apoptosis and mitosis were by and large absent in this phase" (11). Lobular glands at this time are lined by crowded, poorly oriented epithelial cells with little or no lumen formation and secretion. Myoepithelial cells are inconspicuous and difficult to distinguish from epithelial cells. The lobular stroma is relatively dense and hypovascular, with plump fibroblasts ringing lobular glands.

Mitoses and apoptic bodies are inconspicuous in the *follicular phase* (days 8–14). At this stage, the myoepithelial cells have a polygonal shape, clear cytoplasm, and become more apparent. Epithelial cells become columnar, with increasingly basophilic cytoplasm and basally oriented, darkly stained nuclei. An acinar lumen without secretion is evident.

During the *luteal phase*, comprising days 15 through 20, myoepithelial cells become more prominent following increased glycogen accumulation that results in cytoplasmic clearing. The glandular lumen is clearly defined by epithelial cells with basophilic cytoplasm. A small amount of secretion is present in a few glands. Edema and a mixed inflammatory cell infiltrate appear in the intralobular stroma. Mitoses and apoptotic bodies are infrequent.

The *secretory phase* corresponding to days 21 through 27 features heightened secretion with distension of glandular lumens by accumulated secretory material. The epithelium consists of columnar epithelial and myoepithelial cells with progressively clear cytoplasm. It is at this stage that mitoses and apoptotic bodies are most conspicuous with maximal intralobular edema and inflammation.

In the *menstrual phase*, comprising days 28 through 2, the stroma becomes compact with loss of intralobular edema. Lymphocytes, macrophages, and plasma cells are most conspicuous in the lobular stroma at this stage (12). Some glandular lumens remain and others appear collapsed. Mitotic activity is absent.

Improved ability to recognize menstrual cycle–related morphologic changes in the breast may become clinically useful in premenopausal women. At present, evidence suggesting that surgery performed during the luteal phase is prognostically advantageous (14,15) remains controversial

(16,17). These observations have been based on retrospective reviews in which the reporting of menstrual cycle data was variously reliable. The status of breast tissue morphology can serve as a means of corroborating menstrual cycle information provided by the patients in future prospective studies. Needle core biopsy sampling might be used to obtain tissue for this purpose.

Estrogen and progesterone receptors are expressed in the nuclei of epithelial cells in the normal breast. Immunohistochemical staining reveals a higher proportion of positive nuclei in lobular than in ductal cells (18). Considerable heterogeneity exists in nuclear hormone–receptor activity among lobules with maximal expression in the follicular phase (19). No consistent menstrual cycle–related pattern has been found in the expression of estrogen and progesterone receptors in breast carcinomas that arise in premenopausal women (20,21).

Secretory changes associated with *pregnancy* occur unevenly throughout the breast (Fig. 1.3). There is progressive recruitment of lobules with successive pregnancies. Early in pregnancy, terminal ducts and lobules grow rapidly resulting in lobular enlargement with some coincidental depletion of the fibrofatty stroma (22,23). Stromal vascularity increases, accompanied by infiltration by mononuclear inflammatory cells. During the second and third trimesters, lobular growth progresses through the enlargement of cells as well as by cellular proliferation. The cytoplasm of lobular epithelial cells becomes vacuolated and secretion accumulates in lobular glands (Fig. 1.4). Lactation features markedly distended irregularly shaped lobular glands formed by cells with hyperchromatic nuclei (Fig. 1.5).

Hormonal alterations that occur during and after the *menopause* are manifested by a decrease in the cellularity and number of lobules, mainly as a result of epithelial atrophy. Coincidental with the loss of glandular epithelium, there is a tendency toward thickening of lobular basement membranes and collagenization of intralobular stroma.

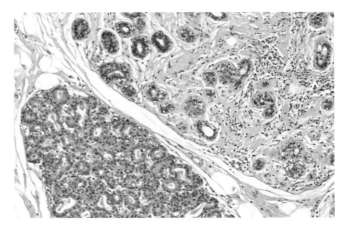

Figure 1.3 Lactational hyperplasia. This needle core biopsy specimen from a 31-year-old woman 34 weeks pregnant shows lactational hyperplasia in one lobule **(lower left)** and another unaltered lobule with fibroadenomatoid change.

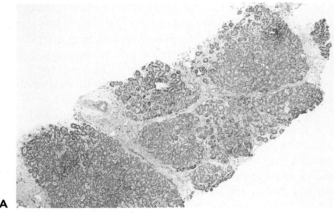

A

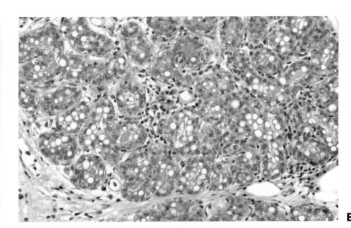

B

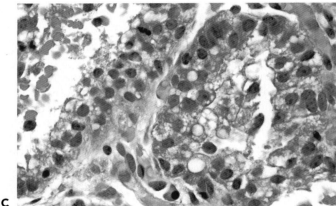

C

Figure 1.4 **Lactational hyperplasia. A:** The patient was 8 months pregnant when the needle core biopsy was performed for a mass that proved to be nodular lactational hyperplasia. **B:** The markedly enlarged lobules are composed of a greatly increased number of glands that should not be mistaken for carcinoma. **C:** Basophilic, vacuolated cytoplasm, luminal secretion, and inconspicuous myoepithelial cells are characteristic features.

The process of menopausal atrophy occurs in a heterogeneous fashion, often leaving some lobules relatively unaffected, by comparison with neighboring glands. Atrophy tends to spare lobular myoepithelial cells that frequently persist even in a late stage of the process. Most lobular glands appear to collapse and shrink but cystic distention

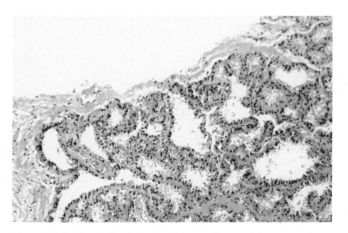

Figure 1.5 **Lactating breast.** This needle core biopsy specimen was obtained from a 36-year-old nursing woman 8 months postpartum. The lactating glands shown here are larger and more irregular in shape than in lactational hyperplasia. The cytoplasm has prominent apical blebs and a frayed appearance at the luminal border. Nuclei are condensed and hyperchromatic.

may also occur and calcifications are sometimes formed in atrophic lobular glands. In many women over 65 years of age, lobular integrity is progressively lost, leaving ducts and glands that may contain calcifications embedded in fibrocollagenous stroma (Fig. 1.6). The relative proportions of fat and stroma vary greatly in the atrophic breast. In advanced atrophy, calcifications may be found in the stroma unaccompanied by epithelium and pronounced elastotic change in the stroma may be a source of calcifications (Fig. 1.7).

Mammographic changes suggestive of physiologic proliferative alterations have been observed in women receiving postmenopausal hormone replacement therapy (24,25). The effect of hormone replacement therapy on the mammographic appearance of the breast is substantially less in women who have undergone prior breast irradiation (26). In the nonradiated breast, the effect of hormone replacement is manifested mainly by increased parenchymal density. This has been observed after treatment with estrogen alone and with an estrogen–progesterone combination therapy. Histologic examination does not reveal a consistent pattern. Some patients have lobular differentiation comparable to the premenopausal state, whereas others have prominent cystic or proliferative alterations of ducts and lobules. The findings suggest that the existing epithelial status of the breast is accentuated by exogenous hormone administration.

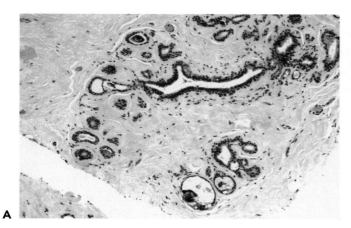
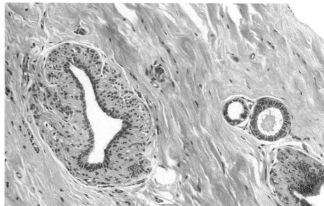
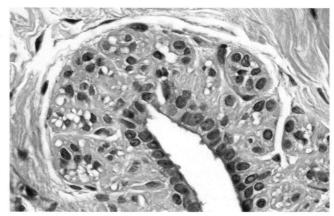

Figure 1.6 **Atrophy. A:** An atrophic lobule with a calcification in inactive glands. The needle core biopsy was performed on a 78-year-old woman with mammographically detected calcifications. **B, C:** Myoid metaplasia of myoepithelial cells is evident around the atrophic duct in this biopsy specimen.

Pregnancy-like change (pseudolactational hyperplasia) is a microscopic alteration characterized by lobules that resemble lactational hyperplasia. It occurs in breast tissue from patients who are neither pregnant nor lactating when the specimen is obtained. Many of the patients are parous, pre- or postmenopausal women, but similar changes have been observed in nulliparous women (27). The reported frequency of pregnancy-like change is 1.7% to about 3% in

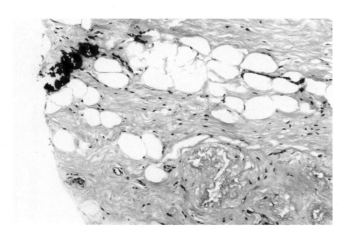

Figure 1.7 **Atrophy.** Calcification is shown in fibrofatty stroma at the edge of a needle core biopsy specimen from a 73-year-old woman. Note the stromal elastotic nodules **(lower right)**.

surgical pathology and autopsy series (27,28). The etiology of pregnancy-like change is unknown.

Glands and terminal ducts with pregnancy-like change usually contain little or no secretion, although they may be dilated (Fig. 1.8). The glandular cells are swollen with abundant pale-to-clear, finely granular, or vacuolated cytoplasm. The nuclei are usually small, uniform, round, and darkly stained. The luminal cytoplasmic borders of glandular cells are frayed, and small cytoplasmic blebs are formed. The nucleus may be contained in a bleb of cytoplasm extruded into the glandular lumen. Diastase-resistant granules that stain positively with periodic acid–Schiff (PAS) are present in the cytoplasm, that is also immunoreactive for α-lactalbumin and S-100 (28). Calcifications can be formed in pregnancy-like change (Fig. 1.9).

In most instances, the epithelium in lobules altered by pregnancy-like change remains one or two cell layers thick. *Pregnancy-like hyperplasia* represents the occurrence of pregnancy-like change in hyperplastic epithelium, that usually has a papillary configuration (Fig. 1.10). The epithelium is arranged in irregular fronds composed entirely of glandular cells. Although the cytologic appearance may duplicate the findings in pregnancy-like change, some of these lesions feature nuclear atypia, manifested in most instances by pleomorphism. Rarely, these atypical cytologic

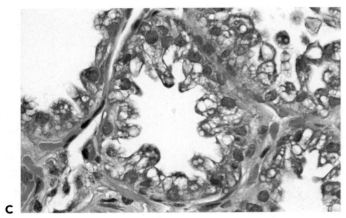

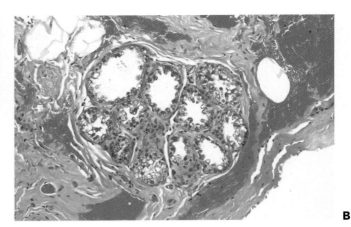

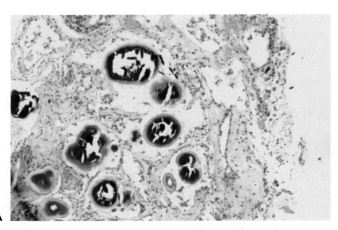

Figure 1.8 **Pregnancy-like change. A:** This lobule was present in a needle core biopsy specimen from a 49-year-old woman with invasive carcinoma. The enlarged lobule is composed of irregularly shaped glandular acini that contain small amounts of secretion. **B, C:** Pregnancy-like change in the atrophic lobule of a 74-year-old woman who had a needle core biopsy performed for calcifications that were localized to columnar cell duct hyperplasia.

changes may warrant a diagnosis of *atypical pregnancy-like hyperplasia* (Fig. 1.11). Atypical changes are more likely to be present when pregnancy-like hyperplasia coexists with cystic hypersecretory hyperplasia (29) (Fig. 1.12). Rarely, carcinoma has been found to arise from pregnancy-like hyperplasia, usually in combination with cystic hypersecretory hyperplasia (30).

Clear cell change is a cytologic alteration in lobular and terminal duct epithelium that has also been referred to as "lamprocytosis," and "hellenzellen," meaning clear cells (31). The affected lobules tend to be larger than adjacent uninvolved lobules. The lobular gland epithelium is composed of swollen cells with abundant clear or pale cytoplasm (Fig. 1.13). The cells have well-defined borders.

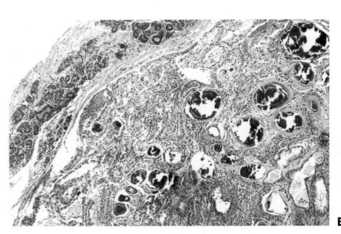

Figure 1.9 **Pregnancy-like change with calcification. A:** Large, laminated calcifications are present in pregnancy-like change shown in this needle core biopsy specimen from a 53-year-old-woman with mammographically detected calcifications. **B:** Lymphocytes are scattered in the stroma of the enlarged lobule with pregnancy-like hyperplasia and calcifications in this needle core biopsy sample from a 34-year-old woman.

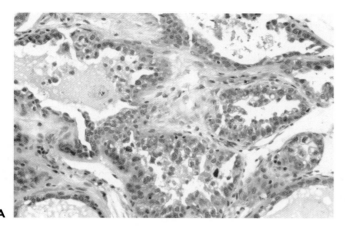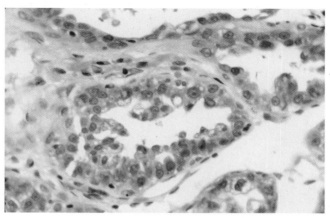

Figure 1.10   Pregnancy-like hyperplasia. A,B: Micropapillary fronds composed of hyperplastic epithelium protrude into some gland lumens. Note the slightly uneven, crowded distribution of nuclei. Some nuclei have prominent nucleoli. Pale eosinophilic secretion is present. This appearance resembles cystic hypersecretory carcinoma in a lobule, but the epithelium does not have the appearance of micropapillary carcinoma and the secretion lacks the intense eosinophilia and linear parallel cracks that characterize a cystic hypersecretory lesion.

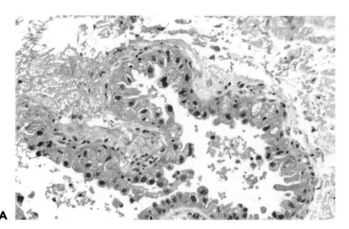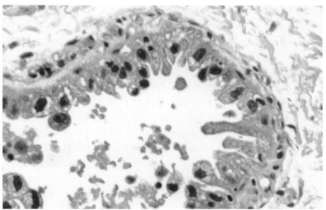

Figure 1.11   Atypical pregnancy-like hyperplasia. A,B: Enlarged, hyperchromatic and pleomorphic nuclei in pregnancy-like change from a needle core biopsy specimen in a 48-year-old woman. Despite the cytologic atypia, the cells tend to be distributed in a single layer. Extrusion of nuclei is shown at the luminal border.

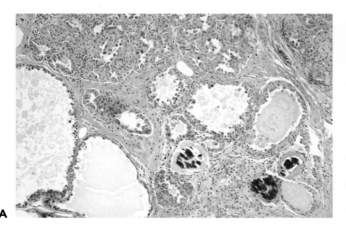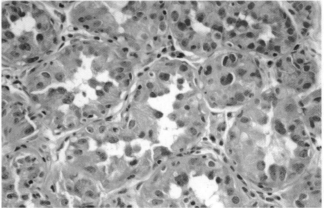

Figure 1.12   Atypical pregnancy-like hyperplasia and cystic hypersecretory hyperplasia. A: This needle core biopsy specimen was obtained for calcifications that proved to be at the junction between cystic hypersecretory hyperplasia **(below)** and atypical pregnancy-like hyperplasia **(above). B:** Magnified view of lobular glands in atypical pregnancy-like hyperplasia.

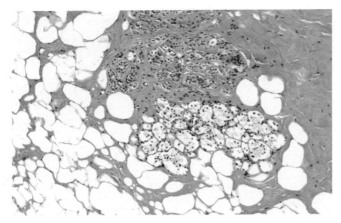

Figure 1.13 Clear cell change. The lower lobule is composed of cells with clear cytoplasm and small dark nuclei in this needle core biopsy specimen from a 54-year-old woman with mammographically detected calcifications that were associated with intraductal carcinoma.

Some glands have dilated lumens in which there is PAS-positive, diastase-resistant secretion, but more often the lobular gland lumina are obliterated by the swollen cells (32). Calcifications are very uncommon in clear cell change. The small, round, and darkly stained nuclei are often displaced toward the center of the gland. The clear cells are immunoreactive for cytokeratin but not for actin.

The etiology of clear cell change is not known. It is encountered in the pre- and postmenopausal women. There is no association with pregnancy or exogenous hormone use (32,33). Foci of clear cell change have been identified retrospectively in breast tissue obtained before exogenous hormones were available. Clear cell change is usually multifocal and can involve both breasts. Viña and Wells reported finding clear cell change in 15 of 934 (1.6%) biopsies (28). Specimens that contain clear cell change may harbor carcinoma or fibrocystic changes, there being no association with any particular breast lesions (28). Rarely, clear cell change and pregnancy-like change may coexist in the same breast (33).

The differential diagnosis of clear cell change includes pregnancy-like change, cytoplasmic clearing in apocrine metaplasia, cytoplasmic clearing in myoepithelial cells, and clear cell forms of carcinoma. Pregnancy-like change is most readily distinguished from clear cell change by the presence of "decapitation" secretion at the luminal borders of the cells in the former. Cytoplasmic clearing in apocrine metaplasia is usually a focal change in epithelium that otherwise has the typical features of apocrine metaplasia. Myoepithelial cells with clear cell change retain their position between the epithelium and basement membrane.

REFERENCES

1. Anbazhagan R, Osin PP, Bartkova J, et al. The development of epithelial phenotypes in the human fetal and infant breast. *J Pathol.* 1998; 184:197–206.
2. Adriance MC, Inman JL, Peterson OW, Bissell MJ,. Myoepithelial cells: good fences make good neighbors. *Breast Cancer Res.* 2005;7:190–197.
3. Sternlicht MD. Key stages in mammary gland development. The cues that regulate ductal branching morphogenesis. *Breast Cancer Res.* 2006;8:201–212.
4. van Winter JT, Noller KL, Zimmerman D, Melton III JL. Natural history of premature thelarche in Olmsted County, Minnesota, 1940 to 1984. *J Pediatr.* 1990;116:278–280.
5. Pasquino AM, Pucarelli I, Passeri F, et al. Progression of premature thelarche to central precocious puberty. *J Pediatr.* 1995;126:11–14.
6. Topper YJ, Freeman CS. Multiple hormone interactions in the developmental biology of the mammary gland. *Physiol Rev.* 1980;60:1049–1106.
7. Lee NA, Rusinek H, Weinreb J, et al. Fatty and fibroglandular tissue volumes in the breasts of women 20–83 years old: comparison of x-ray mammography and computer-assisted MR imaging. *Am J Roentgenol.* 1997;168:501–506.
8. Rosen PP, Tench W. Lobules in the nipple. *Pathol Annu.* 1985;20(pt. 1): 317–322.
9. Davies JD. Pigmented periductal cells (ochrocytes) in mammary dysplasias: their nature and significance. *J Pathol.* 1974;114:205–216.
10. Christov K, Chew KL, Ljung B-M, et al. Proliferation of normal breast epithelial cells as shown by *in vivo* labeling with bromodeoxyuridine. *Am J Pathol.* 1991;138:1371–1377.
11. Ramakrishnan R, Khan S, Badve S. Morphological changes in breast tissue with menstrual cycle. *Mod Pathol.* 2002;15:1348–1356.
12. Longacre TA, Bartow SA. A correlative morphologic study of human breast and endometrium in the menstrual cycle. *Am J Surg Pathol.* 1986;10:382–393.
13. Ferguson DJP, Anderson TJ. Morphological evaluation of cell turnover in relation to the menstrual cycle in the "resting" human breast. *Br J Cancer.* 1981;4:177–181.
14. Donegan W, Shah D. Prognosis of patients with breast cancer related to the timing of operation. *Arch Surg.* 1993;128:309–313.
15. Badwe R, Mittra I, Havaldor R. Timing of surgery during the menstrual cycle and prognosis of breast cancer. *J Biosci.* 2000;25:113–120.
16. Milella M, Nistico C, Ferraresi V, et al. Breast cancer and timing of surgery during menstrual cycle: a 5-year analysis of 248 premenopausal women. *Breast Cancer Res Treat.* 1999;55:259–266.
17. Nomura Y, Kataoka A, Tsuitsui S, et al. Lack of correlation between timing of surgery in relation to the menstrual cycle and prognosis of premenopausal patients with early breast cancer. *Eur J Cancer.* 1999;35:1326–1330.
18. Petersen OW, Hoyer PE, van Deurs B. Frequency and distribution of estrogen receptor-positive cells in normal, nonlactating human breast tissue. *Cancer Res.* 1987;47:5748–5751.
19. Fabris G, Marchetti E, Marzola A, et al. Pathophysiology of estrogen receptors in mammary tissue by monoclonal antibodies. *J Steroid Biochem.* 1987;27:171–176.
20. Markopoulos C, Berger U, Wilson P, et al. Oestrogen receptor content of normal breast cells and breast carcinoma throughout the menstrual cycle. *Brit Med J.* 1988;296:1349–1351.
21. Smyth CM, Benn DE, Reeve TS. Influence of the mentrual cycle on the concentrations of estrogen and progesterone receptors in primary breast cancer biopsies. *Breast Cancer Res Treat.* 1988;11:45–50.
22. McCarty KS Jr, Tucker JA. Breast. In: Sternberg SS, ed. *Histology for Pathologists.* New York: Raven Press; 1992:893–902.
23. Salazar H, Tobon H, Josimovich JB. Developmental gestational and postgestational modifications of the human breast. *Clin Obstet Gynecol.* 1975;18: 113–137.
24. Rand T, Heytmanek G, Seifert M, et al. Mammography in women undergoing hormone replacement therapy. Possible effects revealed at routine examination. *Acta Radiol.* 1997;38:228–231.
25. Laya MB, Gallagher JC, Schreiman JS, et al. Effect of postmenopausal hormonal replacement therapy on mammographic density and parenchymal pattern. *Radiology.* 1995;196:433–437.
26. Margolin FR, Denny SR, Gelfand CA, Jacobs RP. Mammographic changes after hormone replacement therapy in patients who have undergone breast irradiation. *Am J Roentgenol.* 1999;172:147–150.
27. Kiaer HW, Andersen JA. Focal pregnancy-like changes in the breast. *Acta Path Microbiol Scand [A].* 1977;85:931–941.
28. Viña M, Wells CA. Clear cell metaplasia of the breast: a lesion showing eccrine differentiation. *Histopathology.* 1989;15:85–92.
29. Shin SJ, Rosen PP. Pregnancy-like (pseudolactational) hyperplasia: a primary diagnosis in mammographically detected lesions of the breast and its relationship to cystic hypersecretory hyperplasia. *Am J Surg Pathol.* 2000;24: 1670–1674.
30. Shin S, Rosen PP. Carcinoma arising from preexsiting pregnancy-like and cystic hypersecretory hyperplasia lesions of the breast: a clinicopathologic study of 9 patients. *Am J Surg Pathol.* 2004;28:789–793.
31. Skorpil F. Uber das Vorkommen von sog. hellen Zellen (Lamprocyten) in der Milchdruse. *Beitrage zur pathol Anat.* 1943;108:378–393.
32. Barwick KW, Kashigarian M, Rosen PP. "Clear-cell" change within duct and lobular epithelium of the human breast. *Pathol Annu.* 1982;17(pt. 1): 319–328.
33. Tavassoli FA, Yeh IT. Lactational and clear cell changes of the breast in nonlactating, nonpregnant women. *Am J Clin Pathol.* 1987;87:23–29.

Inflammatory and Reactive Tumors

2

FAT NECROSIS

Fat necrosis may result from incidental trauma, but at present the most frequent causes are prior surgery and radiation therapy. Patients typically present with a painless mass located superficially in the breast, accompanied by retraction or dimpling of the overlying skin. Any part of the breast may be affected. The tumors average 2 cm. The clinical problem of distinguishing between fat necrosis and recurrent carcinoma is especially difficult in patients who have undergone breast-conserving surgery and radiation therapy (1). Fat necrosis has been reported after external beam therapy and at the site of iridium implantation (2,3). Hemorrhagic necrosis of the skin, subcutaneous tissue, and breast parenchyma associated with Coumadin anticoagulant treatment is an uncommon form of fat necrosis (4). Pain and breast swelling appear within a week of the start of therapy, usually progressing to gangrene of most of or all the breast (5).

Mammography of fat necrosis usually reveals a spiculated mass that may contain punctate or large irregular calcifications (6). Less frequently, the lesion consists of a circumscribed, oil-filled, partly calcified cyst (7). Both patterns may coexist in a single lesion.

The initial histologic change in fat necrosis is disruption of fat cells and hemorrhage (Fig. 2.1). Evolution of the lesion is marked by the appearance of histiocytes, hemosiderin deposition, and a variable infiltrate of lymphocytes, plasma cells, and sometimes eosinophils (Fig. 2.2). A foreign body giant cell reaction may be elicited (Fig. 2.3). Fibrosis develops peripherally, demarcating the area of necrotic fat, cellular debris, and calcifications (Fig. 2.4). In late lesions, the reactive inflammatory components are replaced by fibrosis and contract into a scar. Loculated, necrotic fat with calcification may persist for months or years within such a scar (Fig. 2.5). Squamous metaplasia may develop in the epithelium of ducts and lobules in the vicinity of fat necrosis. Among patients who develop fat necrosis after breast-conserving surgery and radiotherapy, cytologic changes associated with irradiation can be found in surrounding ducts, lobules, and blood vessels.

Biopsy is required in most instances because the clinical and radiologic features resemble those of carcinoma. When there is a history of trauma or prior surgery and characteristic radiologic findings of a demarcated lesion with typical calcifications, excision need not be performed after the diagnosis has been established by needle core biopsy.

Erdheim–Chester disease, an infrequent xanthomatous form of non-Langerhans cell histiocytosis, rarely involves the breast and can be mistaken for fat necrosis histologically, especially if the initial clinical manifestation is a breast tumor (8). Subcutaneous and osseous lesions are typically present as well. Microscopic examination reveals infiltrates of foamy histiocytes, plasma cells, Touton giant cells, and infrequent epithelioid granulomas. The histiocytes are reactive for CD68 but negative for S-100 and CD1a (8).

BREAST INFARCT

The most frequent form of breast infarct occurs during pregnancy or postpartum. The lesion presents as a discrete, firm mass that can suggest carcinoma clinically. Pain and tenderness are sometimes reported. Hemorrhage and ischemic degeneration with little or no inflammation characterize the histologic appearance of early lesions. Later stages feature fully developed coagulative necrosis.

Infarction also occurs spontaneously in fibroadenomas and benign proliferative lesions. Foci of necrosis may be found in florid sclerosing adenosis, usually during pregnancy, when the epithelium in sclerosing adenosis may also exhibit pronounced hyperplasia, cytologic atypia, and mitotic activity. Papillomas are susceptible to partial or complete infarction, especially in major lactiferous ducts. Infarction can occur in papillomas at any age, but it tends to be more frequent in postmenopausal women, and there is no association with pregnancy (9). Bloody nipple discharge is the most frequent sign of an infarcted or degenerated papilloma.

Acutely infarcted regions in a papilloma exhibit ischemic coagulative necrosis microscopically. Structural integrity is usually maintained in such foci despite progressive loss of cytologic detail (Fig. 2.6). At a late stage, fragmentation of

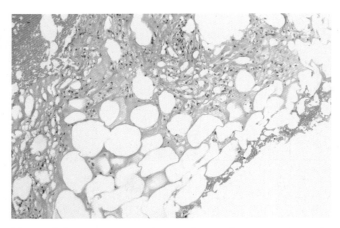

Figure 2.1 **Fat necrosis.** This needle core biopsy specimen obtained from a 1-cm stellate lesion consists of infarcted fat cells, hemorrhage, and histiocytic reaction.

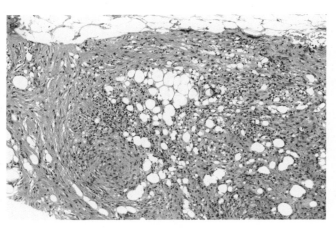

Figure 2.2 **Fat necrosis.** A needle core biopsy specimen from a mammographically detected mass at the site of a prior lumpectomy for intraductal carcinoma. Fibrosis and granulomatous reaction are evident in the fat necrosis. No foreign body material was found.

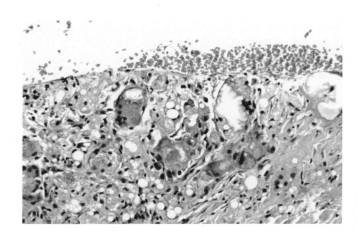

Figure 2.3 **Fat necrosis.** Multinucleated histiocytes with foreign body material are shown in a needle core biopsy specimen from fat necrosis at a prior surgical site.

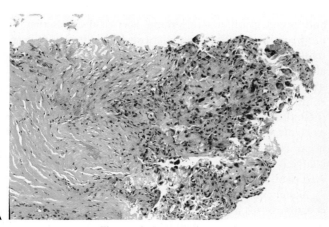

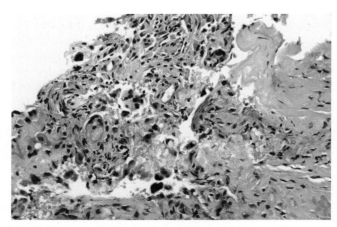

A   B

Figure 2.4 **Fat necrosis. A,B:** Fibrosis is evident around this focus of long-standing fat necrosis in a needle core biopsy specimen.

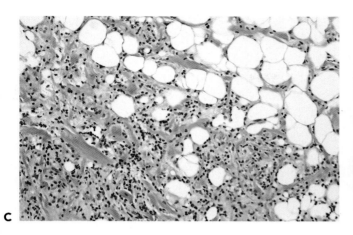

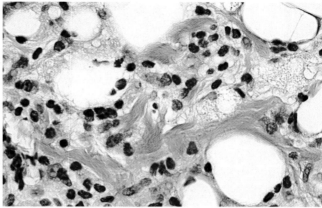

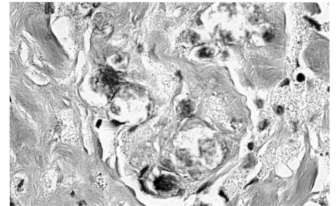

Figure 2.4 *(continued)* **C,D:** Lymphocytes and histocytes in fat necrosis from a 52-year-old woman. **E:** Calcifications in the lesion shown in **(C)** and **(D).**

superficial portions of infarcted regions occurs. Occasionally, an infarcted papilloma is reduced to an inflammatory intraductal polyp consisting of granulation tissue with little or no epithelium. Chronic ischemia and healing of infarcts are marked by fibrosis, that may cause considerable distortion of residual entrapped epithelium, producing a pattern that could be mistaken for carcinoma (9). Squamous metaplasia sometimes develops in the reparative epithelium that

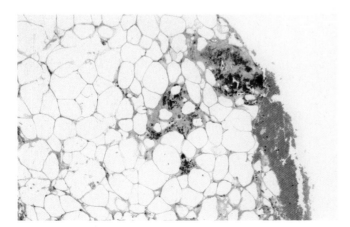

Figure 2.5 **Fat necrosis.** Infarcted fat with calcification in a needle core biopsy specimen. Nuclear detail is absent from the fat cells. The lesion was biopsied after calcifications were found on a routine mammogram.

proliferates in a papilloma after infarction, and calcification may form in the infarcted tissue (9,10). Sometimes infarcted carcinoma can be distinguished from infarction of a benign lesion if there is residual intact in situ or invasive carcinoma (11).

The reliability of immunostains for evaluating infarcted papillary lesions is unpredictable and probably depends on the extent of decomposition. Many of these lesions have a "ghost" architecture that is revealed by the reticulin stain. In some instances, immunoreactivity for cytokeratin and myoepithelial markers, especially p63, is surprisingly well preserved. When this occurs it may be possible to "resurrect" the structure of the lesion to a considerable degree. These procedures can be helpful when trying to distinguish between an infarcted papilloma and papillary carcinoma.

Excisional biopsy is usually necessary for the diagnosis of a mammary infarct, although the findings in a needle core biopsy specimen may be suggestive. In most cases, recognition of the underlying condition hinges on finding a residual uninfarcted component. A reticulin stain is helpful for unmasking the architecture of infarcted tissue or as noted above, immunostains may be useful. Rarely, the diagnosis of a totally infarcted lesion remains enigmatic (Fig. 2.7). If a papillary structure can be demonstrated in this circumstance, the lesion was probably a papilloma rather than a papillary carcinoma because infarction occurs considerably more often in benign papillary tumors than in papillary carcinomas.

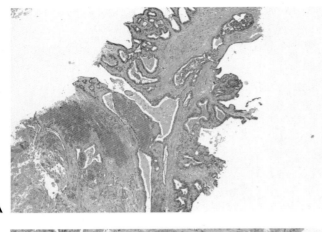

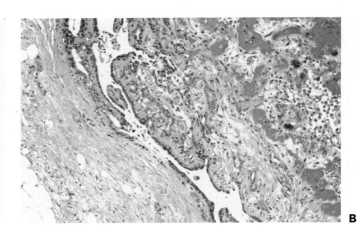

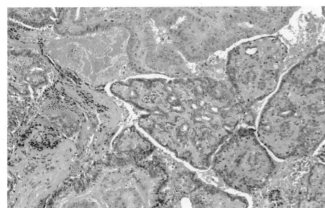

Figure 2.6 **Infarcted papilloma. A:** A needle core biopsy specimen showing an area of hemorrhage and infarction in a papilloma. **B:** A sample from the periphery of the lesion with degenerated papillary tissue fragments. **C:** An area in the excised papilloma showing intact papillary structures and focal necrosis *(upper left)*.

GALACTOCELE

The lesions average about 2 cm in diameter, but galactoceles 5 cm or larger have been described (12). Mammography reveals a circumscribed density that in many instances has a characteristic appearance consisting of a hypodense upper area and a lower region with density close to that of the surrounding tissue (13). The interface tends to remain horizontal as the patient changes position. The two zones consist of lighter lipid-containing components above the water-based constituents of the fluid. Comparable differences in echogenicity are observed on ultrasound examination.

The firm, usually painless tumor may suggest carcinoma clinically. Necrotic cells and nuclear debris, possibly accompanied by inflammatory cells, are seen in a fine-needle aspiration specimen (14). Cells with hyperchromatic,

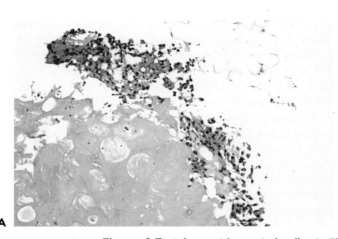

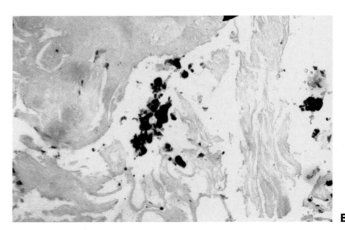

Figure 2.7 **Infarct with atypical cells. A:** This needle core biopsy specimen shows a totally infarcted lesion, possible fat necrosis, and an attached fragment of tissue composed of atypical cells. **B:** The atypical cells proved to be epithelial rather than histocytic with the CAM5.2 cytokeratin immunostain shown here (immunoperoxidase). Excisional biopsy revealed atypical duct hyperplasia near the fat necrosis.

atypical-appearing nuclei may be present. In this inflammatory background these cells could be mistaken for carcinoma. Excisional biopsy is diagnostic and provides adequate therapy if the lesion does not resolve after aspiration of the cyst contents.

A galactocele is composed of cysts lined by smooth cuboidal epithelium. The cysts contain fluid that resembles milk. Inspissated secretion may be present in the form of soft caseous material. Intact cysts are encompassed by a fibrous wall of varying thickness with little or no inflammatory reaction. Leakage from a cyst elicits a chronic inflammatory reaction that may be accompanied by fat necrosis.

PLASMA CELL MASTITIS

In the early phase, patients experience the acute onset of mild pain, tenderness, redness, and nipple discharge consisting usually of thick secretion. After the inflammatory symptoms subside, the skin may be edematous over a firm-to-hard mass several centimeters in diameter that remains at the same site. Nipple discharge usually persists and nipple retraction is observed in the majority of patients. Axillary lymph nodes are often enlarged. Plasma cell mastitis in its acute and mature phases is difficult to distinguish clinically from mammary carcinoma. The radiologic findings may be interpreted as indicative of carcinoma, especially when calcifications are present.

Plasma cell mastitis is a form of periductal mastitis characterized by variable hyperplasia of ductal epithelium and a marked, diffuse plasma cell infiltrate surrounding ducts as well as lobules (Fig. 2.8). A histiocytic reaction to the desquamated epithelium and lipid material in the ducts is responsible for areas that grossly appear to be xanthomatous and for the comedo-like character of the duct contents. Granulomatous features may be present microscopically, especially in areas of necrosis. Lymphocytes and neutrophils are variably present. Periductal

fibrosis and obliterative intraductal proliferation of granulation tissue are not features of plasma cell mastitis. Hyperplastic epithelial cells, that may appear very atypical, can be mistaken for carcinoma in a needle core biopsy sample, leading to an erroneous diagnosis of comedocarcinoma.

MAMMARY DUCT ECTASIA

The earliest symptom is spontaneous, intermittent mainly watery nipple discharge. In more advanced cases, subareolar induration progresses to the formation of a mass. The presence of nipple inversion is generally associated with periductal fibrosis and contracture. In some cases, squamous metaplasia of the terminal lactiferous duct epithelium results in obstruction that contributes to the development of duct ectasia and eventually to the formation of lactiferous duct fistulas (15,16). The mammographic abnormalities include microcalcifications, spiculated masses, and lobulated partially smooth masses. In some instances the mammographic findings suggest carcinoma (17).

The microscopic composition of the duct contents is variable. The most bland form consists of eosinophilic (granular or amorphous) proteinaceous material. Usually, there is an admixture of lipid-containing histiocytic cells and desquamated duct epithelial cells. Cholesterol crystals and calcifications may be found in the intraductal debris (Fig. 2.9). Histiocytes that contain ceroid pigment, termed *ochrocytes* by Davies (18), and foam cells may be found within the epithelial-myoepithelial layer of the duct, in periductal tissue and in the duct lumen (Fig. 2.9). Neutrophils, lymphocytes, and plasma cells within the ducts are usually indicative of a more intense inflammatory reaction (Fig. 2.10). Disruption of ducts is accompanied by discharge of stasis material into the breast, causing periductal inflammation. Plasma cells and granulomas are not conspicuous features of the lesion in most

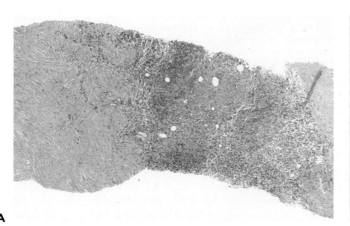

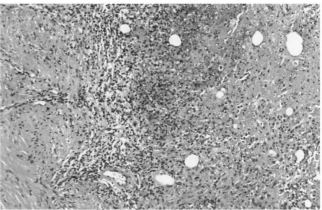

A   **B**

Figure 2.8 **Plasma cell mastitis. A,B:** A needle core biopsy specimen from a patient with a breast mass suspected to be carcinoma. Plasma cells are a prominent element in the reactive cellular infiltrate around the area of necrosis.

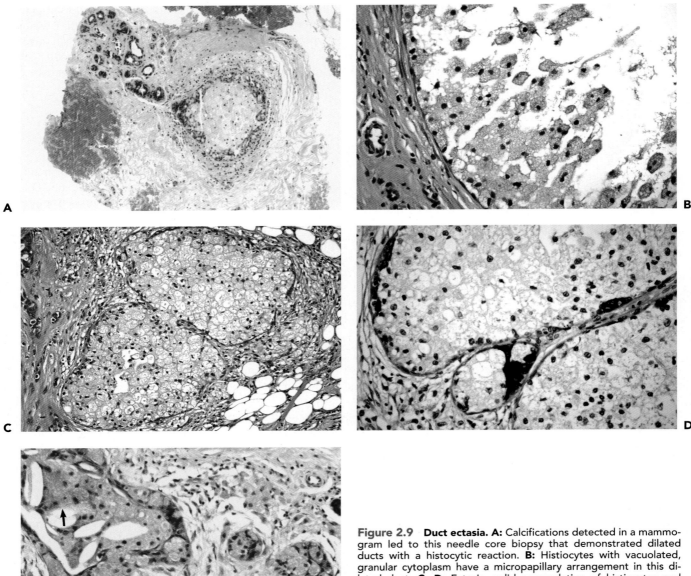

Figure 2.9 Duct ectasia. A: Calcifications detected in a mammogram led to this needle core biopsy that demonstrated dilated ducts with a histocytic reaction. **B:** Histiocytes with vacuolated, granular cytoplasm have a micropapillary arrangement in this dilated duct. **C, D:** Ectasia, solid accumulation of histiocytes and periductal inflammation that mimics clear cell intraductal carcinoma. Residual ductal epithelial cells are highlighted by the cytokeratin immunostain in **D**. The histocytes are cytokeratin-negative (immunoperoxidase). **E:** Histiocytes with finely granular ceroid pigment (*arrow*), so-called ochrocytes, are present in the duct lumen, the epithelium, and the surrounding tissue.

cases. Calcium oxalate crystals may be found when stasis occurs in a duct with apocrine epithelium (Fig. 2.10).

Histocytic cells with clear or "foamy" cytoplasm positioned in the epithelium of ducts can be confused with pagetoid carcinoma cells. In most instances, the distinction is made with little difficulty on the basis of bland nuclear cytology of the cells and the presence of typical inflammatory components of duct ectasia. The histocytic phenotype of these cells can be confirmed by a positive periodic acid–Schiff (PAS) reaction and selected immunostains. Pagetoid foam cells are reactive for CD68. They are negative for cytoplasmic cytokeratin as well as actin but may display misleading surface cytokeratin staining from the cell membranes of contiguous epithelial cells or weak reactivity for adsorbed antigens such as gross cystic disease fluid protein-15 (GCDFP-15) (19).

Periductal fibrosis and hyperelastosis, often with a lamellar distribution, lead to mural thickening in the late phase of mammary duct ectasia (Fig. 2.11). The inflammatory reaction is less conspicuous and the ducts are encased in a thick, laminated layer of hyaline fibrous and elastic tissue (20). The duct lumen may be patulous (Fig. 2.12). In some instances the sclerotic process includes actively proliferating granulation tissue and hyperelastosis, that

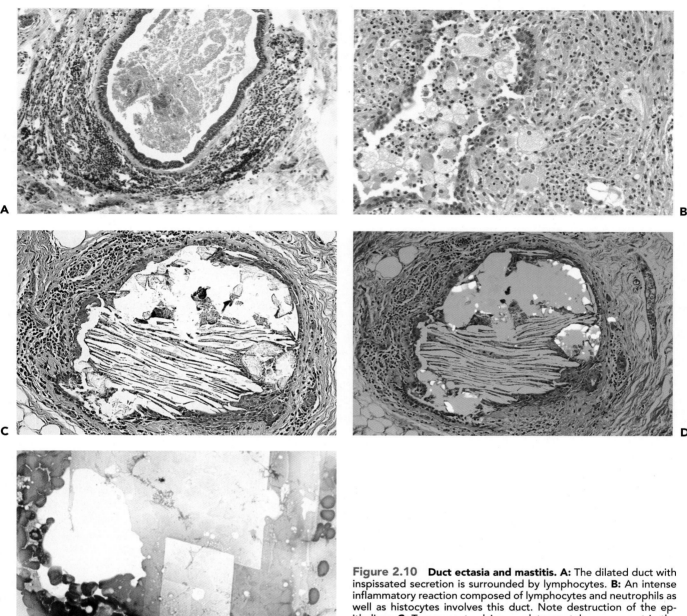

Figure 2.10 **Duct ectasia and mastitis. A:** The dilated duct with inspissated secretion is surrounded by lymphocytes. **B:** An intense inflammatory reaction composed of lymphocytes and neutrophils as well as histocytes involves this duct. Note destruction of the epithelium. **C:** Transparent calcium oxalate crystals are present in the duct lumen. **D:** The calcium oxalate crystals glow when viewed with polarized light. **E:** Calcium oxalate crystals in a needle core biopsy touch preparation. The specimen showed apocrine hyperplasia.

narrows and may totally occlude ducts (21). Remnants of persisting epithelium may proliferate to form secondary glands within the sclerotic duct. When the epithelium is totally absent, the duct is reduced to a fibrous scar.

GRANULOMATOUS MASTITIS

Numerous pathogenic processes responsible for granulomatous inflammation of the breast are included under the generic heading of granulomatous mastitis (22). The differential diagnosis of granulomatous mastitis includes specific agents such as tuberculosis, leprosy, brucellosis

and other bacterial infections, fungi, parasitic infestations, and rheumatoid nodules (22,23). It is necessary to exclude the presence of acid-fast or other bacteria and fungi with cultures, histochemical stains, and appropriate clinical tests. Reactive, sarcoid-like granulomatous inflammation that develops in breast carcinomas is restricted to the tumor, immediately surrounding mammary parenchyma and axillary lymph nodes (24).

Granulomatous lobular mastitis is a clinicopathologic condition characterized by perilobular granulomatous inflammation (25,26). This distribution suggests a cell-mediated reaction to one or more substances concentrated in the mammary secretion or lobular cells, but no specific anti-

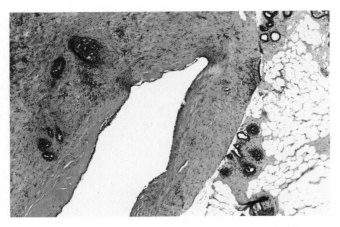

Figure 2.11 **Duct ectasia.** A late stage lesion sampled by needle core biopsy. There is marked periductal fibrosis with minimal inflammation.

gen has been identified. The lesion usually appears an average of 2 years after a pregnancy. The age at diagnosis ranges from 17 to 42 years, with a mean of about 33 years (26). Virtually all patients are parous. The distinct, firm-to-hard mass may involve any part of the breast, but it tends to spare the subareolar region. The breast tumors have reportedly measured from 1 cm to as much as 8 cm, averaging nearly 6 cm. The clinical findings often suggest carcinoma, and mammography has been described as "suspicious" (22). In one report, sonograms were characterized by "multiple clustered, often contiguous tubular hypoechoic lesions" (27).

The primary pathologic change is granulomatous lobulitis (Fig. 2.13). The granulomas are composed of epithelioid histiocytes and Langhans giant cells accompanied by lymphocytes, plasma cells, and occasional eosinophils. Asteroid bodies are unusual and Schaumann bodies have not been reported in the giant cells. While not typically a conspicuous feature, fat necrosis and abscesses containing polymorphonuclear leucocytes are sometimes present, contributing to effacement of the lobulocentric distribution in confluent

lesions. Spaces that develop in the centers of the abscesses contain no foreign material or demonstrable secretion. It is likely that lipid from degenerating cells contained in these spaces is dissolved during histologic processing of the tissues. A narrow zone of neutrophils usually outlines these spaces and neutrophils may accumulate in the lumens. Squamous metaplasia of duct and lobular epithelium is unusual. Vasculitis is not seen. Stains and cultures for bacteria, acid fast organisms, and fungi are negative.

Sarcoidosis usually occurs in the breast of women in their 20s and 30s, reflecting the overall age distribution of sarcoidosis (28,29). Mammary lesions often are detected after the diagnosis has been established on the basis of the typical clinical manifestations of the disease. Only very rarely does sarcoidosis present as a primary breast tumor. In some patients the breast lesion caused by mammary sarcoidosis is a firm-to-hard mass that may be mistaken clinically for carcinoma. Occasionally, sarcoidosis is not apparent clinically, and the granulomas may be discovered when a biopsy of the breast is performed for an unrelated condition.

The mammographic, ultrasound, and magnetic resonance imaging (MRI) characteristics of mammary sarcoidosis are not specific and can be interpreted as suggestive of carcinoma (30), especially if a speculated lesion is seen on mammography (31). Rarely, sarcoidosis produces multiple, bilateral small mammographically detected lesions (32).

Microscopic examination reveals epithelioid granulomas in the mammary parenchyma among lobules and ducts (Fig. 2.14). Multinucleated Langhans giant cells in the granulomas may contain asteroid or Schaumann bodies. The lesions do not have caseous necrosis or calcification, and fat necrosis is not found in the surrounding breast tissue. A lymphoplasmacytic reaction and fibrosis are present in varying amounts. Small, isolated granulomas with a sparse lymphocytic reaction may be found in surrounding breast tissue that appears grossly to be unaffected. These inconspicuous granulomatous foci tend to be associated with ducts or lobules.

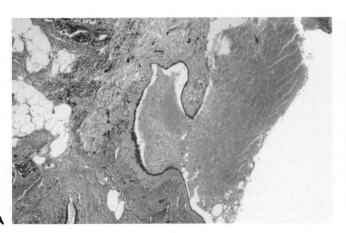

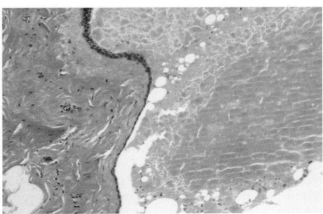

A   B

Figure 2.12 **Duct ectasia and stasis. A,B:** The dilated duct is lined by flat epithelium. There is no inflammation. Acellular proteinaceous material fills the duct lumen.

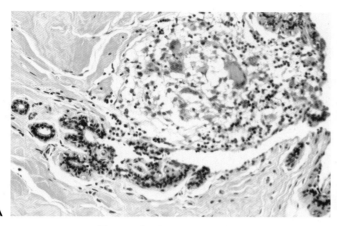

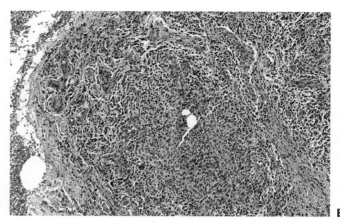

Figure 2.13 Granulomatous lobulitis. A: A granuloma with epithelioid giant cells in a lobule at the edge of a needle core biopsy specimen. No specific etiology was demonstrated in this patient. **B:** This granuloma of undetermined etiology and central necrosis has destroyed much of the lobule in which it resides.

INFLAMMATORY PSEUDOTUMOR

There is no well-characterized lesion of the breast that qualifies for this diagnosis. The diagnosis has been mistakenly used for metaplastic carcinoma, sarcomas with inflammation, granulomatous mastitis, fibromatosis, and infarcts. In most cases, lesions diagnosed as inflammatory pseudotumors were probably the result of fat necrosis or duct ectasia with mastitis (Fig. 2.15). Localized nodular lesions in the breast formed by interlacing bundles of myofibroblastic cells with a prominent infiltrate composed mainly of plasma cells, histocytes and lymphocytes have been diagnosed as inflammatory pseudotumors (33–35). Elevated serum immunoglobulin IgG4 that is associated with sclerosing pancreatitis has been reported in a patient with inflammatory pseudotumor of the breast (36). Immunohistochemistry revealed many IgG4-positive plasma cells in the lesional tissue.

Mammography in one case revealed a 2 cm round mass with ill-defined borders and no calcifications. The tumor was hypoechoic, homogeneous, and lacked acoustic shadowing on ultrasound (35). One patient had a unilateral lesion that did not recur after excision (34). Another patient with bilateral tumors developed recurrences in both breasts (33).

The differential diagnosis includes other lesions rarely encountered in the breast such as Erdheim–Chester disease (8), previously discussed under Fat Necrosis, and adult type "juvenile" xanthogranuloma (37). The latter lesion consists of a prominent spindle cell proliferation associated with multinucleated giant cells, including Touton type cells, lymphocytes, plasma cells, and xanthomatous histocytes. The xanthomatous cells are reactive for KP1, MAC387, and PGM1 but negative for S-100 and CD1a (37).

VASCULITIS

Inflammatory lesions of arteries are encountered in a variety of systemic disorders that are broadly grouped under the heading of collagen-vascular disease. The breasts may be affected as an isolated manifestation or as part of multi-

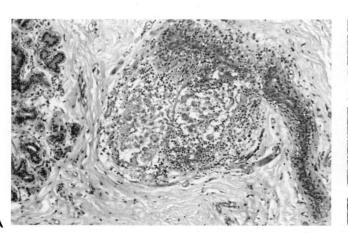

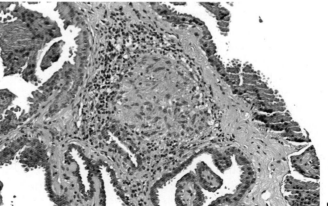

Figure 2.14 Sarcoidosis. A: The discrete granuloma adjacent to a duct does not involve the nearby lobule. **B:** A small granuloma amidst apocrine cysts in a needle core biopsy sample from a 53-year-old woman known to have sarcoidosis.

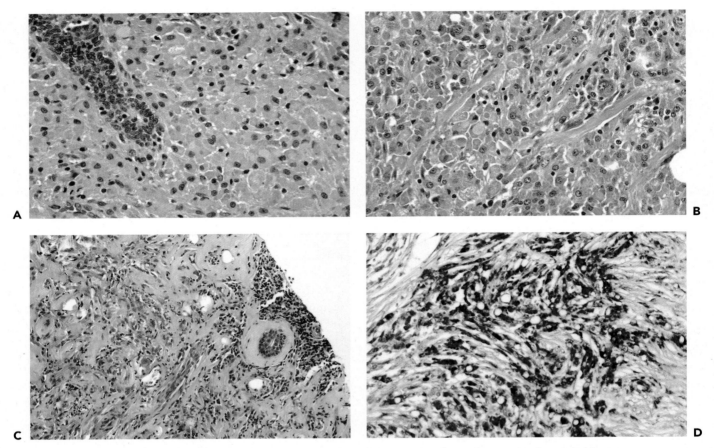

Figure 2.15   Inflammatory pseudotumor. A,B: This specimen is from a 2-cm tumor that probably represents resolving fat necrosis. The lesion is composed of numerous epithelioid histiocytes and sparse fibroblasts and lymphocytes. **C:** A needle core biopsy specimen from another, more fibrotic inflammatory pseudotumor. Note the duct at the border of the specimen. **D:** Histocytes in the lesion shown in **(C)** are highlighted by the MAC immunostain (immunoperoxidase).

organ involvement. The mammary lesions caused by vasculitis often resemble carcinoma clinically. Although there are differences in the histopathologic features of the vasculitides associated with various collagen–vascular diseases, the diagnosis of a specific condition is made on the basis of the clinical and pathologic findings. Some of these conditions may be manifested by a tumorous lesion or mammographically detected calcifications (38).

Giant cell arteritis limited clinically to the breast has been reported in women 52 to 72 years of age who presented with one or more palpable breast tumors (39,40). The lesions were bilateral in nearly 50% of cases. The firm tumors have measured from less than 1 to 4 cm, and carcinoma was suspected in most patients (41). Axillary nodal enlargement has been noted in some cases (40). Systemic symptoms reported by patients with giant cell arteritis of the breast include headache, muscle and joint pain, fever, and night sweats. Mild anemia and an elevated erythrocyte sedimentation rate are found in most cases.

Microscopically, transmural inflammation involves small- and medium-size arteries throughout the affected

tissue (Fig. 2.16). Veins and arterioles are largely spared. Fibrinoid necrosis is not a consistent feature, but fragmentation of the mural elastic fibers is demonstrable with an

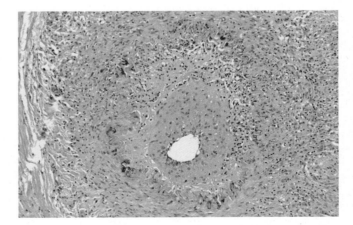

Figure 2.16   Giant cell arteritis. The patient presented with a mass and biopsy revealed fat necrosis due to diffuse arteritis. This artery is almost totally occluded by the inflammatory process. The elastica is fragmented. No giant cells are evident in this particular area.

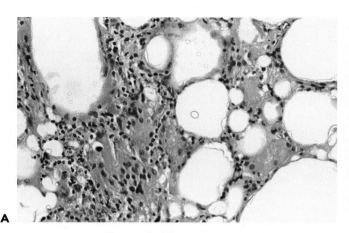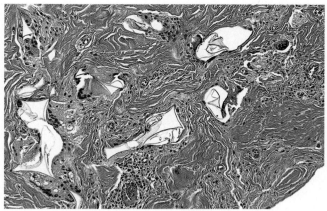

A

B

Figure 2.17 Implant-associated mastitis. A: Chronic inflammation surrounds vacuolar spaces that contain silicone material. **B:** Refractile fragments of polyurethane from the outer surface of a silicone cosmetic breast implant were present in this needle core biopsy sample from a 44-year-old woman who presented with a breast mass.

elastic tissue stain. Multinucleated giant cells tend to be oriented around the disrupted elastic fibers. The vascular lumen may be narrowed or occluded. The surrounding fibrofatty tissue exhibits fibrosis, edema, fat necrosis, and atrophy of glandular elements. The differential diagnosis includes other types of arteritis, phlebitis, infarction related to pregnancy or lactation, and traumatic fat necrosis.

Breast involvement has also been reported in patients with *Wegener granulomatosis* (42), *polyarteritis* (43), *scleroderma* (44), *dermatomyositis* (45), and *lupus erythematosis* (46). The lesions may be manifested by a mass with vascular calcifications or with irregular dystrophic calcifications (38). Biopsy reveals arterial necrosis and a transmural inflammatory reaction. Necrosis of surrounding breast parenchyma is often present. Patients with one of these forms of systemic vasculitis may develop coincidental breast carcinoma in the absence of mammary vasculitis, but there is no evidence that these diseases predispose a patient to breast carcinoma (47–49).

Lupus mastitis is a rare complication of lupus erythematosus (46). In some cases this is manifested by lymphocytic mastopathy distributed mainly in and around lobules but a perivascular component may also be detected. Lupus mastitis is a form of lupus panniculitis characterized clinically by nodular lesions and histologically by fat necrosis in various stages of evolution (50). Concentric perivascular fibrosis and hyalinized stromal fibrosis extending around ducts and lobules were described in a woman who had recurrent lupus mastitis over an 8-year period starting at 40 years of age (51). The patient had clinically documented systemic lupus with elevated serum antinuclear antibody (ANA) titers. Advanced lesions may have considerable calcification. Ig deposits can be demonstrated around blood vessels in the lesional tissue and serum ANAs are present. Clinical findings in the skin may mimic inflammatory carcinoma (52). The radiologic appearance of lupus mastitis has been described (53).

SILICONE MASTITIS

The ability to detect carcinoma by mammography and ultrasound is impaired by mastitis caused by injected silicone or the reaction to a silicone containing implant (54,55). Calcifications caused by silicone mastitis are generally irregular and coarse but finer calcifications resembling those of carcinoma have been reported in silicone mastitis and when present, they should be biopsied (56). Enhanced MRI is reportedly an important procedure for detecting carcinoma in a breast distorted by silicone mastitis (55).

Silicone by itself or with adulterants causes fat necrosis and elicits a foreign body giant cell reaction (Fig. 2.17). The microscopic features of these processes are not specific for silicone injection. Silicone may also enter the lumens of ducts and lobular glands (57). During the processing of histologic sections, some of the silicone is lost from the tissue, leaving clear spaces of varying size. The presence of silicone can be confirmed by electron microscopy, infrared spectroscopy, atomic absorption spectrophotometry, and other procedures (58). The accompanying chronic inflammatory reaction and fibrosis vary in intensity.

DIABETIC MASTOPATHY

The occurrence of tumor-forming stromal proliferations in patients with diabetes mellitus is referred to as diabetic mastopathy (59). The pathologic changes are not entirely specific for insulin-dependent diabetes mellitus (60), and similar lesions have been reported in patients with autoimmune diseases who did not have diabetes (61,62).

With rare exceptions (63), diabetic mastopathy has been limited to females. Most patients were younger than 30 years when type I insulin-dependent diabetes mellitus was diagnosed. Age at the time of breast biopsy ranged from 19 to 63 years, with a mean of 34 to 47 years in six studies. The interval between the onset of diabetes and detection of the breast lesion averages about 20 years. Bilateral lesions have been present in nearly 50% of the cases. The majority of the patients have had complications of juvenile onset diabetes with severe diabetic retinopathy reported in many instances. The initial clinical symptom is a palpable, firm-to-hard tumor that may suggest carcinoma.

The mammogram often reveals localized, increased density or a heterogeneous parenchymal pattern, but no changes have been specifically associated with this condition (64,65). In some patients, the mammographic appearance of the mass resembles carcinoma or a fibroadenoma (61,66). An irregular hypoechoic mass with variable acoustic shadowing is found on sonographic examination. Ultrasound guidance may be the preferred modality for performing a core biopsy procedure (64). Breast density associated with diabetic mastopathy could obscure a coexistent lesion such as carcinoma, a setting in which MRI may be useful (67,68). Spontaneous regression and clinical disappearance of diabetic mastopathy has been described (69).

The lesional tissue consists of collagenous stroma with keloidal features and a variably increased number of stromal cells when compared with the surrounding breast tissue. Polygonal epithelioid cells are found dispersed in the collagen among the spindly stromal cells in most but not all cases. The stromal cells are myofibroblasts with variable fibroblastic and myoid differentiation (Fig. 2.18). Multinucleated stromal giant cells and mitotic activity are not part of this proliferative process. Mature lymphocytes are clustered around small blood vessels throughout the lesion as well as in and around lobules and ducts. Very few plasma cells or leucocytes are present in the perivascular infiltrates. Germinal centers are rarely formed. When studied by immunohistochemistry, the lymphocytes have a B-cell phenotype. The polymerase chain reaction detected no Ig heavy chain gene rearrangements in tissue samples from six patients with diabetic mastopathy (70).

In most instances, diabetic mastopathy has all of the foregoing histologic features, but on occasion, one or more of the typical findings may be absent (71). Infarcts, fat necrosis, granulomas, duct stasis, arteritis, and other inflammatory lesions are not features of diabetic mastopathy. Stromal collagen fibers are sometimes prominent, but they do not have a keloidal appearance. Proliferative epithelial changes may be present coincidentally but they are not an integral component of diabetic mastopathy. The differential diagnosis of diabetic mastopathy includes nonspecific lymphocytic lobulitis (Fig. 2.19) and fibromatosis.

Diabetic mastopathy is a self-limited stromal abnormality. Recurrent tumors have occurred in the ipsilateral breast in a minority of cases, and these patients are prone to asynchronous, as well as synchronous, bilateral involvement.

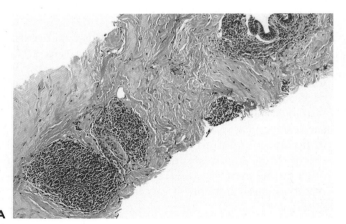

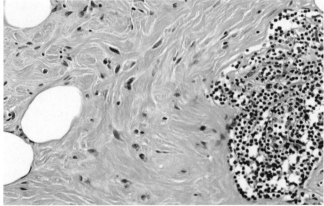

Figure 2.18 Diabetic mastopathy. A,B: Mature lymphocytes are clustered around a small blood vessel and prominent myofibroblastic cells are evident in the stroma. The specimen was obtained from a young woman with juvenile-onset diabetes mellitus who presented with a unilateral breast mass. **C:** Spindly myofibroblasts are CD34-positive (immunoperoxidase).

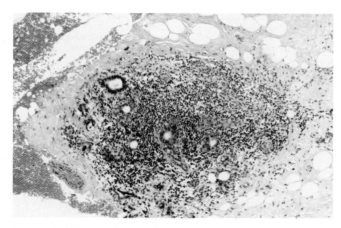

Figure 2.19 Lymphocytic lobulitis. This needle core biopsy was performed to assess a nonpalpable lesion without calcifications. The patient had no known systemic disease. One of several lobules infiltrated by mature lymphocytes is shown here.

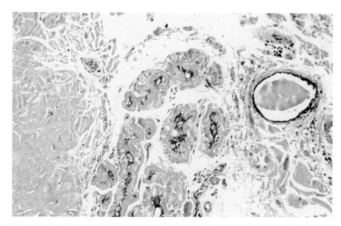

Figure 2.20 Amyloidosis. A thick layer of amyloid has been deposited in the basement membranes of the glands in a lobule next to a nodule of amyloid in the stroma on the left.

Excisional biopsy is adequate treatment. There is no evidence to suggest that diabetic mastopathy predisposes to the development of mammary carcinoma or stromal neoplastic diseases such as fibromatosis. Nonetheless, patients with diabetic mastopathy can coincidentally develop mammary carcinoma, and, therefore, any mass that occurs in these women should be subjected to diagnostic assessment.

AMYLOID TUMOR

Amyloid deposits in the breast have been described in patients with predisposing systemic diseases such as primary amyloidosis, rheumatoid arthritis, and multiple myeloma. Primary amyloid tumors clinically limited to the breast are uncommon (72,73). Age at diagnosis ranges from 45 to 86 years (median 56 years). Bilateral involvement has been described (72,74,75). The tumors have usually been solitary. Clinical examination reveals a discrete, hard tumor that can mimic carcinoma and may contain calcifications on mammography (75–77). Concurrent mammary carcinoma and amyloidosis have been described (78,79).

Histologically, eosinophilic amorphous, homogeneous deposits of amyloid are distributed in fat, fibrocollagenous stroma, and the walls of blood vessels (Fig. 2.20). Deposits of amyloid around ducts and in lobules are associated with atrophy and obliteration of these glandular components. In adipose tissue, thin ribbons of amyloid may be formed around individual fat cells. These so-called amyloid rings are accentuated when Congo red–stained sections are examined with polarized light (80). Varying numbers of plasma cells, lymphocytes, and multinucleated giant cells are usually present in association with the amyloid deposits, that can also have punctate or irregular calcifications and rarely to osseous metaplasia (77,81). Amyloid is stained red-orange with alkaline Congo red and it exhibits apple-green birefringence when the Congo red–stained section is examined with

polarized light. Staining with crystal violet results in a strong metachromatic reaction. Amyloid deposits are immunoreactive for the amyloid P component and variably reactive for κ-light chain, λ-light chain, and other Igs (78).

When limited to the breast, amyloid tumor has proven to be a benign condition that has been treated by excisional biopsy. Most patients have remained well following an excisional biopsy in the limited follow-up thus far reported. However, one woman who presented with bilateral mammary amyloid tumors developed systemic amyloidosis 1 year later (75). The prognosis of patients with mammary lesions and systemic amyloidosis depends on the clinical course of the underlying condition.

REFERENCES

1. Clarke D, Curtis JL, Martinez A, et al. Fat necrosis of the breast simulating recurrent carcinoma after primary radiotherapy in the management of early breast cancer. *Cancer.* 1983;52:442–445.
2. Rostom AY, el-Sayed ME. Fat necrosis of the breast: an unusual complication of lumpectomy and radiotherapy in breast cancer. *Clin Radiol.* 1987;38:31.
3. Girling AC, Hanby AM, Millis RR. Radiation and other pathological changes in breast tissue after conservation treatment for carcinoma. *J Clin Pathol.* 1990;43:152–156.
4. Hogge JP, Robinson RE, Magnant CM, Zuurbier RA. The mammographic spectrum of fat necrosis of the breast. *Radiographics.* 1995;15:1347–1356.
5. Martin BF, Phillips JD. Gangrene of the female breast with anticoagulant therapy: report of two cases. *Am J Clin Pathol.* 1970;53:622–626.
6. Isenberg JS, Tu Q, Rainey W. Mammary gangrene associated with warfarin ingestion. *Ann Plast Surg.* 1996;37:553–555.
7. Bargum K, Moller Nielsen S. Case report: fat necrosis of the breast appearing as oil cysts with fat-fluid levels. *Br J Radiol.* 1993;66:718–720.
8. Barnes, PJ Foyle A, Hache KA, et al. Erdheim-Chester disease of the breast: a case report and review of the literature. *Breast J.* 2005;11:462–467.
9. Flint A, Oberman HA. Infarction and squamous metaplasia of intraductal papilloma: a benign breast lesion that may simulate carcinoma. *Hum Pathol.* 1984;15:764–767.
10. Murad TM, Contesso G, Mouriesse H. Papillary tumors of large lactiferous ducts. *Cancer.* 1981;48:122–133.
11. Jones EL, Codling BW, Oates GD. Necrotic intraduct breast carcinomas simulating inflammatory lesions. *J Pathol.* 1973;110:101–103.
12. Golden GT, Wangensteen SL. Galactocele of the breast. *Am J Surg.* 1972;123:271–273.
13. Salvador R, Salvador M, Jimenez JA, et al. Galactocele of the breast: radiologic and ultrasonographic findings. *Br J Radiol.* 1990;63:140–142.
14. Novotny DB, Maygarden SJ, Shermer RW, Frable WJ. Fine needle aspiration of benign and malignant breast masses associated with pregnancy. *Acta Cytol.* 1991;35:676–686.

15. Habif DV, Perzin KH, Lipton R, Lattes R. Subareolar abscess associated with squamous metaplasia of lactiferous ducts. *Am J Surg.* 1970;119:523–526.

16. Passaro ME, Broughan TA, Sebek BA, Esselstyn Jr CB. Lactiferous fistula. *J Am Coll Surg.* 1994;178:29–32.

17. Sweeney DJ, Wylie EJ. Mammographic appearances of mammary duct ectasia that mimic carcinoma in a screening programme. *Austral Radiol.* 1995;39:18–23.

18. Davies JD. Pigmented periductal cells (ochrocytes) in mammary dysplasias: their nature and significance. *J Path.* 1974;114:205–216.

19. Tashire T, Hirokawa M, Sano T. Are mammary pagetoid foam cells histocytic or epithelial? *Virchows Arch.* 2001;439:102–103.

20. Davies JD. Inflammatory damage to ducts in mammary dysplasia: a cause of duct dilatation. *J Path.* 1975;117:47–54.

21. Davies JD. Hyperelastosis, obliteration and fibrous plaques in major ducts of the human breast. *J Path.* 1973;110:13–26.

22. Fitzgibbons PL. Granulomatous mastitis. *NY State J Med.* 1990;90:287.

23. Cooper NE. Rheumatoid nodule of the breast. *Histopathology.* 1991; 19:193–194.

24. Bässler R, Birke F. Histopathology of tumour associated sarcoid-like stromal reaction in breast cancer. An analysis of 5 cases with immunohistochemical investigations. *Virchows Arch.* [A] 1988;412:231–239.

25. Fletcher A, Magrath IM, Riddell RH, Talbot IC. Granulomatous mastitis: a report of seven cases. *J Clin Pathol.* 1982;35:941–945.

26. Going JJ, Anderson TJ, Wilkinson S, Chetty U. Granulomatous lobular mastitis. *J Clin Pathol.* 1987;40:535–540.

27. Han B-K, Choe YH, Park JM, et al. Granulomatous mastitis: mammographic and sonographic appearances. *Am J Roentgenol.* 1999;173:317–320.

28. Fitzgibbons PL, Smiley DF, Kern WH. Sarcoidosis presenting initially as breast mass: report of two cases. *Hum Pathol.* 1985;16:851–852.

29. Banik S, Bishop PW, Ormerod LP, O'Brien TEB. Sarcoidosis of the breast. *J Clin Pathol.* 1986;39:446–448.

30. Kenzel PP, Hadijuana J, Hosten N, et al. Boeck sarcoidosis of the breast: mammographic, ultrasound, and MR findings. *J Comp Assisted Tomogr.* 1997;21:439–441.

31. Kirshy D, Gluck B, Brancaccio W. Sarcoidosis of the breast presenting as a spiculated lesion. *Am J Roentgenol.* 1999;172:554–555.

32. Nicholson BT, Mills SE. Sarcoidosis of the breast: an unusual presentation of a systemic disease. *Breast J.* 2007;13:99–100.

33. Yip CH, Wong KT, Samuel D. Bilateral plasma cell granuloma (inflammatory pseudotumour) of the breast. *Aust NZ J Surg.* 1997;67:300–303.

34. Pettinato G, Manivel JC, Insabato L, et al. Plasma cell granuloma (inflammatory pseudotumour) of the breast. *Am J Clin Pathol.* 1988;90:627–632.

35. Haj M, Weiss M, Loberant N, Cohen I. Inflammatory pseudotumor of the breast: case report and literature review. *Breast J.* 2003;9:423–425.

36. Zen Y, Kasahara Y, Horita K, et al. Inflammatory pseudotumor of the breast in a patient with a high serum IgG4 level. *Am J Surg Pathol.* 2005;29:275–278.

37. Shin SJ, Scamman W, Gopalan A, Rosen PP. Mammary presentation of adult-type "juvenile" xanthogranuloma. *Am J Surg Pathol.* 2005;29:827–831.

38. Kim SM, Park JM, Moon WK. Dystrophic breast calcifications in patients with collagen diseases. *J Clin Imaging.* 2004;28:6–9.

39. Clement PB, Senges H, How AR. Giant cell arteritis of the breast: case report and literature review. *Hum Pathol.* 1987;18:1186–1189.

40. Lau Y, Mak YF, Hui PK, Achong AK. Giant cell arteritis of the breast. *Aust NZ J Surg.* 1996;66:259–261.

41. Pappo I, Beglaibter N, Amir G. Mammary arteritis mimicking cancer. *Eur J Surg.* 1992;158:191–193.

42. Jordan JM, Rowe TW, Allen NB. Wegener's granulomatosis involving the breast. Report of three cases and review of the literature. *Am J Med.* 1987;83:159–164.

43. Yamashina M, Wilson TK. A mammographic finding in focal polyarteritis nodosa. *Br J Radiol.* 1985;58:91–92.

44. Harrison GO, Elliott RL. Scleroderma of the breast: light and electron microscopy study. *Am Surg.* 1987;53:526–531.

45. Gyves-Ray KM, Adler DD. Dermatomyositis: an unusual cause of breast calcifications. *Breast Dis.* 1989;2:195–201.

46. Cernea SS, Kihara SM, Sotto MN, Vilela MAC. Lupus mastitis. *J Am Acad Dermatol.* 1993;29:343–346.

47. Bonnetblanc JM, Bernard P, Fayol J. Dermatomyositis and malignancy. A multicenter cooperative study. *Dermatologica.* 1990;180:212–216.

48. Sigurgeirsson B, Lindelöf B, Edhag O, Allander E. Risk of cancer in patients with dermatomyositis or polymyositis. A population-based study. *N Engl J Med.* 1992;326:363–367.

49. Kontos M, Fentiman I. Systemic lupus erythematosus and breast cancer. *Breast J.* 2008;14:81–86.

50. Holland NW, McKnight K, Challa VR, Agudelo CA. Lupus panniculitis (Profundus) involving the breast: report of 2 cases and review of the literature. *J. Rheumatol.* 1995;22:344–346.

51. Nigar E, Contractor K, Singhal H, Matin RN. Lupus mastitis- a cause of recurrent breast lumps. *Histopathology.* 2007;51:847–849.

52. Fernandez-Flores A, Crespo LG, Alonso S, Montero MG. Lupus mastitis in the male breast mimicking inflammatory carcinoma. *Breast J.* 2006;12; 272–273.

53. Georgian-Smith D, Lawton TJ, Moe RE, Couser WG. Lupus mastitis: radiologic and pathologic features. *Am J Roentgenol.* 2002;178:1233–1235.

54. Destouet JM, Monsees BS, Oser RF, et al. Screening mammography in 350 women with breast implants: prevalence and findings of implant complications. *Am J Roentgenol.* 1992;159:973–978.

55. Cheung YC, Su MY, Ng SH. Lumpy silicone-injected breasts: enhanced MRI and microscopic correlation. *J Clin Imaging.* 2002;26:397–404.

56. Morgenstern L, Gleischman SH, Michel SL, et al. Relation of free silicone to human breast carcinoma. *Arch Surg.* 1986;120:573–577.

57. Leibman AJ, Kossoff MB, Kruse BD. Intraductal extension of silicone from a ruptured breast implant. *Plast Reconstr Surg.* 1992;89:546–547.

58. Travis WE, Balogh K, Abraham JL. Silicone granulomas: report of three cases and review of the literature. *Hum Pathol.* 1985;16:19–27.

59. Tomaszewski JE, Brooks JSJ, Hicks D, LiVolsi VA. Diabetic mastopathy: a distinctive clinicopathologic entity. *Hum Pathol.* 1992;23:780–786.

60. Seidman JD, Schnaper LA, Phillips LE. Mastopathy in insulin-requiring diabetes mellitus. *Hum Pathol.* 1994;25:819–824.

61. Ashton MA, Lefkowitz M, Tavassoli FA. Epithelioid stromal cells in lymphocytic mastitis—a source of confusion with invasive carcinoma. *Mod Pathol.* 1994;7:49–54.

62. Love JE, Lawton TJ. Diabetic mastopathy in patients with non-diabetic autoimmune disease. *Mod Pathol.* 2005;18(suppl.):41A.

63. Weinstein SP, Conant EF, Orel SG, et al. Diabetic mastopathy in men: imaging findings in two patients. *Radiology.* 2001;219:797–799.

64. Tang DA, Diamond AB, Rogers L, Butler D. Diabetic mastopathy: adjunctive use of ultrasound and utility of core biopsy in diagnosis. *Breast J.* 2000;6:183–188.

65. Camuto PM, Zetrenne E, Ponn T. Diabetic mastopathy. A report of 5 cases and a review of the literature. *Arch Surg.* 2000;135:1190–1193.

66. Byrd BF Jr, Hartmann WH, Graham LS, Hogle HH. Mastopathy in insulin-dependent diabetics. *Ann Surg.* 1987;205:529–532.

67. Gabriel HA, Feng C, Mendelson EB, Benjamin S. Breast MRI for cancer detection in a patient with diabetic mastopathy. *Am J Roentgenol.* 2004; 182:1081–1083.

68. Tuncbilek N, Karakas HM, Okten O. Diabetic fibrous mastopathy: dynamic contrast-enhanced magnetic resonance imaging findings. *Breast J.* 2004; 10:359–362.

69. Bayer U, Horn LC, Schulz HG. Bilateral, tumor-like diabetic mastopathy-progression and regression of the disease during a 5-year follow-up. Case report. *Eur J Radiol.* 1998;26:248–253.

70. Valdez R, Thorson J, Finn WG, et al. Lymphocytic mastitis and diabetic mastopathy: a molecular, immunophenotypic, and clinicopathologic evaluation of 11 cases. *Mod Pathol.* 2003;16:223–228.

71. Morgan MC, Weaver MG, Crowe JP, Abdul-Karim FW. Diabetic mastopathy: a clinicopathologic study of palpable and nonpalpable breast lesions. *Mod Pathol.* 1995;8:349–354.

72. Silverman JF, Dabbs DJ, Norris HT, et al. Localized primary (AL) amyloid tumor of the breast. Cytologic, histologic, immunocytochemical and ultrastructural observations. *Am J Surg Pathol.* 1986;10:539–545.

73. Luo J-H, Rotterdam H. Primary amyloid tumor of the breast: a case report and review of the literature. *Hum Pathol.* 1997:10:735–738.

74. Fleury AM, Buetens OW, Campasi C, Argani P. Pathologic Quiz Case: a 77-year old woman with bilateral breast masses. *Arch Pathol Lab Med.* 2004;128:e67.

75. Hecht AH, Tan A, Shen JF. Case report: primary systemic amyloidosis presenting as breast masses, mammographically simulating carcinoma. *Clin Radiology.* 1991;44:123–124.

76. Liaw Y-S, Kuo S-H, Yang P-C, Luh K-T. Nodular amyloidosis of the lung and the breast mimicking breast carcinoma with pulmonary metastasis. *Eur Respir J.* 1995;5:871–873.

77. Lynch LA, Moriarty AT. Localized primary amyloid tumor associated with osseous metaplasia presenting as bilateral breast masses: cytologic and radiologic features. *Diagn Cytopathol.* 1993;9:570–575.

78. Rocken C, Kronsbein H, Sletten K, et al. Amyloidosis of the breast. *Virchows Arch.* 2002;440:527–535.

79. Munson-Bernardi BD, DePersia LA. Amyloidosis of the breast coexisting with ductal carcinoma in situ. *Am J Roengenol.* 2006;186:54–55.

80. Libbey CA, Skinner M, Cohen AS. The abdominal fat aspirate for the diagnosis of systemic amyloid. *Arch Intern Med.* 1983;143:1549–1552.

81. Yokoo H. Nakazato Y. Primary localized amyloid tumor of the breast with osseous metaplasia. *Pathol Int.* 1998;48:545–548.

Specific Infections

3

FUNGAL INFECTIONS

Infection with *Histoplasma capsulatum* is endemic in some regions of the United States and other nations. Calcified granulomas have not been described in the breast but there have been rare instances of localized mammary *Histoplasma* infection presenting as a solitary unilateral mass that suggested a neoplasm clinically (1,2). Histologically, the lesions consist of confluent necrotizing granulomas in which *H. capsulatum* is demonstrated by a methenamine silver reaction. The granulomatous reaction is histologically similar to that of nonspecific granulomatous lobular mastitis (2). The diagnosis of mastitis caused by *Histoplasma* in a needle core biopsy specimen has been reported (3).

Rare instances of other fungal infections of the breast have also been reported. These include *Cryptococcus* (4,5), *Aspergillus* (6,7), *Coccidioides* (8), and *Blastomyces* (9). *Aspergillus* infection has been reported at the site of breast augmentation implants (6).

PARASITIC INFECTIONS

Mammary *filariasis* caused most frequently by *Wuchereria bancrofti* has been reported from tropical and semi-tropical regions in South America, China, and the Indian Subcontinent, where infection with this organism is endemic. Involvement of the breast occurs in the chronic phase of the disease, sometimes more than a decade after the last exposure to infection.

The patient usually presents with a solitary, nontender, painless unilateral breast mass. Multiple lesions occur in a minority of cases. Many of the lesions involve subcutaneous tissue, and they may be fixed to the skin. The resultant hard mass with cutaneous attachment, sometimes accompanied by inflammatory changes including edema of the skin, appears to be clinically indistinguishable from carcinoma (10). In this setting, axillary nodal enlargement caused by filarial lymphadenitis further complicates the differential diagnosis. Viable microfilariae can be detected in the breast by ultrasound examination if they produce a distinctive pattern of movement referred to as the "filaria

dance sign" (11). Mammographically detected calcifications attributed to *W. bancrofti* and *Loa loa* infection have been described as having a spiral or serpiginous configuration (12). Microscopic examination of fine needle aspiration or tissue biopsy samples reveals adult filarial worms that may be well preserved or in varying stages of degeneration (Fig. 3.1). Microfilariae are not always detected in the peripheral blood (13). Granulomatous reaction with eosinophilia is present in the surrounding tissue. Fully degenerated worms are likely to become calcified. Adult worms and microfilariae may also be found in axillary lymph nodes (14).

Several examples of mammary *cysticercosis,* an infection caused by the larvae of tapeworms, have been described. Most instances of mammary cysticercosis were caused by *Taenia solium* (15). The breast can also be the site of hydatid cyst formation caused by *Echinococcus granulosus.* The lesion typically presents as a firm, discrete mobile mass. Mammography reveals a dense well-circumscribed tumor within which internal ring structures representing air fluid levels may be seen in an overly penetrated view. Ultrasound shows air fluid levels and multiple cysts to better advantage (16). Rarely, mammographically detected calcification of an inapparent cyst have been the first evidence of mammary cysticercosis (17,18). Mammary hydatid disease can be recognized by finding fragments of the adult worm, the hydatid membranes and hooklets in a biopsy specimen or in the aspirated cyst contents (19) (Fig. 3.2A). Needle core biopsy sampling of mammary sparganosis due to the tapeworm *Spirometra* has been described (20) (Fig. 3.2B).

Calcified ova of *Schistosomiasis* can produce a radiologic appearance in mammograms suggestive of carcinoma (21) (Fig. 3.3) or the inflammatory nodule may be mistaken for a fibroadenoma (22). Microcalcifications attributed to *Trichinella* infection have been found in the pectoral muscles by mammography (23).

Cutaneous myiasis caused by larvae of the botfly *Dermatobia hominis* results in a mass lesion accompanied by local inflammation. The mammographic and ultrasound findings in five patients with mammary lesions were reported by de Barros et al. (24). The mammographically ill-defined tumors measured 0.7 to 2.0 cm. Paired linear microcalcifications

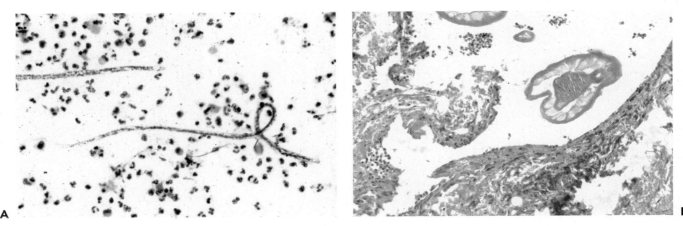

Figure 3.1   Filariasis. A: Microfilariae in a fine needle aspiration specimen with *W. bancrofti* infection. **B:** Biopsy specimen from a filarial abscess showing a microfilaria in cross section and fragments of the surrounding tissue (courtesy of Dr Kusum Kapila).

were visualized in three lesions. Oval larvae outlined by a hypoechoic zone were demonstrated by ultrasound examination. Although the diagnosis of myiasis will be suggested by a history of origin from or a visit to an endemic area, the clinical signs, the ultrasound findings, the presence of an ill-defined mass with calcification, and inflammation may mimic inflammatory carcinoma resulting in a needle core biopsy (25). Another form of cutaneous myiasis that manifests as abscesses with draining sinuses is caused by infestation by larvae of the Tumbu fly (*Cordylobia anthropophaga*), which is found in sub-Saharan West Africa (26).

MYCOBACTERIAL INFECTIONS

Mycobacterium tuberculosis infection of the breast is not an uncommon condition in some regions of the world (27). Tuberculous mastitis has been reported as a manifestation of AIDS and this presentation is encountered with increasing frequency in HIV-positive individuals (28,29).

Mammary tuberculosis not associated with HIV infection is primarily a disease of premenopausal women with a predilection for the lactating breast (30), but it can affect the adult female breast at any age. Infection of the breast may be the primary manifestation of tuberculosis, but the breasts are probably infected secondarily in most patients even when the primary nonmammary focus remains clinically inapparent.

It is difficult to make a diagnosis of tuberculous mastitis because the disease has multiple patterns of clinical presentation. The most common form is nodular mastitis in which the patient develops a slowly growing solitary mass. The mammographic appearance of such lesions resembles carcinoma (31,32). Microcalcifications are typically absent. Advanced nodular lesions become fixed to the skin and may develop draining sinuses (31). A diffuse type of tuberculous mastitis is characterized by the acute development of multiple painful nodules throughout the breast producing a pattern that can be mistaken for inflammatory carcinoma clinically and mammographically (32). A third, sclerosing

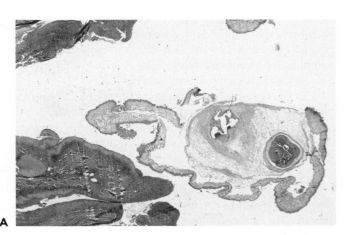
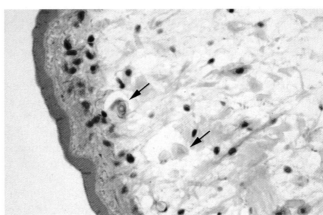

Figure 3.2   Cysticercosis. A: Part of hydatid cyst wall and a cross section of the larval tapeworm (courtesy of Dr Kusum Kapila). **B:** Portion of a sparganum larva obtained by needle core biopsy of the breast. Note the presence of whorled calcifications in the larva (*arrows*) (courtesy of Dr Amy Bik-Wan Chan).

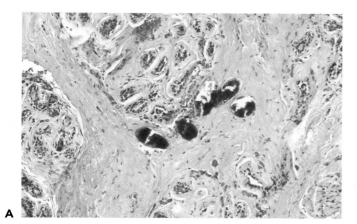

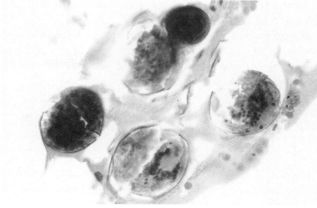

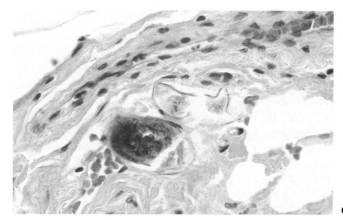

Figure 3.3   Schistosomiasis. This young woman with gastrointestinal symptoms was found to have numerous calcifications in the breast by mammography. **A:** The needle core biopsy sample shown here has five calcified ova of *Schistosoma mansoni* in the stroma next to a lobule. **B:** Five calcified ova in fat from the same specimen. **C:** Magnified view of showing the characteristic spine (courtesy of Dr Rhonda Yantiss).

variety of infection occurs predominantly in elderly women, resulting in diffuse induration of the breast and diffuse increased density on mammography. The clinical distinction between tuberculous mastitis and mammary carcinoma is complicated by the occasional coexistence of the lesions (33).

Microscopically, granulomatous lesions in tuberculous mastitis do not always feature caseous necrosis and in chronic cases, fibrosis may be prominent. The granulomas are associated with ducts and lobules (Fig. 3.4). Acid-fast bacteria are not detected histologically in most cases. Neutrophils can obscure the granulomatous character of the process in specimens from patients with necrotizing abscesses or sinus tracts. Calcifications are uncommon. The finding of necrotizing granulomas in a needle core biopsy specimen may be considered presumptive evidence supporting a diagnosis of mammary tuberculosis in the proper clinical setting. If mammary infection is suspected clinically,

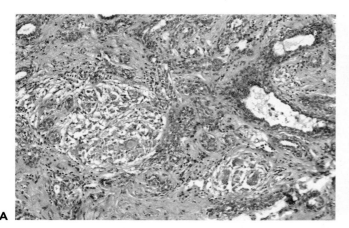

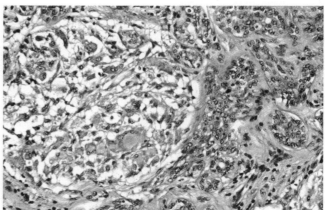

Figure 3.4   Tuberculous mastitis. A, B: Granulomatous inflammation in sclerosing adenosis in a patient with active pulmonary tuberculosis. The needle core biopsy was performed to evaluate a breast mass. No acid-fast bacteria were found with the Ziehl–Neelsen stain.

an aspirate or tissue sample should be reserved for microbiologic study.

Breast abscess formation attributable to *Mycobacterium fortuitum* (34) and *Mycobacterium abscesses* (35) has been observed following nipple piercing. *M. fortuitum* infections have also complicated prosthetic breast implants (36).

NONTUBERCULOUS BACTERIAL INFECTIONS

Patients with HIV/AIDS are susceptible to mastitis attributable to bacteria other than tuberculosis, such as *Salmonella* and *Pseudomonas aeruginosa* (29).

Mammary lesions due to cat-scratch disease caused by *Bartonella* present as a mass with inflammatory signs, often accompanied by axillary nodal enlargement, that may mimic inflammatory carcinoma (37). The mammary lesion is due to infection of an intramammary lymph node.

Actinomycotic infection of the breast typically presents as an abscess beneath or near the nipple and areola. Predisposing factors include breast feeding, corticosteroid therapy, and nipple piercing (38,39). Sinus tracts usually develop following incision and drainage when the specific diagnosis is unsuspected clinically, or with progression of the untreated lesion. A chronic abscess may form, creating a hard mass that simulates carcinoma. Axillary nodal enlargement typically reflects a reaction to the mammary inflammatory process more often than the spread of actinomycosis to the lymph nodes, but actinomycotic axillary lymphadenitis has been reported (38,39). In advanced cases, the infection can spread to the chest wall. Extension of pulmonary actinomycosis to the breast has also been described (40). The diagnosis of mammary actinomycosis is made by demonstrating the gram-positive organism as filaments or colonies (sulfur granules). Organisms isolated from mammary actinomycosis include *Actinomyces meyeri* (41), *A. viscosus* (42), *A. radingae*, *A. turicensis* (39), and *A. israelli* (43). Treatment with penicillin has reportedly been effective (38), but recurrent or advanced infections may require multiple antibiotics (39) and rarely mastectomy.

Rare instances of mammary abscesses due to *Nocardia* (44) and *Salmonella* (45) have been reported.

REFERENCES

1. Salfelder K, Schwarz J. Mycotic "pseudotumors" of the breast. *Arch Surg.* 1975;110:751–754.
2. Osborne BM. Granulomatous mastitis caused by *Histoplasma* and mimicking inflammatory breast carcinoma. *Hum Pathol.* 1989;20:47–52.
3. Farmer C, Stanley MW, Bardales RH, et al. Mycoses of the breast: diagnosis by fine-needle aspiration. *Diagn Cytopathol.* 1995;12:51–55.
4. Ramos-Barbosa S, Guazzelli LS, Severo LC. Cryptoccocal mastitis after corticosteroid therapy. *Rev Soc Bras Med Trop.* 2004;37:65–66.
5. Haddow LJ, Sahid F, Moosa M-YS. Cryptoccocal breast abscess in an HIV-positive patient. Arguments for reviewing the definition of immune reconstitution inflammatory syndrome. *J Infect.* 2008;57:82–84.
6. Williams K, Walton RL, Bunkis I. Aspergillus colonization associated with bilateral silicone mammary implants. *J Surg Pathol.* 1982;71:260–261.
7. Giovindarajan M, Verghese S, Kuruvilla S. Primary aspergillosis of the breast. Report of a case with fine needle aspiration cytology. *Acta Ctyol.* 1993;37:234–236.
8. Bocian JJ, Fahmy RN, Michas CA. A rare case of 'coccidioidoma' of the breast. *Arch Pathol Lab Med.* 1991;115:1064–1067.
9. Propeck PA, Scanlan KA. Blastomycosis of the breast. *Am J Roentgenol.* 1996;166:726.
10. Choudhury M. Bancroftian microfilaria in the breast clinically mimicking malignancy. *Cytopathology.* 1995;6:132–133.
11. Dreyer G, Brandão AC, Amaral F, et al. Detection by ultrasound of living adult *Wuchereria bancrofti* in the female breast. *Mem Inst Oswaldo Cruz.* 1996;91:95–96.
12. Chow CK, McCarthy JS, Neafie R, et al. Mammography of lymphatic filariasis. *Am J Roentgenol.* 1996;167:1425–1426.
13. Parida G, Rout N, Samantaray S, et al. Filariasis of breast simulating carcinoma. *Breast J.* 2008;14:598–599.
14. Chen YH, Qun X. Filarial granuloma of the female breast: a histopathologic study of 131 cases. *Am J Trop Med Hyg.* 1981;30:1206–1210.
15. Kunkel JM, Hawksley CZ. Cysticercosis presenting as a solitary dominant breast mass. *Hum Pathol.* 1987;18:1190–1191.
16. Vega A, Ortega E, Cavada A, Garijo F. Hydatid cyst of the breast: mammographic findings. *Am J Roentgenol.* 1994;162:825–826.
17. Lucarelli AP, Martins MM, de Oliviera VM, et al. A short report: cysticercosis of the breast. *Am J Trop Med Hyg.* 2008;279:864–865.
18. Haholy A, Sonmez G, Karaman M, et al. Unilocular cystic hydatidosis in breast. *Breast J.* 2008;14:393–394.
19. Sagin HB, Kiroglu Y, Aksoy F. Hydatid cyst of the breast diagnosed by fine needle aspiration biopsy. A case report. *Acta Cytol.* 1994;38:965–967.
20. Chan ABW, Wan SK, Leung S-L, et al. Sparganosis of the breast. *Histopathology.* 2004;44:510–511.
21. Sloan BS, Rickman LS, Blau EM, Davis CE. Schistosomiasis masquerading as carcinoma of the breast. *South Med J.* 1996;89:345–347.
22. Elma CA, Cavalcanti AC, Lima MM, Piva N. Pseudoneoplastic lesion of the breast caused by *Schistosoma mansoni. Rev Soc Bras Med Trop.* 2004;37:63–64.
23. Valdes PV, Prieto A, Diaz A, et al. Microcalcifications of pectoral muscle in trichinosis. *Breast J.* 2005;11:150.
24. de Barros N, D'Avila MS, de Pace Bauab S, et al. Cutaneous Myiasis of the breast: mammographic and US features-report of five cases. *Radiology.* 2001;218:517–520.
25. Ugwu BT, Nwadiaro PO. *Cordylobia anthropophaga* mastitis mimicking breast cancer: a case report. *East Afr Med J.* 1999;76:115–116.
26. Adisa CA, Mbanaso A. Furuncular myiasis of the breast caused by the larvae of the Tumbu fly (*Cordylobia anthropophaga*). *BMC Surg.* 2004;4:5.
27. Hale JA, Peters GN, Cheek JH. Tuberculosis of the breast: rare but still extant. *Am J Surg.* 1985;150:620–624.
28. Hartstein M, Leaf HL. Tuberculosis of the breast as a presenting manifestation of AIDS. *Clin Infect Dis.* 1992;15:692–693.
29. Pantanowitz L, Connolly JL. Pathology of the breast associated with HIV/AIDS. *Breast J.* 2002;8:234–243.
30. Alagaratnam TT, Ong GB. Tuberculosis of the breast. *Br J Surg.* 1980;67:125–126.
31. Makanjuola D, Murshid K, Sulaimani A, Al Saleh M. Mammographic features of breast tuberculosis: the skin bulge and sinus tract sign. *Clin Radiol.* 1996;51:354–358.
32. Sopeña B, Arnillas E, Garcia-Vila LM, et al. Tuberculosis of the breast: unusual clinical presentation of extrapulmonary tuberculosis. *Infection.* 1996;24:57–58.
33. Rothman GM, Kolkov Z, Meroz A, Lewinski UH. Breast tuberculosis and carcinoma. *Isr J Med Sci.* 1989;25:339–340.
34. Lewis CG, Wells MK, Jennings WC. *Mycobacterium fortuitum* breast infection following nipple-piercing, mimicking carcinoma. *Breast J.* 2004;10:363–365.
35. Trupiano JK, Sebek BA, Goldfarb J, et al. Mastitis due to *Mycobacterium abscessus* after body piercing. *Clin Infect Dis.* 2001;33:131–134.
36. Haiavy J, Tobin H. *Mycobacterium fortuitum* infection in prosthetic breast implants. *Plast Reconstr Surg.* 2002;109:2124–2128.
37. Povoski SP, Spigos DG, March WL. An unusual case of cat-scratch disease from *Bartonella quintana* mimicking inflammatory breast cancer in a 50-year old woman. *Breast J.* 2003;9:497–500.
38. Jain BK, Sehgal VN, Jagdish S, et al. Primary actinomycosis of the breast: a clinical review and a case report. *J Dermatol.* 1994;21:497–500.
39. Attar KH, Waghorn D, Lyons M, Cunnick G. Rare species of Actinomyces as causative pathogens in breast abscess. *Breast J.* 2007;13:501–505.
40. Pinto MM, Longstreth GB, Khoury GM. Fine needle aspiration of *Actinomyces* infection of the breast. A novel presentation of thoracopleural actinomycosis. *Acta Cytol.* 1991;35:409–411.
41. Allen JN. *Actinomyces meyeri* breast abscess. *Am J Med.* 1987;83:186–187.
42. Capobianco G, Dessole S, Becchere MP, et al. A rare case of primary actinomycosis of the breast caused by *Actinomyces viscosus:* diagnosis by fine-needle aspiration cytology under ultrasound guidance *Breast J.* 2005;11:57–59.
43. Akhlaghi M, Ghazvini RD. Clinical presentation of primary actinomycosis of the breast. *Breast J.* 2009;15:102–103.
44. Simpson AJH, Jumaa PA, Das SS. Breast abscess caused by *Nocardia asteroides. J Infect.* 1995;30:266–267.
45. Asaadi M, Suh EDW. Salmonella infection following breast reconstruction. *Plast Reconstr Surg.* 1995;96:1749–1750.

Benign Papillary Tumors

4

INTRADUCTAL PAPILLOMA

A papilloma is a discrete, benign papillary tumor that arises most often in the central part of the breast from a lactiferous duct, but it can occur in any quadrant. An *intracystic papilloma* is a papilloma in a cystically dilated duct. Solid, noncystic papillomas have been classified as *ductal adenomas* or *solid papillomas*. Papillomas may be *solitary*, consisting of a single papillary tumor in one duct, or *multiple* usually growing in contiguous branches of the ductal system. Intraductal papillomas should be distinguished from *papillomatosis* (epitheliosis), a term that describes microscopic duct hyperplasia. Papillomatosis may, and often does, coexist with solitary or multiple papillomas.

A subareolar mass may be palpable in a patient with a central solitary papilloma, and a palpable tumor can be the first clinical manifestation of a papilloma in one of the quadrants. Cystic papillomas appear to be well circumscribed on mammography (1) (Fig. 4.1). The presence of a cystic component is best appreciated by ultrasonography. Solitary papillomas occur at any age from infancy to the ninth decade. Nipple discharge occurs in most patients with a central papilloma. Bloody discharge, more commonly associated with papillary carcinoma, can be caused by degenerative changes in a papilloma.

Multiple papillomas develop more often peripherally than centrally and typically cause a palpable lesion. These patients tend to be younger on average than women with solitary papillomas, often presenting in their 40s and early 50s.

After a detailed mammographic and sonographic study of 40 papillary tumors that were later excised and examined histologically, Lam et al. (2) concluded that "radiologic features are not sufficiently sensitive or specific to differentiate benign from malignant papillary lesions." By using a combination of both imaging modalities, the authors achieved a sensitivity of 61%, specificity of 33%, a positive predictive value (PPV) of 85% and a negative predictive value (NPV) of 13%.

Part of the mass associated with a solitary papilloma may be the cyst formed by a dilated duct in which the papilloma arose. Some papillomas obliterate the cystic space. These solid papillary lesions are well circumscribed and appear to be enclosed in a capsule formed by the duct wall and accompanying reactive changes. The average size of palpable lesions is 2 to 3 cm. Cystic papillomas can be larger than 10 cm.

The most orderly form of papilloma consists of branching fronds of stroma supporting a layer of epithelium composed of cuboidal to columnar epithelial cells and myoepithelial cells (Fig. 4.2). The papillary stroma may arise from a single base or from several sites in the duct wall. The nonpapillary portion of the duct usually exhibits little or no epithelial hyperplasia in such lesions (Fig. 4.3).

Some papillomas have a more complex structure caused by stromal overgrowth, hyperplasia of the epithelium, or both processes resulting in fusion of papillary fronds. Secondary microlumens are formed within the hyperplastic epithelium and there may be micropapillary epithelial hyperplasia (Fig. 4.4). Proliferation of epithelium in the midst of the fibrovascular stroma results in a pattern resembling sclerosing adenosis (Figs. 4.5–4.7). The most florid form of epithelial hyperplasia is the solid intraductal papilloma, in which virtually all space between fibrovascular stalks is filled by proliferative duct epithelium (Fig. 4.8). Secondary lumens are often formed within the hyperplastic epithelium, resulting in irregular microlumens, micropapillary epithelial fronds, focal solid areas, or heterogeneous combinations of these patterns. Cytologically bland or mildly atypical apocrine epithelium is almost always an indication that a papillary tumor is a papilloma (Fig. 4.9). Rarely, there may be focal intraductal carcinoma in such a papilloma. Apocrine atypia manifested by nuclear pleomorphism and cytoplasmic clearing is more likely to be encountered in sclerosing papillary tumors (3).

In many papillomas, the stroma is limited to a network of slender inconspicuous bands consisting of thin-walled capillaries accompanied by sparse fibroblasts, collagen, and mononuclear cells. Collagenization of the fibrovascular stroma occurs in some papillomas. The presence of histocytes in the stroma of papillary fronds almost always indicates that the lesion is a papilloma (see Fig. 4.3). The papillary architecture is accentuated when sclerosis is limited to the intrinsic papillary structure. If myofibroblastic proliferation accompanies collagenization of the stroma,

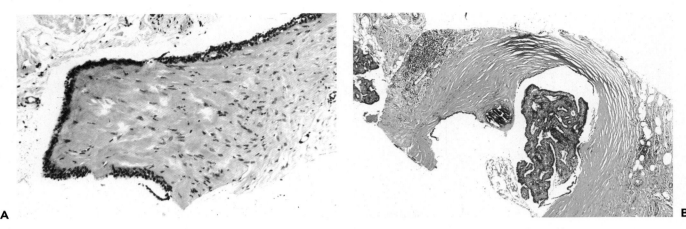

Figure 4.1   Cystic papilloma. A: A fragment of cyst wall around a cystic papilloma obtained in a needle core biopsy procedure. **B:** Part of an intracystic papilloma and the surrounding cyst wall. Note calcification in the cyst wall at the center of the picture.

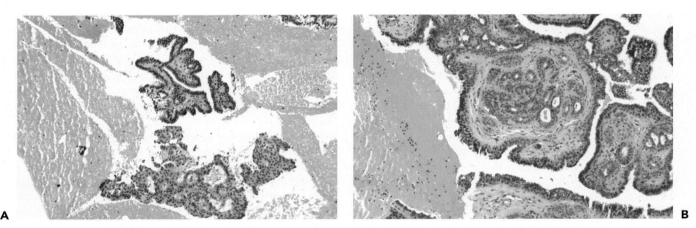

Figure 4.2   Papilloma. A, B: Detached fragments of papillary epithelium in a core biopsy specimen. Samples such as this are usually obtained from a cystic papilloma. Note the simple surface epithelium with minimal hyperplasia, inconspicuous myoepithelial cells, and the distinct fibrovascular stroma.

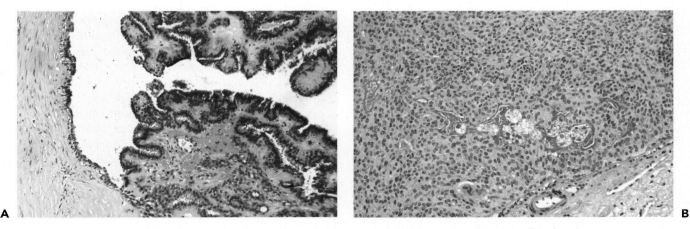

Figure 4.3   Papilloma. A: This needle core biopsy sample shows a cyst wall and papillary fronds extending into the lumen. Epithelium lining the cyst between the papillary fronds is not hyperplastic. **B:** Part of a solid papilloma with histocytes in fibrovascular stroma.

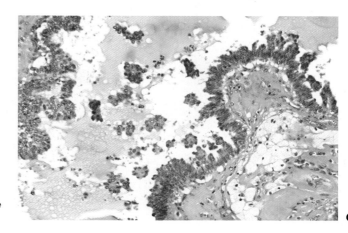

Figure 4.3 (*continued*) **C:** Histiocytes with clear cytoplasm are shown in the fibrovascular stroma of a papilloma.

the papillary arrangement is likely to become distorted (Fig. 4.10). Epithelial elements entrapped in this stroma may simulate invasive carcinoma within the lesion or at the periphery (Fig. 4.11). When immunostains are done to detect myoepithelial cells, it is necessary to distinguish between stromal and myoepithelial reactivity. Fibrous sclerosis can be so severe that it virtually obliterates the papilloma, reducing it to a nodular scar, containing scattered benign glandular elements that may be difficult to distinguish from a fibroadenoma. The myoepithelium may become noticeably attenuated and focally undetectable by immunostains in regions of sclerosis in a

papilloma. This finding, by itself, is not diagnostic of carcinoma in the lesion. The epithelial cells in papillomas typically exhibit strong nuclear immunoreactivity for estrogen receptor.

The epithelium of intraductal papillomas contains a myoepithelial cell layer. Myoepithelial cells are not equally apparent in all portions of a papilloma, and they may be focally absent. The nuclei of quiescent myoepithelial cells are usually inconspicuous and flattened along the basement membrane, whereas hyperplastic myoepithelial cells form a prominent layer of columnar or cuboidal cells that often have relatively clear cytoplasm

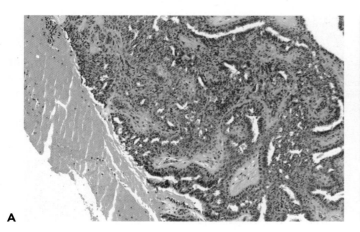

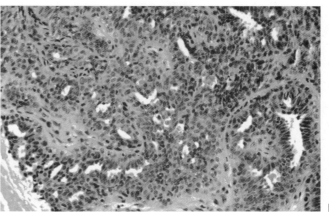

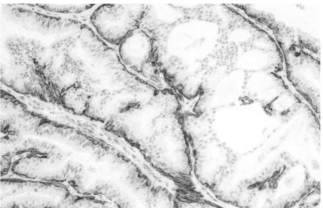

Figure 4.4 Papilloma with ductal hyperplasia. A, B: Hyperplasia in a needle core biopsy sample is manifested by increased thickness of the epithelial layer and bridging of epithelium across spaces between fronds, resulting in the formation of microlumens. **C:** Myoepithelium is demonstrated by reactivity for smooth muscle actin (immunoperoxidase).

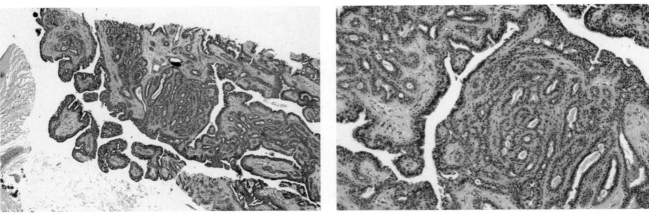

Figure 4.5   Papilloma with adenosis. A, B: Hyperplasia in this needle core sample takes the form of nodular adenosis within the fibrovascular stroma. The surface epithelium is focally hyperplastic.

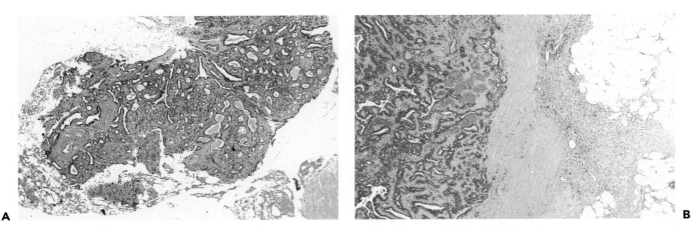

Figure 4.6   Papilloma with adenosis. A: A needle core biopsy sample from a mammographically detected circumscribed papillary tumor. The proliferation consists almost entirely of small adenosis-type glands in the stroma. **B:** The excisional biopsy specimen is shown here. Scarring around the papilloma is due to the needle biopsy procedure.

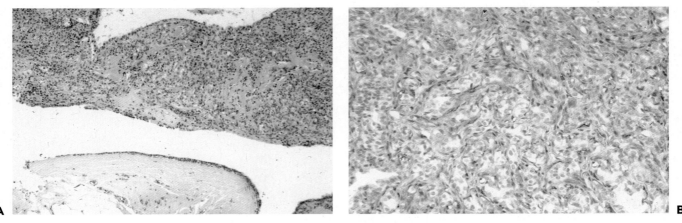

Figure 4.7   Cystic papilloma with florid adenosis. A: The needle core biopsy sample contains a compact proliferation of adenosis glands lacking lumina. Part of the cyst wall is shown at the lower border of the picture. **B:** The immunohistochemical stain for actin highlights myoepithelial cells that appear red-orange in this preparation around the adenosis glands (immunoperoxidase; smooth muscle actin).

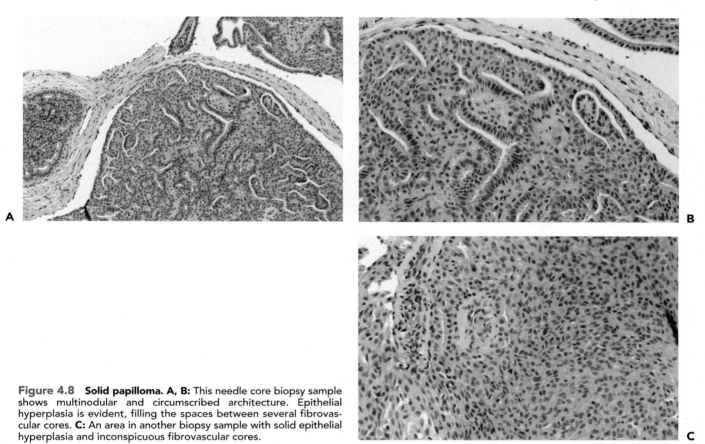

Figure 4.8 Solid papilloma. A, B: This needle core biopsy sample shows multinodular and circumscribed architecture. Epithelial hyperplasia is evident, filling the spaces between several fibrovascular cores. **C:** An area in another biopsy sample with solid epithelial hyperplasia and inconspicuous fibrovascular cores.

(Fig. 4.12). Some papillomas have markedly hyperplastic myoepithelial cells that assume an epithelioid phenotype (Fig. 4.13). Myoepithelial cells are immunoreactive for actin, calponin, myosin, CD10 and p63, and CK5/6 (4) (Fig. 4.14). The p63 immunostain is localized to myoepithelial cell nuclei and infrequently in papillary epithelial nuclei, but it is not reactive with stromal myofibroblasts or vascular structures (5). It is preferable to include the

p63 stain when immunostains are done to detect myoepithelial cells. When there is marked hyperplasia of myoepithelial cells, the differential diagnosis includes adenomyoepithelioma.

Infarction can occur in a papilloma, often without an apparent extrinsic cause (Fig. 4.15). Chronic inflammation and hemosiderin in and around many papillomas suggest that these lesions are prone to intermittent, transient bleed-

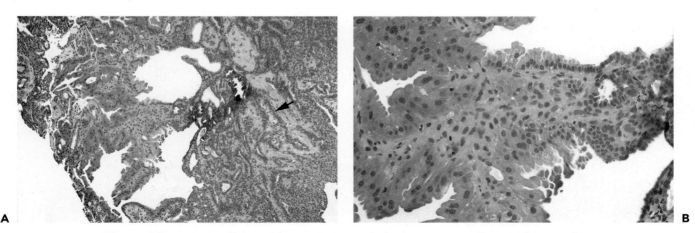

Figure 4.9 A, B: Papilloma with apocrine metaplasia. Apocrine metaplasia is shown in the hyperplastic epithelium of this needle core biopsy sample of a papilloma. No connection in one fibrovascular core (*arrow*) **(A).**

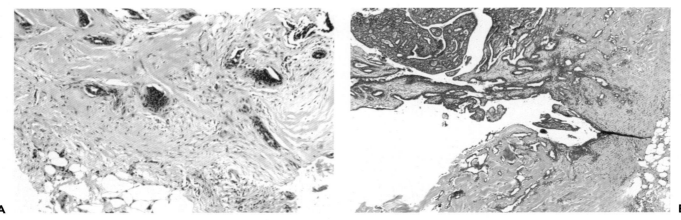

Figure 4.10 **Papilloma with sclerosis. A:** This needle core biopsy sample of a mammographically detected circumscribed mass shows small nests of epithelial cells in collagenized stroma. This pattern is easily mistaken for invasive carcinoma. **B:** The subsequent excisional biopsy revealed a partly cystic papilloma. Mural sclerosis with trapped glandular tissue shown here was the source of the material seen in **(A)**.

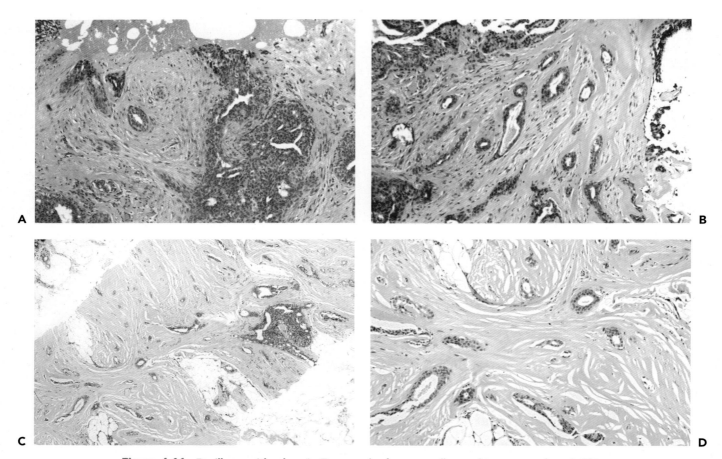

Figure 4.11 **Papilloma with sclerosis.** Two samples from a needle core biopsy procedure. **A:** This tissue has an area of papillary hyperplasia in sclerotic stroma. Note the epithelium cut tangentially as it protrudes into the stroma. This appearance should not be interpreted as invasive carcinoma. **B:** The cords of cells are distributed here largely in parallel arrays between bands of collagenized stroma. The glands with angular contours resemble tubular carcinoma. Myoepithelial cells are inconspicuous in this section stained with hematoxylin and eosin. **C, D:** These needle core biopsy samples from a severely sclerotic papillary lesion were mistakenly interpreted as tubular carcinoma. Immunostains (not shown) revealed myoepithelium around the glandular elements.

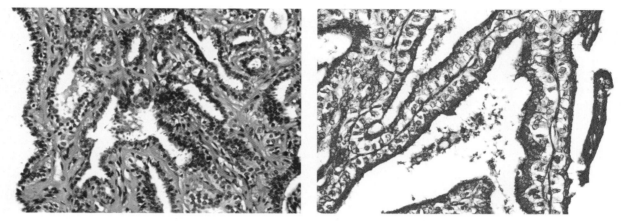

Figure 4.12 **Papillomas with prominent myoepithelial cells. A, B:** Myoepithelial cells with clear cytoplasm are shown outlining glands in these needle core biopsy samples from two papillomas.

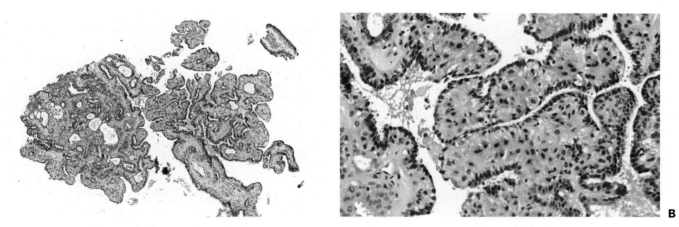

Figure 4.13 **Papilloma with hyperplastic myoepithelial cells. A, B:** Clusters of myoepithelial cells with epithelioid and myoid appearances fill the subepithelial stromal space in this needle core biopsy sample.

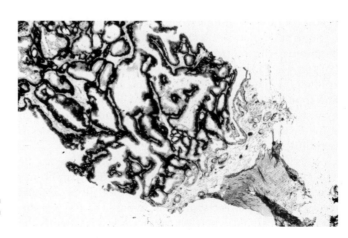

Figure 4.14 **Papilloma with myoepithelial cell hyperplasia.** An exaggerated myoepithelial cell zone is highlighted by an actin immunostain in this sample (immunoperoxidase).

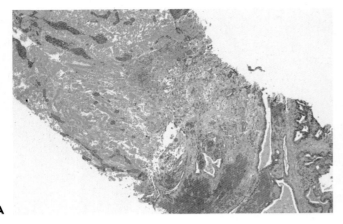

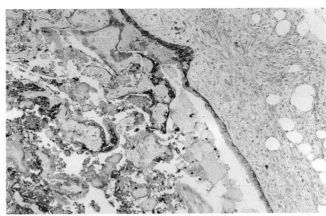

A

B

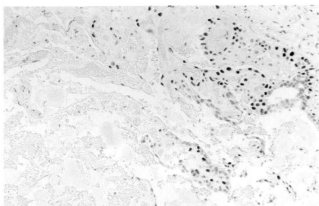

C

Figure 4.15 Papilloma with infarction. This needle core biopsy sample was obtained from a patient with bloody nipple discharge and a mammographically detected nonpalpable mass. No needling procedure was performed before the biopsy. **A:** The ghost architecture of a papillary lesion is evident in this almost completely infarcted sample. **B:** Myoepithelial cells are highlighted around the fibrovascular stroma and at the perimeter of the cystic duct with the CD10 immunostain (immunoperoxidase). **C:** Myoepithelial cell nuclei are reactive for p63 in part of the infarcted lesion. (immunoperoxidase).

ing. Rarely, the entire lesion is infarcted spontaneously or after a needle biopsy procedure. The underlying architecture of an infarcted papilloma can be demonstrated with a reticulin stain in many instances. Sometimes immunoreactivity for cytokeratin and p63 is preserved in infarcted portions of a papilloma (6). If myoepithelium can be demonstrated in the infarcted tissue, the tumor is more likely a papilloma than a papillary carcinoma. Cytologic atypia, manifested by nuclear hyperchromasia and pleomorphism, is commonly found in the partially degenerated epithelium of a papilloma in the vicinity of an infarct. These cytologic abnormalities may lead to an erroneous diagnosis of carcinoma in the needle core biopsy sample from such a lesion.

Squamous metaplasia can occur in the epithelium of a papilloma with infarction or in the absence of infarction (7) (Fig. 4.16). Extension of squamous metaplasia to the epithelium of adjacent ducts is an uncommon finding (8). Entrapped metaplastic epithelium in the stromal reaction may simulate metaplastic or squamous carcinoma and in some instances the distinction between these processes is very difficult (7).

A series of 26 papillary tumors diagnosed by needle core biopsy included 19 papillomas (9). Ten papillomas were classified as atypical. Calcifications were detected more often in lesions classified as atypical than in papillomas without atypia, whereas a mass was less frequently the mammographic abnormality that led to biopsy of atypical

papillomas. Intraductal carcinoma was found in excisional biopsies 3 of 10 (33%) atypical papillomas but not in seven excised papillomas lacking atypia. At a later date, one of the patients with a papilloma without atypia, who did not undergo excisional biopsy, developed invasive carcinoma that arose from residual papilloma.

Subsequently, the foregoing investigators reported a series of 50 papillomas among 3864 lesions (1.3%) subjected to needle core biopsy in which the biopsy diagnosis and imaging studies were "concordant" (10). Follow-up consisting of surgical biopsy (25 cases) or mammography (10 cases) at least 2 years later if excision was not performed was available for 35 (70%) of the patients. Carcinoma was diagnosed in 5 of the 35 patients. Intraductal carcinoma was found in one (4%) of the 25 patients who underwent contemporaneous excision. Four (40%) of the 10 patients with mammographic follow-up developed carcinoma (3 intraductal, 1 invasive ductal) after follow-up of 7 to 25 months (median 22 months). Findings that led to the diagnosis of subsequent carcinoma were interval changes on mammography, bloody nipple discharge, or the appearance of a mass on imaging and palpation. Patients with multiple papillomas were more likely to be found to have carcinoma subsequently. These data led the authors to conclude that "surgical excision may be warranted for percutaneously diagnosed papillomas."

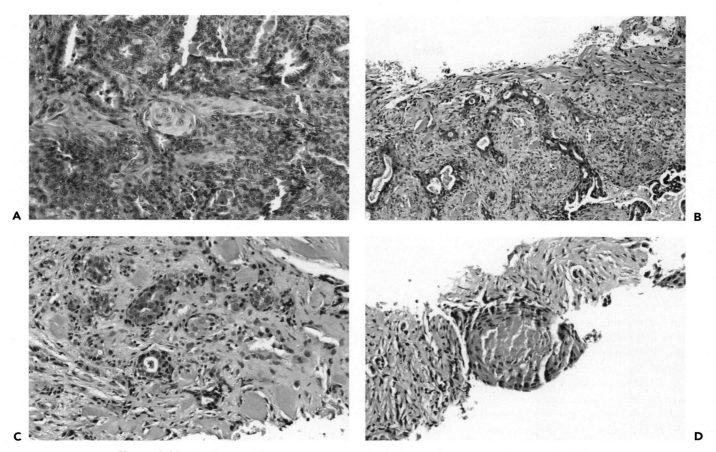

Figure 4.16 **Papilloma with squamous metaplasia. A:** A nest of squamous cells is present in the papillary glandular epithelium with florid hyperplasia. **B–D:** This needle core biopsy sample from a sclerosing papilloma had focal squamous metaplasia **(D).** The biopsy was misinterpreted as infiltrating carcinoma with squamous differentiation.

Several additional studies have correlated the results of core biopsies and subsequent excisional biopsies of papillary lesions. Puglisi et al. (11) reported that prior core biopsies from 5 of 19 lesions proven by excisional biopsy to be papillary carcinomas were interpreted as showing "absent" or "low" "suspicion of malignancy." These authors concluded that the sensitivity of the core biopsy procedure was too low to be reliable for excluding carcinoma and that excisional biopsy should be performed. Ivan et al. (12) described 30 patients reported to have a papilloma in a core biopsy. Excision in six cases (20%) revealed papilloma without atypia. The remaining patients had "no clinical or radiological evidence of disease progression" after follow-up of 1 to 51 months or a mean of 14.7 months. Philpotts et al. (13) studied 16 patients with papillary lesions that were interpreted as benign in needle core biopsy samples. Six patients underwent surgical excision, which revealed intraductal carcinoma in one (17%). Among the 10 who did not have an excisional biopsy, follow-up by mammography for 6 to 34 months documented that the lesions were radiologically "gone" in five cases, "unchanged" in two and "decreased" in three. In a fourth study, Mercado et al. (14) investigated 12 patients with papillary tumors

diagnosed as benign by needle core biopsy. Five of the six who had an excisional biopsy proved to be benign or had no residual lesion, and one (17%) was found to be the site of intraductal carcinoma. Mammographic follow-up in the other six cases revealed decreased size in five and no residual lesion in one case. Excisional biopsies following a diagnosis of papilloma without atypia in 38 consecutive needle core biopsy specimens revealed intraductal carcinoma in three cases (8%) studied by Jacobs et al. (15). The intraductal carcinoma was in or near to the excised residual papillary lesion. Jaffer et al. (16) studied excisional biopsies from 99 patients who had an intraductal papilloma diagnosed in a needle core biopsy specimen and reported finding carcinoma in 8.4% (intraductal, 5; invasive, 3). A larger series was reported by Gendler et al. (17) who identified 152 papillary lesions (2%) among 9310 consecutive needle core biopsy samples. Excisional biopsy documented in 87 (57%), yielded carcinoma, either in situ or invasive, in 15 patients (17%) and atypical hyperplasia in 16 (18%) patients who had an excisional biopsy.

Data from the foregoing studies do not provide definitive guidelines for the management of a papilloma diagnosed by needle core biopsy. A decision on whether

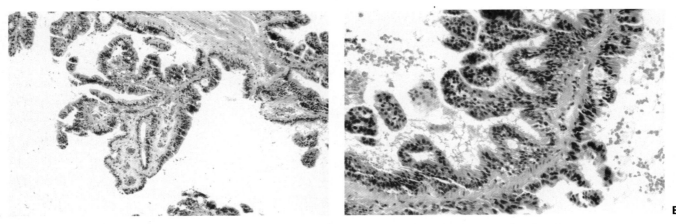

Figure 4.17 **Papilloma with atypical hyperplasia. A:** The epithelium of the papillary fronds in this part of the needle core biopsy sample is composed of an orderly layer of columnar cells. **B:** This frond from the same biopsy sample exhibits atypical micropapillary hyperplasia. Note nuclear condensation at the apical ends of the micropapillae and residual columnar epithelium of the duct between the micropapillae.

surgical excision should be performed will be influenced by factors such as lesion size, the presence of atypia in the core biopsy sample, evidence of persistent tumor post-biopsy, the ease of mammographic follow-up, family history of breast cancer, and patient concerns. In general, surgical excision is recommended for palpable papillomas, and it would be prudent for nonpalpable papillomas when part of the lesion is radiologically evident after the needle core biopsy procedure. Overall, intraductal or invasive carcinoma will be found in 5% to 15% of the excisional biopsy specimens in the absence of atypia in the needle core biopsy sample from a papilloma. Surgical excision should be performed for a papilloma found to have atypical hyperplasia (Figs. 4.17 and 4.18). Agoff and Lawton (18) reported finding in situ or invasive ductal carcinoma in 12 of 25 (48%) of patients with atypical papillary lesions who underwent an excisional biopsy.

Among women recommended for follow-up without an initial surgical excision, some will require surgical biopsy at a later date. In a series studied by Sexton et al. (19), 59

of 78 (75%) of patients with a papilloma diagnosed by needle biopsy did not undergo surgical biopsy and were followed for 3 to 5 years. Subsequent-interval mammographic changes necessitated surgical biopsy in 10 of the 59 (17%), and 2 (3%) had a subsequent needle core biopsy. All subsequent biopsies were reportedly "benign." This study suggests that up to 20% of patients enrolled in follow-up after a needle core biopsy diagnosis of papilloma will undergo another biopsy within 5 years of the initial procedure.

Most follow-up studies of papillomas confirm the low "precancerous" potential of these lesions after complete surgical excision (20–22). The reported frequency of carcinoma subsequent to the excision of a papilloma has been less than 5% (23). MacGrogan and Tavassoli (24) described the follow-up of 119 patients who underwent excision of papillary breast tumors. One of 22 women (4.5%) who had a "papilloma with florid hyperplasia" developed invasive carcinoma after an interval of 104 months. Among 40 women who had a "papilloma with

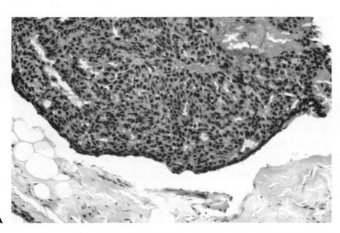

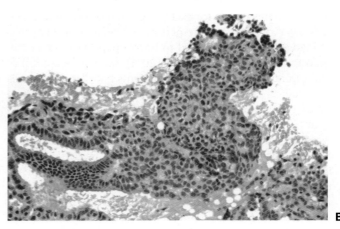

Figure 4.18 **Papilloma with atypical hyperplasia. A, B:** Detached epithelial fragments in a needle core biopsy specimen. Note the tendency of the cells to be oriented around microlumens.

focal atypia," 2 (5%) developed invasive carcinoma 35 and 162 months later. Atypical papillomas, defined as lesions in which 10% to 32% of the "papilloma's entire surface was involved" by atypical epithelium, were found in 24 women. Subsequent carcinomas (2 invasive, 1 intraductal) were diagnosed in 3 (12.5%) after intervals of 28 to 145 months. A greater risk for concurrent (25) or subsequent carcinoma has been demonstrated in women with multiple papillomas than in those with solitary papillomas (25–27), and these women are at risk to develop carcinoma in the contralateral breast.

Lewis et al. (28) examined the follow-up of patients with solitary and multiple papillomas treated at the Mayo Clinic. The distribution of patients with respect to the papilloma group was not significantly related to having history of breast carcinoma. The risk for developing breast carcinoma after the diagnosis of solitary or multiple papilloma was determined by comparison with an age and calendar period matched cohort from Surveillance, Epidemiology, and End Results (SEER) data. Standardized incidence rates (SIRs) of breast carcinoma were higher for women with solitary (5.11) or multiple (7.01) papillomas with atypical hyperplasia than for those with solitary (2.04) or multiple (3.01) papillomas without atypia. The mean time to the diagnosis of carcinoma ranged from 4.8 to 6.2 years, being slightly less in patients with multiple papillomas.

COLLAGENOUS SPHERULOSIS

This structural alteration occurs as an incidental microscopic finding in 1% to 2% of surgical biopsies with hyperplastic duct lesions. When calcification is present in collagenous spherulosis, it may be detected mammographically as a nonpalpable abnormality, leading to sampling in a needle core biopsy procedure. Collagenous spherulosis is formed by deposits or spherules of basement membrane components surrounded by myoepithelial cells within hyperplastic epithelium (29) (Figs. 4.19–4.21). This material is analogous to the cylindromatous deposits found in adenoid cystic carcinoma.

Collagenous spherulosis occurs in benign proliferative lesions including papilloma, papillary duct hyperplasia, atypical duct hyperplasia, and sclerosing adenosis (30–32). It is more often multifocal than unifocal (31). Carcinoma may be present coincidentally in the same specimen and rarely, carcinoma in situ, usually lobular type, replaces the benign epithelium of collagenous spherulosis (Fig. 4.22). The E-cadherin stain is useful for confirming the presence of lobular carcinoma in situ in collagenous spherulosis. Duct hyperplasia and lobular carcinoma in situ with collagenous spherulosis can be mistakenly interpreted as cribriform intraductal carcinoma. There is no evidence to indicate that the presence of collagenous

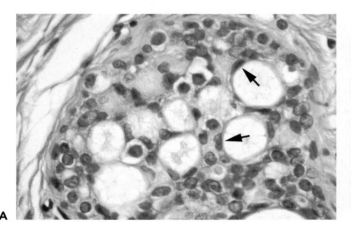

A

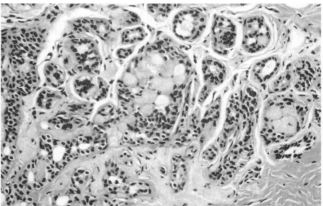

B

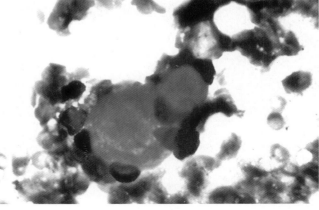

C

Figure 4.19 Collagenous spherulosis. A: Each of the multiple spherules in this duct is outlined by a membrane-like border around which elongated nuclei of myoepithelial cells can be identified (*arrows*). Fibrillar material is present in some spherules. **B:** Collagenous spherulosis consisting of solid eosinophilic intraepithelial nodules in small ducts in sclerosing adenosis in a needle core biopsy sample obtained for calcifications. **C:** Spherules from collagenous spherulosis in a fine needle aspiration cytology specimen (Diff–Quick stain).

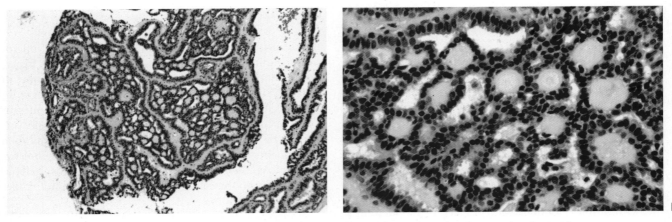

A

B

Figure 4.20 Collagenous spherulosis in a papilloma. A, B: The spherules are round, weakly eosinophilic bodies in the epithelium. Myoepithelial cells are, for the most part, inconspicuous but they can be seen rimming spherules in the lower right corner of **(B).** The true glandular lumens have irregular contours.

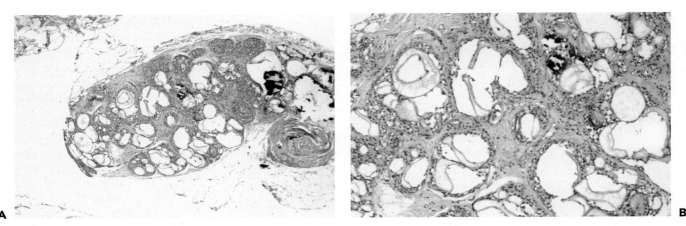

A

B

Figure 4.21 Collagenous spherulosis with degenerative changes. A, B: Degeneration in collagenous spherulosis with detachment of basement membranes that have collapsed into the cystic spherules. The biopsy was performed for mammographically detected nonpalpable calcifications, some of which are shown.

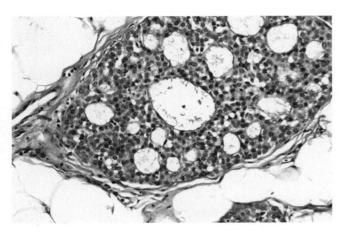

Figure 4.22 Collagenous spherulosis with in situ carcinoma. Lobular carcinoma in situ has expanded and filled the epithelium between spherules. Note the loss of cohesion between the neoplastic cells and the fine filamentous material in some spherules.

spherulosis is a precancerous condition when it occurs in fibrocystic changes.

In lesions with collagenous spherulosis, the hyperplastic epithelium forms true glands and encompasses acellular spherules creating an adenoid cystic structural arrangement. The lumens of the glandular spaces tend to have more irregular shapes than in adenoid cystic carcinoma. Attenuated myoepithelial cells around the spherules are difficult to identify in hematoxylin and eosin (H&E)-stained sections. Immunostains for actin p63, CD10, and calponin highlight the myoepithelial cells.

The spherules measure 20 to 100 μm in diameter and they have various staining patterns. Some are as dense as the cylindromatous deposits in adenoid cystic carcinoma. The center of a spherule is sometimes relatively transparent, and it may be possible to see stellate fibrils that radiate from a central nidus toward the periphery. Degenerative changes in spherules can result in loss of the radial structure and create a lumen-like space. However, at least a thin rim of basement membrane material is always present around the perimeter of the spherule, where it is encompassed by a ring of myoepithelial cells. The myoepithelial cells are highlighted by various immunostains such as p63, actin, and calponin. Constituents in spherules include components of basement membrane: elastin, periodic acid–Schiff (PAS)-positive polysaccharides, and type IV collagen (29,33). However, immunostains for basement membrane proteins are not always reliable, probably because of degenerative changes in the spherule material.

RADIAL SCLEROSING LESIONS

Radial sclerosing lesions (RSLs) have been described by a variety of names. *Radial scar*, a widely employed term for these lesions, is derived from Hamperl's phrase, *strahlige Narben* (34). Use of the word *scar* implies that there is a reparative process in the stroma because the stellate configuration has a cicatrix-like appearance, but it is equally likely that the stromal change is an integral part of the overall proliferative lesion. In this regard, Jacobs et al. (35) compared the "expression of factors involved in vascular stroma formation" in radial scars with the stroma of invasive carcinomas. When compared with normal breast tissue, the stroma of radial scars and invasive carcinomas displayed increased vascularity as well as "focally increased expression" of messenger RNA for collagen type 1, total fibronectin, vascular permeability factor/vascular endothelial growth factor, and other markers. These results provided molecular confirmation for the presence of a vasoproliferative process in both classes of lesions, but they do not identify the mechanism by which this occurs nor do they necessarily indicate that the same mechanism is involved.

The term *radial sclerosing lesion* is preferable because it describes the mammographic and histopathologic appearance of the process without suggesting histogenesis, and it

is sufficiently nonspecific to encompass the many histologic variants included in this category.

Most RSLs are microscopic in size and not detectable by palpation. Multiple microscopic RSLs are not uncommon in one breast, and both breasts can be affected (36,37). RSLs have been detected in 1.7% (38) to 28% (39) of benign breast specimens. These are uncommon before age 30 and most frequent between 40 and 60 years of age.

Clinically apparent RSLs are usually found by mammography. Radiologically, they are stellate or spiculated foci of architectural distortion that usually measure less than 2 cm (40). Typical lesions are characterized by a lucent or dense center, radiating slender strands of tissue and changes in appearance in different imaging projections (41). Microcalcifications are detected in some but not all RSLs (42,43). Although some mammographic features may favor the radiologic diagnosis of a benign RSL over a stellate carcinoma, these are not distinct enough to be the basis for a definitive diagnosis in many cases, and there are no specific imaging criteria that rule out the presence of in situ carcinoma in a RSL (40,43,44).

The proliferative components that are most commonly present in differing proportions in a RSL are sclerosing adenosis, duct hyperplasia, and cysts. The central nidus is a relatively sclerotic zone composed of fibrosis and elastosis (Fig. 4.23). Elastin in the walls of ducts and in the stroma forms dense, sometimes granular eosinophilic or weakly basophilic deposits that can be highlighted by an elastic tissue stain. In an early phase of development, a RSL is composed centrally of branching ductal structures that are surrounded by relatively cellular spindle cell stroma extending along radiating fibrous bands toward the periphery (Fig. 4.24). Many of the stromal cells are myofibroblasts (45). In later stages, the stromal cells are less conspicuous as the tissue becomes more collagenized and elastotic (Fig. 4.25).

A "corona" of ducts, lobules, and cysts is often present at the periphery of the lesion between the bands of radiating sclerotic tissue (Fig. 4.24). This peripheral zone is not seen around every RSL, and, when present, it can appear to be incomplete. The variability in appearance is the result of intrinsic asymmetry of lesions or it may be a consequence of asymmetric sectioning. In some lesions, the "corona" consists predominately of cysts.

Small ductules trapped in the fibrous reaction may be mistaken for invasive carcinoma. This is an important consideration when examining needle core biopsy samples. Nests of epithelium trapped in the stroma at the periphery of a sclerosing papilloma or a RSL simulate invasive carcinoma. The presence of a myoepithelial cell layer that is demonstrated with the p63 or actin immunostains characterizes epithelial entrapment at the periphery of a RSL. Ductules at the center of a RSL may lack myoepithelial reactivity. By itself, this finding is not diagnostic of carcinoma, but it can be misleading in a needle core biopsy sample.

Apocrine metaplasia is frequently observed in RSLs. Clear cell change and nuclear atypia are not uncommon in this

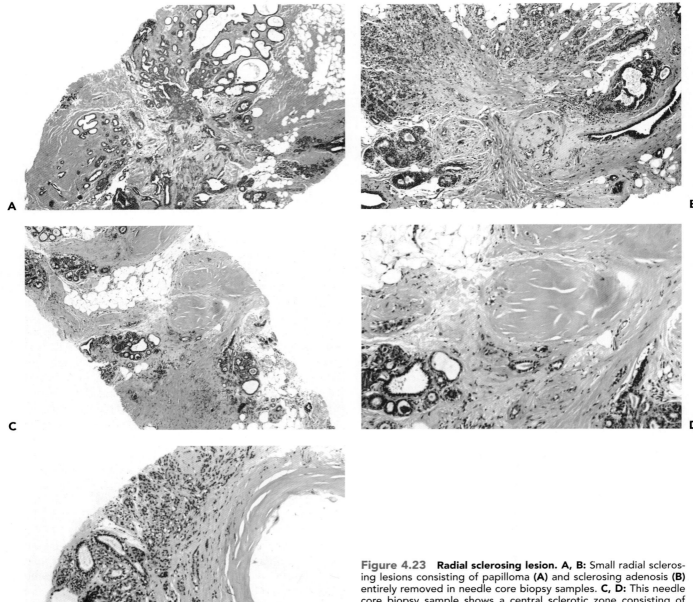

Figure 4.23   **Radial sclerosing lesion. A, B:** Small radial sclerosing lesions consisting of papilloma **(A)** and sclerosing adenosis **(B)** entirely removed in needle core biopsy samples. **C, D:** This needle core biopsy sample shows a central sclerotic zone consisting of dense collagenous tissue and adenosis with calcifications. **E:** A peripheral portion of the same lesion with prominent sclerosing adenosis and a cyst devoid of epithelium. Portions of the adenosis are attenuated and resemble infiltrating lobular carcinoma.

apocrine epithelium. Squamous metaplasia is relatively infrequent in RSLs. Duct hyperplasia in a RSL may be solid, cribriform, micropapillary, or any combination of these structural patterns. Myoepithelial cells can be demonstrated around the perimeter of most hyperplastic ducts by using immunostains for p63, CD10, myosin, or actin. However, in the central part of the lesion myoepithelium may be substantially attenuated and even undetectable in hyperplastic ducts. Focal necrosis occurs in the hyperplastic duct epithelium of about 10% of RSLs. The epithelium with these comedo-like foci is usually indistinguishable from the epithelium in hyperplastic ducts lacking necrosis in the

same RSL. The presence of mitoses or necrosis is evidence of atypical hyperplasia in a RSL. Often, the significant proliferative foci are distributed in multiple tissue fragments in a needle core biopsy specimen. Care should be taken to avoid an erroneous diagnosis of intraductal or invasive carcinoma in this setting (Figs. 4.26 and 4.27). Entrapped nerves are apparently incorporated into RSLs by the same mechanism that is responsible for this phenomenon in other sclerosing lesions (46).

A major consideration in the differential diagnosis of RSLs is tubular carcinoma. The epithelium in tubular carcinoma lacks the myoepithelial layer characteristically present

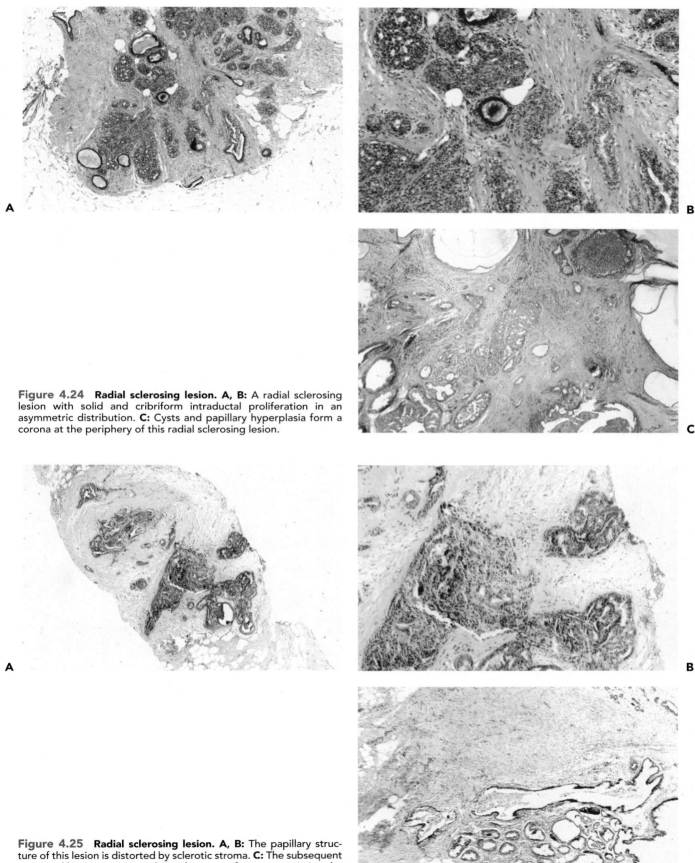

Figure 4.24   Radial sclerosing lesion. A, B: A radial sclerosing lesion with solid and cribriform intraductal proliferation in an asymmetric distribution. **C:** Cysts and papillary hyperplasia form a corona at the periphery of this radial sclerosing lesion.

Figure 4.25   Radial sclerosing lesion. A, B: The papillary structure of this lesion is distorted by sclerotic stroma. **C:** The subsequent excisional biopsy specimen showed an area of scar representing the core biopsy site and sclerosing adenosis. The needle core biopsy had been performed for mammographically detected calcifications.

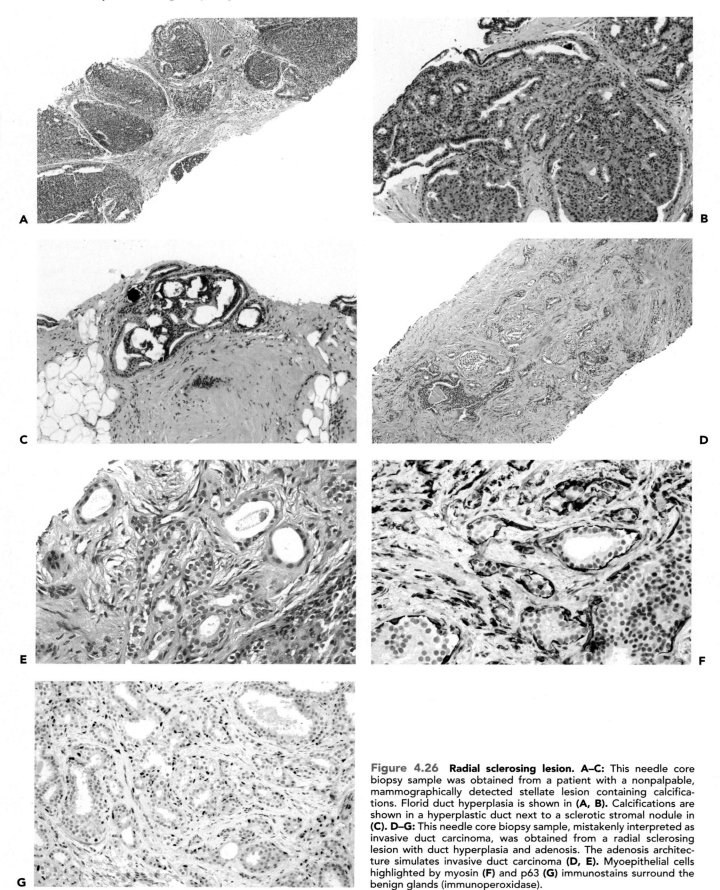

Figure 4.26 Radial sclerosing lesion. A–C: This needle core biopsy sample was obtained from a patient with a nonpalpable, mammographically detected stellate lesion containing calcifications. Florid duct hyperplasia is shown in **(A, B).** Calcifications are shown in a hyperplastic duct next to a sclerotic stromal nodule in **(C). D–G:** This needle core biopsy sample, mistakenly interpreted as invasive duct carcinoma, was obtained from a radial sclerosing lesion with duct hyperplasia and adenosis. The adenosis architecture simulates invasive duct carcinoma **(D, E).** Myoepithelial cells highlighted by myosin **(F)** and p63 **(G)** immunostains surround the benign glands (immunoperoxidase).

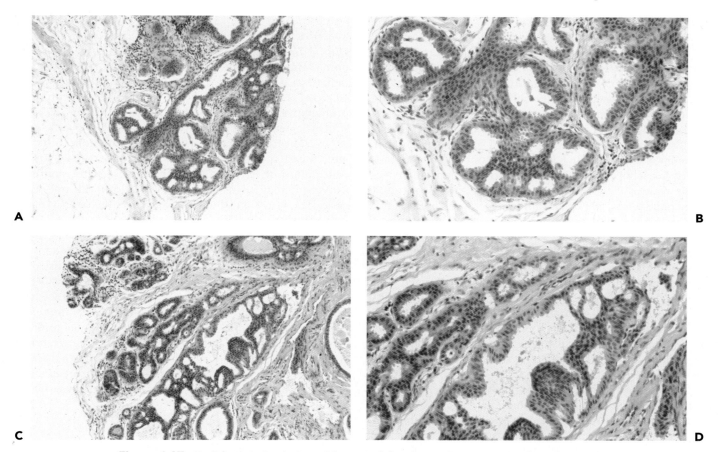

Figure 4.27 **Radial sclerosing lesion with atypical duct hyperplasia. A–D.** Two foci of atypical micropapillary hyperplasia in peripheral portions of a radial sclerosing lesion are seen in these needle core biopsy samples. Note the radial pattern and microcyst at the right border in **(C)**. These findings were initially diagnosed as intraductal carcinoma. A subsequent excisional biopsy showed only reactive changes at the biopsy site. The needle core biopsy specimen was reviewed in consultation, and the diagnoses were revised to atypical hyperplasia.

in hyperplastic component of a RSL. The cystic component of a RSL is absent from a tubular carcinoma unless the carcinoma mingles with fibrocystic changes. However, the origin of carcinoma, including tubular carcinoma, in RSLs has been well documented (47). In one series, 28% of mammographically detected RSLs larger than 1 cm had foci of carcinoma (48). Carcinoma is most frequently found in RSLs larger than 2 cm, and it occurs more often in RSLs from women older than 50 years (49). The most common form of carcinoma arising in a RSL is lobular carcinoma in situ (Fig. 4.28). Intraductal carcinoma and invasive duct carcinoma that may be tubular type are less frequent. Myoepithelium may be detected in the intraductal carcinoma, but it will be absent from invasive carcinoma.

A needle core biopsy procedure provides a tissue sample that is a more reliable basis for the specific diagnosis of a RSL than fine needle aspiration cytology, but ultimately, complete excision is necessary to fully evaluate these lesions for the presence of focal carcinoma. Specimen radiography

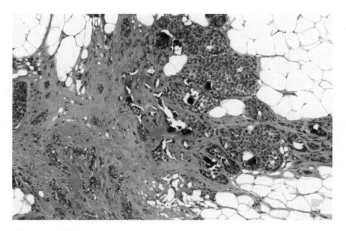

Figure 4.28 **Radial sclerosing lesion with carcinoma.** A mammographically detected stellate lesion with calcifications led to a needle core biopsy. In the sample shown here, lobular carcinoma in situ fills glands with an adenosis pattern in sclerotic tissue in the right portion of the lesion.

should be performed on the excisional biopsy specimen to confirm the excision of a RSL detected by mammography.

A number of studies have investigated the possibility of selectively recommending clinical follow-up rather than surgical excision after the needle core biopsy diagnosis of a RSL. The investigators have typically compared the pathologic findings in the core biopsy specimen with those of the excised lesion in an effort to determine criteria that distinguish between RSL that are most and least likely to harbor carcinoma (50,51). It has been suggested that mammographic follow-up rather than surgical excision can be recommended if the RSL in a core biopsy specimen from a mammographically detected nonpalpable lesion does not have atypical hyperplasia or in situ carcinoma. Additional criteria proposed are that at least 12 core biopsy samples be obtained showing a RSL without atypia (50), and that the radiologic and pathologic findings be concordant. No long-term follow-up studies are available for women with RSLs diagnosed by needle core biopsy that were not surgically excised. On the basis of the currently available data, excisional biopsy would be prudent when a needle core biopsy sample from a palpable or radiologically detected lesion is diagnostic of a RSL. If the RSL does not have an atypical component and there are no concomitant atypical proliferative lesions, the decision about whether to recommend excision or follow-up should be made on a case-by-case basis. Factors to consider are prior biopsy findings and other factors predisposing to increased cancer risk such as family history and ease of clinical or radiologic follow-up.

The presence of carcinoma or atypical hyperplasia in some RSLs has been an important factor in the concern over the precancerous potential of these lesions. RSLs from the breasts of women with carcinoma do not appear appreciably different from comparable lesions not associated with carcinoma (52).

The conflicting data thus far available have created uncertainty as to the risk for the subsequent development of carcinoma in women who have a RSL diagnosed in a needle core biopsy specimen. Many studies have investigated the possibility of selectively recommending clinical follow-up rather than surgical excision after the needle core biopsy diagnosis of RSL. The investigators have typically compared the pathologic findings in the core biopsy specimen with those of the excised lesion in an effort to determine criteria that distinguish between RSLs that are most and least likely to harbor carcinoma (50,51,53). Consequently, these studies have dealt with the immediate issues of coexisting carcinoma rather than the risk for developing carcinoma at a later time, after the RSL has been excised surgically.

A prospective cohort study of the 1396 women with a median follow-up of 12 years after biopsy of a benign breast lesion included that "radial scars" were an independent risk factor for breast carcinoma (54). In this study, "radial scar" was defined by a "fibroelastotic core from which ducts and lobules radiate. These ducts and lobules exhibit various alterations, including cysts and proliferative lesions." As so defined, radial scars were

found in 99 women (7.1%), and these were solitary in 60.6% of affected women with a median size of 4 mm. During follow-up, 255 women developed breast carcinoma. The relative risk for carcinoma in women with a radial scar versus those without radial scar was 1.8 (95% CI, 1.1–2.9). The relative risk was increased by concurrent proliferative changes and was greatest when the radial scar coexisted with atypical hyperplasia (RR 5.8, 95% CI, 2.7–12.7) when compared with women with nonproliferative breast specimens. The mean and median size and distribution of size among radial scars were not significantly different between women who did or did not develop carcinoma and the risk was not influenced by the number of radial scars.

Sanders et al. (55) described a retrospective cohort study of 9556 women among whom 880 (9.2%) were found by review to have one or more "radial scar" lesions. The risk of developing ipsilateral breast carcinoma was directly related to the number of radial scar lesions. When the presence of other proliferative lesions was taken into consideration, it was observed "that this risk can be largely attributed to the category of coexistent" proliferative disease, being greatest when there was atypical hyperplasia. The finding of a radial scar "did not significantly increase the risk of carcinoma due to proliferative disease with atypia or atypical hyperplasia existing without a radial scar."

SUBAREOLAR SCLEROSING DUCT HYPERPLASIA

Sclerosing duct hyperplasia can produce a tumor of the central or subareolar breast parenchyma without involving the substance of the nipple. The term *subareolar sclerosing duct hyperplasia* (56) should be reserved for subareolar lesions that constitute a clinicopathologic entity distinct from florid papillomatosis of the nipple.

The age at diagnosis ranges from 26 to 73 years, averaging about 50 years. The presenting symptom is a mass located beneath the nipple and/or areola or in the breast close to the areola. Erosion or ulceration of the nipple surface is absent. Nipple retraction may occur and some patients have had bloody discharge. The mammographic findings have not been specific for this lesion and may suggest carcinoma. The surgical approach to subareolar sclerosing duct hyperplasia is invariably via a periareolar incision whereas sampling of florid papillomatosis is always through the nipple.

The histologic structure of subareolar sclerosing duct hyperplasia is similar to that of radial sclerosing papillary lesions in other parts of the breast. Sclerosis and elastosis are more pronounced toward the center of the tumor, whereas duct hyperplasia is prominent at the periphery (Fig. 4.29). Cartilaginous metaplasia, a rare occurrence in these lesions, typically occurs in the sclerotic core. Much of the tumor has a rounded margin created by the nodular expansion of confluent large ducts with florid epithelial

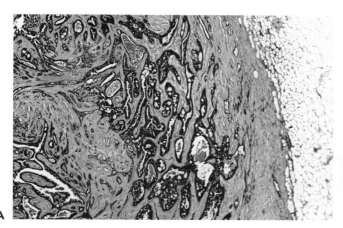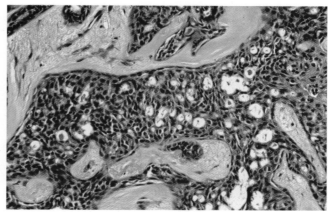

A

B

Figure 4.29 **Subareolar sclerosing duct hyperplasia. A:** The border of the lesion is well circum-scribed. **B:** Florid duct hyperplasia with a fenestrated pattern.

hyperplasia. Scattered mitotic figures may be encountered in the epithelium or in hyperplastic myoepithelial cells. Rarely, focal comedo necrosis is found in the hyperplastic duct epithelium. In contrast to radial sclerosing prolifera-tive lesions elsewhere in the breast, subareolar sclerosing duct hyperplasia generally lacks cysts, cystic and papillary apocrine change, and squamous metaplasia. Carcinoma may arise in subareolar sclerosing duct hyperplasia.

CYSTIC AND PAPILLARY APOCRINE METAPLASIA

Embryologically, the breasts develop from the anlage that gives rise to apocrine glands, but apocrine differentiation is not a constituent of the normal microscopic anatomy of the mammary gland. Any benign proliferative lesion may contain cells with apocrine cytologic features. In their most banal form, metaplastic apocrine cells are indistinguish-able from the cells that comprise normal apocrine glands. Mitoses are almost never seen in ordinary apocrine meta-plasia, and a low proportion of cells are in S-phase (57). There are no clinical features specifically attributable to cystic and papillary apocrine metaplasia.

Microscopic apocrine metaplasia is common in the fe-male breast after age 30, with the highest frequency in the fifth decade (58,59), probably reflecting physiologic alter-ations associated with the menopause. Apocrine cysts and hyperplasia with apocrine metaplasia were more common in the breasts of American women in New York than in Japanese women from Tokyo (60). Haagensen reported finding apocrine metaplasia in 78% of 1169 biopsies per-formed for gross cystic disease (61).

No significant difference in the frequency of apocrine metaplasia is visible when breasts with and without carci-noma are compared (62–64). Some follow-up studies have suggested that apocrine metaplasia is a predictor for the subsequent development of carcinoma. Haagensen et al. (61) reported a 10-fold greater frequency of carcinoma in

women with apocrine metaplasia in a prior biopsy than when apocrine change was absent. When compared with a control population, patients with apocrine metaplasia had 3.5 times the expected frequency of carcinoma, whereas the risk was only 0.3 times expected when apocrine metaplasia was absent. A slight increase in the number of subsequent carcinomas was observed by Page et al. (65) in women with papillary apocrine change in an antecedent benign biopsy when compared with the expected number of carcinomas based on an age-matched comparison with the Third National Cancer Survey. The difference was statis-tically significant only in women older than 45 years when the apocrine lesion was detected. Florid apocrine metapla-sia with atypia often coexists with apocrine carcinoma (66). Short-term follow-up of patients with atypical apoc-rine lesions has not revealed a predisposition to the early onset of carcinoma of apocrine or nonapocrine type (3).

Cystic apocrine metaplasia is composed of flat and cuboidal cells that may form a single cell layer or blunt papillae (Fig. 4.30). The evenly spaced cells have round nu-clei with homogeneous, moderately dense chromatin and a single central small nucleolus. A myoepithelial cell layer is usually visible in hematoxylin and eosin (H&E)–stained sections of cystic and papillary apocrine epithelium. How-ever, there are rare instances where immunostains do not detect myoepithelium in otherwise ordinary, benign apo-crine cysts. The significance of this extraordinary finding is not known.

Florid papillary proliferation produces more elaborate patterns of apocrine hyperplasia that have a micropapillary or a branching, papillary architecture. Cellular crowding results in a thickened epithelium more than one cell in depth and the formation of a papilloma composed entirely of apocrine epithelium (Fig. 4.31). Calcifications associ-ated with cystic and papillary apocrine metaplasia may be coarse, basophilic, easily fractured particles, or birefringent calcium oxalate crystals (Fig. 4.32).

Atypical changes can be encountered in apocrine metaplasia in virtually any proliferative configuration (3).

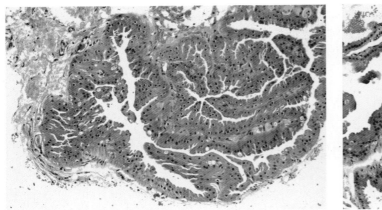
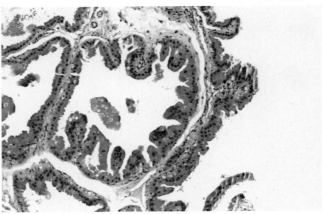

Figure 4.30 Cystic and papillary apocrine metaplasia. A, B: Note the evenly spaced, basally oriented distribution of the nuclei and blunt papillae.

Architectural atypia consists of irregular papillary fronds with little or no stromal support in which the apocrine cells are arranged in a disordered fashion. Epithelial bridges and cribriform areas may be present (Fig. 4.33). Apocrine cells with mild cytologic atypia retain abundant, finely granular eosinophilic cytoplasm. Small, clear vacuoles may be found in the cytoplasm. The nuclei in apocrine atypia are not spaced at regular intervals, and they may not all be basally oriented. Nucleoli are less uniform, they may be eccentric, and an occasional nucleus has more than one nucleolus. The cytoplasm of individual cells may be vacuolated or clear (Fig. 4.34). Nuclear pleomorphism and hyperchromasia can become striking. Prominent, pleomorphic nucleoli characterize the most atypical lesions and apocrine carcinoma.

When atypical apocrine metaplasia is present, the severity of the change is usually not uniform in a given lesion.

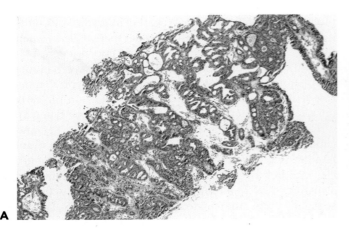
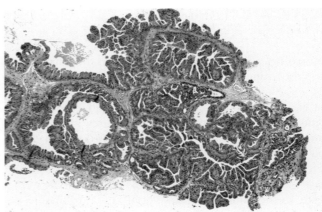

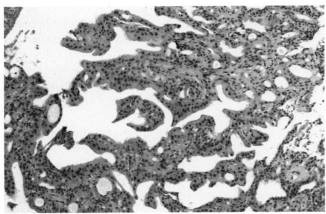

Figure 4.31 Cystic and papillary apocrine metaplasia. A–C: Apocrine metaplasia is present throughout this complex cystic and papillary lesion. The hyperplastic epithelium has micropapillae and cribriform areas. Complex branching papillary fronds and cysts with hyperplastic apocrine epithelium are shown in this needle core biopsy sample.

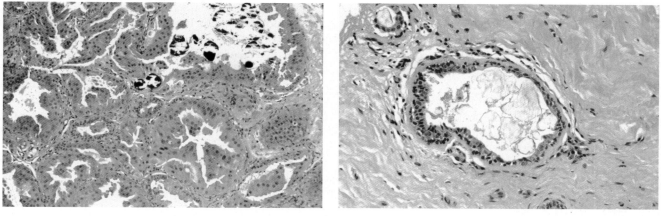

Figure 4.32 Cystic and papillary apocrine metaplasia with calcifications. A: Round basophilic calcifications in a lesion composed of papillary apocrine epithelium. **B:** Platelike, transparent calcium oxalate crystals are shown illuminated with polarized light in a small apocrine cyst.

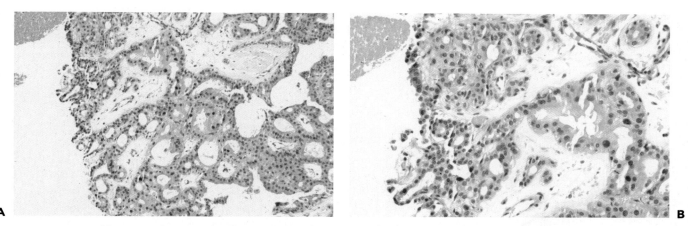

Figure 4.33 Cystic and papillary apocrine metaplasia with atypia. A, B: The epithelium has focal cribriform microlumens and isolated hyperchromatic enlarged nuclei in these needle core biopsy specimens.

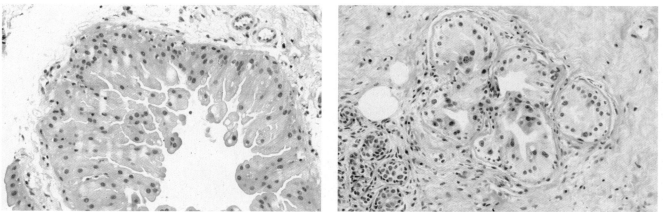

Figure 4.34 Papillary apocrine metaplasia with atypia. A: The small, round nuclei are distributed in a disorderly fashion in these fused papillary fronds. The abundant cytoplasm is vacuolated in some cells. **B:** Apocrine cells with pale cytoplasm and pleomorphic nuclei are shown. Note the presence of relatively large nuclei near the tips of papillary fronds.

Cysts and papillary duct hyperplasia partly or entirely occupied by bland metaplastic apocrine epithelium, are commonly found in the vicinity of atypical apocrine metaplasia. The distinction between atypical apocrine metaplasia and apocrine carcinoma is ordinarily not difficult, but this may be a challenging diagnostic problem in limited needle core biopsy samples. In this setting, a diagnosis of carcinoma is warranted when the cytologically atypical apocrine proliferation has the configuration of one of the conventional forms of intraductal carcinoma (56).

FLORID PAPILLOMATOSIS AND SYRINGOMATOUS ADENOMA OF THE NIPPLE

Because of their superficial location in the nipple, these lesions are ordinarily not subjected to stereotactic needle core biopsy. A brief discussion of each is provided for reference.

Florid Papillomatosis

The majority of patients are 40 to 50 years old. Approximately 15% of patients are younger than 35 years. The most frequent presenting symptom is discharge that is often bloody. Pain, itching, or burning sensations are not unusual (67). In many instances, the nipple appears enlarged and a mass can be palpated. The surface of the nipple may appear granular, ulcerated, reddened, warty, or crusted. The symptoms and clinical findings can be mistaken for Paget disease. The mammographic and sonographic findings may suggest carcinoma (68). Fewer than 5% of the reported examples of florid papillomatosis of the nipple have been in men (67).

The lesions can be grouped according to microscopic growth pattern into four categories. Three subtypes have one structural feature that dominates the lesion or is present exclusively, while the fourth group consists of tumors with two or three of these patterns. No prognostic significance has been attached to these subtypes.

Florid papillomatosis with the *sclerosing papillomatosis pattern* is histologically indistinguishable in many respects from sclerosing papillomas encountered elsewhere in the breast. Exuberant papillary hyperplasia of ductal epithelium is distorted by an accompanying stromal proliferation within and around the affected ducts (Fig. 4.35). Focal comedo type necrosis may be found in the hyperplastic

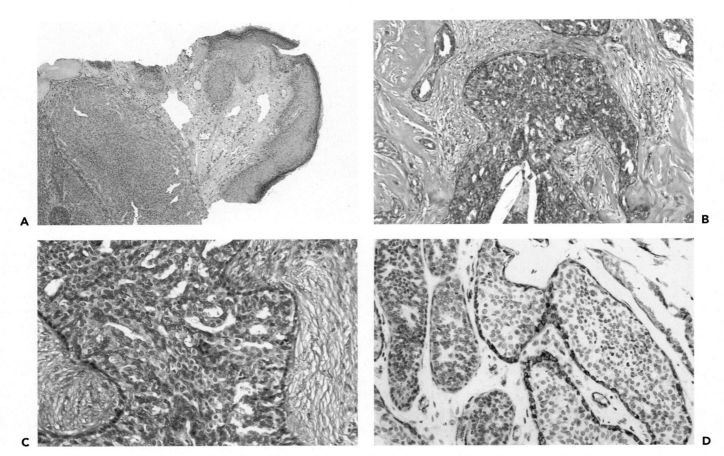

Figure 4.35 Florid papillomatosis of the nipple. A: This needle core biopsy sample taken from a nodule in the nipple shows florid duct hyperplasia just beneath the epidermis. **B:** Hyperplastic epithelium with a fenestrated pattern in sclerotic stroma is commonly present in the sclerosing type of florid papillomatosis. **C:** Myoepithelial cells outline the hyperplastic epithelium. **D:** Myoepithelial cells are accentuated by the immunostain for actin (immunoperoxidase).

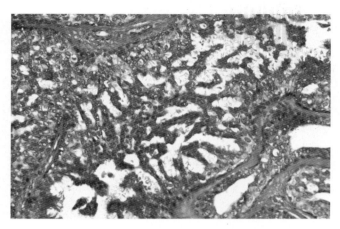

Figure 4.36 **Florid papillomatosis of the nipple.** Micropapillary hyperplasia in a papillomatosis-type lesion.

duct epithelium, sometimes associated with scattered mitoses in epithelial cells. Squamous cysts are commonly formed in the terminal portions of lactiferous ducts.

Lesions with the *papillomatosis pattern* consist of florid papillary hyperplasia of ductal epithelium, causing expansion and crowding of the affected ducts (Fig. 4.36). Focal epithelial necrosis and scattered mitotic figures may be found. These tumors lack the sclerosing stromal proliferation that characterizes the sclerosing papillomatosis type of lesion. Hyperplastic glandular tissue may replace the overlying squamous epithelium over part or the entire apical skin surface of the nipple. Squamous-lined cysts and apocrine metaplasia are not prominent in these lesions.

Florid papillomatosis with the *adenosis pattern* is composed of crowded, glandular structures arranged in a pattern indistinguishable from florid sclerosing adenosis or an adenosis tumor. Myoepithelial hyperplasia accompanies the epithelial proliferation. Prominent apocrine metaplasia, hyperplasia of the squamous epithelium, and superficial squamous cysts may be encountered. Mitotic figures and focal necrosis are uncommon.

The *mixed proliferative type of florid papillomatosis* consists of varying combinations of the other three patterns. Prominent features in most cases include squamous metaplasia of ducts with cysts, apocrine metaplasia, and acanthosis of the overlying epithelium. Cystic dilatation of ducts is not uncommon near the deep margin of the lesion. Focal necrosis may be found in the duct epithelium. Mitotic activity is minimal. Adenosis occurs in about one-third of these lesions.

It can be difficult to detect carcinoma arising in florid papillomatosis of the nipple (69). Hyperplastic areas in the lesions often exhibit atypical features that may include foci with necrosis as well as cribriform and micropapillary growth patterns, mitoses, and cytologic atypia. In the absence of definitive evidence of invasion, Paget disease of the nipple epidermis is the most reliable evidence for a diagnosis of carcinoma arising in florid papillomatosis. The CAM5.2 and CK7 immunostains for cytokeratin are helpful for detecting intraepidermal Paget cells that

are immunoreactive for these markers. Immunostains for myoepithelial markers, especially p63, demonstrate myoepithelium throughout the benign proliferative components of florid papillomatosis. If these immunostains identify ducts that do not have immunoreactive myoepithelium, intraductal carcinoma may be present. However, it should be noted that myoepithelium may be depleted or absent in the central region of a benign sclerosing papillary lesion. If Paget disease or invasive carcinoma is not detected, a diagnosis of carcinoma arising in florid papillomatosis is extremely difficult to substantiate with routine H&E sections.

Incisional biopsy or needle core biopsy is not satisfactory to exclude the possibility of carcinoma arising in florid papillomatosis. Complete excision, which is recommended as definitive treatment, usually requires removal of the nipple. Local recurrence of florid papillomatosis may occur following subtotal excision, but a number of patients have reportedly remained asymptomatic after incomplete excision.

SYRINGOMATOUS ADENOMA

This benign, locally infiltrating neoplasm of the nipple has a close histopathologic resemblance to syringomatous tumors that commonly arise in the skin of the face and other anatomic sites (70,71). The patients range from 11 to 76 years of age at diagnosis, with a mean age of 45 years (72). The initial symptom is a unilateral mass in the nipple and/or subareolar region. The tumors have measured 1.0 to 3.5 cm. Pain, tenderness, redness, itching, discharge, or nipple inversion have been noted in isolated cases. Mammography reveals a dense stellate tumor (73), and ultrasound reveals an indistinct tumor that may be accompanied by dilated ducts (72).

The lesion consists of tubules, ductules, and strands of small, uniform generally basophilic cells infiltrating the dermis of the skin and the stroma of the nipple. Invasion into the smooth muscle bundles of the nipple is very common, and occasionally perineural invasion is observed. The neoplastic glands sometimes appear to be connected with the basal layer of the epidermis. Paget disease is not present.

The ducts formed by one or more layers of cells, have "teardrop," "comma," and branching shapes, with lumina that are usually open and round (Fig. 4.37). Some cells may exhibit cytoplasmic clearing. A distinct layer of myoepithelial cells is not apparent. Mitoses are virtually absent and nuclei lack prominent nucleoli and pleomorphism. The lumens are empty or they contain deeply eosinophilic, retracted secretion. Flattening of cells around the lumina is early evidence of squamous differentiation, which in a fully developed form results in keratotic cysts. A foreign body giant cell reaction may be elicited in the vicinity of ruptured squamous cysts. Calcification is sometimes seen in the keratinized epithelium. Secretion in tubular lumens is PAS-positive and weakly mucicarmine positive (70). Because the

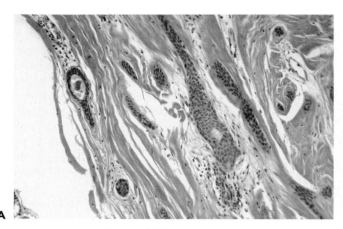
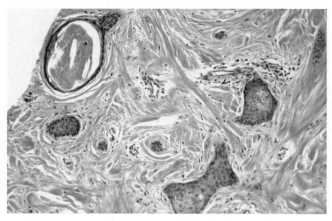

Figure 4.37 **Syringomatous adenoma of the nipple. A:** This area from a needle core biopsy specimen shows elongated, ductlike structures, one of which has an open lumen with secretion. Squamoid differentiation is shown in the center. **B:** An area with cystic dilatation and prominent squamous differentiation.

p63 immunostain is reactive with cells with squamous differentiation, it is not a reliable method for detecting myoepithelium in a syringomatous adenoma. The differential diagnosis of syringomatous adenoma of the nipple includes florid papillomatosis, tubular carcinoma, and low-grade adenosquamous carcinoma (74).

In most cases this benign infiltrative tumor is adequately treated by local excision that may by necessity include the nipple. Local recurrence, reported in 25% to 30% of patients after local excision, is likely to occur are if the margins are involved in the initial procedure (72,75).

REFERENCES

1. Cardenosa G, Eklund GW. Benign papillary neoplasms of the breast: mammographic findings. *Radiology.* 1991;181:751–755.
2. Lam WM, Chu WCW, Tang APY, et al. Role of radiologic features in the management of papillary lesions of the breast. *Am J Roentgenol.* 2006; 186:1322–1327.
3. Carter DJ, Rosen PP. Atypical apocrine metaplasia in sclerosing lesions of the breast. A study of 51 patients. *Mod Pathol.* 1991;4:1–5.
4. Papotti M, Gugliotta P, Eusebi V, Bussolati G. Immunohistochemical analysis of benign and malignant papillary lesions of the breast. *Am J Surg Pathol.* 1983;7:451–461.
5. Stefano D, Batistou A, Nonni A, et al. P63 expression in benign and malignant breast lesions. *Histol Histopathol.* 2004;19:465–471.
6. Judkins AR, Montone KT, LiVolsi VA, van de Rijn M. Sensitivity and specificity of antibodies on necrotic tumor tissue. *Am J Clin Pathol.* 1998;110: 641–646.
7. Flint A, Oberman HA. Infarction and squamous metaplasia of intraductal papilloma: a benign breast lesion that may simulate carcinoma. *Hum Pathol.* 1984;15:764–767.
8. Soderstrom KO, Toikkanen S. Extensive squamous metaplasia simulating squamous cell carcinoma in benign breast papillomatosis. *Hum Pathol.* 1983;14:1081–1082.
9. Liberman L, Bracero N, Vuolo M, et al. Percutaneous large core biopsy of papillary breast lesions. *AJ Roentgenol.* 1999;172:331–337.
10. Liberman L, Tornos C, Huzjan R, et al. Is surgical excision warranted after benign, concordant diagnosis of papilloma in a percutaneous breast biopsy? *Am J Roentgenol.* 2006;186:1328–1334.
11. Puglisi F, Zuiani C, Bazzocchi M, et al. Role of mammography, ultrasound and large core biopsy in the diagnostic evaluation of papillary breast lesions. *Oncology.* 2003;65:311–315.
12. Ivan D, Selinko V, Sahin AA, et al. Accuracy of core needle biopsy diagnosis in assessing papillary breast lesions: histologic predictors of malignancy. *Mod Pathol.* 2004;17:165–171.
13. Philpotts LE, Shaheen NA, Jain KS, et al. Uncommon high-risk lesions of the breast diagnosed at stereotactic core-needle biopsy: clinical importance. *Radiology.* 2000;216:831–837.
14. Mercado CL, Hamele-Bene D, Singer C, et al. Papillary lesions of the breast: Evaluation with stereotactic directional vacuum-assisted biopsy. *Radiology.* 2001;221:650–655.
15. Jacobs TW, Guinee DG, Holden J, et al. Intraductal papillomas without atypia on breast core needle biopsy (CNB): surgical excision is advisable. *Mod Pathol.* 2005;18(suppl):37A.
16. Jaffer S, Nagi CS, Bleiweiss I. Should intraductal papilloma diagnosed on core needle biopsy be excised? *Mod Pathol.* 2005;18(suppl):37A.
17. Gendler LS, Feldman SM, Balassanian R, et al. Association of breast cancer with papillary lesions identified at percutaneous image-guided breast biopsy. *Am J Surg.* 2004;188:365–370.
18. Agoff SN, Lawton TJ. Papillary lesions of the breast with and without atypical ductal hyperplasia. Can we accurately predict benign behavior from core needle biopsy? *Am J Clin Pathol.* 2004;122:440–443.
19. Sexton K, Brill YM, Atkins L, et al. Outcome of benign papillary lesions of the breast diagnosed by needle core and mammotome biopsies with 3 to 5 year follow-up. *Mod Pathol.* 1007;19(suppl);42A.
20. Kilgore AR, Fleming R, Ramos N. The incidence of cancer with nipple discharge and the risk of cancer in the presence of papillary disease of the breast. *Surg Gynecol Obstet.* 1953;96:649–660.
21. Kraus FT, Neubecker RD. The differential diagnosis of papillary tumors of the breast. *Cancer.* 1962;15:444–455.
22. Carter D. Intraductal papillary tumors of the breast. A study of 76 cases. *Cancer* 1977;39:1689–1692.
23. Rosen PP. Arthur Purdy Stout and papilloma of the breast. Comments on the occasion of his 100th birthday. *Am J Surg Pathol.* 1986;10(suppl 1):100–107.
24. MacGrogan G, Tavassoli FA. Central atypical papillomas of the breast: a clinicopathological study of 119 cases. *Virchows Arch.* 2003;443:609–617.
25. Ali-Fehmi R, Carolin K, Wallis T, Visscher DW. Clinicopathologic analysis of breast lesions associated with multiple papillomas. *Hum Pathol.* 2003; 34:234–239.
26. Estabrook A. Are patients with solitary or multiple intraductal papillomas at a higher risk of developing breast cancer? *Surg Oncol Clin North Am.* 1993; 2:45–56.
27. Haagensen CD, Bodian C, Haagensen DE. *Breast Carcinoma: Risk and Detection.* Philadelphia: WB Saunders Co; 1981:146–237.
28. Lewis JT, Hartmann LC, Vierkaut RA, et al. An analysis of breast cancer risk in women with single, multiple and atypical papilloma. *Am J Surg Pathol.* 2006;30:665–672.
29. Clement PB, Young RH, Azzopardi JG. Collagenous spherulosis of the breast. *Am J Surg Pathol.* 1987;11:411–417.
30. Guarino M, Tricomi P, Cristofori E. Collagenous spherulosis of the breast with atypical epithelial hyperplasia. *Pathologica.* 1993;85:123–127.
31. Resetkova E, Albarracin C, Sneige N. Collagenous spherulosis of breast. Morphologic study of 59 cases and review of the literature. *Am J Surg Pathol.* 2006;30:20–27.
32. Stephenson TJ, Hird PM, Laing RW, Davies JD. Nodular basement membrane deposits in breast carcinoma and atypical ductal hyperplasia: mimics of collagenous spherulosis. *Pathologica.* 1994;86:234–239.
33. Grignon DJ, Ro JY, MacKay BN, et al. Collagenous spherulosis of the breast. Immunohistochemical and ultrastructural studies. *Am J Clin Pathol.* 1989; 91:386–392.
34. Hamperl H. Strahlige Narben und obliterierende Mastopathie Beitrage zur pathologischen histologie der Mamma. *Virchows Arch.* [A] 1975;369: 55–68.
35. Jacobs TW, Schnitt SJ, Tan X, Brown LF. Radial scars of the breast and breast carcinomas have similar alterations in expression of factors involved in vascular stroma formation. *Hum Pathol.* 2002;33:29–38.
36. Linell F, Ljungberg O, Anderson I. Breast carcinoma: aspects of early stage, progression and related problems. *Acta Pathol Microbiol Scand.* 1980;(suppl) 272:1–233.

37. Nielsen M, Jensen J, Andersen JA. An autopsy study of radial scar in the female breast. *Histopathology.* 1985;9:287–295.

38. Andersen JA, Gram JB. Radial scar in the female breast: a long-term follow-up study of 32 cases. *Cancer.* 1984;53:2557–2560.

39. Nielsen M, Christensen L, Andersen J. Radial scars in women with breast cancer. *Cancer.* 1987;59:1019–1025.

40. Adler DD, Helvie MA, Oberman HA, et al. Radial sclerosing lesion of the breast: mammographic features. *Radiology.* 1990;176:737–740.

41. Tabar L, Dean PB. Stellate lesions. In: Tabar L, Dean PB, eds. *Teaching Atlas of Mammography.* 2nd rev ed. New York: Georg Thieme Verlag; 1985:87–136.

42. Ciatto S, Morrone D, Catarzi S, et al. Radial scars of the breast: review of 38 consecutive mammographic diagnoses. *Radiology.* 1993;187:757–760.

43. Orel SG, Evers K, Yeh IT, Troupin RH. Radial scar with microcalcification: radiologic-pathologic correlation. *Radiology.* 1992;183:479–484.

44. Mitnick JS, Vazquez MF, Harris MN, Roses DF. Differentiation of radial scar from scirrhous carcinoma of the breast: mammographic-pathologic correlation. *Radiology.* 1989;173:697–700.

45. Battersby S, Anderson TJ. Myofibroblast activity of radial scars. *J Pathol.* 1985;147:33–40.

46. Taylor HB, Norris HJ. Epithelial invasion of nerves in benign diseases of the breast. *Cancer.* 1967;20:2245–2249.

47. Alvarado-Cabrero I, Tavassoli FA. Neoplastic and malignant lesions involving or arising in a radial scar: a clinicopathologic analysis of 17 cases. *BreastJ.* 2000;6:96–102.

48. Caneva A, Bonetti F, Manfrin E, et al. Is radial scar of the breast a premalignant lesion? *Mod Pathol.* 1997;10:17A.

49. Sloane JP, Mayers MM. Carcinoma and atypical hyperplasia in Radial scars and complex sclerosing lesions: importance of lesion size and patient age. *Histopathology.* 1993;23:225–231.

50. Brenner RJ, Jackman RJ, Parker SH, et al. Percutaneous core needle biopsy of radial scars of the breast: when is excision necessary? *Am J Roentgenol.* 2002;179:1179–1184.

51. Cawson JN, Malara F, Kavanagh A, et al. Fourteen-gauge needle core biopsy of mammographically evident radial scars. Is excision necessary? *Cancer.* 2003;97:345–351.

52. Anderson TJ, Battersby S. Radial scars of benign and malignant breasts; comparative features and significance. *J Pathol.* 1985;147:23–32.

53. Elavathil LJ, Mothafar F, Dhamanaskar P. Is excision of all radial scars diagnosed in needle core biopsies necessary? *Mod Pathol.* 2006;19(suppl 1) 26A.

54. Jacobs TW, Byrne C, Colditz G, et al. Radial scars in benign breast biopsy specimens and the risk of breast cancer. *N Engl J Med.* 1999;340:430–436.

55. Sanders ME, Page DL, Simpson JF, et al. Interdependence of radial scar and proliferative disease with respect to invasive breast carcinoma risk in patients with benign breast biopsies. *Cancer.* 2006;106:1453–1461.

56. Rosen PP. Subareolar sclerosing duct hyperplasia of the breast. *Cancer.* 1987;59:1927–1930.

57. Bussolati G, Cattani MG, Gugliotta P, et al. Morphologic and functional aspects of apocrine metaplasia in dysplastic and neoplastic breast tissue. *Ann NY Acad Sci.* 1986;464:262–274.

58. Benigni G, Squartini F. Uneven distribution and significant concentration of apocrine metaplasia in lower breast quadrants. *Tumori.* 1986;72:179–182.

59. Wellings SR, Alpers CE. Apocrine cystic metaplasia: subgross pathology and prevalence in cancer-associated versus random autopsy breasts. *Hum Pathol.* 1987;18:381–386.

60. Schuerch III C, Rosen PP, Hirota T, et al. A pathologic study of benign breast diseases in Tokyo and New York. *Cancer.* 1982;50:1899–1903.

61. Haagensen CD, Bodian C, Haagensen Jr, DE. Apocrine epithelium. In: Haagensen CD, Bodian C, Haagensen Jr DE, eds, *Breast Carcinoma: Risk and Detection.* Philadelphia: W.B. Saunders; 1981:83–105.

62. Foote Jr FW, Stewart FW. Comparative studies of cancerous versus non-cancerous breasts. *Ann Surg.* 1945;12:6–79.

63. McCarty Jr KS, Kesterson GHD, Wilkinson WE, Georigiade N. Histopathologic study of subcutaneous mastectomy specimens from patients with carcinoma of the contralateral breast. *Surg Gynecol Obstet.* 1978;147:682–688.

64. Nielsen M, Thomsen JL, Primdahl L, et al. Breast cancer and atypia among young and middle-aged women: a study of 110 medicolegal autopsies. *Br J Cancer.* 1987;56:814–819.

65. Page DL, Van der Zwaag R, Rogers LW, et al. Relation between component parts of fibrocystic disease complex and breast cancer. *JNCI.* 1978;61:1055–1063.

66. Abati AD, Kimmel M, Rosen PP. Apocrine mammary carcinoma: a clinicopathologic study of 72 cases. *Am J Clin Pathol.* 1990;94:371–377.

67. Rosen PP, Caicco J. Florid papillomatosis of the nipple: a study of 51 patients including nine having mammary carcinoma. *Am J Surg Pathol.* 1986;10:87–101.

68. Fornage BD, Faroux MJ, Pluot M, Bogomoletz W. Nipple adenoma simulating carcinoma. Misleading clinical, mammographic, sonographic and cytologic findings. *J Ultrasound Med.* 1991;10:55–57.

69. Diaz NM, Palmer JO, Wick MR. Erosive adenomatosis of the nipple: histology, immunohistology, and differential diagnosis. *Mod Pathol.* 1992; 179–184.

70. Rosen PP. Syringomatous adenoma of the nipple. *Am J Surg Pathol.* 1983; 7:739–745.

71. Ward BE, Cooper PH, Subramony C. Syringomatous tumor of the nipple. *Am J Clin Pathol.* 1989;92:692–696.

72. Kubo M, Tsuji H, Kunitomo T, Taguchi K. Syringomatous adenoma of the nipple: A case report. *Breast Cancer.* 2004;11:214–216.

73. Slaughter MS, Pomerantz RA, Murad T, Hines JR. Infiltrating syringomatous adenoma of the nipple. *Surgery.* 1992;111:711–713.

74. Rosen PP, Ernsberger D. Low grade adenosquamous carcinoma. A variant of metaplastic mammary carcinoma. *Am J Surg Pathol.* 1987;11:351–358.

75. Carter E, Dyess DL. Infiltrating syringomatous adenoma of the nipple: a case report and 20-year retrospective review. *Breast J.* 2004;10:443–447.

Myoepithelial Neoplasms

5

Myoepithelial cells comprise part of the normal microscopic anatomy of mammary lobules and ducts (1). They participate in many benign proliferative processes, most notably sclerosing adenosis and papillary proliferative lesions of ducts (2,3). Benign tumors composed of myoepithelial cells are termed *myoepitheliomas*. When epithelial and myoepithelial cells participate in the proliferation, the term *adenomyoepithelioma* is appropriate. Malignant neoplasms formed by myoepithelial cells may have an epithelial phenotype (myoepithelial carcinoma), a myoid phenotype (leiomyosarcoma), or both appearances (malignant adenomyoepithelioma) (4–6).

The diagnosis of myoepithelial or adenomyoepithelial neoplasms in needle core biopsy and fine needle aspiration (7) samples of the breast can be a very challenging problem, especially for pathologists who have little experience with the histologic spectrum of these uncommon tumors. Attention is drawn especially to benign myoepithelial tumors with a predominately epithelial appearance, benign adenomyoepitheliomas, in which glandular elements are dispersed amidst spindly myoepithelial cells and tumors that qualify as "pleomorphic adenomas." When seen out of the context of a complete histologic section, needle core biopsy and fine needle aspiration samples from any of these benign lesions can be mistaken for invasive carcinoma (7,8). If the possibility of a myoepithelial or adenomyoepithelial neoplasm is considered in this situation, selected appropriate immunostains will almost always resolve the diagnosis in the needle core biopsy sample.

ADENOMYOEPITHELIOMA

Almost all patients have been women, ranging in age from 26 to 82 years (average approximately 60 years), who presented with a solitary unilateral painless mass. Nipple discharge, pain, and tenderness are infrequent. The mammographic findings may be interpreted as suspicious in some patients (6). Nonpalpable adenomyoepitheliomas measuring 2 cm or less have been detected as well-circumscribed mass lesions by ultrasonography (8) or by mammography (9). Calcifications are sometimes but not always present. One malignant adenomyoepithelioma appeared to be cystic on mammography (10). Berna et al. (11) described a partially cystic circumscribed 2.5 cm adenomyoepithelioma in an 84-year-old man. The tumor was histologically benign with immunoreactivity for actin and cytokeratin.

The majority of adenomyoepitheliomas are variants of intraductal papilloma, but a small number of these tumors appear to arise from a lobular proliferation. Adenomyoepithelioma is closely related to ductal adenoma (12,13) and pleomorphic adenoma (mixed tumor) (14,15). Foci of adenomyoepithelioma can frequently be detected in tubular adenomas and in mammary pleomorphic adenomas. As is the case with sclerosing papillary tumors generally, the needle core biopsy sample obtained from an adenomyoepithelioma can be misinterpreted as invasive carcinoma as reported by Zhang et al. (7).

Microscopically, adenomyoepitheliomas are circumscribed and composed of aggregated nodules (Fig. 5.1). Some nodules consist of a compact proliferation of epithelial and myoepithelial cells, but most lesions have one or more nodules in which there is at least a focal papillary growth pattern. Sometimes the papillary intraductal component extends into ducts outside the gross tumorous lesion. This characteristic may be responsible for local recurrence after a seemingly adequate excision.

The basic microscopic structural unit of the adenomyoepithelioma is a small glandular lumen encompassed by cuboidal epithelial cells. Surrounding the glands are polygonal or spindle-shaped myoepithelial cells with eosinophilic or clear cytoplasm and a basement membrane (Fig. 5.2). The most common microscopic pattern, referred to as the tubular type of adenomyoepithelioma, is a proliferation of tubular glandular elements separated by islands and bands of polygonal myoepithelial cells that have clear cytoplasm. In some lesions myoepithelial cells proliferate between glands in broad bands and trabeculae that are separated by strands of basement membrane and fibrovascular stroma (Figs. 5.3 and 5.4). The contrast between the dark staining cytoplasm of glandular cells and the pale cytoplasm of myoepithelial cells is

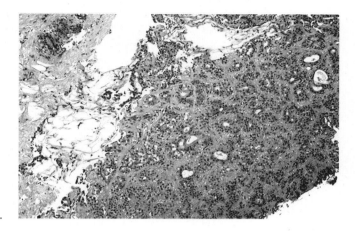

Figure 5.1 Adenomyoepithelioma. A needle core biopsy specimen.

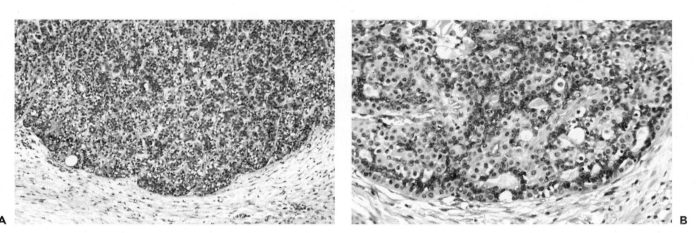

Figure 5.2 Adenomyoepithelioma. A: The lesion has a well-circumscribed border. Darkly stained epithelial cells and myoepithelial cells with clear cytoplasm are apparent. **B:** Glandular elements composed of darkly stained epithelial cells are compressed by myoepithelial cells with an epithelioid phenotype and eosinophilic cytoplasm. There are a few small glandular lumens.

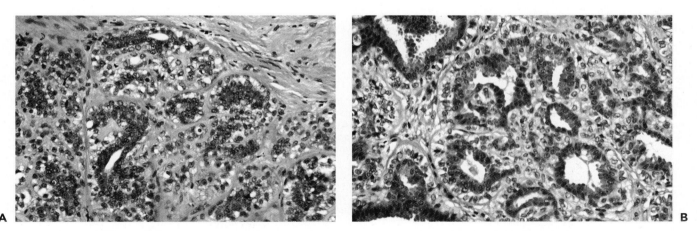

Figure 5.3 Adenomyoepithelioma. A: This tumor has prominent myoepithelial cells with clear cytoplasm that provide a striking contrast to the epithelial cells. **B:** Epithelioid myoepithelial cells form bands between glands composed of hyperplastic epithelial cells. Slender strands of basement membrane and fibrovascular stroma are evident.

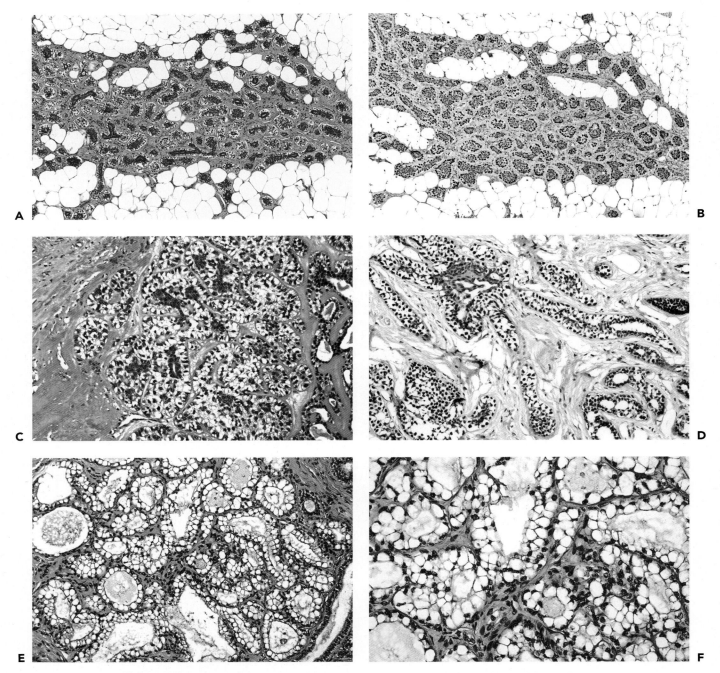

Figure 5.4 **Adenomyoepithelial hyperplasia in adenosis. A:** Myoepithelial cell hyperplasia is manifested by clear cells around the adenosis glands shown in fat. **B:** Myoepithelial cell nuclei are immunoreactive for p63 in the lesion shown in **(A)** (immunoperoxidase). **C:** Clear myoepithelial cell hyperplasia around adenosis glands. **D:** Nuclear p63 reactivity in clear cell myoepithelial hyperplasia (immunoperoxidase). **E, F:** Adenosis consisting entirely of myoepithelial cells with clear cytoplasm.

striking. Fragments of adenomyoepithelioma in needle core biopsy specimens can be mistaken for infiltrating carcinoma (Fig. 5.5).

Apocrine metaplasia may be encountered in the glandular epithelium, particularly in papillary areas and it can be cytologically atypical. Foci of sebaceous, squamous, or mucoepidermoid metaplasia are variably present (Fig. 5.6). Calcifications are occasionally formed in glandular spaces.

Some tumors develop central fibrosis or necrosis due to infarction (Fig. 5.7). A cystic papillary type of adenomyoepithelioma is uncommon. Collagenous spherulosis (16) and cartilaginous metaplasia of the stroma are rarely encountered in adenomyoepitheliomas.

Some adenomyoepitheliomas have foci of myoid growth composed of a mixture of spindle and polygonal cells (Fig. 5.8). Palisading of spindle cells and alveolar

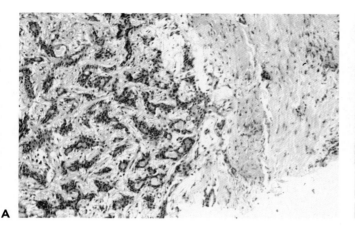

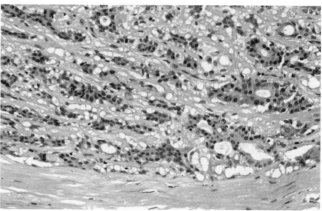

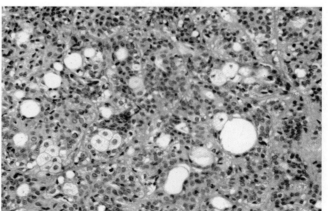

Figure 5.5 Adenomyoepithelioma mistaken for carcinoma. A: This needle core biopsy sample from an adenomyoepithelioma was interpreted as infiltrating duct carcinoma. Markedly vacuolated myoepithelial cells are difficult to recognize between the unevenly shaped glands, resulting in an appearance that simulates infiltrating carcinoma. **B:** The excisional biopsy specimen contained a well-circumscribed adenomyoepithelioma shown here. **C:** Myoepithelial cells are highlighted in this immunostain for smooth muscle actin (immunoperoxidase).

clustering of polygonal myoepithelial cells are common myoid patterns. The glandular elements may be intermixed with myoid areas or they may be largely overgrown by the myoepithelial proliferation (Fig. 5.9). Atypical features include scattered mitotic figures, nuclear pleomorphism, and hyperchromasia and occasional multinucleated cells. Myoid hyperplasia may give rise to areas with leiomyomatous features or a storiform growth pattern (17), and rarely this process produces leiomyosarcoma (3,18).

Origin of a malignant neoplasm in an adenomyoepithelioma has only very rarely been documented. Some lesions were reported to result in local recurrence (5,19), whereas others have produced metastases and a fatal outcome (20–22). Malignant adenomyoepitheliomas may have a biphasic growth pattern at the primary site and in metastases. Simpson et al. (23) described a malignant adenomyoepithelioma with carcinomatous and osteogenic elements. A case report by Jones et al. (22) documents a 3 cm malignant

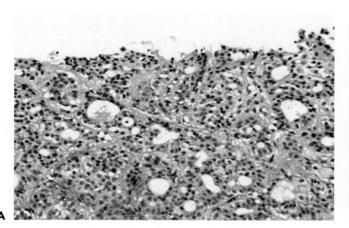

Figure 5.6 Adenomyoepithelioma with sebaceous and squamous differentiation. A, B: In this needle core biopsy sample, the myoepithelial cells with vacuolated cytoplasm have largely overgrown the epithelial cells. Focal sebaceous differentiation is shown in **(B).**

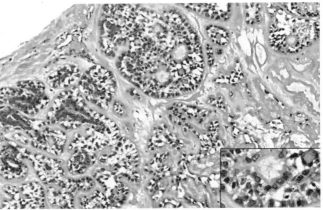

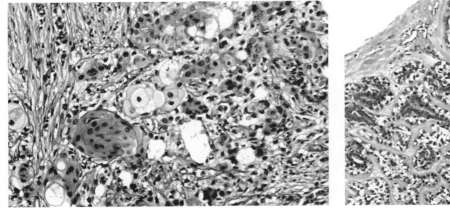

Figure 5.6 *(continued)* **C:** Squamous and sebaceous metaplasia in another adenomyoepithelioma. **D:** Collagenous spherulosis. Two spherules are present in the upper center. Note the central stellate filamentous material in a spherule **(inset).**

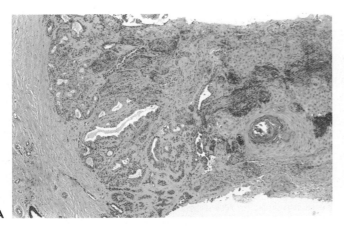

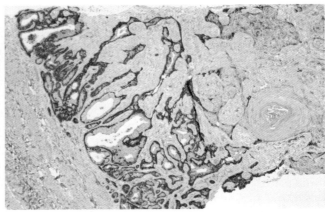

Figure 5.7 **Adenomyoepithelioma with infarction. A:** Most of the tumor in this needle core biopsy specimen is infarcted. **B:** Myoepithelium is highlighted in noninfarcted areas by reactivity for CD10 (immunoperoxidase).

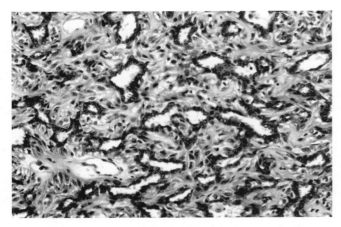

Figure 5.8 **Adenomyoepithelioma with myoid differentiation.** The spindly myoepithelial cells in this lesion have a myoid phenotype characterized by eosinophilic cytoplasm.

adenomyoepithelioma that had a substantial malignant spindle cell component with mitoses and necrosis. The tumor gave rise to multiple liver metastases composed of spindle cells. Comparative genomic hybridization (CGH) analysis revealed progressively more genetic alterations between the glandular and spindle cell elements of the primary tumor and the liver metastases.

Myoepithelial carcinoma with an epithelial phenotype can arise in an adenomyoepithelioma (20,21). Features indicative of myoepithelial carcinoma in this setting are overgrowth by epithelioid myoepithelial cells with clear cytoplasm, nuclear pleomorphism, mitotic activity, and necrosis (Fig. 5.10).

Glands in an adenomyoepithelioma may contain secretion that is positive with periodic acid–Schiff (PAS) or mucicarmine stains, but intracytoplasmic secretion is rarely detectable. The cytoplasm of glandular cells is strongly

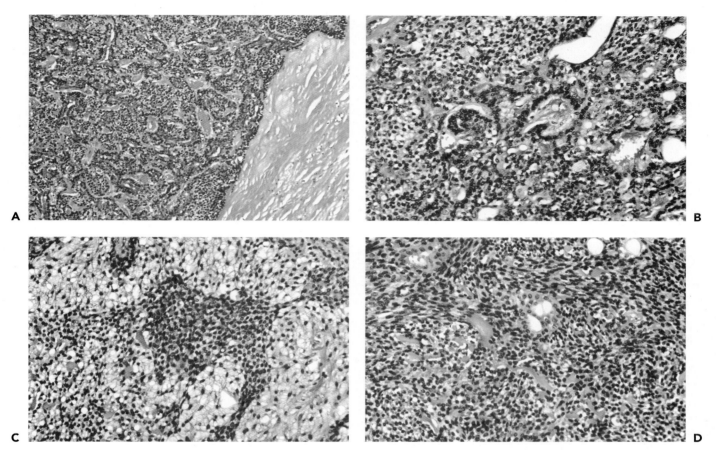

Figure 5.9   Adenomyoepithelioma with myoepithelial cell hyperplasia. A, B: Epithelial cells are distributed in bands and nests with inconspicuous glandular lumina. The myoepithelial cells that have small, punctate nuclei and sparse clear cytoplasm, tend to aggregate in poorly defined alveolar groups. **C:** This part of the tumor shown in **(A)** is composed entirely of myoepithelial cells. The combination of small, compact cells and cells with extremely vacuolated cytoplasm resembles a pattern seen in cellular pleomorphic adenoma (mixed tumor) of salivary gland origin. **D:** Spindle cell myoid differentiation of myoepithelial cells is shown surrounding inconspicuous glands.

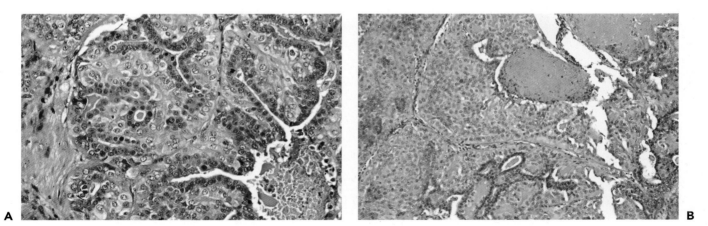

Figure 5.10   Myoepithelial carcinoma arising in adenomyoepithelioma, papilloma, and adenosis. A: Epithelioid myoepithelial cells with large vesicular nuclei are indicative of an atypical proliferation in this adenomyoepithelioma. The epithelial cells are also hyperplastic. Focal necrosis is shown in the lower right corner. **B:** Neoplastic myoepithelial cells surround a focus of comedo-type necrosis. Residual glands are present.

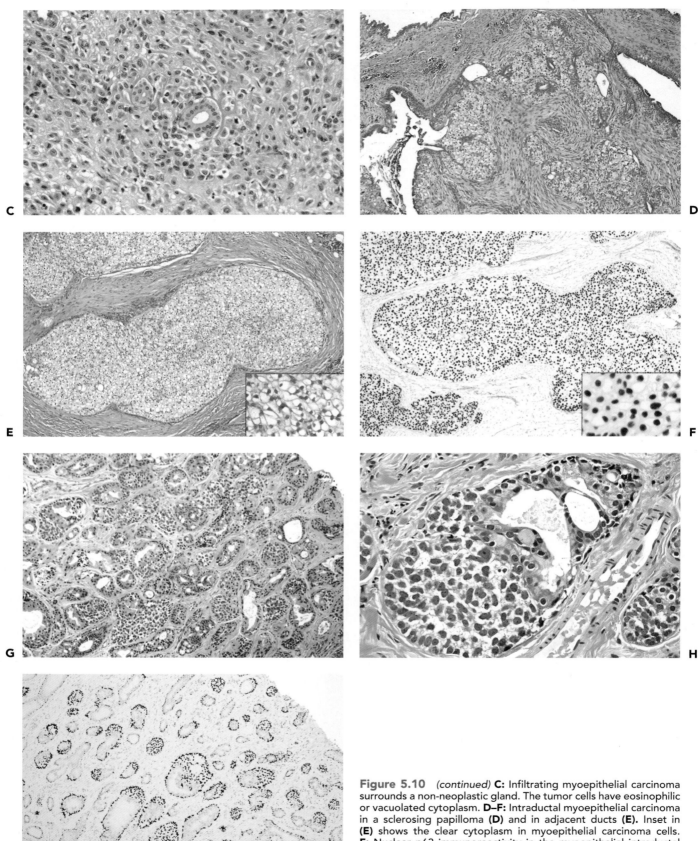

Figure 5.10 *(continued)* **C:** Infiltrating myoepithelial carcinoma surrounds a non-neoplastic gland. The tumor cells have eosinophilic or vacuolated cytoplasm. **D–F:** Intraductal myoepithelial carcinoma in a sclerosing papilloma **(D)** and in adjacent ducts **(E)**. Inset in **(E)** shows the clear cytoplasm in myoepithelial carcinoma cells. **F:** Nuclear p63 immunoreactivity in the myoepithelial intraductal carcinoma (immunoperoxidase). **G–I:** Myoepithelial intraductal carcinoma arising in apocrine adenosis. Nuclear p63 is shown in the myoepithelial cells **(I)** (immunoperoxidase).

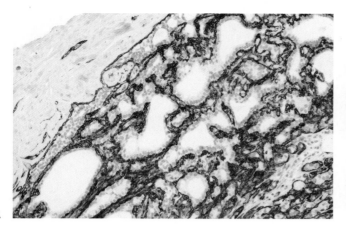

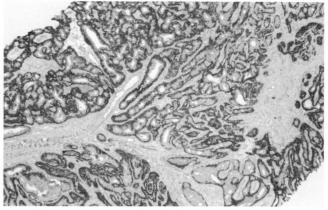

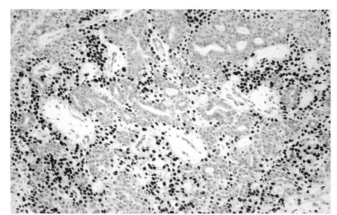

Figure 5.11 Adenomyoepithelioma, immunohistochemistry. A: Myoepithelial cells are highlighted by an immunostain for smooth muscle actin (immunoperoxidase). **B:** The myoepithelium is highlighted here by reactivity for CD10 (immunoperoxidase). **C:** Nuclear reactivity for p63 delineates the distribution of myoepithelial cells in this adenomyoepithelioma (immunoperoxidase).

reactive with antibodies to cytokeratin and the luminal surfaces of these cells are positive for epithelial membrane antigen. Most epithelial cells in adenomyoepitheliomas are S-100 negative, but small groups may be strongly reactive for this antigen. Collagenous spherulosis, a structural feature associated with duct hyperplasia and papillomas has been described in an adenomyoepithelioma (17).

Polygonal and spindle myoepithelial cells are not reactive for epithelial membrane antigen or carcinoembryonic antigen (CEA) and variably reactive for low–molecular weight cytokeratin. Actin staining tends to be more conspicuous in spindle than in clear polygonal myoepithelial cells, and no actin reactivity is found in the epithelial cells. A subset of myoepithelial cells is S-100 positive in virtually all tumors, but the intensity and uniformity of reactivity varies considerably. Because S-100 reactivity is expressed by glandular as well as myoepithelial cells it is not a specific marker for the latter cell type (24). A similar immunophenotype has been reported for the myoepithelial cells of a "pleomorphic adenoma" in the breast (15).

Immunostain markers that are relatively specific for myoepithelial cells include CK5, SMA, CD10, myosin, calponin, p63, and maspin (25,26). p63 is especially helpful because of its nuclear localization that precludes cytoplasmic cross-reactivity in myofibroblasts that occurs sporadically with markers such as myosin, calponin, SMA,

and CD10. (Fig.5.11). The immunophenotype of neoplastic myoepithelial cells is sometimes different from that of their normal counterpart, and they are not necessarily reactive for all markers. Therefore a panel of immunostains should be used to minimize the likelihood of failing to detect the presence of myoepithelial cells.

Adenomyoepithelioma is a benign tumor that can be treated by local excision (6). Local recurrence has been reported, usually more than two years after the initial excision (5,6). The multinodular character of the lesion and peripheral intraductal extension contribute to the risk for local recurrence. Reexcision may be performed when the tumor is incompletely excised, especially for multinodular lesions with peripheral intraductal extension. Mastectomy, breast irradiation, and axillary dissection are not appropriate treatment for benign adenomyoepitheliomas but may be considered in exceptional patients who have malignant or recurrent tumors.

MYOEPITHELIOMA

Myoid transformation of myoepithelial cell is sometimes present in foci of sclerosing adenosis, and it may occasionally dominate the process leading to a leiomyomatous appearance. Myoepithelial neoplasms of the breast are extremely uncommon and reports are limited to case studies. Hamperl's review of the subject in 1970 (3) described lesions composed of epithelioid and spindle-shaped myoepithelial cells.

Spindle cell neoplasms composed entirely of myoepithelial cells consist of interlacing bundles of cells sometimes arranged in a storiform pattern. The cytoplasm is more often eosinophilic than clear. An infiltrative growth pattern may be present. The spindle cells are immunoreactive for actin. Tumors with few or no mitotic figures have had a benign clinical course after relatively short follow-up (27,28), whereas those with multiple mitoses, necrosis, and cellular pleomorphism can result in metastases (22).

Pure spindle cell myoepithelial tumors can be difficult to distinguish by light microscopy from other spindle cell mammary neoplasms. The differential diagnosis includes metaplastic carcinoma, primary spindle cell sarcomas, especially leiomyosarcoma or fibrous histiocytoma, myofibroblastoma, and metastatic tumor such as malignant melanoma. In most cases the issue can be resolved by considering the clinical history, as well as careful histologic and immunohistochemical analysis, but electron microscopy is sometimes required. The distinction between metaplastic carcinoma and spindle cell myoepithelial neoplasms is complicated by the fact that both tumor types express p63 and CK5. In this circumstance, reactivity for other cytokeratins such as CK7, K903, CAM 5.2, or AEl/AE3 will establish the diagnosis of metaplastic carcinoma.

Myoepithelial carcinomas composed entirely of epithelioid polygonal cells have received less attention than spindle cell myoepithelial tumors. Some myoepithelial carcinomas arise in and have remnants of an underlying adenomyoepithelioma (Fig. 5.10). Pure myoepithelial carcinomas typically have an alveolar growth pattern, and most are probably misclassified as examples of clear cell, adenoid cystic, apocrine, secretory, or signet ring cell carcinoma. Most pure myoepithelial duct carcinomas, growing as intraductal carcinoma or as invasive duct carcinoma. Two examples of intralobular myoepithelial carcinoma have been described (29).

Prasad and Zarbo (30) studied 18 patients with myoepithelial carcinomas. The patients were 31 to 72 years old (mean 50 years). Tumor size ranged from 1.4 to 17cm (mean 3.5 cm). The lesions were typically multinodular and had central necrosis. Cytologic appearances included epithelial, clear plasmacytoid, and spindle cells. All tumors were mitotically active and lacked receptors for estrogen or progesterone. Three patients had axillary nodal metastases. Median follow-up of 50 months in 17 cases revealed two recurrences, one of which was fatal.

REFERENCES

1. Gusterson BA, Warburton MJ, Mitchell D, et al. Distribution of myoepithelial cells and basement membrane proteins in the normal breast and in benign and malignant breast diseases. *Cancer Res.* 1982;42:763–770.
2. Ahmed A. The myoepithelium in human breast carcinoma. *J Pathol.* 1974; 112:129–135.
3. Hamperl H. The myoepithelia (myoepithelial cells): normal state; regressive changes; hyperplasia; tumors. *Curr Topics Pathol.* 1970;53:161–213.
4. Cameron NM, Hamperl H, Warambo W. Leiomyosarcoma of the breast originating from myoepithelium (myoepithelioma). *J Pathol.* 1974;114:89–92.
5. Loose JH, Patchefsky AS, Hollander IJ, et al. Adenomyoepithelioma of the breast. A spectrum of biologic behavior. *Am J Surg Pathol.* 1992;16:868–876.
6. Rosen PP. Adenomyoepithelioma of the breast. *Hum Pathol.* 1987;18: 1232–1237.
7. Zhang C, Quddus MR, Sung CJ. Atypical adenomyoepithelioma of the breast: diagnostic problems and practical approaches in core needle biopsy. *The Breast Journal.* 2004;10:154–155.
8. Chang A, Bassett L, Bose S. Adenomyoepithelioma of the breast: a cytologic dilemma. report of a case and review of the literature. *Diagn Cytopathol.* 2002;26:191–196.
9. Weidner N, Levine JD. Spindle-cell adenomyoepithelioma of the breast. A microscopic ultrastructural and immunocytochemical study. *Cancer.* 1988; 62:1561–1567.
10. Trojani M, Guiu M, Trouette H, et al. Malignant adenomyoepithelioma of the breast. An immunohistochemical, cytophotometric and ultrastructural study of a case with lung metastases. *Am J Clin Pathol.* 1992;98:598–602.
11. Berna JD, Arcas I, Ballester A, Bas A. Adenomyoepithelioma of the breast in a male [letter]. *Am J Roentgenol.* 1997;169:917–918.
12. Gusterson BA, Sloane JP, Middwood C, et al. Ductal adenoma of the breast-a lesion exhibiting a myoepithelial/epithelial phenotype. *Histopathology.* 1987;11:103–110.
13. Guarino M, Reale D, Squillaci S, Micoli G. Ductal adenoma of the breast. An immunohistochemical study of five cases. *Pathol Res Pract.* 1993;189: 515–520.
14. Diaz NM, McDivitt RW, Wick MR. Pleomorphic adenoma of the breast: a clinicopathologic and immunohistochemical study of 10 cases. *Hum Pathol.* 1991;22:1206–1214.
15. Reid-Nicholson M, Bleiweiss I, Pace B, et al. Pleomorphic adenoma of the breast. A case report and distinction from mucinous carcinoma. *Arch Pathol Lab Med.* 2003;127:474–477.
16. Reis-Filho JS, Fulford LG, Crebassa B, et al. Collagenous spherulosis in an adenomyoepithelioma of the breast. *J Clin Pathol.* 2004;57:83–86.
17. Tamura G, Monma N, Suzuki Y, et al. Adenomyoepithelioma of the breast in a male. *Human Pathol.* 1993;24:678–681.
18. Zarbo RJ, Oberman HA. Cellular adenomyoepithelioma of the breast. *Am J Surg Pathol.* 1983;7:863–870.
19. Pauwels C, de Potter C. Adenomyoepithelioma of the breast with features of malignancy. *Histopathology.* 1994;24:94–96.
20. Chen PC, Chen C-K, Nicastri AD, Wait RB. Myoepithelial carcinoma of the breast with distant metastasis and accompanied by adenomyoepitheliomas. *Histopathology.* 1994;24:543–548.
21. Michal M, Baumruk L, Burger J, Manhalova M. Adenomyoepithelioma of the breast with undifferentiated carcinoma component. *Histopathology.* 1994;24:274–276.
22. Jones C, Tooze R, Lakhani SR. Malignant adenomyoepithelioma of the breast metastasizing to the liver. *Virchows Arch.* 2003;442:504–506.
23. Simpson RH, Cope N. Skálová A, Michal M. Malignant adenomyoepithelioma of the breast with mixed osteogenic, spindle cell, and carcinomatous differentiation. *Am J Surg Pathol.* 1998;22:631–636.
24. Gilett CE, Bobrow LG, Millis RR. S 100 protein in human mammary tissue-immunoreactivity in breast carcinoma including Paget's disease of the nipple, and value as a marker of myoepithelial cells. *J Pathol.* 1990;160:19–24.
25. Reis-Filho JS, Milanezi F, Schmitt FC. Maspin is expressed in the nuclei of breast myoepithelial cells. *J Pathol.* 2002;197:272–274.
26. Lele SM, Graves K, Gatalica Z. Immunohistochemical detection of maspin is a useful adjunct in distinguishing radial sclerosing lesions from tubular carcinoma. *Appl Immunohistochem Molecul Morphol.* 2000;8:32–36.
27. Erlandson RA, Rosen PP. Infiltrating myoepithelioma of the breast. *Am J Surg Pathol.* 1982;6:785–793.
28. Bigotti G, DiGiorgio G. Myoepithelioma of the breast: histologic, immunologic and electron microscope appearance. *J Surg Oncol.* 1986;32:58–64.
29. Soares J, Tomasic G, Bucciarelli M, Eusebi V. Intralobular growth of myoepithelial cell carcinoma of the breast. *Virchows Arch [A].* 1994;425:205–210.
30. Prasad AR, Zarbo RJ. Myoepithelial carcinoma of the breast: a clinicopathologic study of 18 cases. *Mod Pathol.* 2000;13:46A.

Adenosis and Microglandular Adenosis

6

ADENOSIS

Adenosis is a proliferative lesion largely derived from the terminal duct–lobular unit. Epithelial and myoepithelial cells participate in adenosis, which is characteristically a lobulocentric lesion (Fig. 6.1). Adenosis usually occurs as part of the spectrum of proliferative fibrocystic abnormalities. The entire complex may produce a palpable mass that is usually not attributable only to the adenosis component. When limited to isolated lobules that are not part of fibrocystic change, adenosis is a microscopic lesion that comes to attention clinically if it contains calcifications that are detected by mammography.

A palpable mass formed largely or completely by adenosis occurs when there is fusion of the affected lobules to form an *adenosis tumor* (Fig. 6.2). Patients with an adenosis tumor are almost always premenopausal, averaging about 30 years of age at diagnosis (1,2). The tumor is usually smaller than 2 cm and easily mistaken for a fibroadenoma (1,3). Nonpalpable adenosis tumors that contain calcifications may be detected by mammography. Sonography reveals a solid, well-defined tumor (2).

Adenosis growing as microscopic foci or as a tumor tends to have a more prominent glandular pattern in premenopausal women, whereas sclerosis and loss of gland formation are conspicuous after the menopause. In some patients, there is very little variability in the spectrum of adenosis, whereas others exhibit diverse patterns.

The most cellular type of adenosis, referred to as *florid adenosis*, is the growth pattern usually present in adenosis tumors. Proliferation of ductules and lobular glands severely distorts and usually effaces the architecture of the underlying lobules. The hyperplastic structures elongate, becoming tortuous and entwined in a fashion that results in many more ductular cross sections than are present in an anatomically normal lobule (Fig. 6.3). In the plane of section, the complex proliferative structure has a swirling pattern, punctuated by glands cut transversely that have round, open lumina. The majority of the ductular structures cut tangentially or longitudinally have elongated lumina, usually with rounded, but sometimes with angular contours. Cystic dilation of ductules is not a prominent feature of florid adenosis.

Epithelial cells lining the tubules and glands are flattened, cuboidal, or slightly columnar and arranged in one or two layers surrounded by myoepithelial cells. Increase in cell size and nuclear pleomorphism can be found in florid adenosis, especially during pregnancy or lactation. Intracytoplasmic mucin vacuoles and signet ring cells are not present in the benign glandular epithelium of florid adenosis. Luminal secretion may undergo calcification, but this is usually less common and less extensive than in sclerosing adenosis. Hyperplastic change in the epithelial component of florid adenosis is mirrored in hyperplasia of the myoepithelium. Mitoses in epithelial and myoepithelial cells are very infrequent, but they may be more evident during pregnancy (Fig. 6.4) and rarely in the absence of pregnancy. Apocrine metaplasia occurs in florid adenosis. Florid adenosis may surround nerves in adjacent breast parenchyma.

In *sclerosing adenosis* there is preferential preservation of myoepithelial cells with variable atrophy of epithelial cells accompanied by lobular fibrosis (Fig. 6.5). The swirling lobulocentric pattern encountered in adenosis is retained, but epithelial cells are less conspicuous and the ductules tend to be more attenuated. Some examples of sclerosing adenosis are not limited to a lobulocentric pattern. When this occurs, the proliferating benign glands have an infiltrative pattern in the stroma (Fig. 6.6) and fat (Fig. 6.7) that can be mistaken for invasive carcinoma (Fig. 6.8), especially in fragmented needle core biopsy samples that lack the orientation provided by surrounding tissue in sections from a surgical biopsy. Epithelial cells may be markedly reduced in number, or even absent, leaving compressed elongated myoepithelial cells surrounded by basement membranes. The persisting myoepithelial cells with a pronounced spindle shape or myoid phenotype

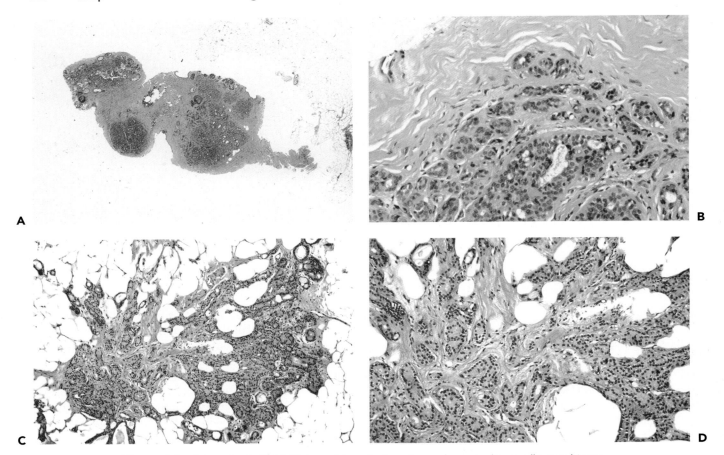

Figure 6.1 **Adenosis. A, B:** Multiple nodules of adenosis are shown in this needle core biopsy specimen. Larger nodules are the result of coalescent lobules, such as the one shown in **(B). C, D:** This needle core biopsy specimen shows sclerosing adenosis in fat.

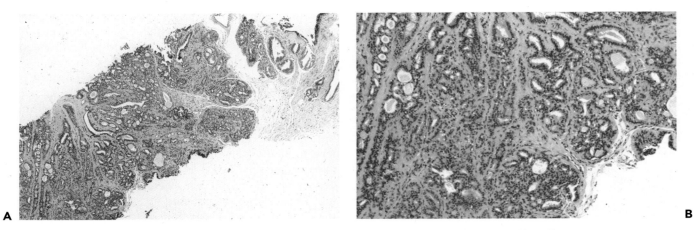

Figure 6.2 **Adenosis tumor. A, B:** Traces of the underlying lobular structure are visible in this needle core biopsy specimen. The adenosis glands vary in size and some are elongated or tubular.

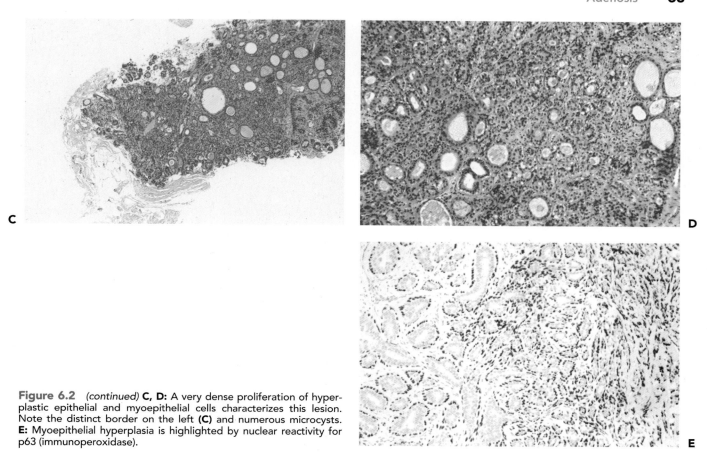

Figure 6.2 *(continued)* **C, D:** A very dense proliferation of hyperplastic epithelial and myoepithelial cells characterizes this lesion. Note the distinct border on the left **(C)** and numerous microcysts. **E:** Myoepithelial hyperplasia is highlighted by nuclear reactivity for p63 (immunoperoxidase).

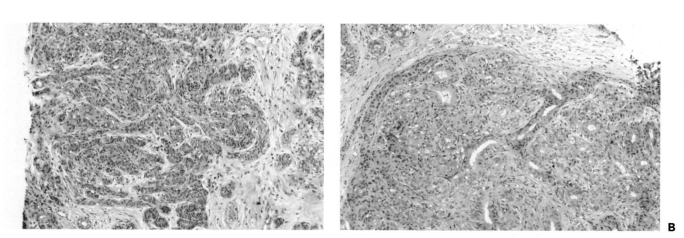

Figure 6.3 **Florid adenosis. A, B:** Elongated, hyperplastic entwined adenosis glands and myoepithelium are shown in a needle core biopsy specimen.

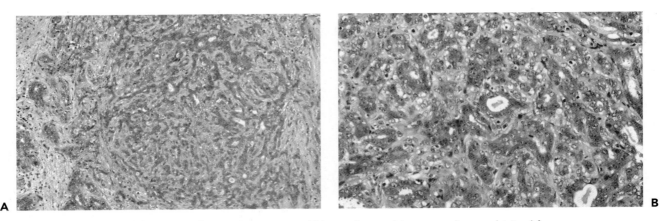

Figure 6.4 **Florid adenosis in pregnancy.** This needle core biopsy sample was obtained from a palpable tumor in a 35-year-old woman who was 9 weeks pregnant. **A, B:** There is marked hyperplasia of epithelial and myoepithelial cells in this example of florid adenosis. Mitoses are present in both cell types.

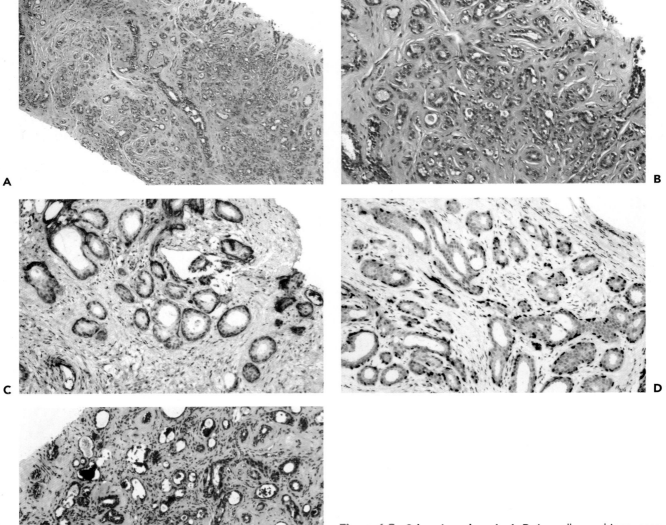

Figure 6.5 **Sclerosing adenosis. A, B:** A needle core biopsy specimen from a confluent lesion showing stromal fibrosis, thickened periglandular basement membranes, and atrophy of some glands. **C:** Myoepithelium is highlighted by cytoplasmic reactivity for CD10 (immunoperoxidase). **D:** Myoepithelium around adenosis glands is identified by nuclear p63 reactivity (immunoperoxidase). **E:** Another lesion with abundant calcifications.

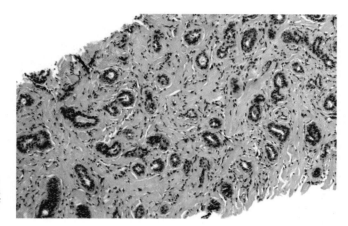

Figure 6.6 Adenosis with a dispersed pattern. Glands with round, angular, and tubular shapes are dispersed in collagenous stroma that exhibits pseudoangiomatous hyperplasia. This type of adenosis resembles tubular carcinoma.

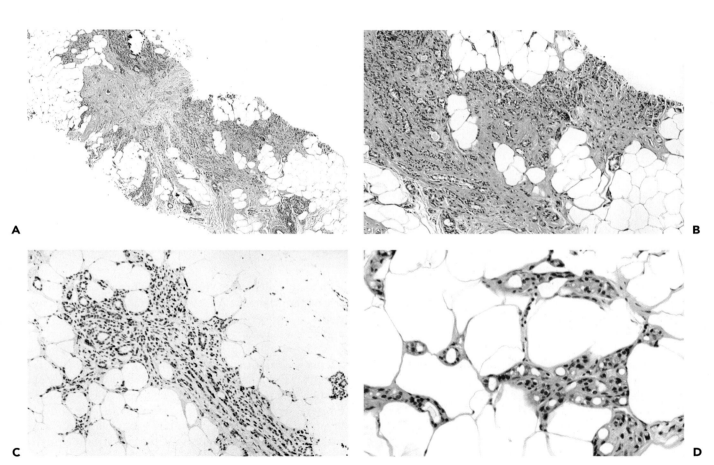

Figure 6.7 Sclerosing adenosis with an invasive pattern. A, B: Sclerosing adenosis in this needle core biopsy specimen extends into fat in a pattern that resembles invasive carcinoma. Note the fibrous stroma that uniformly surrounds the adenosis glands. **C:** Nuclear p63 in myoepithelial cells is shown (immunoperoxidase). **D:** Another needle core biopsy sample in which fat cells are surrounded by sclerosing adenosis and isolated glands are present in the fat.

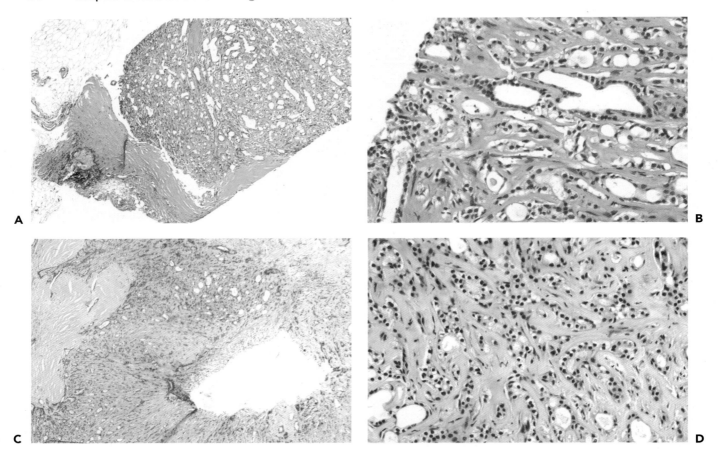

Figure 6.8 **Sclerosing adenosis mistaken for carcinoma. A, B:** This needle core biopsy sample of a palpable adenosis tumor was interpreted as invasive well-differentiated duct carcinoma. The lesion has a well-circumscribed border and lacks lobulocentric architecture. Myoepithelial cells with clear cytoplasm are evident at high magnification. **B, C, D:** The subsequent excisional biopsy specimen revealed a circumscribed focus of sclerosing adenosis with a defect in the center at the site of the previous needle core biopsy. The glands are outlined by thin basement membranes and myoepithelial cells with clear cytoplasm.

(Fig. 6.9) are strongly immunoreactive with cytoplasmic markers of smooth muscle differentiation such as actin and calponin and for the nuclear marker p63. Calcifications become more numerous with increasing sclerosis and thickening of basement membranes (Fig. 6.10). Microcystic ductular dialatation is variably present in sclerosing adenosis.

Apocrine metaplasia is relatively common in adenosis, a configuration that has been referred to as *apocrine adenosis* (3,4) (Fig. 6.11). The cytologic appearance of apocrine adenosis is quite varied (5). In some cases, the cells have conventional pink, finely granular apocrine cytoplasm and round, regular nuclei. Atypical features include clearing or vacuolization of the cytoplasm as well as prominent nucleoli, nuclear pleomorphism, and hyperchromasia (Fig. 6.12). Mitotic figures are very uncommon in atypical apocrine adenosis. If mitoses are identified in a needle core biopsy sample from apocrine adenosis, there is a greater likelihood that apocrine carcinoma is present and excisional biopsy should be performed (5,6). Severe cytologic atypia

with readily identifiable mitotic activity and/or a proliferative pattern characteristic of intraductal carcinoma are necessary to make a diagnosis of carcinoma in atypical apocrine adenosis.

Oncoprotein expression has been found in apocrine adenosis, including c-erbB2 (55.6%), p53 (27.8%), Bax (33.3%), and c-myc (100%) (7). None of the 18 samples studied was reactive for Bcl-2. Reactivity for these markers was seen in apocrine adenosis with and without atypia. It has not been determined that oncoprotein expression in apocrine adenosis is associated with a predisposition to develop carcinoma independent from the presence of histologic atypia. Very unusual variants of sclerosing adenosis can show clear cell change and collagenous spherulosis.

Perineural invasion has been found in 1% to 2% of breast specimens composed of proliferative fibrocystic changes, including sclerosing adenosis (Fig. 6.13) (8,9). Adenosis glands can be found within the perineurium and even within nerves. Myoepithelial cells are evident in

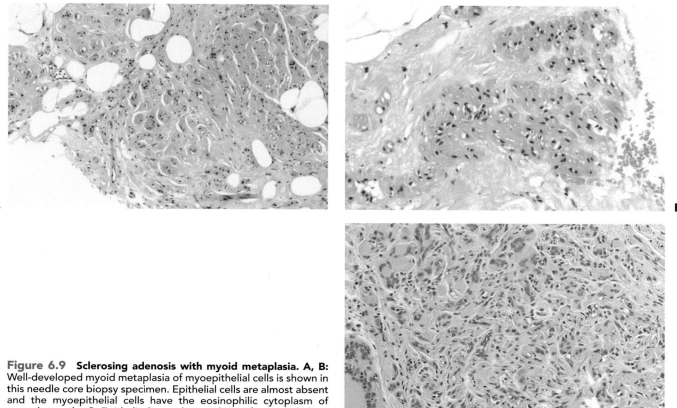

Figure 6.9 **Sclerosing adenosis with myoid metaplasia. A, B:** Well-developed myoid metaplasia of myoepithelial cells is shown in this needle core biopsy specimen. Epithelial cells are almost absent and the myoepithelial cells have the eosinophilic cytoplasm of smooth muscle. **C:** Epitheliod myoid metaplasia of myoepithelium in sclerosing adenosis.

nearly all foci of perineural or intraneural invasion by sclerosing adenosis.

Tubular adenosis is composed of ductules arranged so that the majority are cut longitudinally in the plane of section (Fig. 6.14). The proliferation lacks the lobulocentric distribution of florid or sclerosing adenosis, and the ductules extend in a seemingly haphazard pattern into fibrous mammary stroma and fat. In some instances, there is dense proliferation of tubular structures that appear to be entwined. Secretion that may calcify is variably present in the ductules. The tubular structures have basement membranes and an outer myoepithelial cell layer (7). These features are important in the distinction between tubular carcinoma and tubular adenosis.

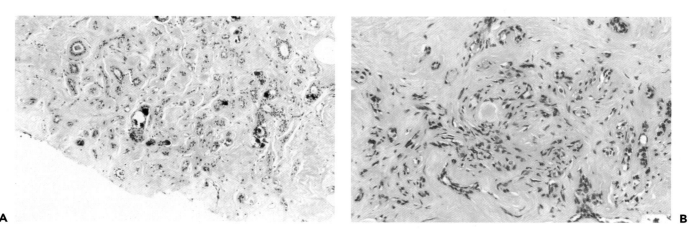

Figure 6.10 **Sclerosing adenosis with atrophy. A:** Thickened basement membranes, glandular atrophy, and calcifications characterize atrophic sclerosing adenosis in this lobule. **B:** Severe atrophy of glandular cells, leaving swirling elongated myoepithelial cells, characterizes this lesion.

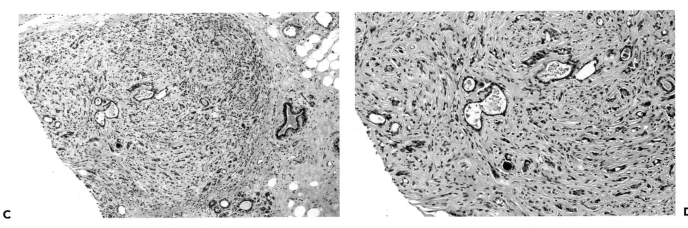

Figure 6.10 *(continued)* **C, D:** This needle core biopsy sample shows nodular, atrophic sclerosing adenosis that resembles invasive lobular carcinoma.

The florid and sclerosing forms of adenosis occur in fibroadenomas, sometimes accompanied by other proliferative changes such as cystic and papillary apocrine metaplasia. Adenosis may be localized to one part of a fibroadenoma or it may be diffuse, obscuring the underlying fibroepithelial structure. A needle core biopsy of adenosis in a fibr-oadenoma may simulate the appearance of invasive carcinoma. A fibroadenoma with sclerosing adenosis or other components of fibrocystic change is termed a *complex of fibroadenoma* (see Chapter 7).

Atypical hyperplasia (Fig. 6.15) and in situ carcinoma may occur in sclerosing adenosis and in tubular adenosis.

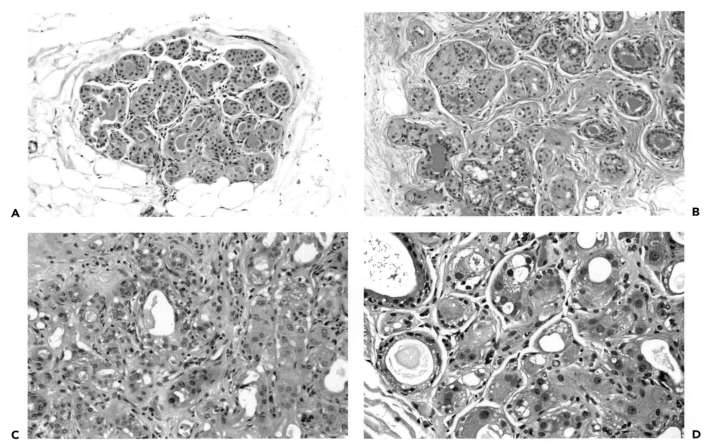

Figure 6.11 **Apocrine adenosis with atypia. A:** Apocrine metaplasia in a lobule. **B:** Apocrine metaplasia in adenosis. **C:** A more complex example of apocrine adenosis. **D:** Apocrine adenosis with nuclear atypia.

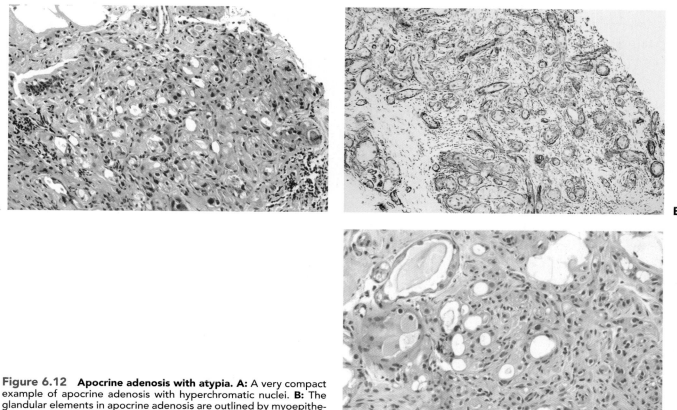

Figure 6.12 Apocrine adenosis with atypia. A: A very compact example of apocrine adenosis with hyperchromatic nuclei. **B:** The glandular elements in apocrine adenosis are outlined by myoepithelial cells shown here to be reactive for smooth muscle actin (immunoperoxidase). **C:** Apocrine adenosis with nuclear atypia **(left).**

The majority of carcinomas that develop in adenosis are of the lobular type (10) (Fig. 6.16). Lobular carcinoma in situ causes expansion of the epithelial component in adenosis, but in some foci of sclerosing adenosis, the neoplastic process is manifested by a pagetoid distribution of poorly cohesive cells (11). Lobular carcinoma in situ in adenosis often has signet ring cells (Fig. 6.17). Signet ring cells and stainable intracytoplasmic mucin are not a feature of benign epithelium in adenosis. Pagetoid lobular carcinoma in situ in sclerosing adenosis can be identified with the E-cadherin stain because the neoplastic cells are not reactive for this marker. It is not unusual to find lobular carcinoma in situ in other lobules, unaffected by sclerosing adenosis, in the same specimen.

Intraductal carcinoma arises less often in adenosis than does lobular carcinoma in situ (Fig. 6.18). Intraductal

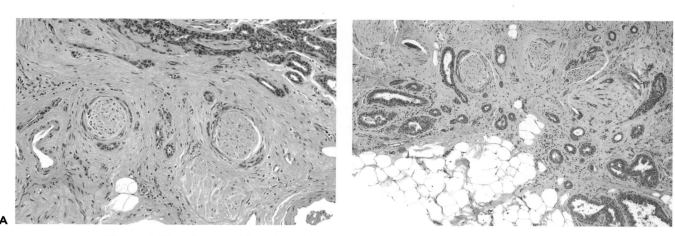

Figure 6.13 Adenosis with perineural invasion. A: Two nerves are shown surrounded circumferentially by adenosis glands. **B:** Adenosis glands encircle nerves at the perimeter of a radial sclerosing lesion in this needle core biopsy specimen.

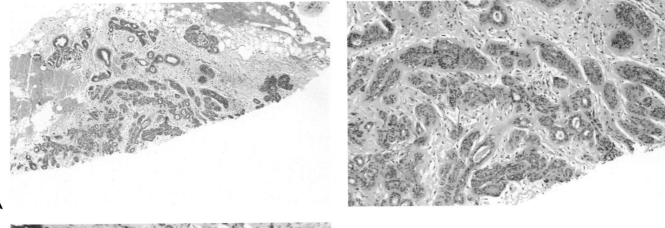

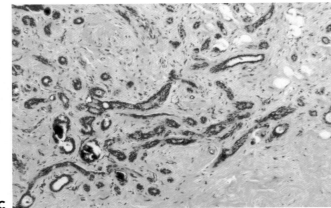

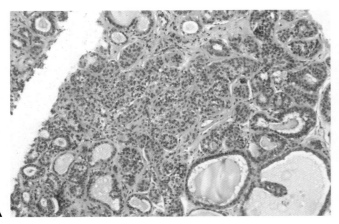

Figure 6.14 **Tubular adenosis. A, B:** Elongated adenosis glands that resemble tubules with epithelial hyperplasia and thick basement membranes are present in this needle core biopsy sample from a premenopausal woman. **C:** Epithelial atrophy, calcifications, and stromal fibrosis in a biopsy specimen from a postmenopausal patient.

carcinoma can be identified in adenosis when comedo necrosis is present, if the proliferation is solid, cribriform, or papillary, and when there is substantial cytologic atypia in an expanded epithelial component (3). Despite considerable cytologic atypia, apocrine metaplasia in adenosis should not be interpreted as carcinoma unless there is sufficient epithelial proliferation to form one of the conventional structural patterns of intraductal carcinoma (5,12) (Fig. 6.19).

The underlying architecture and structure of the glands is preserved when in situ lobular or intraductal carcinoma arises in adenosis. The integrity of individual glands, sometimes difficult to ascertain in these complex proliferative lesions, may be confirmed with a reticulin stain and immunohistochemical studies for basement membrane or myoepithelial cells (13,14). The p63 immunostain that highlights myoepithelial cell nuclei is preferable to

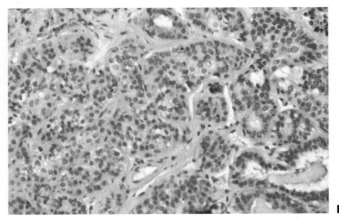

Figure 6.15 **Adenosis with atypical lobular hyperplasia. A, B:** Monomorphic small cells are apparent in some adenosis glands in this needle core biopsy specimen. The biopsy was performed for nonpalpable, mammographically detected calcifications. Note the microcystic dilatation of some glands and a small calcification near the center **(B).**

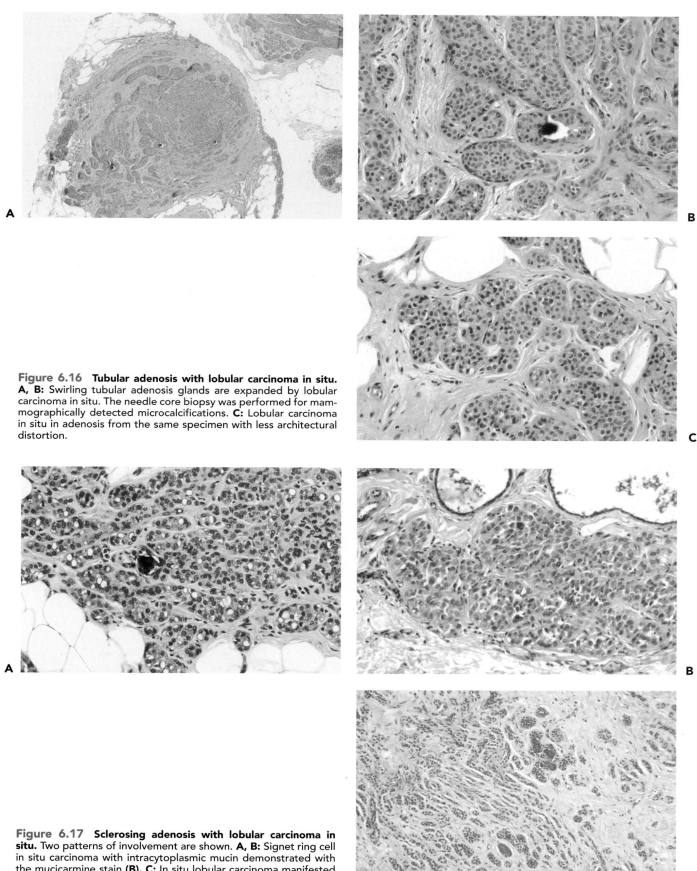

Figure 6.16 Tubular adenosis with lobular carcinoma in situ. A, B: Swirling tubular adenosis glands are expanded by lobular carcinoma in situ. The needle core biopsy was performed for mammographically detected microcalcifications. **C:** Lobular carcinoma in situ in adenosis from the same specimen with less architectural distortion.

Figure 6.17 Sclerosing adenosis with lobular carcinoma in situ. Two patterns of involvement are shown. **A, B:** Signet ring cell in situ carcinoma with intracytoplasmic mucin demonstrated with the mucicarmine stain **(B). C:** In situ lobular carcinoma manifested by cellular discohesion in a severely sclerotic lesion (hematoxylin–phloxine–eosin stain).

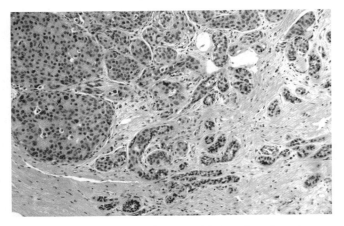

Figure 6.18 Sclerosing adenosis with intraductal carcinoma. The glands on the left are markedly enlarged by intraductal carcinoma that has a solid growth pattern. Remnants of adenosis are evident on the right.

cytoplasmic myoepithelial markers in this situation because it avoids cross-reactivity with stromal cells, but satisfactory results can often be obtained with stains for CD10, calponin, myosin, and actin. Even when basement membranes and a myoepithelial layer appear discontinuous, it is usually not possible to diagnose invasion in adenosis with confidence. The most convincing evidence for a diagnosis of invasive carcinoma arising in adenosis is the finding of invasive foci extending beyond the adenosis lesion. The glands or cells interpreted as invasive carcinoma should not be accompanied by myoepithelial cells. Basement membrane is largely or completely absent and the invasive elements should have a growth pattern that differs from the adjacent adenosis. Double immunolabelling for cytokeratin and actin or for cytokeratin and p63 can detect isolated invasive carcinoma cells in areas of sclerosing adenosis that are involved by carcinoma by identifying epithelial cells that are not accompanied by myoepithelium (15) (Fig. 6.20).

When adenosis is diagnosed in a stereotactic needle core biopsy specimen, surgical excision of the lesional area is recommended to rule out an associated carcinoma if the lesion has radiographically suspicious calcifications, a spiculated contour, an associated radial sclerosing complex, or if there is florid or atypical epithelial hyperplasia (16). In the absence of the foregoing features, clinical follow-up may be suggested when the core biopsy of a circumscribed tumor, or "nonpalpable indistinctly marginated masses" yields sclerosing adenosis (16).

If carcinoma is associated with adenosis, it may also be present in the surrounding breast tissue (10,11). Some investigators have reported an increased risk of subsequent carcinoma after previously diagnosed sclerosing adenosis. The relative risk in comparison with control populations for subsequent carcinoma to develop in women with sclerosing adenosis ranges from 2.1 (17) to 2.5 (17–19). Overall, the breast carcinoma risk associated with usual sclerosing adenosis, without atypia, is very small for an individual patient and no intervention is required beyond clinical surveillance unless there are extenuating clinical circumstances.

MICROGLANDULAR ADENOSIS

Microglandular adenosis (MGA) differs substantially in its structural features from lesions conventionally termed *adenosis*. It is included in this chapter because no more suitable placement is readily evident and the word adenosis is used to name the lesion.

MGA is a proliferative glandular lesion that mimics carcinoma clinically and pathologically (20–22). All reported patients with MGA have been women. They ranged in age from 28 to 82 years, with the majority 45 to 55 years old. The presenting symptom in most instances is a mass or "thickening" in the breast. Mammography may reveal increased density and is sometimes "suspicious," but there are no specific radiologic changes. The tumor usually has measured 3 to 4 cm, but lesions as large as 20 cm have been described. Very rarely nonpalpable MGA has been detected

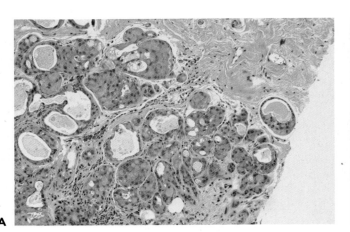

A

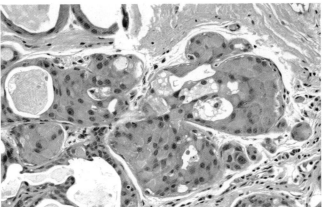

B

Figure 6.19 Sclerosing adenosis with apocrine intraductal carcinoma. A, B: The adenosis glands in this needle core biopsy specimen are expanded by apocrine carcinoma composed of cells with abundant eosinophilic cytoplasm and pleomorphic nuclei.

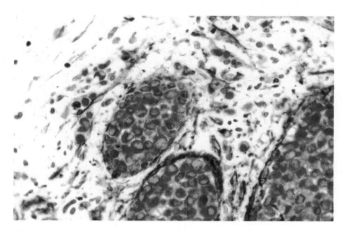

Figure 6.20 Sclerosing adenosis with microinvasive lobular carcinoma. Double immunolabelling has been used to detect microinvasive lobular carcinoma in this specimen in which in situ lobular carcinoma involves sclerosing adenosis. Epithelial cells stained crimson are evident in the stroma outside glands bounded by actin-positive myoepithelial cells stained brown (immunoperoxidase: AE1/AE3; alkaline phosphatase: smooth muscle actin).

mammographically or by ultrasonography at the site of an ill-defined density with calcifications. These lesions may be sampled by needle core biopsy.

MGA is an infiltrative proliferation of small glands in fibrous or fatty mammary stroma. Most often, the distribution seems disorderly. The round glands are lined by a single layer of flat to cuboidal epithelial cells (Fig. 6.21). Each cell has a single round nucleus with an inconspicuous or absent nucleolus. The cytoplasm tends to be clear or amphophilic, but pronounced eosinophilia may be encountered. Secretion forms distinct deeply stained eosinophilic globules in the glands. This material is usually positive for periodic acid–Schiff (PAS) and mucicarmine, and it may calcify.

Cells forming MGA are strongly immunoreactive for some cytokeratins, S-100 protein, E-cadherin, and cathepsin D. They have proven to be negative for CK5/6, nuclear estrogen and progesterone receptors, c-kit, nuclear p53 oncogene expression, and for HER2/neu (23,24). Moderate reactivity for epidermal growth factor receptor (EGFR) has been found in usual MGA (24). Eusebi et al. (25) reported that MGA lacks immunoreactivity for gross cystic disease fluid protein-15 (GCDFP-15) and for epithelial membrane antigen (EMA). The absence of EMA might be helpful in distinguishing MGA from tubular carcinoma, which is often EMA positive.

Myoepithelial cells are not evident in MGA stained with hematoxylin and eosin or with immunohistochemical stains for actin, calponin, CD10, and p63. A basement membrane is demonstrable by immunoreactivity for laminin and type IV collagen (23,25), and the glands are typically invested by a reticulin ring that can be highlighted by silver impregnation and PAS stains. In some instances, the glands are surrounded by a thick collar of collagen and reticulin.

Substantial variation in the growth pattern and cytologic appearance of the glands can be encountered in MGA. In some lesions, the cells lining the glands tend to be pleomorphic with varying amounts of cytoplasm that is clear or exhibits eosinophilia (Fig. 6.21). Prominent, coarse, deeply eosinophilic cytoplasmic granules are present in a minority of cases. Lesions classified as "atypical" MGA have elements of MGA in its uncomplicated form as well as foci with a more complex structure and cytologic atypia (26). Atypical lesions have a heterogenous mixture of connected microacini and larger glands. Ordinary MGA may have crowded, "back-to-back" glands, but each acinus remains separate. The more florid epithelial proliferation of the atypical lesion produces interconnected, budding glandular units with microcribriform nests (Fig. 6.22). When luminal bridging occurs, the monolayered epithelium is replaced by a stratified proliferation that evolves into solid nests of cells. A few mitoses may be found. Chondroid or cartilaginous metaplasia occurs in atypical MGA and in MGA with carcinoma.

When carcinoma arises in MGA, transitions from atypical MGA to carcinoma are usually observed (23,24,26,27). Duct-forming carcinomatous areas have the acinar budding pattern of atypical MGA, but they exhibit frequent mitoses, substantial cytological abnormalities, necrosis, and a desmoplastic stromal reaction. A chronic inflammatory infiltrate often accompanies the development of carcinoma. Chondromyxoid metaplasia or matrix-producing stroma has been described in a minority of cases (24,26).

Many carcinomas arising in MGA have an alveolar growth pattern (Fig. 6.23). The fully developed lesion is usually composed of malignant cells growing in solid nests. The carcinomas may have some clear cells and a few tumors are entirely composed of such cells or of cells with prominent eosinophilic cytoplasmic granularity. These cells are immunoreactive for substances that are found in acinic cell carcinoma, such as amylase, lysozyme, and α-1-antichymotrypsin as well as the protein S-100 (27). Some authors who failed to appreciate the underlying MGA in these lesions have classified such tumors as acinic cell carcinoma of the breast (28,29). A more appropriate momenclature that recognizes origin in MGA would be carcinoma with acinic cell differentiation arising in MGA.

Carcinomas that arise in MGA tend not to express estrogen and progesterone receptors and HER2/neu (24). They express EGFR as does MGA without carcinoma, and have a high Ki67 index (24). Progression from MGA to atypical MGA and to carcinoma arising in MGA is characterized by increasing expression of Ki67 and p53 (24).

Invasive carcinoma arising in MGA usually forms microscopic solid tumor masses that are appreciably larger than the surrounding alveolar MGA glands filled by in situ carcinoma. The invasive foci are typically enveloped by a conspicuous lymphocytic reaction, necrosis may be present, and these are usually regions with readily apparent mitotic activity. It often appears that invasive foci are formed by

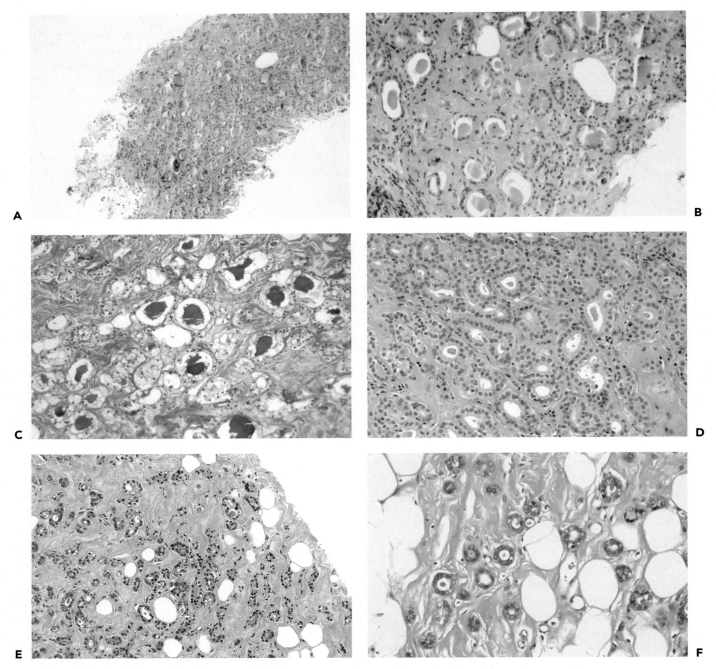

Figure 6.21   Microglandular adenosis. A–C: This needle core biopsy specimen shows small haphazardly distributed glands in fibrous stroma. A few glands contain secretion. The secretion and basement membranes are highlighted with the periodic acid–Schiff (PAS) reaction in **(C).** Note the cytoplasmic clearing (PAS without diastase). **D:** In this surgical biopsy specimen obtained 5 years later, microglandular adenosis was present in the same breast as the lesion show in **(A–C). E, F:** Microglandular adenosis shown here in fibrofatty stroma could be mistaken for infiltrating carcinoma.

the coalescent growth of expanding aleveolar in situ carcinoma elements.

Unusual forms of carcinoma are rarely found in association with MGA. These include carcinoma with secretory differentiation, carcinoma with squamous metaplasia, adenoid cystic carcinoma, and basaloid carcinoma.

Using comparative genomic hybridization and MYC chromogenic in situ hybridization on microdissected sam-

ples of MGA, atypical MGA, and carcinoma arising in MGA, Shin et al. (27) were able to demonstrate genetic alterations indicative of progression from MGA to carcinoma.

The histologic differential diagnosis of MGA includes tubular carcinoma and sclerosing adenosis. Tubular carcinoma is usually composed of angular glands of varying size, and the lesion often has a stellate or radial configuration with central sclerosis and elastosis. Elastosis is not a

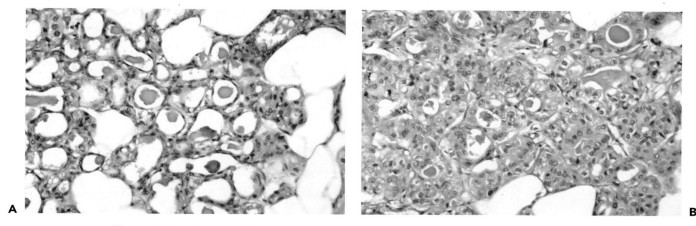

Figure 6.22 Microglandular adenosis with atypia. A: The glands are crowded in this otherwise ordinary example of microglandular adenosis. **B:** Marked cellular crowding and overgrowth has obscured most of the gland lumina in this atypical lesion.

feature of MGA, but it is often present in tubular carcinoma. Myoepithelial cells and a basement membrane are both absent in tubular carcinoma, whereas basement membranes are retained in MGA. Occasionally, the glands in tubular carcinoma are rounded and the cells have clear

or apocrine cytoplasm, making it difficult to distinguish them from MGA in hematoxylin and eosin-stained sections, especially in the limited sample of a needle core biopsy. A thorough search for intraductal carcinoma and stains for basement membranes may be helpful in this

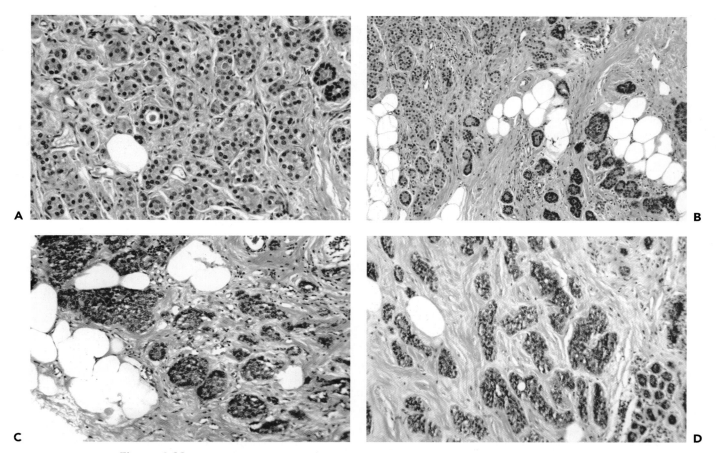

Figure 6.23 Microglandular adenosis with carcinoma. A: Most of this focus is composed of glands with increased cellularity, representing mild atypia. **B:** Atypical glands are shown on the left with transitions to in situ carcinoma in glands on the right grouped around fat cells. **C, D:** Solid masses of poorly differentiated cells that fill the enlarged glands in this biopsy specimen from another patient illustrate the appearance of intraductal carcinoma in microglanduar adenosis. The distorted glandular pattern resembles invasive carcinoma.

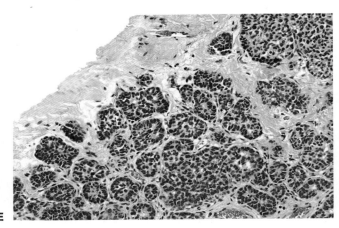

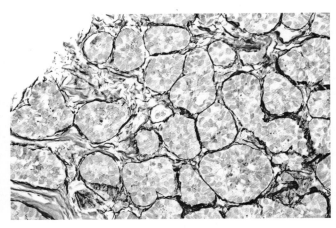

Figure 6.23 *(continued)* **E, F:** A needle core biopsy specimen with another example of intraductal carcinoma in microglandular adenosis. Basement membranes are highlighted by the reticulin stain **(F).**

situation. Sclerosing adenosis features myoepithelial proliferation that often has a spindle cell configuration. The process is commonly lobulocentric and the compressed glands tend to be arranged in a whorled or laminated fashion within the lobular nodules.

Excisional biopsy is necessary if MGA is diagnosed in a needle core biopsy. Re-excision should be considered if the margins of a lumpectomy are found to be microscopically involved. Little is known about the long-term course of incompletely excised lesions. In one case, a patient was treated by lumpectomy for intraductal and invasive duct carcinoma arising in MGA (30). The lumpectomy margins were involved by MGA but not by carcinoma. She received no radiation or chemotherapy. Ten years later, a mass detected in the same region proved to be intraductal carcinoma in residual MGA.

Invasive carcinomas arising in MGA have resulted in axillary nodal and systemic metastases (22–24). It would be prudent to predicate the treatment of carcinoma arising in MGA on the stage of disease in the individual patient. Because of the insidiously invasive character of MGA, carcinoma arising in this condition is likely to extend microscopically well beyond the grossly apparent tumor. It may therefore be difficult to achieve negative margins in some instances. When breast conservation is selected, radiotherapy should be added. Adjuvant chemotherapy is recommended for patients with axillary lymph node metastases or with invasive tumors in the absence of nodal metastases.

REFERENCES

1. Urban JA, Adair FE. Sclerosing adenosis. *Cancer.* 1949;2:625–634.
2. Markopoulous C, Kouskoe E, Philipidis T, Floros D. Adenosis tumor of the breast. *Breast J.* 2003;9:255–256.
3. Nielsen BB. Adenosis tumour of the breast—a clinicopathological investigation of 27 cases. *Histopathology.* 1987;11:1259–1275.
4. Simpson JF, Page DL, Dupont WD. Apocrine adenosis—a mimic of mammary carcinoma. *Surg Pathol.* 1990;3:289–299.
5. Carter DJ, Rosen PP. Atypical apocrine metaplasia in sclerosing lesions of the breast. A study of 51 patients. *Mod Pathol.* 1991;4:1–5.
6. Seidman JD, Aston M, Lefkowitz M. Atypical apocrine adenois of the breast. A clinicopathologic study of 37 patients with 8.7-year follow-up. *Cancer.* 1996;77:2529–2537.
7. Selim AGA, El-Ayat G, Wells CA. Expression of c-erbB2, p53, Bcl-2, Bax, c-myc and Ki=67 in apocrine metaplasia and apocrine change within sclerosing adenosis of the breast. *Virchows Arch.* 2002;441:449–455.
8. Taylor HB, Norris HJ. Epithelial invasion of nerves in benign diseases of the breast. *Cancer.* 1967;20:2245–2249.
9. Davies JD. Neural invasion in benign mammary dysplasia. *J Pathol.* 1973;109:225–231.
10. Oberman HA, Markey BA. Non-invasive carcinoma of the breast presenting in adenosis. *Mod Pathol.* 1991;4:31–35.
11. Fechner RE. Lobular carcinoma in situ in sclerosing adenosis. A potential source of confusion with invasive carcinoma. *Am J Surg Pathol.* 1981;5:233–239.
12. Abati AD, Kimmel M, Rosen PP. Apocrine mammary carcinoma: a clinicopathologic study of 72 cases. *Am J Clin Pathol.* 1990;94:371–377.
13. Lee K-C, Chan JKC, Gwi E. Tubular adenosis of the breast. A distinctive benign lesion mimicking invasive carcinoma. *Am J Surg Pathol.* 1996;20:46–54.
14. Eusebi V, Collina G, Bussolati G. Carcinoma in situ in sclerosing adenosis of the breast: an immunocytochemical study. *Semin Diagn Pathol.* 1989;6:146–152.
15. Prasad ML, Osborne MP, Hoda SA. Observations on the histopathologic diagnosis of microinvasive carcinoma of the breast. *Anat Pathol.* 1998;3:209–232.
16. Gill HK, Ioffe OB, Berg WA. When is a diagnosis of sclerosing adenosis acceptable at core biopsy? *Radiology.* 2003;228:50–57.
17. Jensen RA, Page DL, DuPont WD, Rogers LW. Invasive breast cancer risk in women with sclerosing adenosis. *Cancer.* 1989;64:1977–1983.
18. Bodian CA, Perzin KH, Lattes R, et al. Prognostic significance of benign proliferative breast disease. *Cancer.* 1993;71:3896–3907.
19. Krieger N, Hiatt RA. Risk of breast cancer after benign breast diseases, variation by histologic type, degree of atypia, age at biopsy, and length of follow-up. *Am J Epidemiol.* 1992;136:619–631.
20. Clement PB, Azzopardi JG. Microglandular adenosis of the breast. A lesion simulating tubular carcinoma. *Histopathology.* 1983;7:169–180.
21. Rosen PP. Microglandular adenosis. *Am J Surg Pathol.* 1983;7:137–144.
22. Tavassoli FA, Norris HJ. Microglandular adenosis of the breast. *Am J Surg Pathol.* 1983;7:731–737.
23. James BA, Cranor ML, Rosen PP. Carcinoma of the breast arising in microglandular adenosis. *Am J Clin Pathol.* 1993;100:507–513.
24. Khalifeh I, Albarracin C, Wu Y, et al. Clinical, histopathologic and immunohistochemial features of microglandular adenosis and transition into in situ and invasive carcinoma. *Am J Surg Pathol.* 2008;32:544–552.
25. Eusebi V, Faschini MP, Betts CM, et al. Microglandular adenosis, apocrine adenosis and tubular carcinoma of the breast. An immunohistochemical comparison. *Am J Surg Pathol.* 1993;17:99–109.
26. Rosenblum MK, Purrazzella R, Rosen PP. Is microglandular adenosis a precancerous disease? A study of carcinoma arising therein. *Am J Surg Pathol.* 1986;10:237–245.
27. Shin SJ, Simpson PT, DaSilva L, et al. Molecular evidence for progression of microglandular adenosis (MGA) to invasive carcinoma. *Am J Surg Pathol.* 2009;33:496–504.
28. Damiani S, Pasquinelli G, Lamovec J, et al. Acinic cell carcinoma of the breast: an immunohistochemical and ultrastructural study. *Virchows Arch.* 2000;437:74–81.
29. Coyne JD, Dervan PA. Primary acinic cell carcinoma of the breast. *J Clin Pathol.* 2002;55:545–547.
30. Resetkova E, Flanders DJ, Rosen PP. Ten-year follow-up of mammary carcinoma arising in microglandular adenosis treated with breast conservation. *Arch Pathol Lab Med.* 2003;127:77–80.

Fibroepithelial Neoplasms

7

FIBROADENOMATOID MASTOPATHY (SCLEROSING LOBULAR HYPERPLASIA)

This benign proliferative lesion usually presents as a localized tumor with a mean diameter of 4 cm, but asymptomatic lesions have been detected by mammography (1,2). The most frequent mammographic finding is a well-defined mass. Microcalcifications are not commonly present. The imaging characteristics are not sufficiently specific to distinguish sclerosing lobular hyperplasia from a fibroadenoma. Patients range in age from 14 to 46 years, with a mean age of about 32 years (1,2).

Microscopic examination reveals enlarged lobules composed of an increased number of intralobular glands (Fig. 7.1). The intralobular stroma is collagenized, and there is variable sclerosis of the interlobular stroma. Individual lobules and groups of lobules sometimes have the appearance of miniature fibroadenomas with a prominent glandular component (Fig. 7.2). Secretory activity is variably present or absent and calcifications are not formed. Fibroadenomatoid mastopathy is found in breast tissue surrounding about 50% of fibroadenomas or phyllodes tumors (PTs) (1). Because the fibroadenoma or PT produces a dominant mass, associated sclerosing lobular hyperplasia may be overlooked. Excisional biopsy of the palpable tumor is adequate therapy. This condition may rarely contribute to this syndrome of multiple recurrent fibroadenoms.

FIBROADENOMA

These benign tumors arise from the epithelium and stroma of terminal duct–lobular units. They account for about one-fifth of all benign breast masses and approximately 10% of breast lesions in postmenopausal patients. Dupont et al. (3) found that an increased relative risk for subsequent breast carcinoma was dependent on the presence of proliferative changes in the fibroadenoma (complex fibroadenoma) itself or in the surrounding breast, and a family history of breast carcinoma.

The age distribution of fibroadenomas ranges from childhood to more than 70 years, with a mean age of about 30 and a median around 25 years (4). The most frequent presenting symptom is a self-detected painless, firm, well-circumscribed solitary tumor. A growing proportion of fibroadenomas are nonpalpable tumors that are detected by imaging studies. Multiple fibroadenomas occur in about 15% of patients, with equal proportions found synchronously and metachronously in the same or opposite breast. An uncommon syndrome occurring in adolescence is the metachronous and synchronous development of multiple fibroadenomas, usually in both breasts (5). The intervening breast tissue often manifests extensive fibroadenomatoid mastopathy.

Patients who received cyclosporin A for immunosuppression after organ transplantation are reported to be predisposed to develop fibroadenomas (6–8). The tumors are typically bilateral and multiple. The duration of cyclosporin A treatment before detection of the fibroadenomas is generally more than a year with a mean interval in one study of 4.4 ± 1.7 years (range 1.7–7.1 years) (8). When compared with fibroadenomas found in control women who did not undergo transplantation or cyclosporin A treatment, cyclosporin A–related tumors were significantly larger and had a lower longitudinal to anterior–posterior ratio (8).

Coarse calcifications are not uncommon in fibroadenomas after the menopause (Fig. 7.3). In one series, only 10% of fibroadenomas measured more than 4.0 cm (4). Tumors larger than 4 cm are significantly more frequent in patients 20 years or younger than in patients older than 20 years (4). Fibroadenomas that involve most or all of the breast, often referred to as adolescent giant fibroadenomas, develop as solitary or multiple tumors shortly after puberty (5).

More than 90% of fibroadenomas are of the adult type, with the remainder fulfilling criteria for other, unusual types of fibroadenoma. *Tubular adenoma* or *adenofibroma* is a variant of fibroadenoma composed of closely approximated round or oval glandular structures consisting of a single layer of epithelium supported by myoepithelial cells (9). Foci with the adenofibroma pattern can be encountered within an otherwise ordinary fibroadenoma. Other so-called adenomas are unrelated to the fibroadenoma category. *Apocrine adenoma* is a localized nodular focus of prominent papillary and cystic apocrine metaplasia (10). Nodular foci of sclerosing

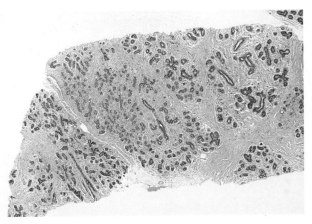

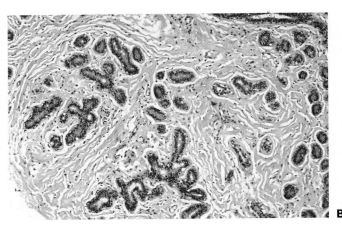

A

B

Figure 7.1   **Fibroadenomatoid mastopathy. A, B:** This needle core biopsy specimen was obtained from one of multiple bilateral breast nodules in a 16-year-old girl. The biopsy specimen shows enlarged lobules with sclerotic stroma.

adenosis with apocrine metaplasia have been variously termed *apocrine adenoma* and *apocrine adenosis. Ductal adenoma* (11) and *pleomorphic adenoma* (12) are variants of intraductal papilloma and adenomyoepithelioma, respectively.

The histologic hallmark of a fibroadenoma is concurrent proliferation of glandular and stromal elements derived from lobules. The majority of adult fibroadenomas have growth patterns that have been described as either intracanalicular or pericanalicular (Fig. 7.4). The former pattern is produced when the abundant stroma compresses ducts into elongated linear branching structures with slit-shaped lumens. When the ducts are not compressed by the stroma, the architecture is described as having a pericanalicular pattern. These structural features are of no known prognostic or clinical significance, and some tumors have both components. A fibroadenoma with a prominent intracanalicular pattern may be mistaken for a benign phyllodes tumor (PT), especially in a needle core biopsy specimen.

The appearance of the stroma varies from one fibroadenoma to another, but it is relatively homogeneous

in any given lesion. The average fibroadenoma in adults has evenly distributed similar proportions of epithelium and stroma throughout the tumor. The density of stromal cellularity is not related to tumor size. Fibroadenomas from women less than 20 years of age tend to have more proliferative epithelium and more cellular stroma as a group than tumors from older women (Fig. 7.5). Mitotic figures are very unusual in fibroadenomatous stroma.

Uncommon types of stroma encountered in a minority of fibroadenomas include smooth muscle metaplasia, derived from myoid metaplasia of myoepithelial cells or myofibroblasts in the fibroadenoma (13) and adipose differentiation (14). Giant cells, sometimes with multiple hyperchromatic nuclei, are found in the stroma of fibroadenomas as well as in phyllodes tumors (15) and in other benign tumors (16). These cells do not influence the clinical course of the lesion. A tumor that has the structural features of a fibroadenoma should not be classified as a phyllodes tumor solely because the stroma contains a few multinucleated giant cells. Osteochondroid metaplasia is very uncommon and almost always occurs in a fibroadenoma from a postmenopausal woman (17). The stroma of a fibroadenoma can undergo marked myxoid change, and in extreme cases, the needle core biopsy from such a tumor could be mistaken for mucinous carcinoma (Fig. 7.6).

Squamous metaplasia, cysts, duct hyperplasia, adenosis, and apocrine metaplasia (Fig. 7.7) can develop in the epithelial component of a fibroadenoma. Sclerosing adenosis in a fibroadenoma can be mistaken for infiltrating carcinoma (Fig. 7.8), and it can develop calcifications (Fig. 7.9). Fibroadenomas with adenosis, papillary apocrine hyperplasia, cysts, or epithelial calcifications have been designated "complex" (3). At least one of these components of proliferative fibrocystic change must be present to achieve a diagnosis of "complex" fibroadenoma. A review of 396 fibroadenomas from a single institution revealed "complex histologic features" in 40.4% of the tumors. These patients tended to be older than women whose fibroadenomas were not complex (18). Marked

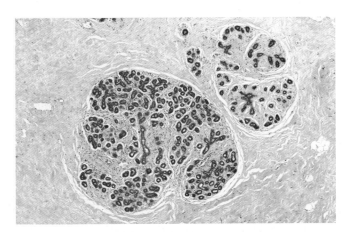

Figure 7.2   **Fibroadenomatoid mastopathy.** The lobules resemble small fibroadenomas.

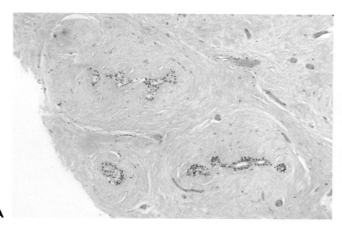
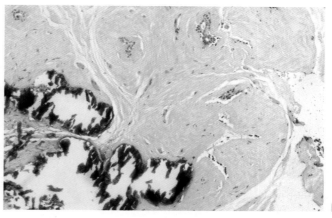

Figure 7.3   Fibroadenoma with sclerosis and calcification. A, B: This needle core biopsy specimen is from a nonpalpable, calcified lesion in a 74-year-old woman.

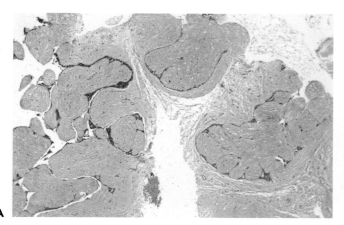
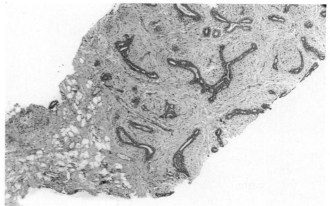

Figure 7.4   Fibroadenomatous growth patterns. A: The intracanalicular growth pattern is formed by compressed epithelial lined spaces. **B:** A pericanalicular lesion in which the stroma is arranged in a circumferential nodular pattern around ductules with focal epithelial hyperplasia.

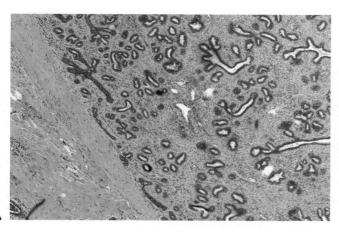
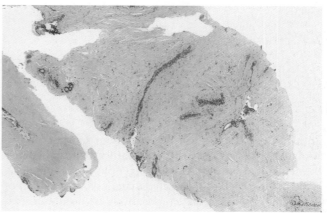

Figure 7.5   Fibroadenomas in young and elderly women. A: Well-formed lobular glands and evenly distributed cellular stroma are present in this tumor from a 23-year-old woman. **B:** This needle core biopsy specimen from a nonpalpable lesion in a 71-year-old woman shows marked fibrosis and sparse, atrophic epithelial elements.

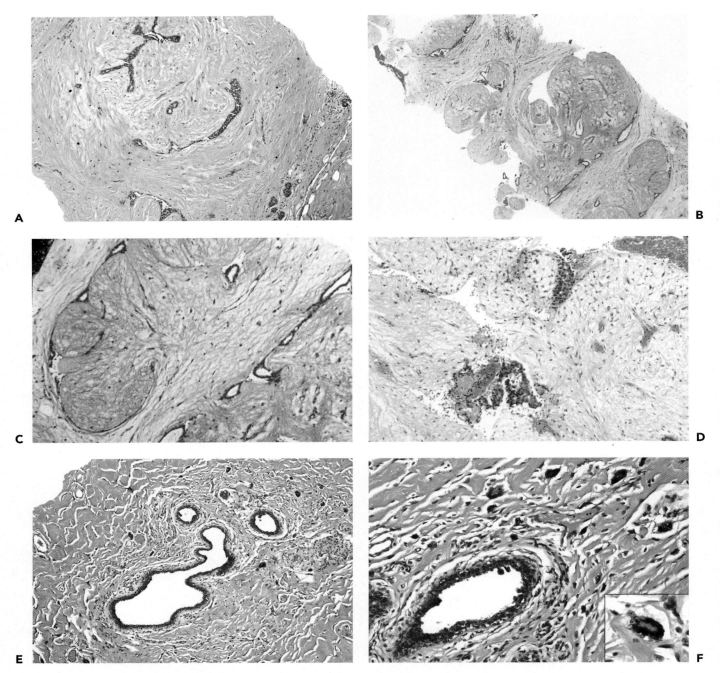

Figure 7.6 Fibroadenomas with myxoid and pseudoanigomatous stroma. A: A needle core biopsy sample showing myxoid stroma in a fibroadenoma. **B, C:** Needle core biopsy specimens in which the epithelium is compressed into slender cords and small glands by myxoid stroma. **D:** Detached fragments of myxoid fibroadenoma and epithelium. **E, F:** Pseudoangiomatous stroma with multinucleated giant cells **(inset)** in a fibroadenoma.

epithelial hyperplasia can be encountered in a complex fibroadenoma (Fig. 7.10). These proliferative changes are not dependent on exposure to exogenous hormones (19).

Sklair-Levy et al. (20) reported that 63 of 401 (15.7%) of fibroadenomas diagnosed consecutively by needle or excisional biopsy were classified as complex. Complex fibroadenomas were associated with older age (median 47 years) than usual fibroadenomas (median, 28.5 years) and smaller size (complex average 1.3 cm; usual average 2.5 cm).

Excision was performed in 40 patients. Twenty-three complex fibroadenomas were not excised. After short-term follow-up, the only carcinoma detected in this series was a 4-mm invasive lobular carcinoma adjacent to a fibroadenoma excised 2 months after a needle core biopsy diagnosis of complex fibroadenoma with atypical lobular hyperplasia.

Estrogen receptor activity is largely localized in the epithelium of fibroadenomas when examined by immunohistochemistry, whereas progesterone receptor is reportedly

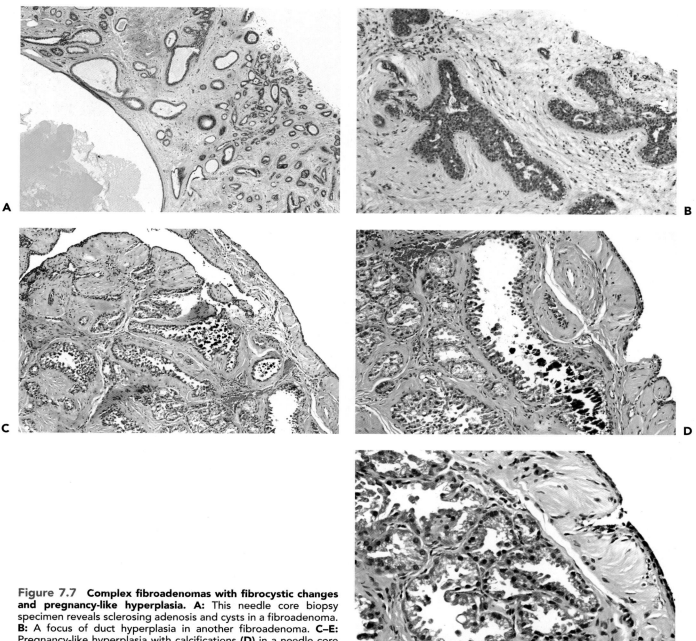

Figure 7.7 **Complex fibroadenomas with fibrocystic changes and pregnancy-like hyperplasia. A:** This needle core biopsy specimen reveals sclerosing adenosis and cysts in a fibroadenoma. **B:** A focus of duct hyperplasia in another fibroadenoma. **C–E:** Pregnancy-like hyperplasia with calcifications **(D)** in a needle core biopsy sample from a 27-year-old woman.

localized in the stroma as well as in the epithelium (21,22). Secretory hyperplasia sometimes occurs diffusely in fibroadenomas during pregnancy. Fibroadenomas with secretory hyperplasia should be distinguished from the tumor commonly referred to as *lactating adenoma,* which is a compact aggregate of lobules exhibiting secretory hyperplasia during pregnancy or post partum. Ultrasonography of lactating adenomas reveals one or more hypoechoic well-defined masses (23). Pregnancy-like hyperplasia is rarely encountered in a fibroadenoma removed from a woman who is neither pregnant nor lactating.

Juvenile fibroadenomas account for less than 5% of all fibroadenomas with the majority of the patients younger than 20 years (24). Tumors with the histologic features of juvenile fibroadenoma have been found in adult women as old as 72 years (25). Juvenile fibroadenomas are characterized microscopically by stromal cellularity and epithelial hyperplasia (Fig. 7.11). The architecture is more often pericanalicular than intracanalicular or a mixture of these patterns. The cellular density of the stroma is variable in any given tumor. Mitoses are few or absent from the stroma and epithelium. Little or no atypia and pleomorphism are encountered in the bipolar fibroblastic stromal cells. Epithelial elements are usually distributed uniformly in the tumor without the stromal overgrowth that characterizes PTs. Most juvenile fibroadenomas feature conspicuous epithelial

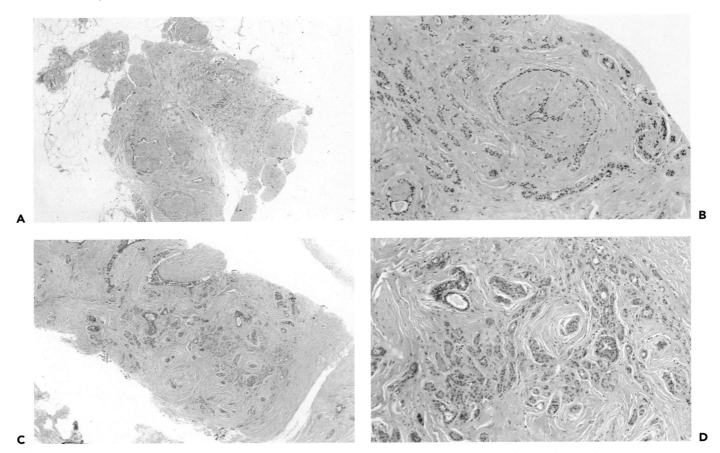

Figure 7.8 **Complex fibroadenomas with sclerosing adenosis misinterpreted as carcinoma. A, B:** A needle core biopsy specimen showing sclerosing adenosis in a fibroadenoma. This specimen was erroneously interpreted as infiltrating lobular carcinoma. **C, D:** This needle core biopsy specimen with sclerosing adenosis in a fibroadenoma was diagnosed as invasive tubular carcinoma.

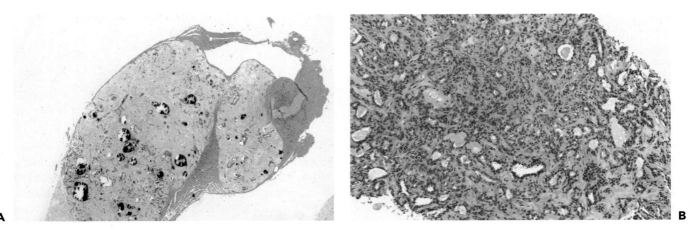

Figure 7.9 **Complex fibroadenomas with sclerosing adenosis. A:** The needle core biopsy specimen from a 70-year-old woman contained this tissue fragment from a fibroadenoma with many calcifications. The excised tumor was a sclerotic fibroadenoma with atrophic sclerosing adenosis. **B:** This needle core biopsy specimen from a 39-year-old woman reveals the dense glandular proliferation characteristically found in an adenosis tumor. The pattern shown here could be mistaken for infiltrating carcinoma. Other portions of the excised tumor displayed features of a fibroadenoma.

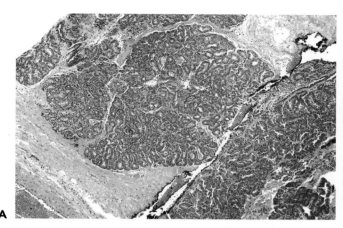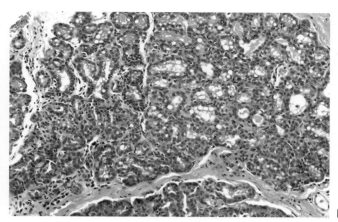

A   **B**

Figure 7.10   Lactating adenoma. A, B: Enlarged lobules with lactational secretory hyperplasia in needle core biopsy samples from a breast tumor in a pregnant 37-year-old woman.

hyperplasia that may have a ductal, lobular, or combined ductal–lobular configuration (26). Several epithelial growth patterns can be found including papillary, solid, and cribriform. Usually more than one pattern is present in a given tumor. The myoepithelium is usually hyperplastic.

The epithelium of a fibroadenoma can develop neoplastic changes. This is more often manifested as lobular carcinoma in situ than as intraductal carcinoma (Fig. 7.12). Invasive carcinoma is extremely uncommon in fibroadenomas.

In most instances, the microscopic diagnosis of an excised fibroadenoma is accomplished without difficulty when the tumor has a sharply defined border and the pericanalicular or intracanalicular growth pattern. However, the distinction between some variants of fibroadenoma, especially those with cellular stroma and benign PTs, is sometimes problematic and unclear. In these situations, it may be helpful to review the characteristic cytologic features of fibradenomas in formulating the diagnosis. Unfortunately, neoplasms that ultimately recur with the histologic and clinical features of a PT may present in a form that is histologically not distinguishable from a fibroadenoma.

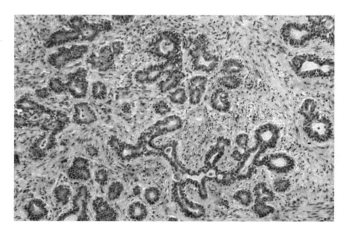

Figure 7.11   Juvenile fibroadenoma. The lesion features a balanced proliferation of glands and stroma.

Many fibroadenomas can be reliably diagnosed in needle core biopsy specimens and do not require excision. Management consists of clinical follow-up for evidence of growth. Gordon et al. (26) concluded that fibroadenomas diagnosed by fine needle aspiration biopsy "may be safely followed up if volume growth rate is less that 16% per month in those younger than 50 years and less than 13% per month in those 50 years or older." Small fibroadenomas measuring 1.5 cm or less may be completely excised in the course of vacuum-assisted ultrasound-guided biopsy (27).

Jacklin et al. (28) summarized the clinical observations that raise concern for PT in a patient considered clinically to have a fibroadenoma. These included the following: growth of a preexisting tumor, tumor larger than 3 cm in a patient older than 35 years, rounded or lobulated mammographic contour, and ultrasonography showing attenuation or cystic areas in a solid mass.

If the core biopsy sample has features that raise concern about a possible PT, excisional biopsy is recommended (Fig. 7.13). Abnormalities that suggest an indeterminate diagnosis in a needle core biopsy sample include an ill-defined border, noteworthy stromal cellularity, tissue fragmentation, mitoses, and atypia of stromal cells (29,30) (Fig. 7.14). In two studies of seven (31) and nine (32) patients, the final diagnosis reached by repeated needle core or excisional biopsies was PT in three (43%) and two (22%) of cases, respectively. Usually, the initial needle core biopsy sample showed an indeterminate fibroepithelial tumor.

Markers of stromal proliferative activity may prove useful in the diagnosis of indeterminate fibroepithelial tumors (30). This possibility has been investigated by using MIB-1, a monoclonal antibody that detects the Ki67 antigen produced by proliferating cells. MIB-1 reactivity is expressed in terms of an index, calculated as the number of immunoreactive nuclei in 10 high-power fields (HPFs). Ridgway et al. (33) reported that the mean MIB-1 index of benign PTs (33.31 ± 6.73; range 1–91) was significantly higher than the mean MIB-1 index of fibroadenomas (1.29 ± 0.69, range 0–6).

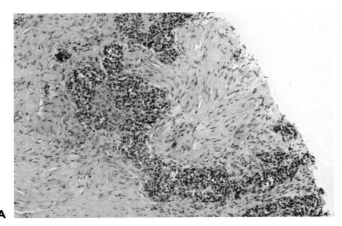

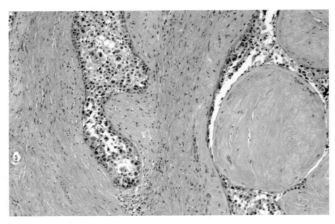

A

B

Figure 7.12   Fibroadenomas with in situ carcinoma. A: A needle core biopsy specimen with lobular carcinoma in situ in a fibroadenoma. **B:** Intraductal carcinoma is present in this sclerotic fibroadenoma.

When the needle core biopsy findings suggest a complex fibroadenoma or atypical features are noted in the fibroadenomatous epithelium, excision of the tumor with sampling of the surrounding tissues should be performed to assess the epithelial component for evidence of occult carcinoma.

Despite substantial epithelial proliferation, sometimes with considerable atypia and stromal cellularity, follow-up of children and adults with juvenile fibroadenomas has not revealed a predisposition to develop PT or carcinoma subsequently in either breast (24,25). Excision should be carried out to preserve as much breast tissue as possible. Near-normal breast development may occur even if removal of very large or multiple tumors leaves a minimal amount of residual uninvolved tissue in young patients (24).

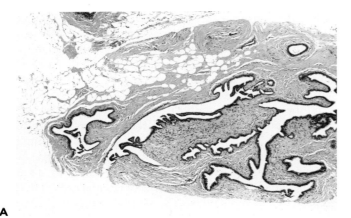

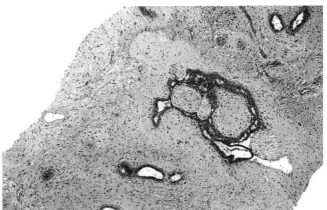

A

B

C

Figure 7.13   Fibroadenoma versus phyllodes tumor. A: This needle core biopsy specimen shows a fibroepithelial tumor with mildly cellular stroma and an exaggerated intracanalicular growth pattern suggestive of a phyllodes tumor. The excised tumor was classified as a fibroadenoma. **B, C:** This needle core biopsy sample shows a fibroepithelial tumor with moderately cellular stroma that proved to be a benign phyllodes tumor.

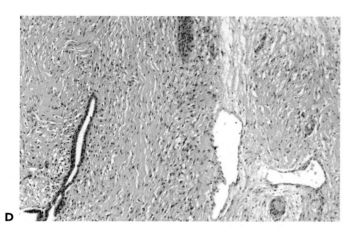

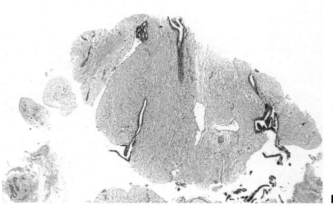

Figure 7.13 *(continued)* **D, E:** These needle core biopsy samples are from a benign phyllodes tumor, a diagnosis suggested by the moderately cellular stroma and epithelium-lined clefts.

Cryoablation has been investigated as a method for treating fibroadenomas without surgical excision (34,35). A registry of 444 tumors treated by this method revealed that 75% of the lesions were clinically palpable before treatment (35). The mean pretreatment tumor diameter was 1.8 cm. After follow-up of 6 and 12 months, there was a palpable abnormality in 46% and 35% of patients, respectively. Persistent palpability was related to initial tumor size, being present more often in women with tu-

mors larger than 2 cm than in those with smaller tumors (35). In some instances, patients have elected to have the residual palpable abnormality excised surgically (34).

Percutaneous excision of fibroadenomas with an ultrasound-guided 8-gauge vacuum-assisted instrument has also been described (36,37). Grady et al. (37) reported 69 consecutive ultrasonographically visible fibradenomas measuring up to 3 cm treated by this method. The procedure was considered to be complete when all ultrasonographic evidence

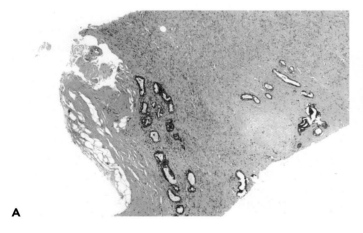

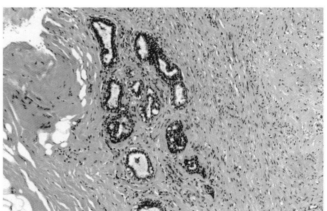

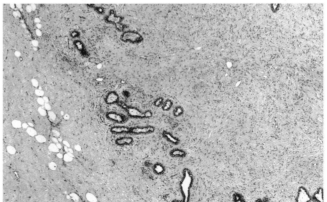

Figure 7.14 **Fibroadenoma versus phyllodes tumor. A, B:** This needle core biopsy specimen reveals stromal overgrowth and an ill-defined junction with the adjacent breast tissue. **C:** The excisional biopsy specimen shown here duplicates the findings in the needle biopsy specimen and is diagnostic of a benign phyllodes tumor. The stroma of the tumor consists of uniform spindle cells.

of the tumor had been removed. Recurrences demonstrated by ultrasonography were detected at the sites of 13 lesions in eight patients after a median follow-up of 22 months (range 7–59 months). The recurrence rate was 15% (8/52 lesions with follow-up), and the actuarial recurrence rate was 33% at 59 months. All recurrences were associated with tumors that measured 2.1 to 2.8 cm. It was concluded that recurrences resulted from residual portions of the fibroadenoma that were too small to detect by ultrasonography and that this was more likely to occur after percutaneous excision of a fibroadenoma larger than 2.0 cm.

PHYLLODES TUMOR

There are no specific clinical features that reliably distinguish between a fibroadenoma and a PT (38). A diagnosis of PT may be favored if the tumor is larger than 4 cm or if there is a history of rapid growth. PT usually occurs as a solitary unilateral mass. Rarely, multifocal PTs have been detected in one breast, or both breasts may be affected (39). Coexistent fibroadenomas, which are found histologically in nearly 40% of cases, are not always apparent clinically (39), and there is often fibroadenomatoid lobular hyperplasia in the surrounding breast tissue.

PTs have been reported in patients ranging in age from 10 to 86 years, with a median and mean age of about 45 years, approximately 20 years older than the median age of patients with fibroadenomas. PTs occur rarely in children and adolescent females (40). The majority of PTs in young patients have been classified as benign but a few examples of malignant PT have been described in this age group (40). The reported average size of PT is 4 to 5 cm (38–41). Although malignant PTs tend to be larger than benign variants, there have been exceptional high-grade malignant lesions smaller than 2 cm and some very large histologically benign tumors. Rare instances of PT in men have been reported (42,43), and PT may occur during pregnancy (44).

Mammography reveals a round or lobulated, sharply defined opaque mass in most instances. Indistinct borders are seen in a minority of cases. The tumor also appears to be well-circumscribed with ultrasound but may be inhomogeneous due to cysts and epithelium-lined clefts (45). Cystic components were evident by ultrasound slightly more frequently in malignant tumors in one study (46). Calcifications are uncommon and occur with equal frequency in benign and malignant lesions (46,47). It is not possible to reliably distinguish between benign and malignant cystosarcomas by mammography and ultrasonography (47–49) or by magnetic resonance imaging (MRI) (48).

PTs arise from periductal rather than intralobular stroma and typically contain sparse lobular elements. PTs typically have a heterogenous histologic appearance, and only a minority of the lesions actually resemble the tumor conventionally described as having the exaggerated structure of an intracanalicular fibroadenoma with increased stromal cellularity. In a number of cases, the intracanalicular pattern of clefts is obscured by hyperplasia of ductal epithelium. In exceptional cases, lobular differentiation may be present, and rarely this gives rise to a pronounced adenosis structure that can obscure the true nature of the tumor. Most PTs are characterized by expansion and increased cellularity of the stromal component. In some tumors, cellularity is denser in the periductal stroma and mitoses may be accentuated in this zone (Fig. 7.15), but a substantial number of PTs have little or no zonal stromal distribution (Fig. 7.16). A subset of PTs with a nodular structure have prominent periductal stromal proliferation. These have been referred to as "periductal stromal tumors" and subclassified as periductal stromal hyperplasia or periductal stromal sarcoma (49). These tumors are capable of recurrence with phyllodes features expressed in the recurrent tumor.

Epithelial-lined clefts are found in many, but not all, PT (Fig. 7.17). Marked expansion of these spaces can result in the formation of cysts and a papillary appearance (Fig. 7.18). The intracanalicular architecture of some fibroadenomas bears a superficial resemblance to the clefted structure of benign PT and occasionally the distinction between the two tumor types may be difficult in a needle core biopsy specimen.

Myxoid change occurs in the stroma of fibroadenomas and PTs. It tends to be homogeneously distributed in fibroadenomas but may be patchy and undergo degenerative changes in PTs. Pseudoangiomatous stromal hyperplasia (PASH) occurs in PT, and in some instances, PASH is a prominent feature of the lesion. Rarely, multinucleated stromal giant cells are found in a PT with PASH stroma. These cells can exhibit lymphophagocytosis. They may express histiocytic immunomarkers as well as p53 and Ki67.

The stroma in many PT is heterogeneous. Foci indistinguishable from a fibroadenoma may abut sharply on much more cellular regions. Such areas can suggest that the PT arose from a fibroadenoma, when in fact this is an intrinsic characteristic of some PT. This structural variability can create substantial difficulty in the accurate classification of lesions sampled by needle core biopsy. Reported instances of malignant clinical behavior or metastases from a "benign" PT are probably a reflection of inaccurate classification of the tumor because of incomplete sampling. Ultimately, excisional biopsy is required to grade a PT, a determination based on stromal cellularity, mitotic activity, and the microscopic character of the tumor border.

A benign PT is characterized by few or no stromal mitoses, rarely more than two per 10 HPFs and modest stromal cellular overgrowth (Fig. 7.19). Epithelial hyperplasia is variably present in the average benign PT. The border of the tumor is more often circumscribed than invasive. Sometimes invasion

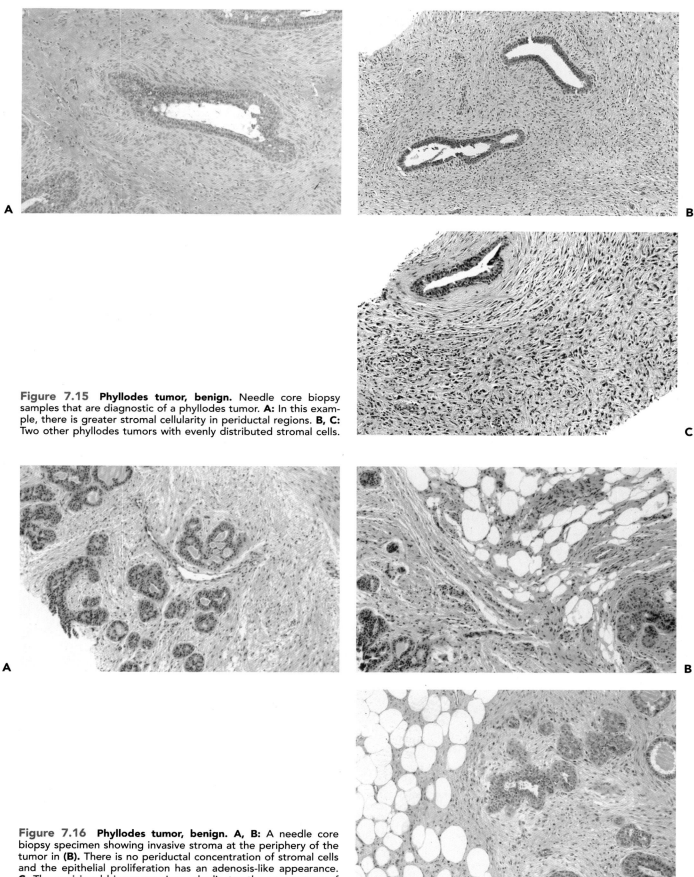

Figure 7.15 Phyllodes tumor, benign. Needle core biopsy samples that are diagnostic of a phyllodes tumor. **A:** In this example, there is greater stromal cellularity in periductal regions. **B, C:** Two other phyllodes tumors with evenly distributed stromal cells.

Figure 7.16 Phyllodes tumor, benign. A, B: A needle core biopsy specimen showing invasive stroma at the periphery of the tumor in **(B)**. There is no periductal concentration of stromal cells and the epithelial proliferation has an adenosis-like appearance. **C:** The excisional biopsy specimen duplicates the appearance of the sample obtained in the needle core biopsy procedure.

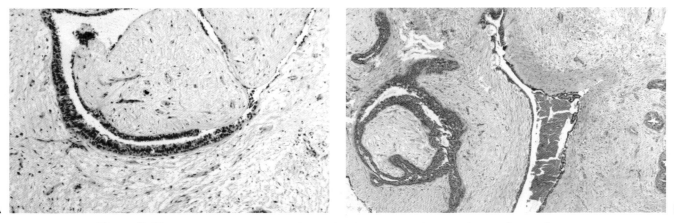

Figure 7.17   Phyllodes tumor. A: Epithelium-lined spaces are shown in this needle core biopsy specimen that is consistent with a fibroadenoma or a phyllodes tumor. **B:** The excisional biopsy specimen shown here has epithelium-lined spaces with focal hyperplasia and hemorrhage caused by the needle core biopsy procedure in a benign phyllodes tumor with midly cellular stroma.

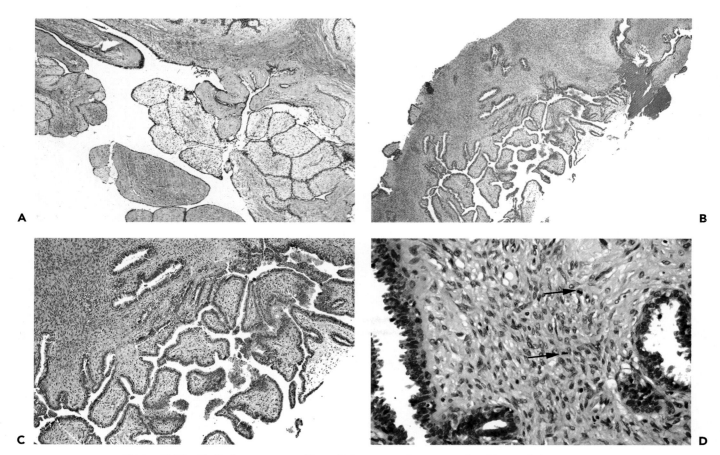

Figure 7.18   Phyllodes tumor, papillary. A: Exaggerated spaces outlined by epithelium create a cystic papillary appearance in this benign tumor. **B–D:** This needle core biopsy sample shows a benign phyllodes tumor with papillary structure and moderately cellular stroma. Mitoses are present (*arrows*).

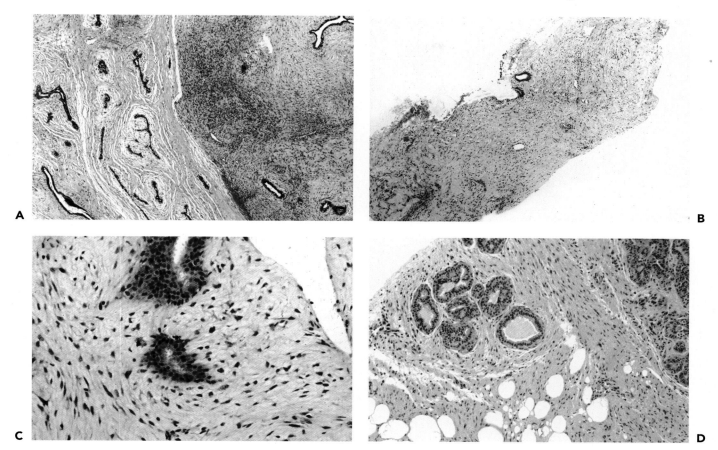

Figure 7.19   Phyllodes tumor, benign. A: Heterogeneity in a benign tumor. The region on the left resembles a fibroadenoma. **B, C:** A needle core biopsy specimen. The border of the lesion is not included in this sample that exhibits stromal overgrowth. **D:** A needle core biopsy specimen from another lesion with an invasive border.

takes the form of secondary, peripheral fibroepithelial nodules (Fig. 7.20). Adipose (Fig. 7.21) and osseous metaplasia can occur in the stroma of a benign PT and stromal cells with multiple hyperchromatic nuclei may be present (Fig. 7.22). Pseudoangiomatous hyperplasia of the stroma occurs in benign and malignant PT (Fig. 7.23).

A high-grade malignant PT is characterized by hypercellular stromal overgrowth that results in substantial separation of epithelial elements with proliferative activity in the stroma (exceeding five mitoses per 10 HPF), and usually an invasive tumor border (Fig. 7.24). Stromal cellular pleomorphism is common in these lesions. Rarely,

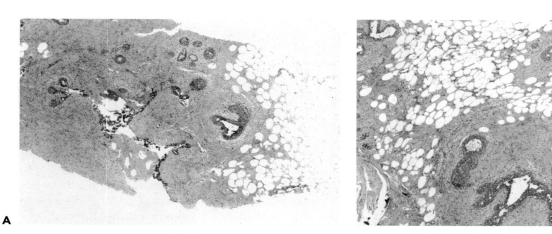

Figure 7.20   Phyllodes tumor, benign. A: A needle core biopsy specimen showing an invasive border. **B:** The invasive growth pattern was also present in the excisional biopsy specimen shown here. Secondary nodules are present in the fat.

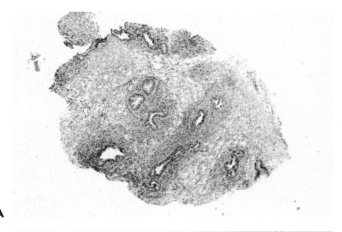

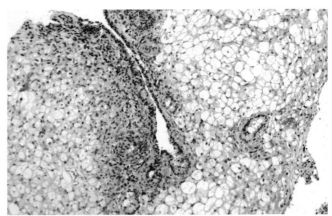

A

B

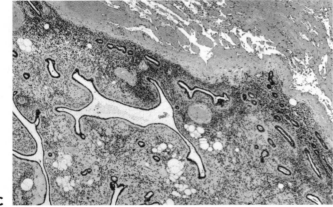

C

Figure 7.21 **Phyllodes tumor, benign with adipose differentiation. A, B:** A needle core biopsy specimen in which the stroma consists of adipose tissue. Mitoses were absent. **C:** The excisional biopsy specimen of the tumor with patches of adipose differentiation. There is angiomatous transformation adjacent to the tumor in the organizing hematoma resulting from the prior needle core biopsy procedure.

the stroma contains heterologous sarcomatous elements such as angiosarcoma, osteosarcoma, liposarcoma, or myosarcoma (14,50,51).

A borderline (low-grade malignant) PT usually has a microscopically invasive border, 2 to 5 mitoses per 10 HPF and moderate stromal cellularity that is often heterogeneously distributed in the midst of hypocellular areas. The spindle cell stroma in most of these lesions resembles fibromatosis or low-grade fibrosarcoma, and it often displays pseudoan-

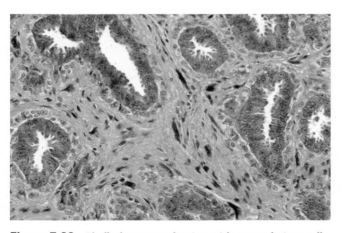

Figure 7.22 **Phyllodes tumor, benign with stromal giant cells.** Multinucleated giant cells are present in the stroma.

giomatous hyperplasia (Fig. 7.25). Infrequent instances of cartilaginous, osseous, and lipomatous metaplasia have been reported in borderline PT. An unusual benign PT in a 42-year-old woman had stromal cells that contained intracytoplasmic inclusion bodies of the type found in infantile digital fibromatosis (52). The inclusions were actin positive.

Many PT have foci of epithelial hyperplasia that results in increased thickness of the cuboidal or columnar epithelium lining the slitlike spaces. Myoepithelial cells participate in this process that may progress to papillary or cribriform hyperplasia (Fig. 7.26). There is a general tendency for the severity of epithelial hyperplasia to parallel the cellularity and mitotic activity of the stroma, but many exceptions to this rule are encountered (Fig. 7.27). Grimes (39) found "marked epithelial hyperplasia" in one-third of benign PT, including four (13%) with atypia, and in 26% of malignant PT. Atypical epithelial hyperplasia is sometimes extreme, leading to consideration of the diagnosis of intraductal carcinoma (Fig. 7.28). The PT character of the tumor may be overlooked if the stromal component is interpreted as reactive rather than as an intrinsic part of the neoplasm. However, the epithelial proliferation rarely reaches a level acceptable as intraductal carcinoma, and the diagnosis of intraductal or invasive ductal carcinoma in a PT is very infrequent (53) (Fig. 7.29). In situ or invasive lobular carcinoma can also develop in a PT (54). Squamous metaplasia of ductal epithelium, which occurs in benign and malignant PT, is

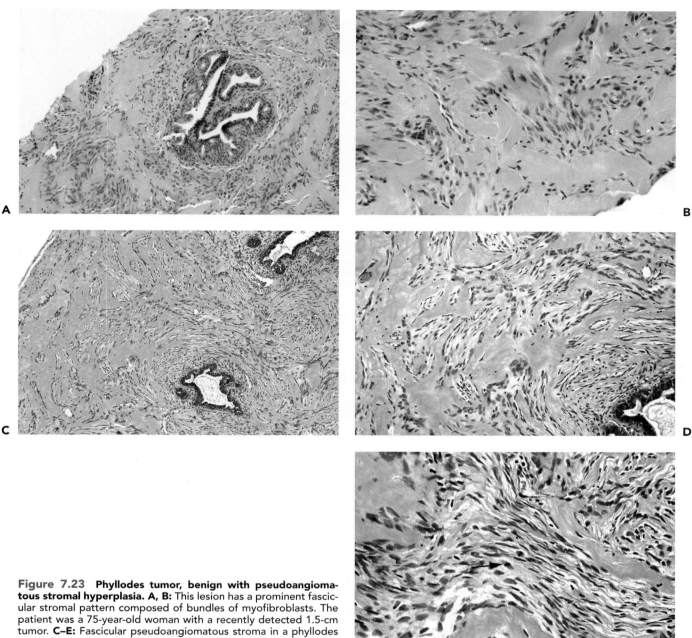

Figure 7.23 Phyllodes tumor, benign with pseudoangioma-tous stromal hyperplasia. A, B: This lesion has a prominent fascicular stromal pattern composed of bundles of myofibroblasts. The patient was a 75-year-old woman with a recently detected 1.5-cm tumor. **C–E:** Fascicular pseudoangiomatous stroma in a phyllodes tumor from a 15-year-old girl. A mitosis (*arrow*) is shown in a fascicular region **(E).**

found in about 10% of PT (39). Apocrine metaplasia has also been reported in the epithelium of PT (39,55).

Lobules are occasionally included in or formed in PTs, and they may exhibit proliferative changes including sclerosing adenosis, pregnancy-like hyperplasia, lactation, and lobular neoplasia. The presence of lobules can lead to an erroneous diagnosis of fibroadenoma, especially when there is lobular hyperplasia and stromal cellularity is not greatly increased. In rare instances, the epithelial proliferation in the form of adenosis or papillary hyperplasia can be so extreme that it obscures the underlying PT that may not be recognized until the tumor recurs.

Ductal elements may be present in locally recurrent PT in the breast or chest wall, and with rare exception, metastatic PT at distant sites consists entirely of the stromal component. Because most malignant PTs are high-grade spindle cell tumors with a fibrosarcomatous pattern, this is the most common appearance encountered in metastatic lesions. Rarely, locally recurrent or metastatic lesions exhibit heterologous differentiation that was not apparent in the primary tumor (56). Uncommon heterologous sarcomatous elements in the primary tumor such as liposarcoma (14,39), chondrosarcoma (39), osteosarcoma (39), and leiomyosarcoma (39) can be expressed in metastases.

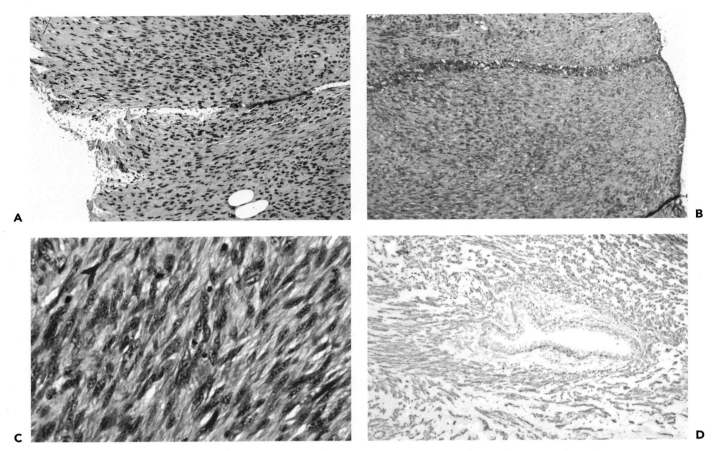

Figure 7.24 **Phyllodes tumor, malignant, high grade. A:** This needle core biopsy specimen is from a fibrosarcomatous phyllodes tumor. **B–D:** The epithelial-lined cleft in **(B)** is virtually obliterated in this needle core biopsy specimen from a tumor with leiomyosarcomatous differentiation. The tumor cells are immunoreactive for smooth muscle actin in **(D)** (immunoperoxidase).

The stroma of PT is vimentin positive. Actin and desmin reactivity are present in the stroma of a variable proportion of tumors that exhibit myoid or pseudoangiomatous differentiation of myofibroblasts (57). The stromal cells are rarely S-100 positive. Tse et al. (58) studied the expression of c-kit, a proto-oncogene that encodes a tyrosine kinase re-

ceptor (CD117), in the stroma of PT. They observed a significantly higher frequency of c-kit immunoreactivity in high-grade malignant (46%) than in benign tumors (17%). Carvalho et al. (59) reported finding c-kit expression in 12 of 19 (63%) benign PT and all 6 malignant PT that they studied. It has also been reported that vascular endothelial

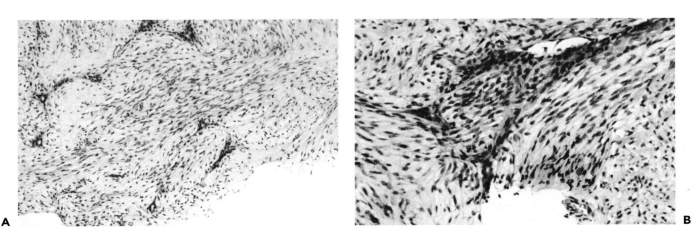

Figure 7.25 **Phyllodes tumor, malignant, low grade. A, B:** A needle core biopsy specimen showing moderately cellular stroma and tightly compressed epithelial slits.

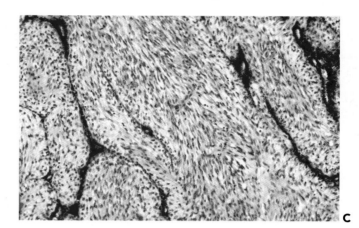

Figure 7.25 *(continued)* **C:** The excisional biopsy specimen showing low-grade fibrosarcomatous stroma. Rare mitotic figures were present.

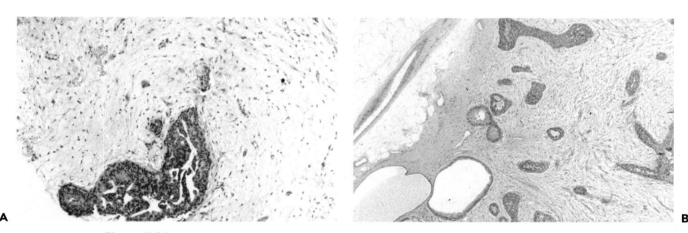

Figure 7.26 **Phyllodes tumor, benign with epithelial hyperplasia. A:** Duct hyperplasia is evident in this needle core biopsy specimen. **B:** The excisional biopsy specimen shows cysts and duct hyperplasia.

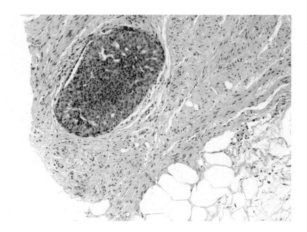

Figure 7.27 **Phyllodes tumor, benign with florid ductal epithelial hyperplasia.** The stromal component in this needle biopsy specimen is not notably cellular in the region of the hyperplastic epithelium.

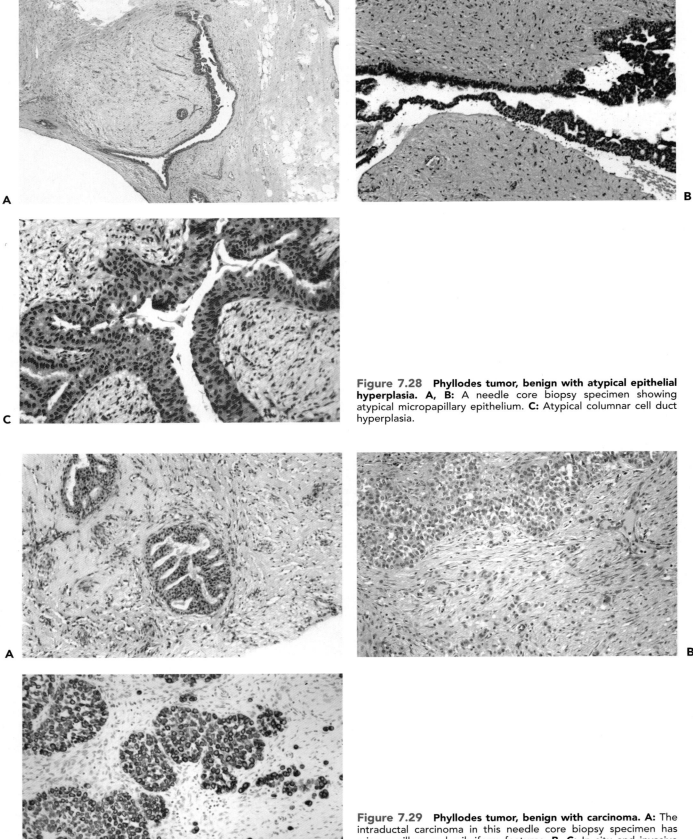

Figure 7.28   Phyllodes tumor, benign with atypical epithelial hyperplasia. A, B: A needle core biopsy specimen showing atypical micropapillary epithelium. **C:** Atypical columnar cell duct hyperplasia.

Figure 7.29   Phyllodes tumor, benign with carcinoma. A: The intraductal carcinoma in this needle core biopsy specimen has micropapillary and cribriform features. **B, C:** In situ and invasive lobular carcinoma in a benign tumor. The invasive carcinoma cells are highlighted by the CK7 cytokeratin immunostain in **(C)** (immunoperoxidase).

growth factor (VEGF) expression is an indicator of the grade of a PT. Tse et al. (60) found significantly more intense VEGF reactivity in the stroma of malignant than benign PT. VEGF expression was absent from 82% of benign PT and 41% of malignant PT. Expression of p53 in greater than 10% of stromal cells has been reported in 5 of 50 (10%) benign PTs and in 9 of 13 (69%) of malignant PTs, a difference that was statistically significant (61). The fact that these markers can be found in benign as well as malignant PT, and absence of these markers from some malignant PT, means that they cannot be used solely as a basis for classifying these lesions.

Markers of stromal proliferative activity may prove to be useful not only in the distinction between fibroadenomas and PT but also in the classification of PT. Ridgway et al. (33) reported that the mean MIB-1 index of benign PT (33.31 ± 6.73) was significantly lower in low-grade than in high-grade malignant PT. Ki67 expression in more than 10% of stromal cells has been reported in 8 of 50 (16%) benign PT and in 11 of 13 (85%) of malignant PT, a statistically significant difference (61). Further study is needed to investigate the heterogeneity of Ki67 expression in PT to determine whether a needle core biopsy specimen is a reliable basis for assessing these markers.

The classification of a PT as benign and low- or high-grade malignant reflects an estimate of the probable clinical course as determined by the histologic appearance of the tumor. A benign PT will not metastasize and has a low probability (approximately 20%) for local recurrence after excision (62). A borderline or low-grade malignant PT has a slight probability (<5%) of metastasis, but such a tumor is more likely than a benign PT (>25%) to recur locally unless widely excised. Recurrences occur earlier with high-grade malignant PT than after initial treatment of benign or low-grade malignant tumors. Metastases occur in about 25% of high-grade malignant PT, and these lesions are also very prone to local recurrence. Less than 1% of high-grade PT give rise to axillary lymph node metastases (39,63).

Barth (64) summarized breast recurrence data based on an extensive literature review. Classification of PT as benign, low-grade malignant (borderline) and high-grade malignant correlated with local breast recurrence in women who did not undergo mastectomy. Of the literature reviewed, 20 published studies provided information about patients treated by "local excision" or lumpectomy. Breast recurrences were reported in 111/540 (21%), 18/39 (46%), and 26/40 (65%) of patients who had benign, low-grade malignant, and high-grade malignant tumors, respectively. Thirteen studies had data for women treated by "wide local excision" with "at least 1 to 2 cm of normal tissue around the tumor." Overall, breast recurrences were reported in 17/212 (8%), 20/68 (29%), and 16/45 (36%) of patients with benign, low-grade malignant, and high-grade malignant tumors, respectively. Combined survival data from the published studies indicated deaths due to disease in 2/600 (0.3%), 7/107 (6.6%), and 48/240 (20%) of patients with

benign, low-grade malignant, and high-grade malignant tumors, respectively. Analysis of 821 patients with malignant PT recorded in the Surveillance, Epidemiology, and End Results (SEER) program with median follow-up of 5.7 years revealed disease-specific survival of 91%, 89%, and 89% at 5, 10, and 15 years, respectively (65). Disease-specific survival was not significantly different between patients treated by excisional surgery and mastectomy.

The fundamental principle of therapy is complete excision to prevent local recurrence (63,66–68). Features that predispose to local recurrence are incomplete excision, an invasive tumor border, and secondary tumor nodules at the periphery. Primary tumor size may be a factor in the success of local excision because a more generous margin may be possible when tumors are small (66). Local recurrence is deleterious, especially because of the tendency of some PTs to have a higher grade in recurrent lesions than in the corresponding primary tumor and the risk of chest wall invasion. The most common sites of distant metastases are the lungs, bone, and heart (69). Virtually any organ may be found to have metastases, but many of these sites are not apparent antemortem.

The overall 5-year survival rate for PT is about 90% (39). Local recurrences, which occur in about 30% of cases, and metastases that develop in about 20% of cases, are usually detected within 3 years of primary treatment (39,41,67,70), although occasional instances of late recurrence have been reported (39). Most deaths due to metastatic PT occur within 5 years of diagnosis (39,71). Virtually all fatalities occur in patients who primarily have high-grade tumors, or who develop recurrences that are high grade (72).

Metastatic PT is not responsive to most currently available chemotherapy or to radiotherapy, but palliation may be achieved with combination of chemotherapy and radiation (73).

REFERENCES

1. Kovi J, Chu HB, Leffall Jr L. Sclerosing lobular hyperplasia manifesting as a palpable mass of the breast in young black women. *Hum Pathol.* 1984;15: 336–340.
2. Poulton TB, Shaw de Pardes E, Baldwin M. Sclerosing lobular hyperplasia of the breast: imaging features in 15 cases. *Am J Roentgenol.* 1995;165:291–294.
3. Dupont WD, Page DL, Parl FF, et al. Long-term risk of breast cancer in women with fibroadenoma. *N Engl J Med.* 1994;331:10–15.
4. Foster ME, Garrahan N, Williams S. Fibroadenoma of the breast: a clinical and pathological study. *J R Coll Surg Edinb.* 1988;33:16–19.
5. Oberman HA. Breast lesions in the adolescent female. *Pathol Annu.* 1979;14: 175–201.
6. Baildam AD, Higgans RM, Hurley E, et al. Cyclosporin A and multiple fibroadenomas of the breast. *Br J Surg.* 1996;83:1755–1757.
7. Weinstein SP, Orel SG, Collazzo L, et al. Cyclosporin A-induced fibroadenomas of the breast: report of five cases. *Radiology.* 2001;220:465–468.
8. Son EJ, Oh KK, Kim EK, et al. Characteristic imaging features of breast fibroadenomas in women given cyclosporin A after renal transplantation. *J. Clin Ultrasound.* 2004;32:69–77.
9. Moross T, Lang AP, Mahoney L. Tubular adenoma of breast. *Arch Pathol Lab Med.* 1983;107:84–86.
10. Tesluk H, Amott T, Goodnight JE. Apocrine adenoma of the breast. *Arch Pathol Lab Med.* 1986;110:351–352.
11. Gusterson BA, Sloane JP, Middwood C, et al. Ductal adenoma of the breast—a lesion exhibiting a myoepithelial/epithelial phenotype. *Histopathology.* 1987;11:103–110.
12. Chen KTK. Pleomorphic adenoma of the breast. *Am J Clin Pathol.* 1990; 93:792–794.

13. Goodman ZD, Taxy JB. Fibroadenomas of the breast with prominent smooth muscle. *Am J Surg Pathol.* 1981;5:99–101.
14. Powell CM, Rosen PP. Adipose differentiation in cystosarcoma phyllodes. *Am J Surg Pathol.* 1994;18:720–727.
15. Powell CM, Cranor ML, Rosen PP. Multinucleated stromal giant cells in mammary fibroepithelial neoplasms. A study of 11 patients. *Arch Pathol Lab Med.* 1994;118:912–916.
16. Ryska A, Reynolds C, Keeney GL. Benign tumors of the breast with multinucleated stromal giant cells. Immunohistochemical analysis of six cases and review of the literature. *Virchows Arch.* 2001;439:768–775.
17. Meyer JE, Lester SC, DiPiro PJ, et al. Occult calcified fibroadenomas. *Breast Dis.* 1995;8:29–38.
18. Kuijper A, Mommers ECM, van der Wall E, van Diest PJ. Histopathology of fibroadenoma of the breast. *Am J Clin Pathol.* 2001;115:736–742.
19. Fechner RE. Fibroadenomas in patients receiving oral contraceptives: a clinical and pathologic study. *Am J Clin Pathol.* 1970;53:857–864.
20. Sklair-Levy M, Sella T, Alweiss T, et al. Incidence and management of complex fibroadenomas. *Am J Roentgenol.* 2008;190:214–218.
21. Mechtersheimer G, Kruger KH, Born IA, Moller P. Antigenic profile of mammary fibroadenoma and cystosarcoma phyllodes. A study using antibodies to estrogen and progesterone receptors and to a panel of cell surface molecules. *Pathol Res Pract.* 1990;186:427–438.
22. Rao BR, Meyer JS, Fry CG. Most cystosarcoma phyllodes and fibroadenomas have progesterone receptor but lack estrogen receptor: a stromal localization of progesterone receptor. *Cancer.* 1981;47:2016–2021.
23. Tobin CE, Hendrix TM, Geyer SJ, et al. Breast imaging case of the day. *Radiographics.* 1996;16:1225–1226.
24. Pike A, Oberman HA. Juvenile (cellular) adenofibromas. A clincopatholgic study. *Am J Surg Pathol.* 1985;9:730–736.
25. Mies C, Rosen PP. Juvenile fibroadenoma with atypical epithelial hyperplasia. *Am J Surg Pathol.* 1987;11:184–190.
26. Gordon PB, Gagnon FA, Lanzkowsky L. Solid breast masses diagnosed as fibroadenoma at fine-needle aspiration biopsy: acceptable rates of growth at long-term follow-up. *Radiology.* 2003;229:233–238.
27. Sperber F, Blank A, Metser U, et al. Diagnosis and treatment of breast fibroadenomas by ultrasound guided vacuum-assisted biopsy. *Arch Surg.* 2003;138:796–800.
28. Jacklin RK, Ridgway PE, Ziprin P, et al. Optimizing preoperative diagnosis in phyllodes tumors of the breast. *J Clin Pathol.* 2006;59:454–459.
29. Jacobs TW, Chen Y-Y, Guinee Jr DG, et al. Fibroepithelial lesions with cellular stroma on breast needle core biopsy. Are there predictors of outcome on surgical excison? *Am J Clin Pathol.* 2006;124:342–354.
30. Yohe S, Yeh I-T. "Missed" diagnoses of phyllodes tumor on breast biopsy: pathologic clues to its recognition. *Int J Surg Pathol.* 2008;16:137–142.
31. Dershaw DD, Morris EA, Liberman L, et al. Non-diagnostic stereotoxic core breast biopsy: results of surgical excision. *Radiology.* 1996;198:323–325.
32. Meyer JB, Smith DN, Lester SC, et al. Large-needle core biopsy of nonmalignant breast abnormalities evaluated with surgical excision or repeat core biopsy. *Radiology.* 1998;206:717–720.
33. Ridgway PF, Jacklin RK, Ziprin P, et al. Perioperative diagnosis of cystosarcoma phyllodes of the breast may be enhanced by MIB-1 index. *J Surg Res.* 2004;122:82–88.
34. Littrup PJ, Freeman-Gibb L, Andea A, et al. Cryotherapy for breast fibroadenomas. *Radiology.* 2005;234:63–72.
35. Nurko J, Mabry CD, Whitworth P, et al. Interim results from the Fibroadenoma Cryoablation Treatment Registry. *Am J Surg.* 2005;190:647–652.
36. Fine RE, Whitworth PW, Kim JA, et al. Low-risk palpable breast masses removed using a vacuum-assisted hand-held device. *Am J Surg.* 2003;186:362–367.
37. Grady I, Gorsuch H, Wilburn-Bailey S. Long-term outcome of benign fibroadenomas treated by ultrasound-guided percutaneous excision. *Breast J.* 2008;14:275–278.
38. Cohn-Cedermark G, Rutqvist LE, Rosendahl I, Silverswürd C. Prognostic factors in cystosarcoma phyllodes. A clinicopathologic study of 77 patients. *Cancer.* 1991;68:2017–2022.
39. Grimes MM. Cystosarcoma phyllodes of the breast: histologic features, flow cytometry analysis, and clinical correlations. *Mod Pathol.* 1992;5:232–239.
40. Rajan PB, Cranor ML, Rosen PP. Cystosarcoma phyllodes in adolescent girls and young women: a study of 45 patients. *Am J Surg Pathol.* 1998;22:64–69.
41. Reinfuss M, Mitus J, Smolak K, Stelmach A. Malignant phyllodes tumours of the breast. A clinical and pathological analysis of 55 cases. *Eur J Cancer.* 1993;29A:1252–1256.
42. Nielsen VT, Andreasen C. Phyllodes tumor of the male breast. *Histopathology.* 1987;11:761–765.
43. Reingold IM, Ascher GS. Cystosarcoma phyllodes in a man with gynecomastia. *Am J Clin Pathol.* 1970;53:852–856.
44. Way JC, Culham BA. Phyllodes tumor in pregnancy: a case report. *Can J Surg.* 1998;41:407–409.
45. Buchberger W, Strasser K, Heim K, et al. Phyllodes tumor: findings on mammography, sonography, and aspiration cytology in 10 cases. *Am J Roentgenol.* 1991;157:715–719.
46. Liberman L, Bonaccio E, Hamele-Bena D, et al. Benign and malignant phyllodes tumors: mammographic and sonographic findings. *Radiology.* 1996;198:121–124.
47. Cosmacini P, Zurrida S, Veronesi P, et al. Phyllode tumor of the breast: mammographic experience in 99 cases. *Eur J Rad.* 1992;15:11–14.
48. Yabucchi H, Soeda H, Matsuo Y, et al. Phyllodes tumor of the breast: correlation between MR findings and histologic grade. *Radiology.* 2006;241:702–709.
49. Burga AM, Tavassoli FA. Periductal stromal tumor. A rare lesion with low-grade sarcomatous behavior. *Am J Surg Pathol.* 2003;27:343–348.
50. Barnes L, Pietruszka M. Rhabdomyosarcoma arising within a breast and its mimic. An immunohistochemical and cystosarcoma phyllodes. *Am J Surg Pathol.* 1978;2:423–429.
51. Silver SA, Tavassoli FA. Osteosarcomatous differentiation in phyllodes tumors. *Am J Surg Pathol.* 1999;23:815–821.
52. Hiraoka N, Mukai M, Hosoda Y, Hata J-I. Phyllodes tumor of the breast containing the intracytoplasmic inclusion bodies identical with infantile digital fibromatosis. *Am J Surg Pathol.* 1994;18:506–511.
53. Knudsen PJ, Ostergaard J. Cystosarcoma phyllodes with lobular and ductal carcinoma in situ. *Arch Pathol Lab Med.* 1987;111:873–875.
54. Kodama T, Kameyama K, Mukai M, et al. Invasive lobular carcinoma arising in phyllodes tumor of the breast. *Virchows Arch.* 2003;442:614–616.
55. Salisbury JR, Singh LN. Apocrine metaplasia in phyllodes tumors of the breast. *Histopathology.* 1986;10:1211–1215.
56. Graadt van Roggen JF, Zonderland HM, Welvaart K, et al. Local recurrence of phyllodes tumor of the breast presenting with widespread differentiation to a telangiectatic osteosarcoma. *J Clin Pathol.* 1998;51:706–708.
57. Aranda FI, Laforga JB, Lopez JI. Phyllodes tumor of the breast. An immunohistochemical study of 28 cases with special attention to the role of myofibroblasts. *Path Res Pract.* 1994;190:474–481.
58. Tse GMK, Putti TC, Lui PCW, et al. Increased c-kit (CD117) expression in malignant mammary phyllodes tumors. *Mod. Pathol.* 2004;17:827–831.
59. Carvalho S, e Silva AO, Milanezi F, et al. c-KIT and PDGFRA in breast phyllodes tumors: overexpression without mutations? *J Clin Pathol.* 2004;57:1075–1079.
60. Tse GMK, Lui PCW, Lee CS, et al. Stromal expression of vascular endothelial growth factor correlates with tumor grade and microvessel density in mammary phyllodes tumors: a multicenter study of 185 cases. *Hum Pathol.* 2004;35:1053–1057.
61. Chan YJ, Chen BF, Chang CL, et al. Expression of p53 protein and Ki-67 antigen in phyllodes tumor of the breast. *J Chin Med Assoc.* 2004;67:3–8.
62. Reinfuss M, Mitus J, Duda K, et al. The treatment and prognosis of patients with phyllodes tumor of the breast. An analysis of 170 cases. *Cancer.* 1996;77:910–916.
63. Treves N, Sunderland DA. Cystosarcoma phyllodes of the breast: a malignant and a benign tumor. A clinicopathological study of seventy-seven cases. *Cancer.* 1951;4:1286–1332.
64. Barth Jr RJ. Histologic features predict local recurrence after breast conserving therapy of phyllodes tumors. *Breast Cancer Res Treat.* 1996;57:291–295.
65. Macdonald OK, Lee CM, Twarl JD, et al. Malignant phyllodes tumor of the female breast. Association of primary therapy with cause-specific survival from the Surveillance, Epidemiology and End Results (SEER) Program. *Cancer.* 2006;107:2127–2133.
66. Bartoli C, Zurrida S, Veronesi P, et al. Small sized phyllodes tumor of the breast. *Eur J Surg Oncol.* 1990;16:215–219.
67. McGregor GI, Knowling MA, Este FA. Sarcoma and cystosarcoma phyllodes tumors of the breast—a retrospective review of 58 cases. *Am J Surg.* 1994;167:477–480.
68. Salvadori B, Cusumano F, Del Bo R, et al. Surgical treatment of phyllodes tumors of the breast. *Cancer.* 1989;63:2532–2536.
69. Kessinger A, Foley JF, Lemon HM, Miller DM. Metastatic cystosarcoma phyllodes: a case report and review of the literature. *J Surg Oncol.* 1972;4:131–136.
70. Hines JR, Murad TM, Beal JM. Prognostic indicators in cystosarcoma phyllodes. *Am J Surg.* 1987;153:276–280.
71. Pietruszka M, Barnes L. Cystosarcoma phyllodes. A clinicopathologic analysis of 42 cases. *Cancer.* 1978;41:1974–1983.
72. Hawkins RE, Schofield JB, Fisher C, et al. The clinical and histologic criteria that predict metastases from cystosarcoma phyllodes. *Cancer.* 1992;69:141–147.
73. Burton GV, Hart LL, Leight GS, et al. Cystosarcoma phyllodes. Effective therapy with cisplatin and etoposide chemotherapy. *Cancer.* 1989;63:2088–2092.

Ductal Hyperplasia and Intraductal Carcinoma

8

DUCTAL HYPERPLASIA: USUAL AND ATYPICAL

The distinction between intraductal hyperplasia and intraductal carcinoma is important for patient management (1). In most instances, intraductal proliferations are readily classified by pathologists on the basis of generally accepted histopathologic features as either hyperplasia or in situ carcinoma (2). There exists a small subset for which assignment to either of these categories is less certain. The existence of these "borderline" lesions, which may be diagnosed as atypical hyperplasia or in situ carcinoma, depending upon which criteria are employed, is not a compelling reason for abandoning the existing practice of distinguishing pathologically and clinically between ductal hyperplasia and in situ duct carcinoma. Studies of interobserver differences in the diagnosis of highly selected examples of these lesions have focused attention on this troublesome diagnostic problem that applies to a small percentage of proliferative breast changes (3–5).

There are no clinical features specifically associated with ductal hyperplasia. The alterations caused by epithelial proliferation in individual ducts or in groups of ducts are microscopic in dimension and usually often not palpable. Ductal hyperplasia in various forms is a frequent constituent of "fibrocystic changes" that may be detected by mammography or form a palpable tumor. The lesion complex can also include sclerosing adenosis, cystic and papillary apocrine metaplasia, duct stasis, fibrosis or pseudoangiomatous stromal hyperplasia, and lobular hyperplasia. An important corollary to the lack of clinical indicators of ductal hyperplasia is the inability to determine the duration of these lesions. The date on which ductal hyperplasia was biopsied is customarily used as if it were the date of "onset." This practice, which is a consequence of inability to determine the preclinical duration of hyperplastic ductal lesions, could be a source of bias in assessing the precancerous significance of proliferative lesions in individual patients.

The mammographic manifestations of duct hyperplasia include altered duct patterns, parenchymal distortion, nonpalpable mass lesions, calcification, and asymmetry when both breasts are compared. Calcifications are the most frequent mammographic indication of atypical ductal hyperplasia in the absence of a palpable abnormality (6–8). Lesions described on mammography as radial scars often have a component of ductal hyperplasia. Some but not all radial scar lesions contain microcalcifications. In the era that preceded the widespread use of mammography, when the indication for biopsy was a palpable abnormality, ductal hyperplasia was found in 25% or fewer of specimens obtained (9,10). Not more than 5% of these biopsies had atypical ductal hyperplasia. The frequency of these atypical abnormalities is higher among mammographically directed biopsies including surgical excisions and needle core biopsies (11,12). The yield of atypical ductal hyperplasia in magnetic resonance imaging (MRI)-directed vacuum-assisted core biopsies ranged from 3% to 8% in several studies (13–15).

Ductal hyperplasia can be found in female patients at virtually any age. In patients younger than 30 years, most examples of ductal hyperplasia occur either as juvenile papillomatosis (16) or as one of the group of lesions referred to as papillary duct hyperplasia in children and young women (17). The majority of women with ductal hyperplasia are between 35 and 60 years of age. After age 60, ductal hyperplasia becomes less frequent, and when present the growth pattern is usually less florid than in younger women. However, occasionally, a woman older than 60 years may be found to have extensive proliferative changes with florid ductal hyperplasia. Use of exogenous estrogens can be documented in some but not all of these cases.

Ductal hyperplasia describes a proliferative condition that is manifested histologically as an increase in the cellularity of epithelium in ducts. Because the normal resting epithelium consists of a continuous monolayer of cuboidal-to-columnar epithelial cells supported by a discontinuous layer of myoepithelial cells, an increase in the cellularity of this two-layer configuration constitutes hyperplasia. The increased thickness of the epithelial layer results in partial or complete obstruction of the duct lumen at the site of the proliferative abnormality. If intraductal hyperplasia is traced in serial sections, it is often possible to observe the discontinuous and multifocal nature of the condition. Various distortions of the basic ductal architecture occur when hyperplastic ducts become more sinuous or are incorporated into complex proliferative lesions, such as papillomas or "radial scars." Ductal hyperplasia can extend into the smallest branches of the duct system, and it may involve the epithelium of terminal duct–lobular units.

The histologic criteria for the diagnosis of duct hyperplasia are the same for needle core biopsy samples and surgical excision specimens. However, needle core biopsy samples present disconnected portions of the lesional area and therefore lack the helpful contextual information provided by intact samples from a surgical biopsy. This situation can lead to overinterpretation of individual ducts seen in isolation.

Pathology of Usual Ductal Hyperplasia

When individual cell borders are inconspicuous, the cellular proliferation in ductal hyperplasia often has a syncytial appearance. Cytoplasmic vacuolization may occur. True intracytoplasmic microlumens that contain secretion that stains positively with the mucicarmine or alcian blue–PAS (periodic acid–Schiff) stains are extremely uncommon in hyperplastic ductal epithelium (18). The presence of intracytoplasmic mucin-containing microlumens is an atypical feature that should result in careful consideration of a diagnosis of intraductal carcinoma or pagetoid lobular carcinoma in situ (LCIS). In duct hyperplasia, nuclear spacing is uneven so that in some areas the cells appear crowded and the nuclei seem to overlap. Nuclei are round, ovoid to spindly, or reniform, depending on the plane of section. Nucleoli are inapparent or inconspicuous unless there is a

prominent element of apocrine metaplasia. Mitotic figures are very infrequent, and when present they have a regular configuration.

Ductal hyperplasia of the usual type has been subdivided on the basis of qualitative and quantitative criteria, into the categories of mild, moderate, and severe or florid. The application of this classification is limited by the fact that disordered epithelial growth with varied structural patterns is a characteristic feature of ductal hyperplasia. As a consequence, hyperplastic epithelium is not uniformly distributed in a stratified fashion that permits easy determination of the number of cell layers. Epithelial thickness is also difficult to judge in tangentially sectioned ducts. The criteria for making these distinctions based largely on the thickness of the epithelium are difficult to apply to ductules and terminal ducts. In these structures, the lumen is relatively small, and it can be filled when there is little increase in epithelial thickness. Degrees of hyperplasia based on epithelial thickness are meaningful only when applied to selected nontangential sections of duct structures of sufficient diameter to manifest diagnostic features. Consequently, the classification of ductal hyperplasia based on epithelial thickness has significant limitations and may not be applicable in many instances.

Mild hyperplasia may affect the entire epithelium circumferentially in a duct cross section or only a segment of the duct. It occurs as an increase in the amount of epithelium, which rarely exceeds three cells in thickness. The epithelium may be focally papillary (Fig. 8.1).

In moderate hyperplasia, the epithelium tends to be more than 3 cells in thickness. Intraluminal proliferation is more pronounced than in mild hyperplasia, resulting in the formation of secondary glandular lumina (Fig. 8.2). Part of the duct lumen may remain as a crescentic space or spaces at the edge of the duct in cribriform hyperplasia (Fig. 8.3). Micropapillary hyperplasia is part of the spectrum of mild and moderate ductal hyperplasia (Fig. 8.4). The papillae are blunt or slender, irregularly shaped fronds

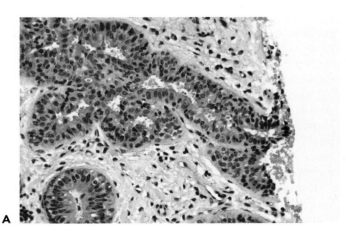
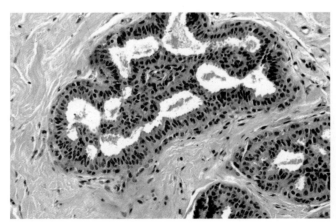

A   **B**

Figure 8.1   Ductal hyperplasia, mild. A: The ducts in this needle core biopsy specimen are lined by epithelium that is one or two cells in thickness. **B:** Minimal papillary hyperplasia is shown in another needle core biopsy specimen. Hyperplasia of myoepithelial cells is also evident.

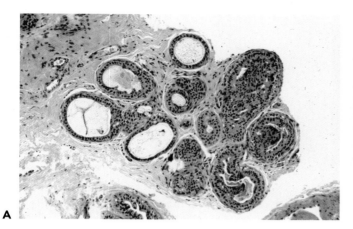

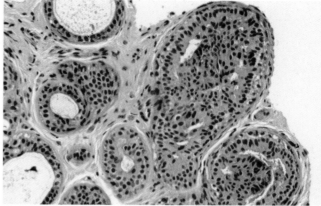

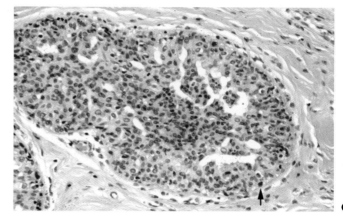

Figure 8.2 Ductal hyperplasia, moderate. A, B: This needle core biopsy specimen shows duct hyperplasia in an enlarged duct-lobular complex. Note the persistent columnar duct epithelium at the periphery of hyperplastic ducts. **C:** This duct from another specimen is nearly filled with hyperplastic epithelium. Note condensation of the cells with diminished cytoplasm in the center of the duct and a mitotic figure *(arrow)*.

of hyperplastic epithelium in which the apical cells are smaller and have more condensed nuclei than those in the underlying basal epithelium.

The nuclei in moderate hyperplasia are often overlapping, irregularly shaped, and may be distributed in a "streaming" fashion (Fig. 8.5). Streaming refers to a growth pattern in which the nuclei of hyperplastic epithelial cells are oriented parallel to the long axes of the cells (Fig. 8.6).

Because the cytoplasmic borders of these cells are often indistinct, streaming is usually detected as a parallel orientation of oval or spindle-shaped nuclei. Streaming occurs in most structural patterns of usual and atypical intraductal hyperplasia. The association of the streaming pattern with ductal hyperplasia has been confirmed by computerized morphometric analysis of the orientation of nuclei in proliferative duct lesions (19).

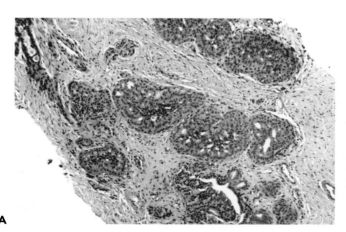

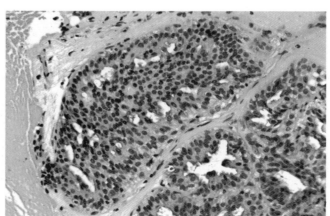

Figure 8.3 Ductal hyperplasia, moderate. A, B: Hyperplastic epithelium fills the ducts in this needle core biopsy specimen forming a cribriform pattern. Cells in the center of the duct have small, condensed nuclei and scant cytoplasm. Columnar epithelium is present at the periphery of the affected duct **(B)**.

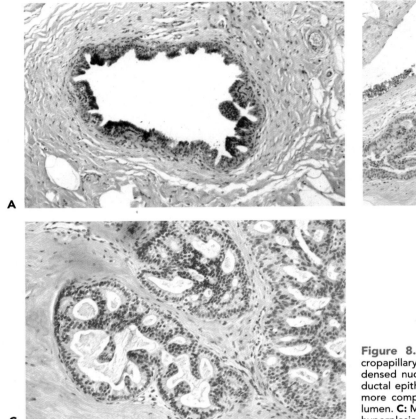

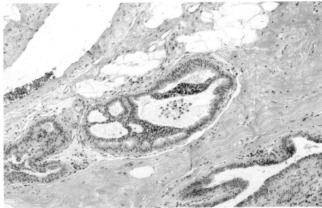

Figure 8.4 Ductal hyperplasia, micropapillary. A: The micropapillary epithelium consists of columnar cells with dark, condensed nuclei and scant cytoplasm. **B:** Well-preserved columnar ductal epithelium is present at the periphery of this duct, with a more complex mildly atypical micropapillary proliferation in the lumen. **C:** Mixed moderately atypical micropapillary and cribriform hyperplasia.

The distinction between moderate and florid hyperplasia is not sharp, but lesions are generally placed in the latter category when the affected ducts are appreciably enlarged in comparison with nonhyperplastic counterparts. Florid hyperplasia has the papillary and bridging growth patterns that are encountered in moderate hyperplasia but the overall proliferation tends to be more cellular and complex than in moderate hyperplasia (Fig. 8.7). Foci of florid hyperplasia are more likely to fill the entire duct lumen in a solid or fenestrated (cribriform) fashion.

Necrotic cellular debris is rarely present in hyperplastic ducts, and when found it is usually associated with florid sclerosing papillary hyperplasia (Fig. 8.8). In such lesions, the hyperplastic ducts with necrosis are indistinguishable cytologically and structurally from adjacent ducts with non-necrotic hyperplastic epithelium. Histiocytes or foam

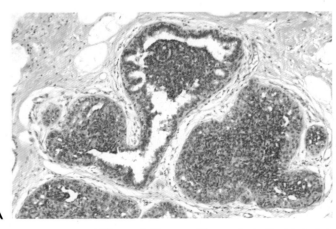

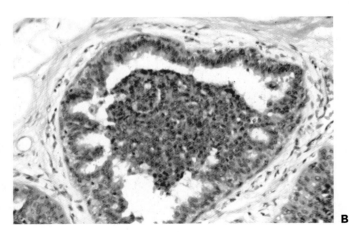

Figure 8.5 Ductal hyperplasia, florid. A, B: In this needle core biopsy specimen, the dense, overlapping cellular proliferation has solid and papillary patterns. Columnar cell and micropapillary hyperplasia are shown in **(B)** at the periphery of the duct.

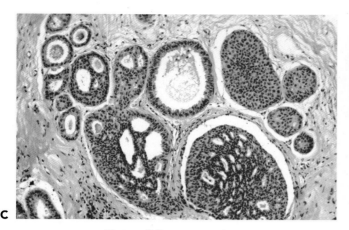

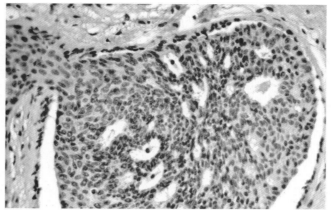

Figure 8.5 *(continued)* **C, D:** Solid and cribriform florid hyperplasia is seen in these lesions. The epithelium in the duct in **(D)** has a streaming pattern. Note the loss of cytoplasm and nuclear condensation in cells in the centers of the ducts.

cells are found relatively often in the lumens of hyperplastic ducts, and the presence of these cells should not be mistaken for necrosis (Fig. 8.9).

The fenestrated growth pattern that occurs in moderate and florid ductal hyperplasia results from the formation of epithelial bridges that become joined as they traverse the duct lumen. The fenestrations represent portions of the original duct lumen that has been passively subdivided by the complex arborizing epithelial proliferation.

Using a serial section, three-dimensional reconstruction method, Ohuchi et al. (20) demonstrated that the lumina that appear to be separated from each other in a two-dimensional histologic section of papillary intraductal hyperplasia were actually part of a network of channels representing the original duct lumen surrounded by the proliferating epithelium. By contrast, three-dimensional reconstruction of intraductal carcinoma revealed that the fenestrations in these lesions were newly formed,

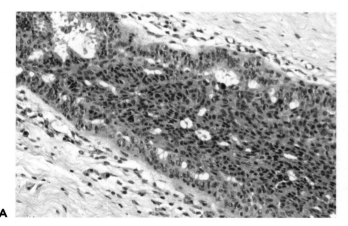

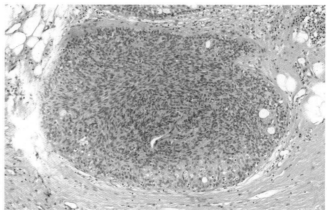

Figure 8.6 Ductal hyperplasia, florid with streaming. A: The hyperplastic epithelium in the lumen of this duct is composed of cells with a streaming pattern. Note the persistent columnar ductal epithelium and microlumens at the border of the duct. **B, C:** This solid papillary ductal hyperplasia, with fibrovascular stroma is composed of spindle cells with a streaming pattern. Microlumina are present at the perimeter of the duct.

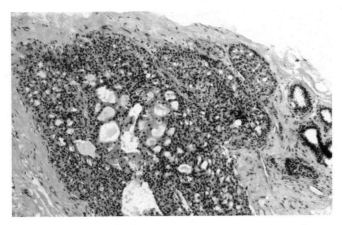

Figure 8.7 **Ductal hyperplasia, florid.** The hyperplastic duct in this needle core biopsy specimen is enlarged and filled by epithelium with solid and cribriform areas. Apocrine metaplasia is present in the center of the duct.

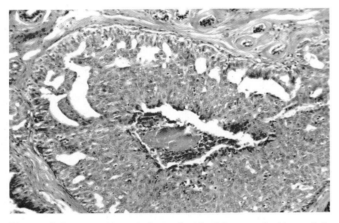

Figure 8.8 **Ductal hyperplasia, florid with necrosis.** Necrosis is present in the center of this hyperplastic duct that was part of sclerosing papillary duct hyperplasia. Columnar epithelium can be seen at the periphery of the duct, where there are microlumina of various sizes and shapes.

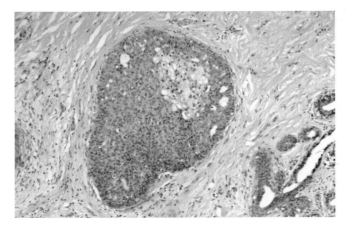

Figure 8.9 **Ductal hyperplasia, florid with histiocytes.** The epithelial proliferation in this enlarged duct is solid with peripheral fenestrations. Histiocytes are present in the duct.

disconnected spaces bordered by polarized neoplastic cells.

The spaces that are found in histologic sections of fenestrated intraductal hyperplasia have distinctive features. The secondary lumens tend to be larger and more numerous at the periphery of the duct than centrally, but the reverse distribution may be encountered. Cells outlining these spaces are distributed in a haphazard fashion except at the edge of the duct, where residual columnar or cuboidal duct epithelium composed of cells with more regularly oriented nuclei may persist. The spaces in a given hyperplastic duct usually have varied shapes (ovoid, crescentic, irregular, or serpiginous) rather than being rounded as occurs in cribriform carcinoma (Figs. 8.3, 8.5–8.7, 8.10). The spaces formed in intraductal hyperplasia may be empty or they may contain secretion and histiocytes. Fine calcifications can develop in the glandular lumina of intraductal hyperplasia.

A layer of myoepithelial cells is often evident at the edge of a hyperplastic duct in H&E sections (Fig. 8.11). These cells may accompany the proliferation into the duct lumen when the fibrovascular stromal framework of papillary hyperplasia is present. Immunohistochemical stains are useful for highlighting the myoepithelium in proliferative ductal lesions. Experience has led to the conclusion that the reactivity of individual markers is unpredictable in a given case and that it is advantageous to employ at least three myoepithelial markers.

p63 is the only marker currently available that is localized specifically in the nuclei of myoepithelial cells. It is not reactive with myofibroblasts or blood vessels (21). p63 is rarely reactive with scattered epithelial cell nuclei in papillary lesions and duct hyperplasia. These epithelial cells can be distinguished from myoepithelial cells by their cytologic appearance or their position. Nuclear staining produces a string of dots between the epithelium and the basement membrane in benign ducts and lobules.

Several cytoplasmic markers are available for highlighting the myoepithelium: smooth muscle actin (SMA), smooth muscle myosin-heavy chain (SM M-HC) calponin, and CD 10. These markers exhibit variable cross reactivity with myofibroblasts or blood vessels (21–24). Because of the variable reactivity of these reagents with myoepithelial cells, it is prudent to employ two or more cytoplasmic markers as well as p63 to evaluate the myoepithelium in a given case.

Myoepithelium is highlighted with immunostains in normal ducts and lobules. When proliferative fibrocystic changes occur in these structures, such as adenosis or duct hyperplasia, the myoepithelium is usually uniformly present. Attenuation of myoepithelial cells that occurs in some hyperplasias, especially sclerosing papillary lesions and duct hyperplasia with atypia, results in increased space between p63 reactive nuclei when compared with the staining pattern in normal structures. In this situation the integrity of the myoepithelium can usually be demonstrated with one of the cytoplasmic markers for these cells. Because of the stromal proliferations that accompany many of these lesions, care must be taken not to mistake myofibroblastic reactivity for myoepithelium. Because myoepithelium per-

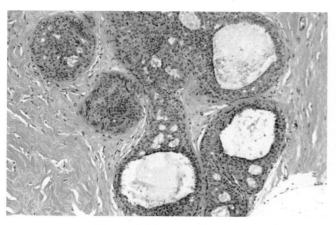

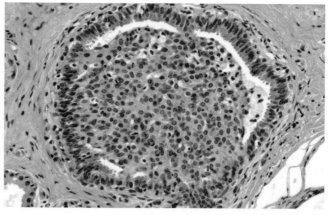

Figure 8.10   Ductal hyperplasia, florid. A: Microlumina and the main duct lumina are apparent in these ducts in a needle core biopsy specimen. **B:** Polypoid florid duct hyperplasia is focally anchored to persisting columnar cell epithelium at the perimeter of this duct.

sists in some examples of intraductal carcinoma, where it can be attenuated or hyperplastic, the presence of this cell layer is not helpful for distinguishing between hyperplasia and intraductal carcinoma. With the exception of some sclerosing papillary lesions, an intraductal proliferation devoid of myoepithelium that is confirmed with more than one marker, in the presence of positive internal controls, is almost certainly in situ carcinoma.

Collagenous spherulosis is a special form of duct hyperplasia wherein myoepithelial cells contribute to the formation of nodular subepithelial deposits of basement membrane material akin to those found in adenoid cystic carcinoma (Fig. 8.12). The center of the spherule may be degenerated so that it resembles a glandular lumen. Immunostains will demonstrate myoepithelial cells around spherules and distinguish these structures from coexisting

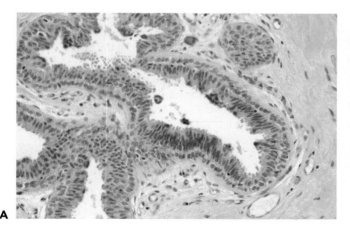

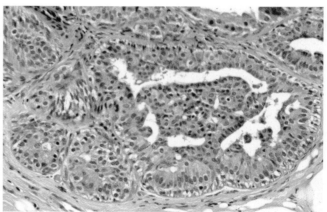

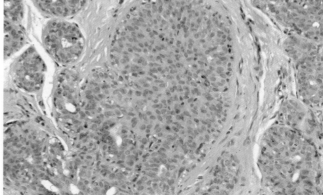

Figure 8.11   Ductal hyperplasia with myoepithelial cells. Three different samples with progressively more florid epithelial hyperplasia and diminishing myoepithelial cell hyperplasia. **A:** Columnar cell hyperplasia with prominent myoepithelium. **B:** Papillary hyperplasia with persisting myoepithelium. **C:** Solid hyperplasia with inconspicuous myoepithelium.

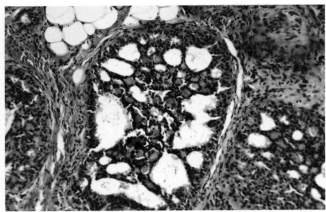

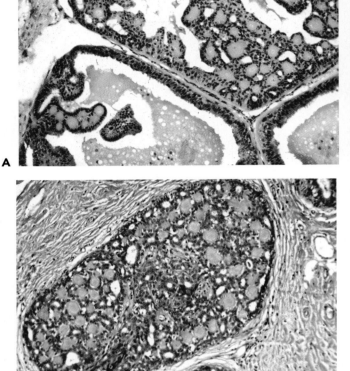

Figure 8.12 **Ductal hyperplasia with collagenous spherulosis.** Three patterns of hyperplasia with collagenous spherulosis. **A:** Papillary growth with prominent eosinophilic spherules. **B:** Cribriform hyperplasia with small spherules amidst the microlumina. **C:** Solid papillary hyperplasia with prominent spherules.

true glandular lumina in cribriform hyperplasia and from the lumina in cribriform intraductal carcinoma.

Pathology of Atypical Ductal Hyperplasia

There is broad agreement on the general description of atypical ductal hyperplasia as a proliferative lesion that fulfills some but not all criteria for a diagnosis of intraductal carcinoma. The difficulty in arriving at a more crisp definition lies in the specifics. In general, these can be considered under two headings: quantitative and qualitative. The former refers to the amount of a proliferative abnormality while the latter is concerned with microscopic structural and cytologic details.

Quantitative criteria for distinguishing between ductal hyperplasia and intraductal carcinoma have been based on the number of duct cross sections that exhibit the abnormality or the dimension of the affected area. Some investigators have classified proliferative lesions limited to a single duct as atypical ductal hyperplasia, even if the abnormality is qualitatively consistent with intraductal carcinoma (10). On the basis of a criterion requiring at least two fully involved duct cross sections for a diagnosis of intraductal carcinoma, cases are arbitrarily assigned to the category of atypical hyperplasia when only one qualitatively diagnostic duct is present.

Another scheme emphasizes the microscopic dimensions of a lesion as one of the bases for a diagnosis of atypical ductal hyperplasia (25). According to this criterion, foci measuring less than 2 mm are diagnosed as atypical ductal hyperplasia, regardless of the number of duct cross sections, even if the individual ducts qualify as intraductal carcinoma. The 2-mm criterion was selected because ". . . it was at the level of one or more small ducts or ductules measuring around 2 mm in aggregate cross-sectional diameter that most pathologists felt hesitant in diagnosing a lesion as intraductal carcinoma" (26). Another explanation offered by the proponents of this criterion was that "questions about quantity are raised generally when dispersed lesions add up to from 1.6 to 2.7 mm in aggregate size. Therefore, we arbitrarily chose 2 mm as a cutoff point" (25).

No scientific studies have compared the clinical significance of different quantitative criteria for the diagnosis of atypical duct hyperplasia. There is no *a priori* reason for choosing two duct cross sections or 2 mm as critical decision points in relation to risk. For example, no data exist for the risk to develop subsequent carcinoma in patients whose biopsies contained proliferative lesions qualitatively consistent with intraductal carcinoma limited to one, two, or three duct cross sections, respectively. Regarding the dimensions of these lesions, no analysis comparing foci measuring 1.5 mm, 2.0 mm, 2.5 mm, or larger has been reported.

A number of technical issues hamper the application of quantitative criteria, especially in the diagnosis of needle core biopsy findings. What appear to be two contiguous cross sections may prove in serial sections to be part of a single duct, or deeper sections of what appears to be a single

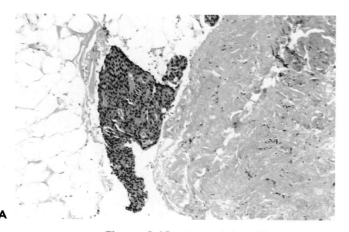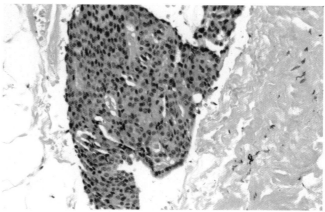

Figure 8.13 **Atypical ductal hyperplasia. A, B:** This needle core biopsy specimen included a detached fragment of nearly solid proliferative duct epithelium.

duct lesion may uncover additional involved duct cross sections. How close must two duct cross sections be to be considered contiguous? Is stroma between duct cross sections included in the measurement? Quantitative criteria assume that the ducts in question have been sectioned perpendicular to their long axis. How to assess ducts cut longitudinally has not been adequately addressed. If the longitudinal dimension of a duct in a section exceeds 2 mm but the transverse diameter is 1 mm, should this focus be considered intraductal carcinoma when employing the 2-mm criterion?

Others have rejected quantitative factors in the diagnosis of atypical ductal hyperplasia. This position was elaborated by Fisher et al. (27) who stated that "our definition of atypical ductal hyperplasia consists of a ductal epithelial alteration approximating but not unequivocally satisfying the criteria for a diagnosis of DCIS. It does not include arbitrarily established quantities of unequivocal DCIS (less than 2.0 mm or 2 'spaces')." In their study of the prognostic significance of proliferative breast "disease," Bodian et al.

(9) reported that "during the course of many years, intraductal carcinoma has been diagnosed if the characteristic features are present in only one ductal space."

The role of quantitative factors in the diagnosis of proliferative ductal lesions seems to lie between these extremes. The use of rigid criteria such as 2 duct cross sections or 2 mm, can be justified in a research setting to ensure a homogeneous study group or to assess a particular criterion, but the strict application of these arbitrary rules in a clinical setting is difficult for technical reasons stated earlier and poorly substantiated by existing data. Given the limitations of current methods for diagnosing intraductal lesions, quantitative factors sometimes play a role in the assessment of a particular lesion in material obtained in a needle core biopsy. This situation arises when the biopsy specimen contains detached fragments of cytologically atypical epithelium (Fig. 8.13), or when only part of one duct with changes suggestive of intraductal carcinoma is represented (Figs. 8.14–8.17). The same issue arises when

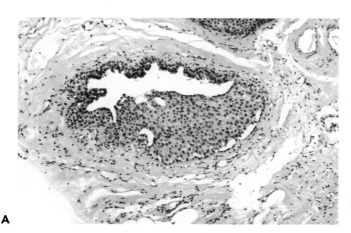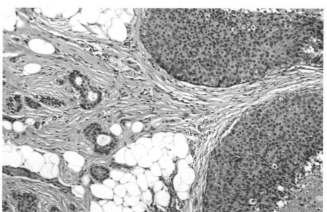

Figure 8.14 **Atypical ductal hyperplasia. A:** The needle core biopsy specimen from this patient contained this duct that is partly occupied by a solid epithelial proliferation of monomorphic cells. Myoepithelial cells are apparent around the upper perimeter of the duct. This partially involved duct is insufficient evidence for a diagnosis of intraductal carcinoma in a needle core biopsy specimen. **B:** The excisional biopsy specimen revealed intraductal and infiltrating duct carcinoma. The area of intraductal carcinoma shown here has a denser and cytologically more atypical cellular population than does the duct in **(A)**.

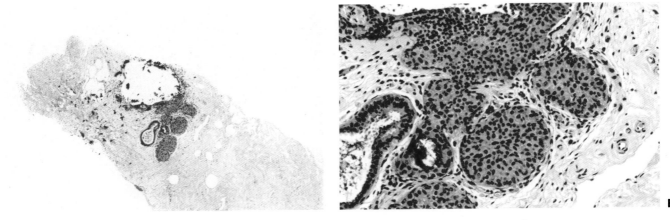

Figure 8.15   Atypical ductal hyperplasia. A, B: This needle core biopsy specimen of mammographically detected calcifications shows solid atypical duct hyperplasia with calcification. The large intraductal calcification was fractured in preparing the slide causing blue-stained fragments to be deposited on the adjacent breast stroma.

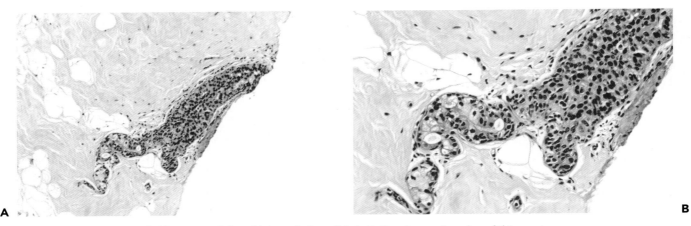

Figure 8.16   Atypical ductal hyperplasia, solid. A, B: The duct at the edge of this specimen was the only significant abnormality in this needle core biopsy specimen. Note the overlapping, hyperchromatic, pleomorphic nuclei and transition to clear cell apocrine change in the narrowest part of the duct. Excisional biopsy yielded a 3-mm focus of atypical duct hyperplasia similar to this duct.

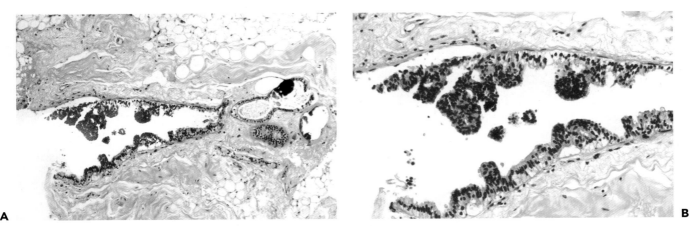

Figure 8.17   Atypical ductal hyperplasia, micropapillary. A, B: Mammographically detected calcifications led to this needle core biopsy specimen. The micropapillae are composed of cells with small, overlapping, hyperchromatic nuclei.

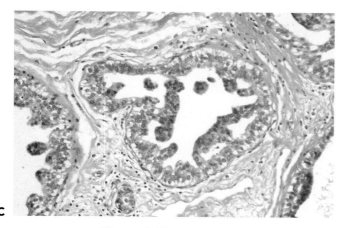

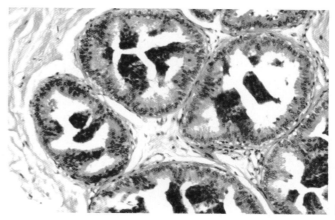

C

D

Figure 8.17 *(continued)* **C, D:** Two other examples of atypical micropapillary hyperplasia with condensation of nuclei in the micropapillae.

a process that suggests lobular extension of ductal carcinoma is present (Fig. 8.18).

In many instances, the diagnosis of atypical duct hyperplasia depends upon the presence of structural elements of intraductal carcinoma mingling with hyperplasia. Architecturally, this may be manifested by a cribriform pattern partially involving a duct (Figs. 8.19 and 8.20). These foci feature sharply defined round to ovoid spaces outlined by cells with distinct borders and a rigid arrangement. Atypical duct hyperplasia can have a solid growth pattern. Micropapillary and true papillary foci involving hyperplastic ducts constitute other architectural manifestations of atypical ductal hyperplasia (Fig. 8.21). Atypical hyperplasia can be encountered in ducts exhibiting apocrine metaplasia (Figs. 8.21 and 8.22). Cytologic atypia may involve individual cells, groups of cells, or the entire population of a proliferative lesion. Atypical features include nuclear enlargement with an increased nuclear-to-cytoplasmic ratio,

nuclear hyperchromasia, an irregular chromatin pattern, mitoses, and the presence of enlarged, pleomorphic nucleoli (Fig. 8.23).

The most challenging atypical ductal proliferations, sometimes referred to as "borderline" lesions, feature marked cytologic and architectural atypia. Most of these foci retain a minor characteristic of hyperplasia, such as persistent columnar ductal epithelium or nuclear overlap, with a structure otherwise typical of intraductal carcinoma (Figs. 8.23–8.25). These slight variations will be disregarded by observers who classify the lesions as intraductal carcinoma, whereas others may diagnose atypical hyperplasia. Similarly, those who place credence in quantitative criteria will diagnose atypical hyperplasia because the extent of a lesion is not sufficient, while others, not adhering to these rules, will diagnose intraductal carcinoma.

Insufficient emphasis has been placed on diagnosing specific proliferative lesions in the context of the overall spectrum

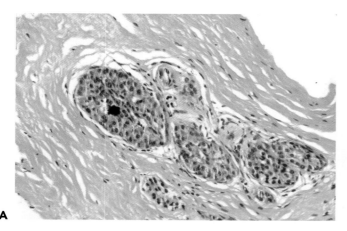

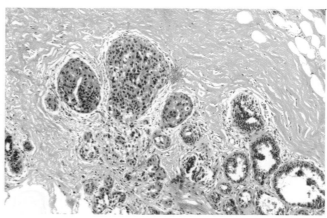

A

B

Figure 8.18 **Atypical ductal hyperplasia, lobular extension.** Shown are two foci of intralobular proliferation that raise concern about lobular extension of intraductal carcinoma. **A:** A thin layer of persistent glandular epithelium outlines a narrow, slit-shaped lumen next to a calcification in the largest lobular gland. Solid intraductal carcinoma was found in the excisional biopsy specimen. **B:** An irregular proliferation of cells with apocrine differentiation fills three lobular glands in this needle core biopsy specimen. Excisional biopsy revealed foci of atypical apocrine ductal hyperplasia.

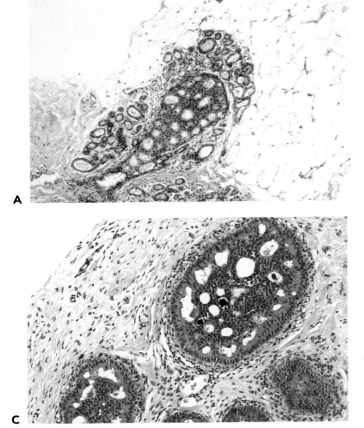

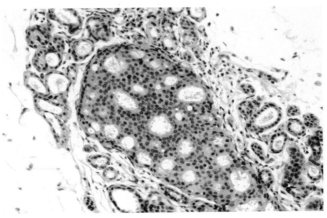

Figure 8.19 Atypical ductal hyperplasia, cribriform. A, B: The only proliferative abnormality in the needle core biopsy specimen in this case was one focus of cribriform proliferation in an intralobular duct. Part of the duct shown **(A)** is not involved by the hyperplasia, (lower left) and it does not extend into lobular glands. Sclerosing adenosis with calcifications was found in the excisional biopsy specimen. **C:** Atypical cribriform hyperplasia with calcifications in another case.

of histologic changes in a biopsy specimen. In a research setting, a pathologist can be required to make a diagnosis that is based only on one or more selected foci on a single slide. This situation, duplicated to a large extent in assessing needle core biopsies, is different from the circumstances under which the various diagnostic criteria were originally developed by reviewing multiple histologic sections (10,25,27). When faced with an atypical ductal proliferative lesion in a needle core biopsy specimen, the pathologist should obtain serial sections of the specimen and, if they are available, slides from previous biopsy

samples should be reviewed for comparison. The diagnosis of "borderline" intraductal proliferations is best made in the context of the spectrum of pathologic changes present in current and prior specimens. A focus of concern may be found to be substantially more atypical and different qualitatively from the overall proliferative level in a given case, or it may prove to be part of a spectrum of changes lacking distinct histologic boundaries. The former situation would tend to support a diagnosis of intraductal carcinoma in the lesional area, whereas the latter suggests atypical hyperplasia.

Columnar Cell Lesions

Proliferative alterations of the duct–lobular complex have become the subject of closer scrutiny as a result of the widespread use of needle core biopsy procedures to sample mammographically detected lesions. Lubelsky et al. (28) reported that 21% of needle core biopsy specimens obtained for calcifications in mammographically screened women had columnar cell lesions (CCLs). These abnormalities are now recognized as being part of a spectrum of lesions described by the terms *columnar cell change* (CCC) *or columnar cell hyperplasia* (CCH) (29,30) and flat epithelial atypia (FEA) (31). Other more cumbersome names that have been offered include atypical cystic lobules (32), cancerization of lobules and atypical ductal hyperplasia adjacent to ductal carcinoma in situ (DCIS) (33), and columnar alteration with prominent apical snouts and secretions (CAPSS) (34).

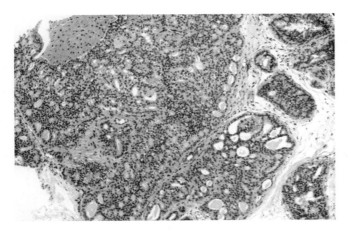

Figure 8.20 Atypical ductal hyperplasia, cribriform. The florid atypical hyperplasia in this needle core biopsy specimen from a solid papillary lesion has areas of cribriform microlumen formation.

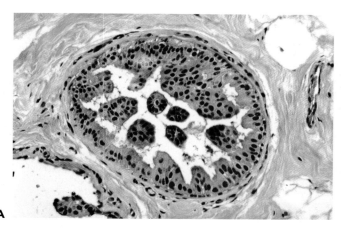
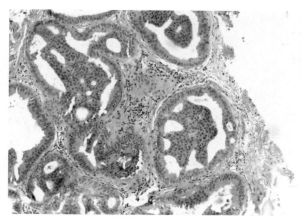

Figure 8.21   Atypical ductal hyperplasia, micropapillary, and cribriform. A: Crowded, multilayered cells in atypical columnar cell duct hyperplasia. Crowding and hyperchromasia of shrunken nuclei at the tips of some micropapillae is apparent in this duct. The cells have apocrine cytoplasm and, there is a ring of evenly spaced ductal cell nuclei at the periphery of the duct. **B:** A monomorphic population of cells forms bridges across these ducts, creating cribriform microlumens. Epithelium at the perimeter of each duct consists of cuboidal or low columnar cells with evenly spaced, basally oriented nuclei.

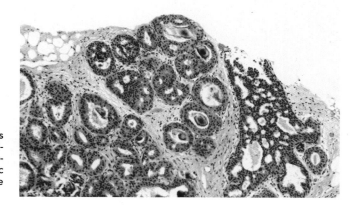

Figure 8.22   Atypical columnar cell ductal hyperplasia. This needle core biopsy procedure was performed for mammographically detected clustered calcifications. The atypical ductal hyperplasia with a columnar cell–cribriform pattern and hyperplastic epithelium in lobular glands shows apocrine differentiation. There are calcifications in the lobular glands.

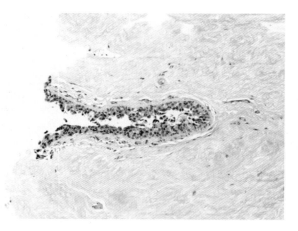
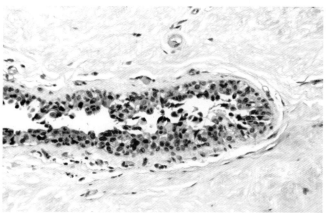

Figure 8.23   Atypical ductal hyperplasia with severe cytologic atypia. A, B: The only proliferative abnormality in this needle core biopsy specimen was this duct at the edge of one tissue sample. The epithelial layer is thickened and composed of cells distributed in a disordered pattern. Many nuclei are hyperchromatic, especially at the luminal border, and there is some nuclear overlap. The proliferation has micropapillary traits.

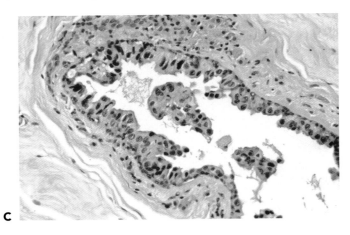

C

Figure 8.23 *(continued)* **C:** The subsequent surgical excision revealed micropapillary intraductal carcinoma with marked nuclear pleomorphism. Periductal reactive changes and vascularity are more pronounced than around the duct in **(B)**, and there is a fully developed micropapillary structure. Note the persistent myoepithelium at the perimeter of the intraductal carcinoma.

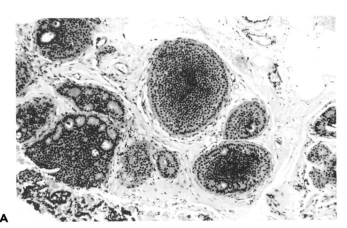

A

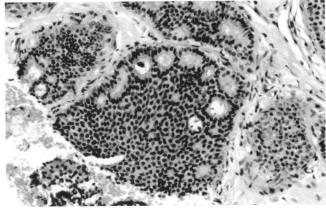

B

Figure 8.24 **Atypical ductal hyperplasia, borderline. A, B:** The ducts in this needle core biopsy specimen have a solid central population of small, monomorphic cells. Microlumina outlined by cells oriented around the rounded fenestrations are present at the periphery of some ducts.

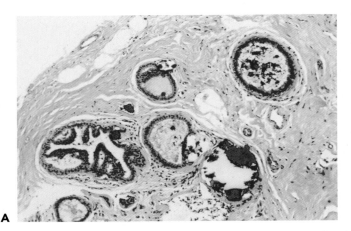

A

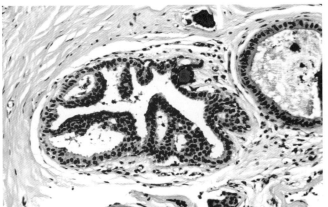

B

Figure 8.25 **Atypical ductal hyperplasia, borderline. A, B:** The needle core biopsy that yielded the specimen containing this lesion was performed for clustered microcalcifications. Calcifications are present in microcysts and the stroma. The proliferation has a micropapillary structure and is composed of cells with condensed, hyperchromatic nuclei. The nonpapillary peripheral epithelium consists of regular cuboidal cells that are indistinguishable from cells lining the adjacent nonproliferative cysts. The micropapillary abnormality was limited to this site.

CCH is a multifocal process that may also be bilateral. It is most often encountered in women 35 to 50 years of age, but CCH can also be present after menopause. CCH rarely produces a palpable abnormality, and it is usually detected mammographically because calcifications are frequently formed, becoming the target of needle core biopsy sampling. The fundamental lesion is localized in terminal duct–lobular units that become enlarged as a result of cystic dilatation.

The simplest form of this process features a thin, flat epithelial layer composed of cuboidal to tall columnar cells distributed in a relatively uniform pattern. Because the nuclei tend to be relatively large, the cells appear crowded and dark. The apical cell surface usually has an apocrine-type cytoplasmic protrusion ("snout") and in some cases this is a prominent feature. In the most banal CCL, that is best termed *columnar cell change*, the epithelium is one to two cells deep and there is little nuclear pleomorphism. Nucleoli and mitotic figures are very rarely found or absent (Fig. 8.26). When present, calcification is in the form of amorphous granular material or discrete basophilic deposits (Fig. 8.27).

The cytologic features of CCLs suggest apocrine differentiation. The cells express gross cystic disease fluid protein-15, an apocrine marker. Ki67 immunoreactivity is low or absent, even in hyperplastic foci (35). The epithelium is also immunoreactive for bcl-2 and estrogen receptor protein that are typically absent in benign apocrine change (35).

CCH is present when the epithelium is more than two cells thick. This is most readily apparent when cellular crowding becomes pronounced and nuclei are not distributed in a single plane relative to the basement membrane. This tendency toward "stacking" of nuclei is usually accompanied by increased nuclear chromasia, and small mounds may be formed in the most cellular regions (Fig. 8.28).

More complex columnar cell-proliferative foci comprise lesions described as *CCH with atypia*. Mild atypia is usually manifested by the presence of small and often isolated foci of micropapillary growth in a background of otherwise usual CCH (Fig. 8.29). The presence of more elaborate growth patterns as well as cytologic atypia characterize CCH with moderate to marked atypia that in its most severe form approaches the appearance of intraductal carcinoma (Figs. 8.30 and 8.31). In some instances, cytologic atypia is more pronounced than the structural abnormalities (Fig. 8.32). When carcinoma arises in CCH, the growth pattern is usually one of the characteristic forms of intraductal carcinoma (Figs. 8.33 and 8.34), but rarely so-called "flat micropapillary" intraductal carcinoma with relatively little epithelial complexity is encountered (Fig. 8.35). Atypical lobular hyperplasia and LCIS frequently accompany columnar cell abnormalities and tubular carcinoma may also be present (Fig. 8.36). Hence, CCLs are part of a triad

Text continues on page 116

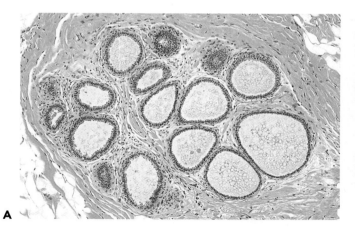

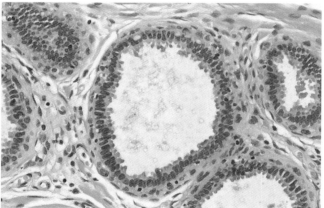

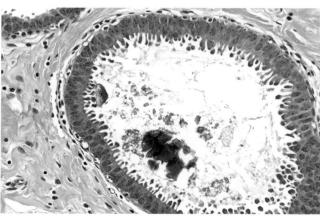

Figure 8.26 Columnar cell change. A: Cystic dilatation of lobular ductules lined by cuboidal and columnar cells with closely approximated, basally oriented nuclei, and luminal cytoplasmic tufts ("snouts"). The dilated structures are embedded in loose, vascularized intralobular stroma. **B:** A magnified view showing the crowded epithelial cells, myoepithelium, and stroma. (From Rosen PP. Ductal hyperplasia: ordinary and atypical. In: Rosen PP, ed. *Breast Pathology*. 2nd ed. Philadelphia, PA: Lippincott, Williams & Wilkins, 2001, with permission.) **C:** Microcystic columnar cell change with luminal cytoplasmic tufts and calcifications.

A

B

C

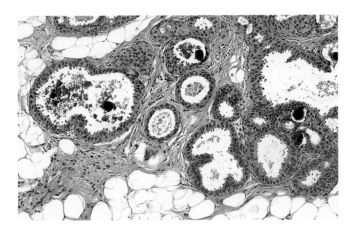

Figure 8.27   Columnar cell change with calcifications. Granular and punctate basophilic calcifications are shown. (From Rosen PP. Ductal hyperplasia: ordinary and atypical. In: Rosen PP, ed. *Breast Pathology*. 2nd ed. Philadelphia, PA: Lippincott, Williams & Wilkins, 2001, with permission.)

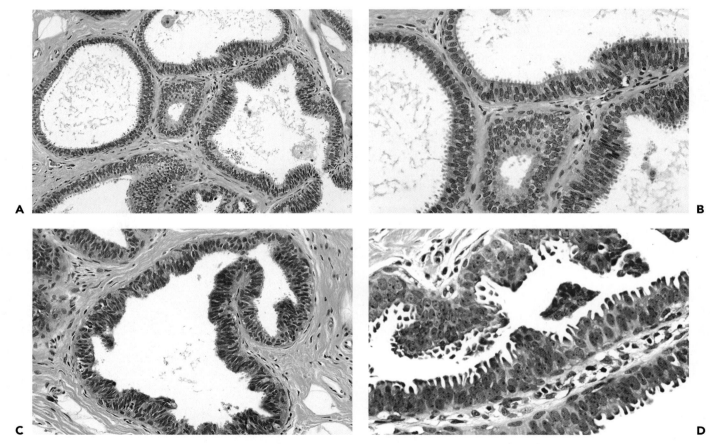

Figure 8.28   Columnar cell hyperplasia. A, B: The thickened epithelium is composed of crowded, columnar cells with overlapping nuclei. **C, D:** Small mounds are formed in the epithelium. (From Rosen PP. Ductal hyperplasia: ordinary and atypical. In: Rosen PP, ed. *Breast Pathology*. 2nd ed. Philadelphia, PA: Lippincott, Williams & Wilkins, 2001, with permission.)

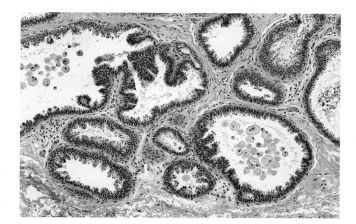

Figure 8.29   Columnar cell hyperplasia, mild atypia. Focal blunt micropapillary proliferation of the hyperplastic columnar cell epithelium. Histiocytes are present in the lumens. (From Rosen PP. Ductal hyperplasia: ordinary and atypical. In: Rosen PP, ed. *Breast Pathology.* 2nd ed. Philadelphia, PA: Lippincott, Williams & Wilkins, 2001, with permission.)

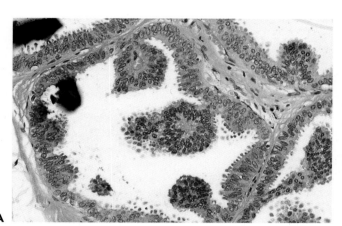

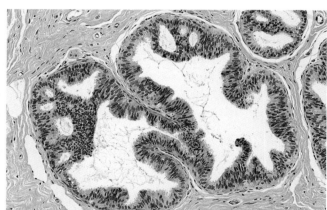

A   B

Figure 8.30   Columnar cell hyperplasia, moderate atypia. A: Atypical micropapillary hyperplasia with calcifications. **B:** Cribriform atypical hyperplasia. (From Rosen PP. Ductal hyperplasia: ordinary and atypical. In: Rosen PP, ed. *Breast Pathology.* 2nd ed. Philadelphia, PA: Lippincott, Williams & Wilkins, 2001, with permission.)

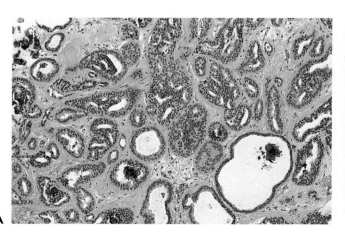

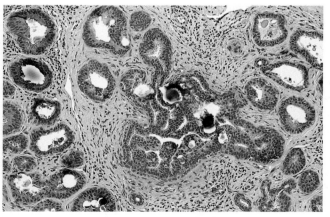

A   B

Figure 8.31   Columnar cell hyperplasia, moderate atypia. A: Cribriform epithelium in ducts surrounded by glands with columnar cell hyperplasia and calcifications. **B:** Papillary hyperplasia in a duct with punctate calcifications. (From Rosen PP. Ductal hyperplasia: ordinary and atypical. In: Rosen PP, ed. *Breast Pathology.* 2nd ed. Philadelphia, PA: Lippincott, Williams & Wilkins, 2001, with permission.)

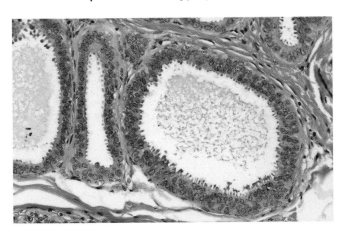

Figure 8.32 Columnar cell hyperplasia with cytologic atypia. The epithelial cells display cytologic atypia. There are no structural abnormalities and no mitoses. (From Rosen PP. Ductal hyperplasia: ordinary and atypical. In: Rosen PP, ed. *Breast Pathology*. 2nd ed. Philadelphia, PA: Lippincott, Williams & Wilkins, 2001, with permission.)

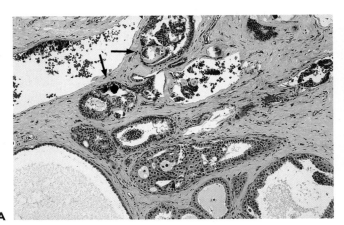

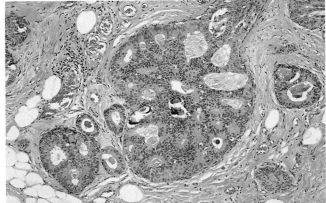

A B

Figure 8.33 Intraductal carcinoma and atypical columnar cell hyperplasia. This needle core biopsy specimen was obtained from a focus of nonpalpable mammographically detected calcifications. **A:** Basophilic and ossifying-type calcifications *(arrows)* are associated with atypical hyperplasia (hematoxylin–phloxine–safranin). **B:** Cribriform intraductal carcinoma was present in the subsequent excisional biopsy specimen. (From Rosen PP. Ductal hyperplasia: ordinary and atypical. In: Rosen PP, ed. *Breast Pathology*. 2nd ed. Philadelphia, PA: Lippincott, Williams & Wilkins, 2001, with permission.)

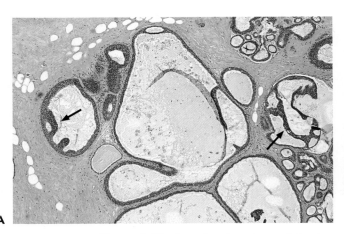

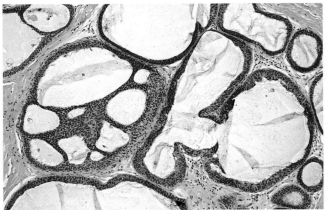

A B

Figure 8.34 Intraductal carcinoma following atypical columnar cell duct hyperplasia. A: An excisional biopsy revealed multifocal, predominantly cystic columnar cell hyperplasia with focal atypia, shown here with micropapillary architecture *(arrows)*. **B:** Four years later, repeat biopsy of the same breast performed for calcifications revealed columnar cell hyperplasia with severe atypia.

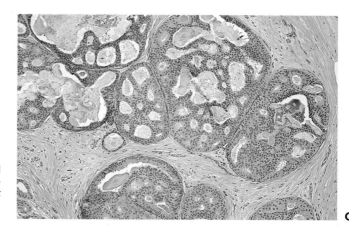

Figure 8.34 *(continued)* **C:** The biopsy specimen also contained this focus of cribriform intraductal carcinoma. (From Rosen PP. Ductal hyperplasia: ordinary and atypical. In: Rosen PP, ed. *Breast Pathology.* 2nd ed. Philadelphia, PA: Lippincott, Williams & Wilkins, 2001, with permission.)

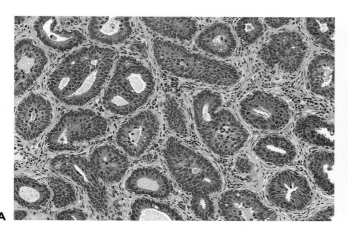

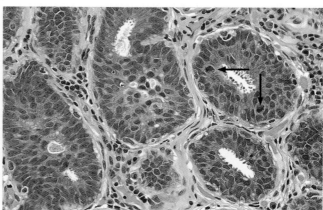

Figure 8.35   Intraductal carcinoma associated with columnar cell duct hyperplasia. A, B: Flat and cribriform intraductal carcinoma with mitoses *(arrows).*

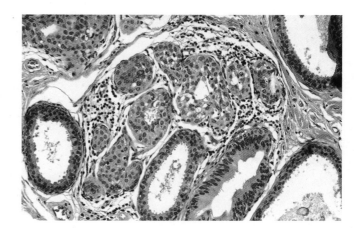

Figure 8.36   Lobular carcinoma in situ associated with columnar cell change. Lobular carcinoma in situ is surrounded by cystic columnar cell change.

that includes lobular neoplasia and tubular carcinoma. All components of this triad are not present in every case.

CCLs develop calcifications that are formed in multiple glands in many of the proliferative sites. Two types of calcifications are encountered: crystalline and ossifying. The crystalline type, usually associated with lesions with less atypia, is deeply basophilic, opaque, round, or angular and prone to fragmentation in the process of histologic sectioning (Figs. 8.27, 8.30, 8.31, 8.33). An ossifying type of calcification usually has a rounded, well-defined contour and an internal structure that resembles an ossifying nodule in which basophilic granular calcific deposits are embedded in lacunar-like spaces within an orangophilic or eosinophilic matrix (Figs. 8.33, 8.37). Ossifying type calcifications occur throughout the range of CCHs, and they appear to develop in the proliferative epithelium, whereas basophilic crystalline deposits are predominantly intraluminal. Both types of calcification can be found in one specimen, and they may occur together in a single proliferative focus.

The proliferative activity of CCLs has been evaluated in the form of Ki67 reactivity (36). The Ki67 index was signif-icantly lower in CCC (mean 0.1%) and CCH without atypia (mean 0.76%) than in normal terminal duct–lobular units (mean 2.4%). The Ki67 indices of CCH with flat atypia (mean 8.2%) and low-grade intraductal carcinoma (8.9%) were not significantly different. The highest Ki67 index was found in intermediate to high-grade intraductal carcinoma (mean 25.5%). If confirmed in a substantially larger series of cases, the Ki67 index could be a helpful adjunctive tool for distinguishing CCH with atypia from some forms of low-grade intraductal carcinoma that arise in CCLs.

Dabbs et al. (37) studied molecular changes in selected microdissected CCLs and found "a gradient of progressive mutational change" between CCC and invasive carcinoma arising in a background of CCLs. Mutational changes manifested as loss of heterozgyosity (LOH) at selected loci were absent from CCC and only rarely found in CCH. Increasing LOH was detected across the spectrum of atypical CCH, intraductal carcinoma, and invasive carcinoma. These results parallel those obtained in noncolumnar cell-proliferative duct lesions (38) and appear to support the concept that atypical duct hyperplasia may, in situations

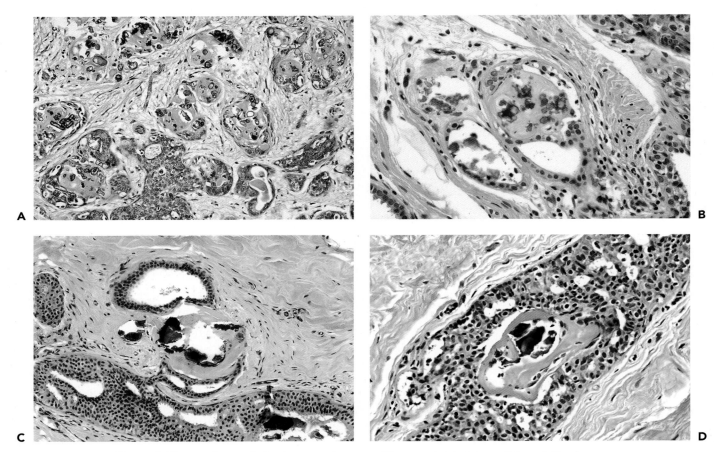

Figure 8.37   Ossifying calcifications in columnar cell lesions. A: Multiple ossifying calcifications in a single proliferative focus. **B:** Fine granules of basophilic calcification are present in the discrete subepithelial eosinophilic nodule. **C:** Basophilic nodular calcification in discrete, subepithelial eosinophilic matrix. (From Rosen PP. Ductal hyperplasia: ordinary and atypical. In: Rosen PP, ed. *Breast Pathology.* 2nd ed. Philadelphia, PA: Lippincott, Williams & Wilkins, 2001, with permission.) **D:** Ossifying calcification in atypical cribriform ductal hyperplasia.

yet to be defined, be a precursor to intraductal and invasive duct carcinoma. The pattern of LOH also parallels the distribution of Ki67 proliferative indices in CCLs.

The management of CCLs found in needle core biopsy specimens obtained for mammographically detected calcifications is uncertain (39). Two issues need to be considered. The first concern is the likelihood that the core biopsy sample is not fully representative of the findings at the time of biopsy. This has been investigated in several studies. Guerra-Wallace et al. (40) evaluated patients who underwent surgical excision after a CCL was found in a needle core biopsy specimen. They reported finding carcinoma in 10 of 135 (7.4%) of women with CCH without atypia and in 11 of 60 (18.3%) with coexisting atypical hyperplasia. Chivukula et al. (41), who referred to atypical CCH as "flat epithelial atypia" (FEA), reported that FEA was detected in 301 of 8054 (3.7%) of needle core biopsy specimens obtained in a 2-year period. Excisional biopsies performed in 270 (90%) of the cases revealed invasive carcinoma in 18 patients (7%) and intraductal carcinoma in 23 (8.5%) patients. Piubello et al. (42) reported that 2 of 10 (20%) excisional biopsies from patients with FEA and atypical duct hyperplasia in a needle core biopsy obtained for calcifications yielded intraductal carcinoma and that invasive carcinoma was found in a third (10%) of patients. In this study, no carcinoma was detected in excisional biopsies from 20 women who had FEA without atypical duct hyperplasia in a prior needle core biopsy specimen. Intraductal carcinoma was found in 1 of 51 (2%) of excisional biopsies performed after a needle core biopsy diagnosis of CCH or FEA without atypical duct hyperplasia reported by Senetta et al. (43).

Intraductal carcinomas associated with CCH and atypical CCH tend to have low nuclear grade, micropapillary, and cribriform architecture and lack necrosis (44). Atypical CCH is significantly related to atypical lobular hyperplasia and LCIS (29,44), and it has been associated with invasive lobular carcinoma (45) as well as tubular carcinoma (29,45,46).

The second issue is the long-term risk for CCLs to evolve into carcinoma. The role of CCLs as precursors to mammary carcinoma was reviewed by Turashvili et al. (47) who concluded that "the natural history of CCLs is currently uncertain in any given patient." In the only currently available long-term follow-up study of a large series of patients with CCLs, Boulos et al. (48) reported a statistically significant slight increased relative risk (RR) for developing breast carcinoma (1.47) when compared with controls with neither proliferative fibrocystic changes nor CCLs. In this study, the RR was not significantly affected by the presence or absence of atypical hyperplasia in the CCL.

With respect to immediate clinical management, the foregoing data support a recommendation to perform an excisional biopsy in a patient found to have a CCL with atypical ductal hyperplasia in a needle core biopsy sample. An excisional biopsy would also be prudent if a needle core biopsy reveals LCIS or atypical lobular hyperplasia coexisting with a CCL without atypical duct hyperplasia.

Clinical circumstances such as the extent and character of mammographically detected calcifications, the presence of a palpable lesion, or a family history of breast carcinoma may play a role in deciding whether to recommend a surgical biopsy if a needle core biopsy reveals a CCL without atypical ductal hyperplasia.

The long-term significance of CCLs with or without atypical ductal hyperplasia for the later development of intraductal or invasive carcinoma remains to be determined. Unfortunately, most studies of the cancer risk attributable to atypical ductal hyperplasia discussed later in this chapter did not distinguish between atypical ductal hyperplasia with and without CCLs. Hence, it is not certain that the elevated cancer risk associated with atypical ductal hyperplasia generally applies equally to CCLs with and without atypical hyperplasia. If the results presented by Boulos et al. (48) are confirmed by other investigators, CCLs may prove to be in a relatively low-risk category. Presently, clinical follow-up with no other intervention is appropriate for the patient whose only abnormality is a nonatypical CCL diagnosed by a needle core biopsy and confirmed by an excisional biopsy or if a nonatypical CCL is found in a needle core biopsy and there are no indications to perform an excisional biopsy. If the needle core biopsy and/or excisional biopsy show atypical ductal hyperplasia or LCIS in conjunction with a CCL, treatment with an antiestrogen may be considered as part of a follow-up program.

Diagnosis of Atypical Ductal Hyperplasia by Needle Core Biopsy

Atypical ductal hyperplasia has been diagnosed in less than 10% of patients subjected to needle core biopsy (7,8,49–52). In four studies consisting of 323 to 900 patients who underwent a needle core biopsy of mammographically detected lesions, the frequencies of atypical ductal hyperplasia were 6.7%, 4.7%, 4.5%, and 4.3% (53–56). Follow-up surgical biopsies were performed on most of the women atypical hyperplasia in these reports. Among women who underwent a surgical biopsy, the reported frequencies of intraductal carcinoma in the excision specimen were 27%, 12.5%, 33%, and 36%. Invasive carcinoma was found in 14%, 12.5%, 0%, and 11% of patients. In these reports, approximately 25% of surgical biopsies revealed additional foci of atypical duct hyperplasia. The yield of significant lesions in the excisional biopsy specimen may be somewhat lower after a needle core biopsy diagnosis of atypical duct hyperplasia if the entire radiologically detected lesion was removed by core biopsy procedure (57). The high frequency of carcinoma detected after a diagnosis of atypical ductal hyperplasia in a needle core biopsy sample dictates that surgical excision should be performed promptly in this setting (8,58).

The reported frequency of atypical duct hyperplasia in vacuum-assisted MRI-directed core biopsies ranges from 3% to 8% (13–15). Among patients with atypical duct hyperplasia detected in vacuum-assisted core biopsy specimens who undergo surgical biopsy, the yield of carcinoma has averaged 34% (15). The higher yield of subsequent carcinoma, sometimes termed *underestimation of atypical ductal hyperplasia*, found in MRI-detected lesions than in mammographically directed biopsies probably reflects the tendency to employ MRI predominantly in women at higher risk for carcinoma. Almost all of the carcinomas found after atypical duct hyperplasia was detected by MRI-directed core biopsy have been intraductal carcinomas.

Because of the limited and often fragmented nature of needle core biopsy specimens, added weight is given to quantitative criteria in assessing these specimens. Pathologists should avoid overinterpreting small biopsy samples because of the expectation that more lesional tissue remains at the biopsy site. In the evaluation of needle core biopsy specimens of breast lesions, especially those which are only evident by mammography, it must be anticipated that the material seen in the needle biopsy sample may be the most extreme and potentially the only abnormality present. Atypical ductal hyperplasia may be diagnosed if detached fragments of abnormal epithelium suggest carcinoma, or if only part of a duct with features of carcinoma is contained in the sample. The importance of quantitative criteria and adequate sampling was documented by Jackman et al. (7) who "progressively increased the average number of core samples obtained per lesion and have found a decrease in both the number of ADH (atypical duct hyperplasia) lesions and the discordance of ADH lesion." The greater success in diagnosis was attributable to more lesions being diagnosed as intraductal carcinoma rather than as atypical ductal hyperplasia as a result of more complete sampling (7). Wagoner et al. (58) reported that the following features of atypical ductal hyperplasia in a needle core biopsy specimen were predictive of finding intraductal carcinoma in the subsequent excision: micropapillary atypical hyperplasia, more than 2 foci of atypical hyperplasia, atypical hyperplasia in multiple samples, and residual mammographic calcifications.

Atypical Ductal Hyperplasia and Breast Carcinoma Risk

The major clinical concern related to usual and atypical intraductal hyperplasia is the risk for the subsequent development of carcinoma. In a minority of women with biopsy findings classified as nonproliferative or proliferative, carcinoma subsequently develops in either breast. The overall proportion of women in whom carcinoma later develops rarely exceeds 10%, even with follow-up of two decades or more. Bodian et al. (9) detected subsequent breast carcinoma in 139 of 1521 patients (9.1%) with biopsy-proven proliferative changes, and in 18 of 278 (6.5%) with nonproliferative biopsies within a follow-up period of 21 years. Overall, 8.7% of the patients developed breast carcinoma. In other reports involving at least 1000 patients, the proportions of women in whom carcinoma developed were 2.2% (59),

4.1% (60), and 4.9% (61). The proportion of patients with subsequent carcinoma tends to increase with the length of follow-up, being highest after follow-up of more than a decade (60,61). This observation is consistent with the rising risk for developing breast carcinoma with advancing age.

The risk for the development of carcinoma subsequent to unilateral biopsy-proven proliferative changes affects both breasts. The bilaterality of risk was noted by Davis et al. (62) in a review of 297 patients with "cystic disease." These authors also tabulated data from 11 articles with at least 100 patients, to show that carcinoma subsequently developed in 0.7% to 4.9% of patients, with 50% of the carcinomas in the contralateral breast.

Krieger and Hiatt (61) found that only 56% of subsequent carcinomas occurred in the previously sampled breast with benign proliferative changes (61). Laterality of subsequent carcinoma was not significantly influenced by the type of antecedent proliferative change or the age at biopsy. The mean interval to subsequent ipsilateral carcinomas (11.2 years) was less than for contralateral carcinomas (14 years). Page et al. (63) reported that 8 of 18 (44%) carcinomas subsequent to atypical duct hyperplasia occurred in the contralateral breast. Involvement of the contralateral breast in a similar proportion of patients was also described by Connolly et al. (64).

The chances for the development of breast carcinoma are influenced by factors that can modify the level of risk associated with benign proliferative changes. Age at diagnosis is inversely related to subsequent risk. Carter et al. (65) found that the rate of subsequent breast carcinoma, when compared with that of normal women, was increased 3.7-fold in women with atypical hyperplasia who were 46–55 years of age and 2.3-fold in women older than 55 years. London et al. (66) also observed an inverse relationship of age and risk, in which the RR increased 2.6-fold among premenopausal women who had biopsy-proven atypia in comparison with postmenopausal subjects.

A history of breast carcinoma among first-degree female relatives is a particularly strong additive factor in women who have atypical hyperplasia. Page et al. (63) and Dupont and Page (67) found that the risk associated with atypical duct hyperplasia in women with a positive family history was more than double that of women without this factor. London et al. (66) also reported that the increased risk associated with family history was strongest in patients with atypical hyperplasia. The RR was not increased by a positive family history in women with nonproliferative biopsies.

Among women who have had a benign result on breast biopsy, the risk for developing subsequent carcinoma is related to the histologic components of the antecedent biopsy. When assessed independently, sclerosing adenosis has been associated with an increased risk in several studies (59,67,68). Some of these investigators reported a greater increase in risk for relatively small groups of women who had atypical hyperplasia coexisting with sclerosing adenosis (67,69).

The proportion of patients who develop carcinoma is highest in the group of women with atypical ductal hyperplasia, intermediate in those with proliferative ductal changes without atypia, and least when there are no proliferative changes. Proliferative changes were identified in 152 (85%) of 1799 biopsies studied by Bodian et al. (9). Moderate-to-severe atypia was present in 70 specimens, representing 3.8% of all cases and 4.6% of specimens with proliferative changes. Follow-up revealed that the RR for the development of carcinoma (in comparison with the general population, represented by the Connecticut Tumor Registry) was higher in women with any proliferative changes (RR of 2.2) than in those with nonproliferative findings on biopsy (RR of 1.6). The RR associated with severe ductal atypia was 3.9. Page et al. (63) found the RR to be 4.7 for women with atypical ductal hyperplasia in comparison with women who had nonproliferative biopsy results. The RR for women with atypical duct hyperplasia and a family history of breast carcinoma was increased further in comparison with women with nonproliferative biopsies and a positive family history (63). Ma and Boyd (68) undertook a meta-analysis of studies that investigated the association between atypical hyperplasia and breast cancer risk. Fifteen reports between 1960 and 1992 fulfilled the authors' requirements for inclusion in the study, resulting in a total sample size of 182,980 women. The overall odds ratio in comparison with controls for the development of carcinoma in women with atypical hyperplasia was 3.67 (95% CI, 3.16–4.26).

INTRADUCTAL CARCINOMA

Frequency of Intraductal Carcinoma

A 1996 review of data included in the National Cancer Institute's Surveillance, Epidemiology, and End Results (SEER) Program demonstrated a striking increase in the incidence of intraductal carcinoma after 1983 (70). Among women 30 to 39 years of age, the average annual increase in the incidence rate changed from 0.3% between 1973 and 1983 to 12.0% between 1983 and 1992. Similar increases were found for women 40 to 49 years (0.4–17.4%) and for women 50 years and older (5.2–18.1%). The estimated total number of cases of intraductal carcinoma in 1992 was 200% higher than expected based on 1983 rates. Further analysis of the SEER data indicated that the estimated number of new cases of intraductual carcinoma in 1993 was 23,275 (71). Review of the records of the Connecticut Tumor Registry revealed a yearly increase in the number of cases in intraductal carcinoma reported (72). In 1979, the 33 diagnoses of intraductal carcinoma represented 1.8% of breast carcinomas, and in 1988 the 200 cases constituted 7.4% of breast carcinomas (72).

The increased age-adjusted incidence of in situ breast carcinoma in the United States coincides with a leveling off in the overall age-adjusted incidence of invasive carcinoma and of localized carcinoma, and a decline in the incidence

of invasive carcinoma classified as "regional" (73). These changes in incidence by stage have been accompanied by a significant decline in age-adjusted breast cancer mortality (73,74). The beneficial effects of mammography as a diagnostic or screening modality and of improved systemic therapy are reflected in these trends.

Clinical Diagnosis of Intraductal Carcinoma

Mammography is a sensitive diagnostic procedure for detecting intraductal carcinoma, a substantial proportion of which is not palpable. Among nonpalpable carcinomas detected by mammography 25% to 30% are intraductal lesions (75–77). Mammographically detected calcifications are found in at least 70% of intraductal carcinomas (76,77). Other radiologic findings that lead to the detection of a lesser proportion of intraductal carcinomas are densities and asymmetric soft-tissue changes, sometimes with microcalcifications. Calcifications alone are more likely to be the mammographic indicator of intraductal carcinoma in women younger than 50 years, whereas coexistent soft-tissue abnormalities are evident more often in women older than 50 years, a distinction that probably results from differences in breast density between these age groups rather than from intrinsic tumor differences (77).

Calcifications associated with intraductal carcinoma are generally described as linear "casts" or as granular in mammograms. Round or oval, well-circumscribed calcifications are less common in intraductal carcinoma. The majority of intraductal carcinomas have five or more calcifications (77).

The mammographic distribution of calcifications has been used as a guide to the extent of intraductal carcinoma or the dimensions of the involved area. However, these measurements may underestimate the size of the lesion when compared with careful histologic sampling (78). When the extent of lesions was measured both mammographically and pathologically, discrepancies were found more often between the interpretations for cases that are predominantly cribriform or micropapillary than for intraductal comedo carcinomas. A discrepancy of more than 20 mm was found in 44% of pure cribriform-micropapillary lesions, in 12% of pure comedo carcinomas, and in 50% of cases with both patterns (78). The likelihood of detecting multifocal intraductal carcinoma radiologically and pathologically is related to the size of the lesion as determined by either procedure. Multifocality is appreciably more frequent in lesions larger than 2.0 to 2.5 cm than in smaller foci of intraductal carcinoma (79).

The mammographic appearance of microcalcifications bears some relationship to the histologic type of the lesion, but as noted by Stomper and Connolly (80), "there is considerable overlap, and the predominant histologic subtype cannot be predicted on the basis of the microcalcification type with a high degree of accuracy." Predominantly linear or "casting-type" calcifications are found significantly more often in comedo carcinomas than in cribriform, papillary, or solid types, which typically contain granular calcifications

(78,80). Nonetheless, 22% of linear calcifications were associated with non-comedo carcinomas, and 47% of granular calcifications occurred in comedo carcinomas in one series (80). The presence of extensive casting-type microcalcifications occupying more than one quadrant in a mammogram was associated with high-grade intraductal carcinoma, multifocal invasive duct carcinoma, and axillary nodal metastases in 33% of 12 patients who had lymph node examined (81).

Abnormal mammogram findings without calcifications are more likely to call attention to intraductal carcinoma of the small cell type than the large cell type, regardless of the growth pattern (solid, cribriform, or mixed) of the lesion (82). Linear calcifications are a marker of necrosis, and small punctate or granular calcifications are associated with intraductal carcinoma without necrosis (82). Intraductal carcinomas that overexpress the HER2/*neu* oncogene are more likely to have calcifications detected by mammography than are HER2/*neu*-negative carcinomas (83).

Intraductal carcinoma in women occurs throughout the age range of breast carcinoma generally. The mean age at diagnosis of patients in multiple studies is between 50 and 59 years. There are no significant differences in the age distribution of structural subtypes of intraductal carcinoma (84).

MRI has proven to be an effective method for detecting intraductal carcinomas especially those that lack calcifications. Menell et al. (85) found that MRI was more sensitive than mammography for detecting intraductal carcinoma overall and for detecting multifocal intraductal carcinoma. Lesion detection is based on the finding of contrast enhancement in breast parenchyma after injection of a gadolinium contrast agent when compared with the preinjection image (86–88). Orel et al. (89) described three patterns of enhancement associated with intraductal carcinoma: ductal, regional, and a peripherally enhancing mass. The mean size of MRI-detected intraductal carcinomas was 10 mm. Correlation of immunohistochemical studies for vascularity and MRI image characteristics of the lesions suggested that tumor angiogenesis contributed to MRI enhancement in one series (86). Contrast-enhanced MRI has proven to be an effective method for the detection of concurrent, unsuspected contralateral carcinoma in women with ipsilateral intraductal carcinoma (90).

Frozen-section Diagnosis of Intraductal Carcinoma

Intraductal carcinoma can be recognized in frozen-section samples from a surgical biopsy but if any difficulty is encountered, the decision should be immediately deferred to permanent sections because there is a significant risk of trimming away the lesional area as more sections are made (Fig. 8.38). In one study of intraductal carcinomas, 50% of

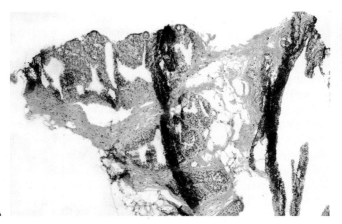

A

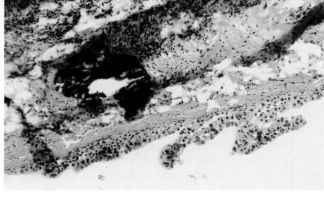

B

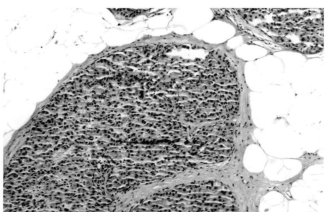

C

Figure 8.38 Intraductal carcinoma, frozen section. The patient had a needle core biopsy procedure for nonpalpable calcifications, and the needle core biopsy sample was submitted for frozen section. **A:** The frozen-section slide has folds and tears. **B:** A displaced calcification is present near the center and a band of atypical cells is present at the lower border of the tissue in the frozen section. The diagnosis was deferred. **C:** Solid intraductal carcinoma with frozen-section artefact in a slide from the paraffin-embedded tissue after examination by frozen section.

the lesions were diagnosed at the time of frozen section, 36% were reported to be benign, 8% were deferred, 5% were diagnosed as atypical hyperplasia, and 1 case was diagnosed as invasive (91). Approximately 3% of biopsies reported to be benign at frozen section prove to contain carcinoma when paraffin sections are examined (92). Because the amount of tissue that can be examined by frozen section during surgery is limited, approximately 20% of patients with a frozen-section diagnosis of intraductal carcinoma prove to have invasion when it is possible to examine multiple paraffin sections of the same biopsy specimen (93). Frozen section is not recommended for the diagnosis of needle core or surgical biopsies of mammographically detected, nonpalpable lesions, unless there are exceptional clinical circumstances.

Pathology of Intraductal Carcinoma

The microanatomic site of origin of many intraductal carcinomas appears to be in the terminal duct–lobular unit, or TDLU. Evidence for this conclusion originally came from the subgross microdissection studies of Wellings et al. (94). Recently characterized CCLs, described earlier in this chapter, lend support to this conclusion. A histologic correlate of this is the presence of the neoplastic process in the epithelium of lobular glands, termed lobular cancerization (Fig. 8.39). Greatly expanded terminal duct–lobular units sometimes resemble primary or secondary segmental ducts, but their lobular origin is suggested by the excessive number of duct structures within a low-power microscopic field and sometimes by the accompanying stroma. The relative frequency of origin from the TDLU and from larger duct structures, and the clinical significance of this distinction remain to be determined.

In standard histologic sections, intraductal carcinoma appears confined within the lumina of ducts and lobules involved in the process. When studied by immunohistochemistry, basement membranes in intraductal carcinomas are intact or focally discontinuous (95). The diagnosis of intraductal carcinoma alone does not apply to lesions in

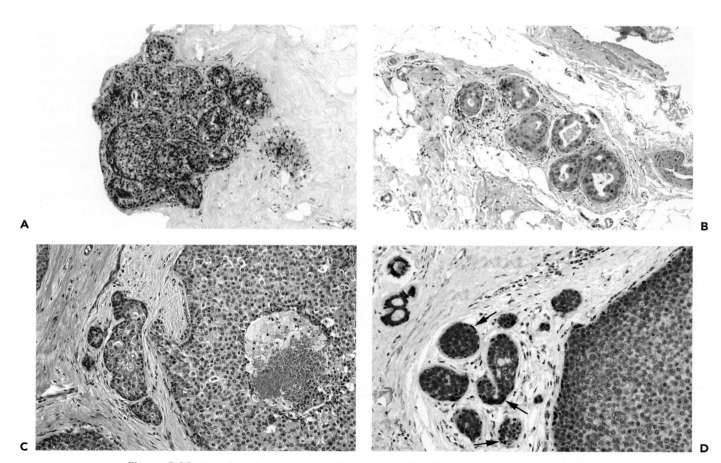

Figure 8.39 **Intraductal carcinoma, lobular extension (lobular cancerization). A:** This enlarged lobular complex at the border of a needle core biopsy specimen is involved by intraductal carcinoma, solid type with poorly differentiated nuclear grade. **B:** Lobular involvement by apocrine intraductal carcinoma in another needle core biopsy specimen. **C, D:** Intraductal carcinoma with central necrosis extending into a lobule in periductal fibrosis. This pattern can be mistaken for microinvasion. In **(D)** myoepithelial cells in the lobules are highlighted by p63 immunostain *(arrows)* (p63: immunoperoxidase; cytokeratin: alkaline phosphatase).

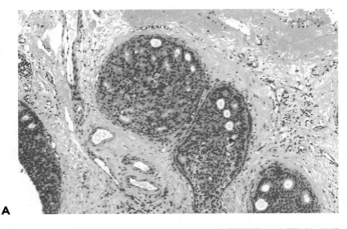

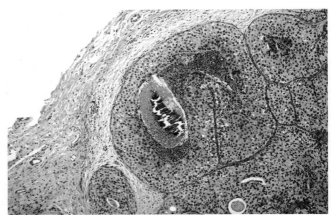

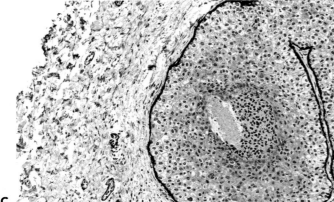

Figure 8.40 Intraductal carcinoma and myoepithelial cells. A: Myoepithelial cells are evident at the perimeter of the flask-shaped duct cross section involved by cribriform intraductal carcinoma. **B, C:** In this needle core biopsy specimen comedo intraductal carcinoma is encircled by myosin-positive **(C)** myoepithelial cells (immunoperoxidase).

which invasive foci are also present, even if the later comprise a minimal portion of the lesion.

The presence or absence of mitotic figures is not a definitive feature in the diagnosis of intraductal carcinoma because infrequent mitoses may also be found in normal lobules and in duct hyperplasia. The finding of numerous mitoses, such as one or more per high power field strongly suggests intraductal carcinoma. Myoepithelial cells are variably retained but attenuated and occasionally hyperplastic at the periphery of a duct involved by intraductal carcinoma (Fig. 8.40). Carcinoma cells at the periphery of the duct exhibit loss of basal polarity as a manifestation of cellular crowding. Rarely, remnants of nonneoplastic normal or hyperplastic duct epithelium persist in ducts involved by intraductal carcinoma (Fig. 8.41).

A range of cell types are found in intraductal carcinomas. Certain distinct variants have been identified and described by specific names. *Signet ring cells*, usually associated with lobular carcinoma, also occur in intraductal carcinomas, most often in the papillary and cribriform types (Fig. 8.42). Signet ring cells have eccentric nuclei that may be often indented by a cytoplasmic mucin vacuole. A minute droplet of secretion may be apparent in the vacuole. Intracytoplasmic mucin sometimes imparts a diffuse pale blue color to the cytoplasm without forming distinct vacuoles (Fig. 8.43). Clear holes in the cytoplasm can be mistaken for signet ring vacuoles. These cytoplasmic

defects, sometimes the site of glycogen accumulation, are not reactive with the mucicarmine stain, they do not indent the nucleus, and there is ordinarily no secretion evident in the lumen.

Clear cell intraductal carcinoma is a poorly defined variant typically encountered with solid and comedo patterns. Some clear cell intraductal carcinomas are composed of cells with an arrangement described as *mosaic* because of the appearance created by sharply defined cell borders (Fig. 8.44). A subset of lesions that are classified under this

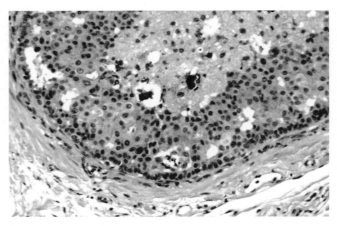

Figure 8.41 Intraductal carcinoma. Microlumina are present at the perimeter of the duct with central necrosis and calcifications.

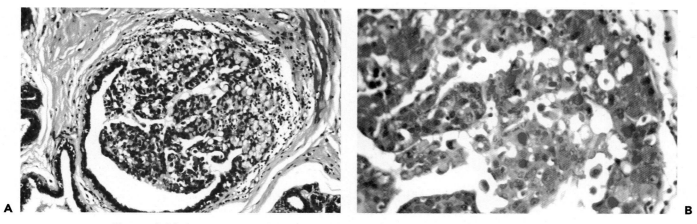

Figure 8.42 Intraductal carcinoma, signet ring cells. A: Papillary intraductal carcinoma with signet ring cells. **B:** The intracytoplasmic mucin is stained magenta with the mucicarmine stain.

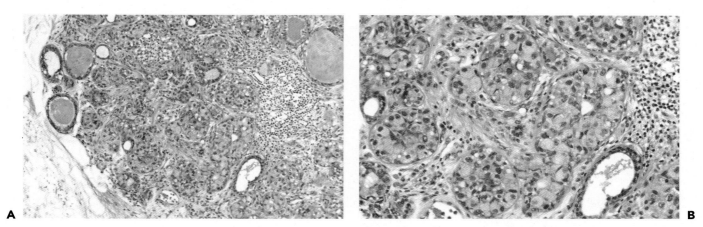

Figure 8.43 Intraductal carcinoma, intracytoplasmic mucin. A, B: Intraductal carcinoma in sclerosing adenosis in a needle core biopsy specimen. The cells have pale blue cytoplasm that was reactive with the mucicarmine stain.

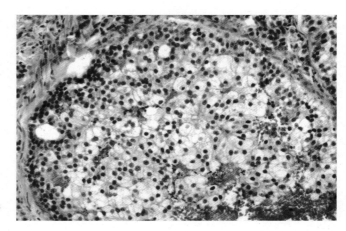

Figure 8.44 Intraductal carcinoma, clear cell type. The cells have sharply defined borders and low-grade nuclei.

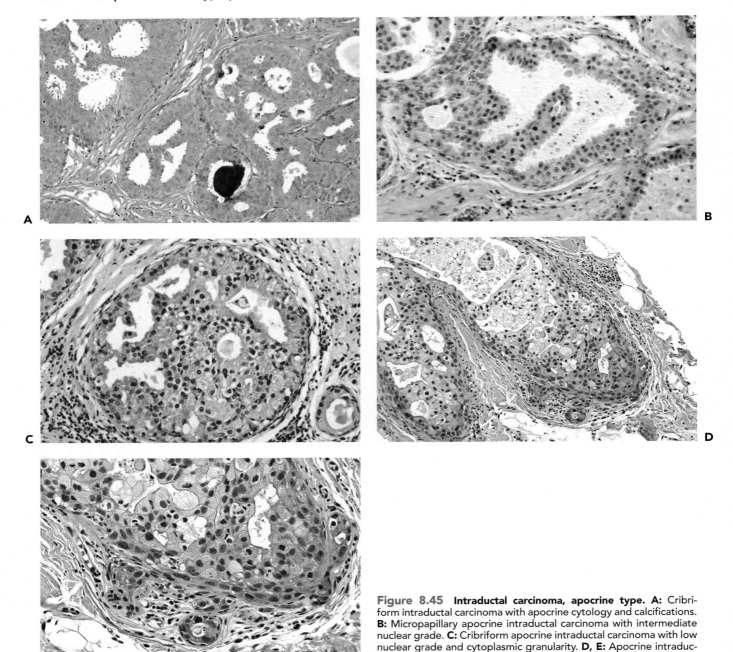

Figure 8.45 Intraductal carcinoma, apocrine type. A: Cribriform intraductal carcinoma with apocrine cytology and calcifications. **B:** Micropapillary apocrine intraductal carcinoma with intermediate nuclear grade. **C:** Cribriform apocrine intraductal carcinoma with low nuclear grade and cytoplasmic granularity. **D, E:** Apocrine intraductal carcinoma with clear cell change and lobular extension.

heading are a form of apocrine carcinoma. Occasionally, clear cell intraductal carcinomas have strongly mucicarmine positive cytoplasm. The presence of a monomorphic clear cell population in a ductal proliferative lesion is highly suggestive of intraducal carcinoma. Other clear cell lesions are the in situ forms of lipid-rich or glycogen-rich carcinomas discussed in Chapter 20. *Apocrine* cytology is encountered in all of the structural types of intraductal carcinoma (Figs. 8.39, 8.45). These cells have abundant cytoplasm that ranges from granular and eosinophilic to vacuolated or clear. There is variable nuclear pleomorphism, sometimes manifested by prominent nucleoli.

Spindle cell intraductal carcinomas may express neuroendocrine markers such as chromogranin, synaptophysin, and neuron specific enolase (96) (Fig. 8.46). The swirling growth pattern of cells in spindle cell intraductal carcinoma mimics "streaming" that is characteristically found in usual duct hyperplasia. Spindle cell intraductal carcinoma often coexists with cribriform intraductal carcinoma.

The expression of neuroendocrine markers can be found in intraductal carcinomas with non-spindle cell cytology and with various growth patterns. Kawasaki et al. (97) found neuroendocrine marker expression in 20 of 294 (6.8%) of intraductal carcinomas. The diagnosis of

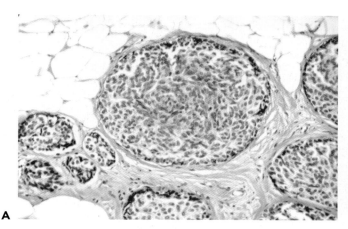
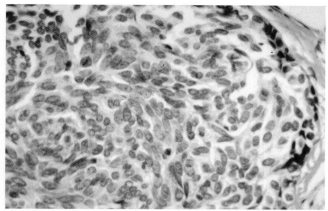

Figure 8.46 **Intraductal carcinoma, spindle cell type. A, B:** The swirling spindle cell proliferation mimics the streaming pattern of ductal hyperplasia. The monomorphic spindle cells extend to the perimeter of the duct in this needle core biopsy specimen.

neuroendocrine intraductal carcinoma was made when at least 50% of the tumor cells expressed chromogranin A and/or synaptophysin. Neuroendocrine intraductal carcinomas had a significantly higher frequency of presentation with bloody nipple discharge (72%) than non-neuroendocrine intraducal carcinomas (5%). Most of the lesions had solid papillary or papillary architecture with low nuclear grade in 90% and an absence of calcifications in 75%. Neuroendocrine intraductal carcinomas tended to express estrogen and progesterone receptors and not to overexpress HER2/neu.

Small cell intraductal carcinoma is extremely uncommon (Fig. 8.47). The growth patterns are typically cribriform and solid or a mixture of these forms. When present by itself, the solid pattern can be distinguished from LCIS with the E-cadherin immunostain. Membrane reactivity will be present in intraductal carcinoma and absent or fragmented and weak in the lobular lesion.

The cellular composition of intraductal carcinomas is usually described as *monomorphic*, a term applied especially to cribriform, solid, and micropapillary carcinomas. In this context, monomorphic means that there is overall homogeneity in the cytologic appearance of the lesion, although the cells are not always identical in such features as the amount of cytoplasm or nuclear size. Cell and nuclear shape may be altered by the presence or absence of crowding in one or another part of the duct. The presence of a myoepithelial cell layer is not a consideration in judging whether a ductal proliferation is monomorphic. Dimorphic variants of intraductal carcinoma, consisting of two distinctly different populations of cells, are unusual (Fig. 8.47).

Intraductal carcinoma in a given patient can have more than a single microscopic structural, cytologic, or immunocytochemical phenotype (84). Mixed histologic patterns are found in 30% to 40% of cases. Whereas some structural combinations, such as papillary– or micropapillary–

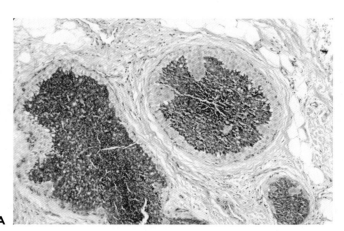
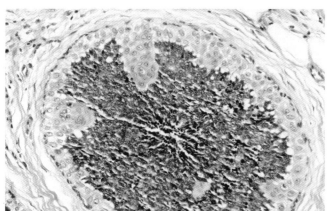

Figure 8.47 **Intraductal carcinoma, small cell type. A, B:** This extraordinary lesion consists of a central nearly syncytial mass of small undifferentiated carcinoma cells and an outer zone of larger polygonal cells. Two protruding mounds of large cells show apical traces of squamous differentiation, a feature that was more pronounced in other ducts. Persistent myoepithelial cells that were immunoreactive for actin are represented by the small dark elongated nuclei at the outer border of the duct.

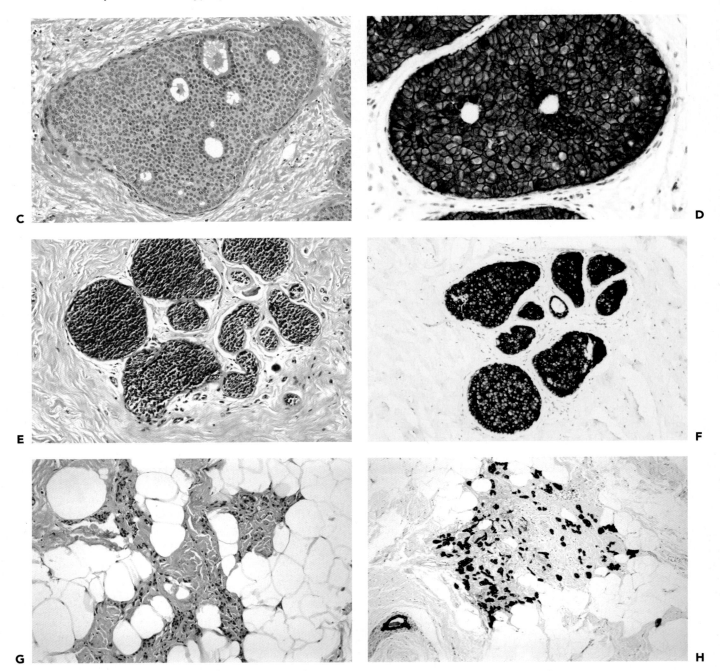

Figure 8.47 *(continued)* **C, D:** Solid, small cell intraductal carcinoma with cribriform microlumina. This growth pattern and cytologic appearance could be mistaken for pagetoid spread of lobular carcinoma in situ in a duct. All cells were strongly E-cadherin positive **(D)** (immunoperoxidase). **E–H:** Small cell intraductal carcinoma in a lobule **(E)** with microinvasion **(G)** that resembles lobular carcinoma. The in situ **(F)** and invasive **(H)** components were E-cadherin positive (immunoperoxidase).

cribriform and solid–comedo, occur relatively more often than others, there is considerable heterogeneity with respect to growth patterns (98). The probability of structural variability increases with the size of the lesion, a phenomenon that must be considered in using needle core biopsy for the subclassification of a mammographically detected intraductal carcinoma.

Cytologic features, especially at the nuclear level, tend to be more homogeneous than the growth pattern in a given case. Some combinations of growth patterns and cytologic appearances occur more frequently, such as classic comedo intraductal carcinoma, composed of poorly differentiated, pleomorphic cells with necrosis, or the low nuclear grade typically present in micropapillary intraductal carcinoma. However, the considerable range of heterogeneity is illustrated by lesions composed of small, cytologically low-grade nuclei growing in a solid pattern with central comedo necrosis, and others having a micropapillary pattern composed of cells with high-grade nuclei found in some examples of clinging intraductal carcinoma.

In a 1997 consensus report (99), nuclear grade was stratified into three categories (Table 8.1). Pleomorphic nuclei of similar size were not consistent with low nuclear grade. The pathology report should reflect the highest nuclear grade but may indicate the relative proportions of grade when there is heterogeneity. *Necrosis* was defined as the "presence of ghost cells and karyorrhectic debris" (Table 8.2). Five architectural patterns were identified: micropapillary, cribriform, solid, comedo, papillary. It was specified that comedo referred "to solid intraepithelial growth within the basement membrane with central (zonal) necrosis. Such lesions are often but not invariably high nuclear grade".

Micropapillary intraductal carcinoma consists of ducts lined by a layer of neoplastic cells that give rise intermittently to slender papillary fronds or arcuate formations that protrude into the duct lumen (Figs. 8.40, 8.45, 8.48). The papillae are variable in appearance, ranging from blunt bumps or mounds to pronounced slender, elongated processes. They almost all lack a fibrovascular core and are composed of cytologically homogenous carcinoma cells. Arcuate structures, commonly referred to as "Roman bridge arches," occur when microlumens are formed beneath adjacent coalescent fronds or within a mound of neoplastic cells. These fenestrations resemble the lumens formed in cribriform intraductal carcinoma. In conjunc-

TABLE 8.1
CONSENSUS COMMITTEE RECOMMENDATION FOR NUCLEAR GRADING OF INTRADUCTAL CARCINOMA

Low nuclear grade (NG1)
Monomorphic (monotonous) appearance
Size of duct epithelial nuclei or 1.5–2.0 normal red blood cells
Chromatin diffuse, finely dispersed
"Occasional nucleoli and mitoses"
Cells usually polarized
High nuclear grade (NG3)
"Markedly pleomorphic"
Size usually more than 2.5 duct epithelial nuclei
Chromatin vesicular with irregular distribution
"Prominent, often multiple nucleoli"
"Mitoses may be conspicuous"
Intermediate nuclear grade (NG2)
"Nuclei that are neither NG1 nor NG3"

Based on The Consensus Conference Committee. Consensus Conference on the classification of ductal carcinoma in situ. *Cancer* 1997;80:1798–1802, with permission.

TABLE 8.2
CONSENSUS COMMITTEE RECOMMENDATION FOR REPORTING NECROSIS IN INTRADUCTAL CARCINOMA

Comedo necrosis

"Central zone necrosis within a duct, usually exhibiting a linear pattern within ducts if sectioned longitudinally"

Punctate

"Nonzonal type necrosis (foci of necrosis that do not exhibit a linear pattern if longitudinally sectioned)"

Based on The Consensus Conference Committee. Consensus Conference on the classification of ductal carcinoma in situ. *Cancer* 1997;80:1798–1802, with permission.

tion with micropapillae, they are a feature of micropapillary intraductal carcinoma (Table 8.3).

The appearance of the micropapillary fronds varies somewhat with the plane of individual histologic sections. Whereas some micropapillae are cut perpendicular to their long axis, others are seen sectioned tangentially or transversely, resulting in irregular nests of seemingly detached cell clusters in the duct lumen (Fig. 8.48). Aside from the epithelial proliferation, ducts with low nuclear grade micropapillary intraductal carcinoma are usually relatively free of cellular debris or inflammatory cells, but they may contain calcifications.

Micropapillary intraductal carcinoma is usually composed of cytologically low-grade, small homogeneous cells with a high nuclear-to-cytoplasmic ratio and dark nuclei (Fig. 8.48). The nuclei typically vary little in size and chromatin density between cells at the base and tip of micropapillae. They may be slightly smaller and darker at the surface, but marked disparity in these characteristics is a feature of micropapillary hyperplasia. At the margin of the duct, between papillary and arcuate structures, the neoplastic cells typically form a thin layer one to not more than three or four cells deep. Persistent nonneoplastic epithelium between micropapillae is a feature of micropapillary hyperplasia rather than micropapillary carcinoma. Mitoses are rarely evident in low-grade micropapillary intraductal carcinoma. In most instances, the cells are so crowded that their individual borders and cytoplasm cannot be identified. Occasionally, the cells have slightly more abundant cytoplasm, with apocrine-type protrusions at the luminal border. In one variant of this cell type, the nuclei of the tumor cells are contained in cytoplasmic blebs that are extruded into the duct lumen. Clear cell change and squamous metaplasia are rarely seen in micropapillary intraductal carcinoma.

A minority of carcinomas with a micropapillary structural phenotype are composed of cells with intermediate- or high-grade (poorly differentiated) cytologic characteristics (see Figs. 8.45, 8.48). This type of micropapillary carci-

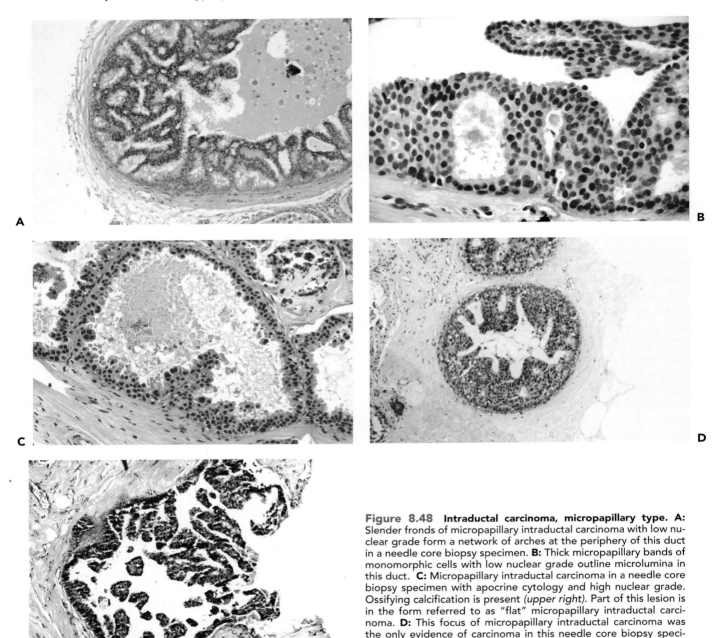

Figure 8.48   Intraductal carcinoma, micropapillary type. A: Slender fronds of micropapillary intraductal carcinoma with low nuclear grade form a network of arches at the periphery of this duct in a needle core biopsy specimen. *(upper right)*. **B:** Thick micropapillary bands of monomorphic cells with low nuclear grade outline microlumina in this duct. **C:** Micropapillary intraductal carcinoma in a needle core biopsy specimen with apocrine cytology and high nuclear grade. Ossifying calcification is present *(upper right)*. Part of this lesion is in the form referred to as "flat" micropapillary intraductal carcinoma. **D:** This focus of micropapillary intraductal carcinoma was the only evidence of carcinoma in this needle core biopsy specimen. **E:** Micropapillary intraductal carcinoma at the inked margin of a needle core biopsy specimen.

noma tends to occur in women 35 to 50 years of age. It is multifocal and sometimes bilateral. The microscopic foci are mainly localized in terminal duct–lobular units. Cells forming this type of carcinoma differ from those in conventional micropapillary lesions in that they are larger, with more abundant cytoplasm. Nuclei are also correspondingly larger, and nucleoli may be apparent. Mitoses can be seen in this epithelium, and the cells often have a distinctly apocrine appearance. This cytologically high-grade form of micropapillary intraductal carcinoma is more likely to have calcifications than the low-grade variant, and necrotic cellular debris may be found in the duct

lumen. Florid micropapillary proliferation tends to result in fusion of the epithelial fronds and the formation of cribriform microlumina. Consequently, it is not unusual to find intraductal carcinomas with a combination of micropapillary and cribriform features.

Two unusual subtypes of micropapillary intraductal carcinoma have been given specific designations. *Cystic hypersecretory intraductal carcinoma* is discussed in Chapter 19. The term *flat micropapillary carcinoma* (clinging carcinoma) refers to intraductal carcinoma with the cytologic appearance of the micropapillary lesion that is lacking in fully developed epithelial fronds. Lesions composed entirely of flat

TABLE 8.3

SCORING SYSTEM FOR THE VAN NUYS PROGNOSTIC INDEX

	Score		
Variable	1	2	3
Size (mm)	≤15	16–40	≥41
Margin (mm)	≥10	1–9	<1
Pathology	Not HG; necrosis absent	Not HG; necrosis present	HG; necrosis present/absent

Abbreviation: HG, high nuclear grade.
Based on Silverstein MJ, Weisman JR, Gierson ED, et al. Radiation therapy for intraductal carcinoma: is it an equal alternative? *Arch Surg.* 1991;126:424–426, with permission.

micropapillary intraductal carcinoma are very uncommon, and more often one or more epithelial fronds or bridges are present. In the absence of calcification or necrosis, flat micropapillary intraductal carcinoma is easily overlooked microscopically. This type of intraductal carcinoma is most often found in a background of CCH which is encountered mainly in women 35 to 55 years of age. The lesions are typically multifocal or multicentric and can be bilateral. Calcifications with distinctive crystalline, ossifying, and laminated appearances tend to occur in CCH, leading to mammographic detection. Patients with CCH may have tubular carcinoma, LCIS, and invasive lobular carcinoma, as well as micropapillary intraductal carcinoma.

Cribriform intraductal carcinoma is a fenestrated epithelial proliferation in which microlumina are formed in the neoplastic epithelium that bridges most or all of the duct lumen (Fig. 8.49). Extension into lobular epithelium (so-called lobular cancerization) or into the main lactiferous ducts of the nipple is uncommon. Dilated ducts with cribriform intraductal carcinoma can be mistaken for adenoid cystic carcinoma or a complex papilloma. Collagenous spherulosis, that is usually associated with hyperplastic duct lesions that may be secondarily involved by LCIS, can be mistaken for cribriform intraductal carcinoma.

The presence of collagenous spherulosis can be confirmed with an actin immunostain that will highlight myoepithelial cells at the perimeter of spherules or immunostains for basement membrane components. The distinction between intraductal carcinoma and LCIS in collagenous spherulosis depends on cytologic features of the lesion and can be confirmed with the E-cadherin stain. The appearance of coexisting in situ carcinoma not in collagenous spherulosis can also be helpful.

The secondary lumina in cribriform intraductal carcinoma tend to be round or oval, with smooth edges bordered by cuboidal cells. The distribution of microlumina is variable. In some instances, the spaces are spread across the entire duct, but in others they are concentrated toward the center or rarely in a zone largely at the periphery of the duct. Microlumina surrounded by a homogeneous cell population that is uniformly distributed throughout the duct are a hallmark of cribriform intraductal carcinoma. The microlumina may contain secretion, small numbers of degenerated or necrotic cells, and punctate calcifications.

Bands of neoplastic cells between and around the microlumina are described as *rigid*, a term that refers to the uniform, not overlapping distribution of polygonal cells, in contrast to the streaming pattern of overlapping, frequently oval cells in duct hyperplasia. Polarization of the cells in a radial fashion around the microlumina contributes to the rigid appearance. The most orderly type of cribriform intraductal carcinoma is composed of cytologically low-grade cuboidal-to-low columnar monomorphic cells. Nucleoli are inconspicuous or absent, and mitoses are rarely encountered. The cells usually have sparse cytoplasm. Cribriform intraductal carcinoma can be composed of cells with intermediate to high-grade nuclei. Necrosis may be present in such foci.

Solid intraductal carcinoma is formed by neoplastic cells that fill most or all of the duct space (Fig. 8.50). Microlumina and papillary structures are absent, but calcifications may be present. Patients with comedo carcinoma often have coexistent foci of nonnecrotic solid intraductal carcinoma. The polygonal cells are typically of a single type with low to intermediate nuclear grade. The cytoplasm has a spectrum of cytologic appearances including clear, granular, amphophilic, and apocrine.

Intraductal comedo carcinoma is composed of carcinoma cells with poorly differentiated nuclei, central necrosis with calcification, and in many cases, a high mitotic rate (Fig. 8.51). The myoepithelial cell layer is sometimes completely eliminated by the carcinomatous proliferation, but in other instances it may be hyperplastic and produce a distinct ring. The latter configuration is usually accompanied by accentuation of the basement membrane itself, as well as a circumferential periductal collar of desmoplastic stroma. A "cocktail" of antibodies to SM M-HC and p63 is especially sensitive for detecting myoepithelium in high-grade intraductal carcinoma (100). Neovascularity in many instances is represented by a partial or complete ring of capillaries immediately external to the basement membrane (101). A variable inflammatory infiltrate is present in the periductal stroma, with a granulomatous reaction in foci where the

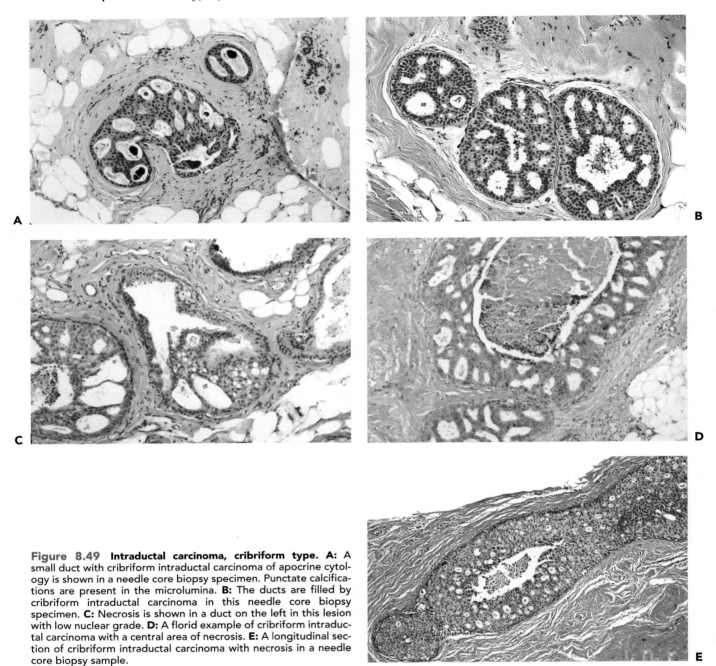

Figure 8.49 Intraductal carcinoma, cribriform type. A: A small duct with cribriform intraductal carcinoma of apocrine cytology is shown in a needle core biopsy specimen. Punctate calcifications are present in the microlumina. **B:** The ducts are filled by cribriform intraductal carcinoma in this needle core biopsy specimen. **C:** Necrosis is shown in a duct on the left in this lesion with low nuclear grade. **D:** A florid example of cribriform intraductal carcinoma with a central area of necrosis. **E:** A longitudinal section of cribriform intraductal carcinoma with necrosis in a needle core biopsy sample.

duct wall is partially disrupted, and it appears that necrotic contents of the duct have been discharged into the stroma. Calcification can also be found in the stroma (Fig. 8.52).

It is important to distinguish between comedo necrosis and the accumulation of secretion accompanied by an inflammatory reaction that occurs in duct stasis. Both conditions are prone to the formation of microcalcifications. Cellular necrosis is rarely seen in duct stasis, and when present, the degenerated cells are usually histiocytes. The duct contents in comedo intraductal carcinoma consist of necrotic carcinoma cells represented by ghost cells and karyorrhectic debris with little or no intraductal inflammation.

There is typically a sharp demarcation between viable carcinoma cells and the necrotic core. A space may be formed between the surviving and dead elements. Dying cells at the inner edge of the viable zone have pyknotic nuclei and frayed cytoplasmic borders. The outlines of necrotic cells may be visible in the center of the duct (ghost cells) (Fig. 8.53).

Calcification develops in the necrotic core when there is comedo necrosis. The calcification can be finely granular and mixed with cellular debris in some instances or, it forms more solid irregular masses that correspond to casting calcifications on mammography. Calcifications in comedo intraductal carcinoma almost always consist of

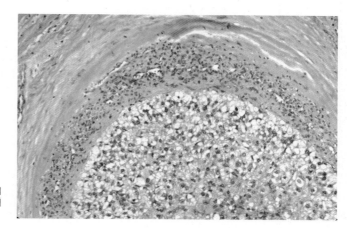

Figure 8.50 Intraductal carcinoma, solid type. An unusual example of solid, clear cell intraductal carcinoma with very marked periductal angiogenesis.

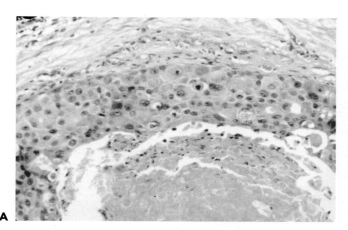

A

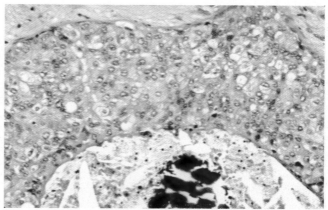

B

Figure 8.51 Intraductal carcinoma, solid comedo-type. A: Solid growth with a high nuclear grade is present at the perimeter of a duct with comedo-type central necrosis. Angiogenesis is evident in the periductal tissue. **B:** Calcification and comedo necrosis are apparent in this duct with solid intraductal carcinoma.

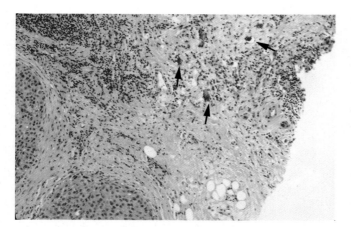

Figure 8.52 Intraductal carcinoma, solid comedo-type with stromal calcification. Fine calcifications *(arrows)* are present in the stroma in an area of lymphocytic reaction in this needle core biopsy specimen with intraductal comedo carcinoma.

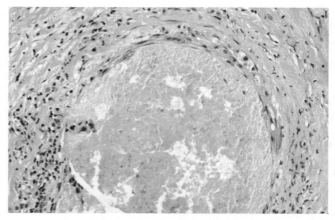

Figure 8.53 Intraductal carcinoma, solid comedo-type with severe central necrosis. The intraductal carcinoma is almost totally necrotic in this needle core biopsy specimen. A few degenerating tumor cells are visible. The ghost architecture of the intraductal carcinoma is evident.

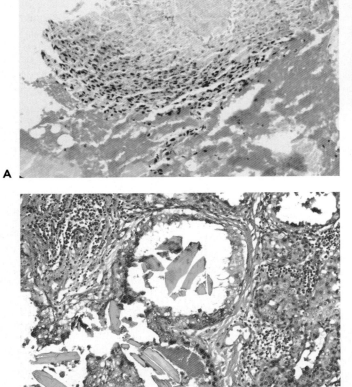

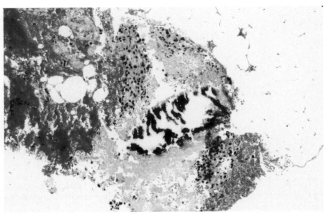

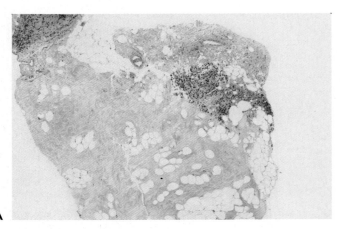

Figure 8.54 Probable intraductal carcinoma, solid comedo-type. A, B: The needle core biopsy specimen had these fragments of calcification, comedo-type necrosis, and atypical cells. A needle core biopsy specimen such as this is an indication for prompt excisional biopsy to determine if comedo carcinoma is present. **C:** Crystalloids in intraductal carcinoma. These protein precipitates are almost always associated with intraductal carcinoma.

calcium salts, mainly calcium phosphate, rather than crystalline calcium oxalate, that is typically found in benign apocrine lesions. In routine hematoxylin and eosin (H&E)-stained sections calcium phosphate calcifications are magenta to purple, whether in comedo carcinoma or other varieties of intraductal carcinoma. Calcifications and necrotic debris may become dislodged in a needle core biopsy specimen and rarely this material is the only component of the lesion found in the specimen. When dislodged calcifications are present in a needle core biopsy specimen, serial sections of the biopsy specimen should be prepared. An excisional biopsy is indicated even if no epithelial elements are found in the needle core biopsy sample that contains dislodged calcifications or crystalloids (Fig. 8.54). If a dislodged fragment of carcinoma becomes embedded in stroma or fat in a needle core biopsy, the resulting appearance can be mistaken for invasive carcinoma (Fig. 8.55).

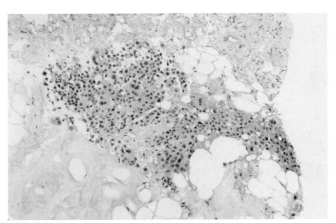

Figure 8.55 Displaced epithelium mistaken for invasive carcinoma in a needle core biopsy sample. A, B: This fragment of carcinoma displaced in fibrofatty tissue was interpreted as invasive carcinoma.

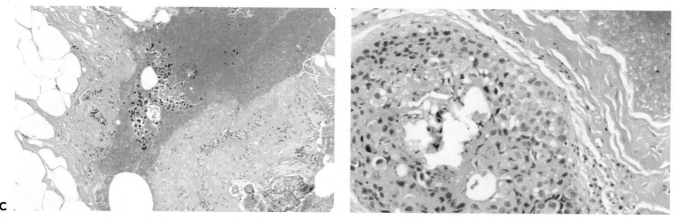

Figure 8.55 *(continued)* **C:** The subsequent excisional biopsy specimen had similar fragments of carcinoma such as one shown here in an area of hemorrhage caused by the needle core biopsy procedure. **D:** The excisional biopsy specimen contained intraductal comedo carcinoma with no intrinsic invasion. Note hemorrhage caused by the needle core biopsy procedure in the upper right corner.

Marked periductal fibrosis can on occasion be associated with extensive obliteration of ducts that contain comedo intraductal carcinoma, a process referred to as *healing* by Muir and Aitkenhead (102). Severe necrosis of the intraductal lesion (see Fig. 8.53) can contribute to this process. The residual ductal structures typically consist of round-to-oval scars composed of circumferential layers of collagen and elastic tissue (Fig. 8.56). The core of the scar, representing the center of the duct, is often less dense, and it may contain a few residual carcinoma cells, histiocytes, fragments of calcification, and granulation tissue. End-stage scars of periductal mastitis are not distinguishable from those of obliterated comedo carcinoma (103). When this type of scar is found in a needle core biopsy specimen, serial sections should be obtained since small foci of carcinoma cells may be detected in the scar. The very limited histologic evidence for carcinoma found in some of these cases may result in a diagnosis of atypical ductal hyperplasia.

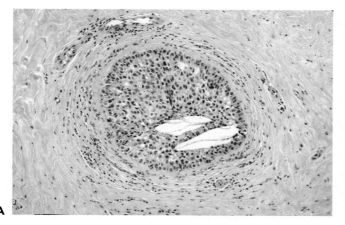

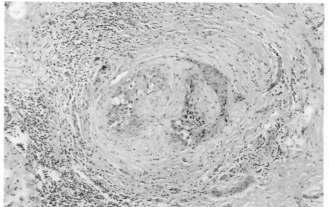

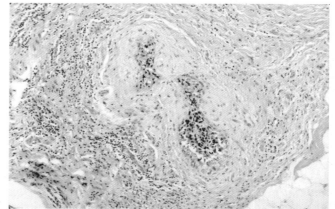

Figure 8.56 Intraductal carcinoma, with obliterative sclerosis. A–C: Different areas in a needle core biopsy specimen arranged in a sequence that suggests the progressive replacement of degenerating intraductal carcinoma by circumferential sclerosis of the ducts.

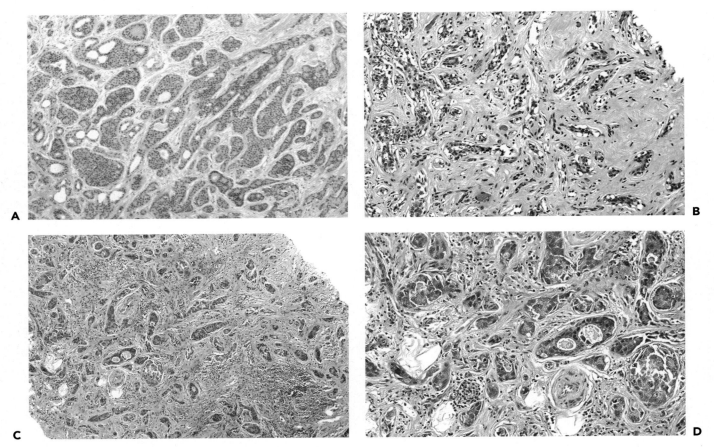

Figure 8.57   Intraductal carcinoma in sclerosing adenosis. A: The carcinoma has solid and cribriform growth patterns with low nuclear grade. Some of the underlying architecture is tubular adenosis. **B–D:** A needle core biopsy specimen showing sclerosing adenosis **(B)** that was involved by intraductal carcinoma **(C, D)**.

Some high-grade intraductal carcinomas exhibit the triple negative basal-like immunophenotype (no reactivity for estrogen and progesterone receptors and for HER2/*neu*). This form of intraductal carcinoma is the putative precursor to invasive basal-like ductal carcinoma (104,105). Bryan et al. (104) found the basal-like immunophenotype in 4 of 55 (6%) of intraductal carcinomas with high nuclear grade. These intraductal carcinomas expressed basal cytokeratins and/or epidermal growth factor receptor (EGFR) significantly more often than high-grade intraductal carcinomas which did not have the basal-like immunophenotype. The intraductal carcinoma may be of the solid, flat, or micropapillary type (105).

Papillary intraductal carcinoma is distinguished by the presence of a fibrovascular stromal architecture supporting one or more of the foregoing structural patterns. Papillary intraductal carcinoma is discussed in Chapter 11. Spindle cell intraductal carcinoma is sometimes a variant of papillary intraductal carcinoma, but spindle cell growth also occurs in nonpapillary intraductal carcinoma.

Intraductal carcinoma arising in sclerosing adenosis assumes the structural configuration of the underlying adenosis and may be mistaken for invasive carcinoma

(106–108). Because sclerosing adenosis is fundamentally a lesion formed by altered lobules, this presentation can be viewed as a form of intralobular extension of the ductal lesion (Fig. 8.57). The condition usually occurs focally but it can be diffuse. The growth patterns of the intraductal carcinoma are usually solid and cribriform. An organoid appearance can be formed when there is alveolar expansion of lobular structures in the adenosis. Microcalcifications may be present in the underlying adenosis or as part of the intraductal carcinoma. Intraductal carcinoma can be limited to the sclerosing adenosis, or there may be additional intraductal foci in the surrounding breast (107).

The underlying architecture of sclerosing adenosis can be appreciated with stains for basement membranes such as PAS, reticulin, or laminin and immunostains to identify myoepithelial cells such as p63, calponin, CD10, and SMA (107). Invasive carcinoma arising in sclerosing adenosis is very difficult to detect unless the invasive component has clearly grown beyond the area of adenosis and has an architectural pattern that differs from the adenosis. Double immunostaining for cytokeratin and actin may be useful in this setting. Nerves can be incorporated in sclerosing adenosis when no carcinoma is present (109). The pres-

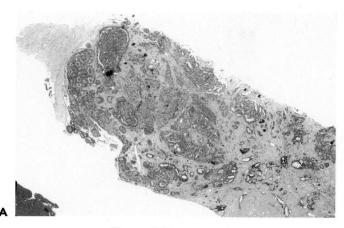
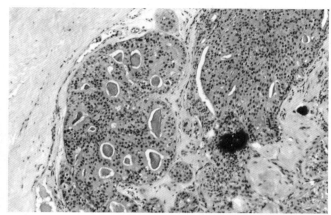

A

B

Figure 8.58 **Intraductal carcinoma in a radial sclerosing lesion. A:** Cribriform intraductal carcinoma is present in the upper left portion of this needle core biopsy specimen. Atypical duct hyperplasia occupies the mid-portion, and sclerosing adenosis is present on the lower right. **B:** The area of cribriform intraductal carcinoma.

ence of this unusual finding coexisting with intraductal carcinoma in the adenosis is not indicative of invasion. Neural entrapment has also been observed in areas of sclerosing papillary intraductal carcinoma not associated with sclerosing adenosis (110).

Intraductal carcinoma in radial sclerosing lesions may be difficult to distinguish from atypical duct hyperplasia. The presence of an underlying radial scar is indicated by the overall configuration of the lesion, and usually by the presence of fibrocystic components such as cysts, sclerosing adenosis, and apocrine metaplasia (Fig. 8.58). Incomplete samples of radial scar lesions obtained in a needle core biopsy specimen are difficult to assess for the presence of intraductal carcinoma or for invasion, and they are likely to be reported as atypical hyperplasia.

Concurrent intraductal and in situ lobular carcinoma are present when there are separate foci of carcinoma with these histologic features in the breast. This is illustrated by instances in which the lobular lesion with the classical small cell phenotype of lobular carcinoma is limited to lobular terminal duct units that are separate from ducts with the classical features of comedo, papillary, or cribriform intraductal carcinoma.

In some instances, the distinction is less clear, especially when the proliferation in the ducts and lobules is composed of uniform cells with cytologically well to moderately differentiated nuclei. The difficulty presented by these lesions is whether they should be classified as entirely intraductal carcinoma with "lobular cancerization," or as LCIS with duct extension. The E-cadherin stain will display strong membrane reactivity if the lesion is intraductal carcinoma. E-cadherin staining will be reduced and fragmented or absent in LCIS. The presence of the cribriform pattern suggests intraductal carcinoma with lobular extension. Cells with apocrine differentiation are more consistent with ductal carcinoma. Ultimately some difficult cases defy classification even after careful consideration of all features and a diagnosis of combined intraductal and in situ lobular carcinoma

may be made, accompanied by a description of the diagnostic issues presented in the particular instance.

Coexistent intraductal and in situ lobular carcinoma in a single duct-lobular unit constitutes one of the most unusual microscopic patterns of noninvasive breast carcinoma (111). This diagnosis depends upon finding carcinoma with two distinctly different cytologic and structural patterns in a single duct. In these combined lesions, LCIS with the conventional small cell cytology is typically present within lobular glands as well as in a pagetoid distribution in the duct epithelium. The duct lumen contains a papillary, solid, or cribriform proliferation composed of more pleomorphic cells typically found in an intraductal carcinoma. Coexistent in situ lesions have been found in association with invasive duct and invasive lobular carcinoma. This pattern of in situ carcinoma should be distinguished from lobular extension of intraductal carcinoma, so-called lobular cancerization. In the latter condition, the nonneoplastic lobular epithelium is displaced by carcinoma cells with the same cytologic appearance as the intraductal carcinoma. The E-cadherin stain can be used to identify LCIS in intraductal carcinoma in combined lesions.

Grading of Intraductal Carcinoma

The grade of intraductal carcinoma has been investigated for predicting the risk of breast recurrence after conservation therapy. When an invasive element is associated with intraductal carcinoma, both components tend to have similar nuclear grades (112). Grading schemes consisting of two categories (high grade and all others) and three categories (high, intermediate, and low grade) have been devised. The determination of grade is based in part upon nuclear cytology. Nuclear grade tends to be relatively constant in a given patient, even when substantial variation in architectural pattern is noted (112). The presence or absence of necrosis, and the architecture of the intraductal carcinoma are also to be considered in grading.

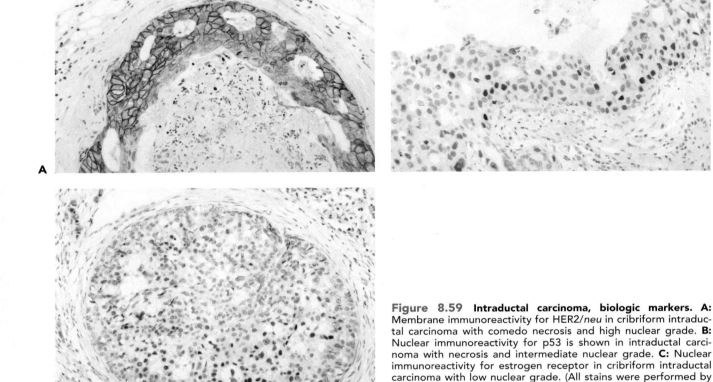

Figure 8.59 Intraductal carcinoma, biologic markers. A: Membrane immunoreactivity for HER2/*neu* in cribriform intraductal carcinoma with comedo necrosis and high nuclear grade. **B:** Nuclear immunoreactivity for p53 is shown in intraductal carcinoma with necrosis and intermediate nuclear grade. **C:** Nuclear immunoreactivity for estrogen receptor in cribriform intraductal carcinoma with low nuclear grade. (All stains were performed by the immunoperoxidase method.)

Comedo carcinoma is "high" grade by definition. Poorly differentiated nuclei, sometimes accompanied by necrosis, are infrequently encountered in papillary, micropapillary, and cribriform intraductal carcinomas (112). Intraductal carcinoma is considered to be in the intermediate grade category when it has a cribriform, solid, or papillary pattern with necrosis but lacks the nuclear anaplasia of comedo carcinoma, or if one of these growth patterns is composed of high-grade carcinoma cells in the absence of necrosis. Any pattern of intraductal carcinoma composed of uniform cells without atypia or necrosis is classified as low grade. A case is usually classified on the basis of the highest grade present (99).

Grading has been a component of most attempts to develop classification schemes for assessing the effectiveness of breast conservation therapy in the treatment of intraductal carcinoma. Several classifications have been proposed (113). These have been based on some or all of the following features: architecture, nuclear grade, presence or absence of necrosis, lesion size, and cell polarity. Most classifications have emphasized nuclear grade, necrosis, and architecture. Generally, three grades have been proposed: high, intermediate, and low grade. There is a significant correlation between the grade of intraductal carcinoma and a corresponding invasive component, if present, regardless of grading system (113). The grading categories also have significant associa-

tions with biologic characteristics of intraductal carcinoma, especially lesions classified as high and low grade. High-grade lesions typically exhibit the following features: absence of estrogen and progesterone receptor expression, aneuploidy, high proliferative rate, periductal angiogenesis, membrane reactivity for HER2/*neu*, nuclear reactivity for p53, and abnormal bcl-2 expression (Fig. 8.59). Low-grade intraductal carcinomas are characterized by the following: presence of estrogen and progesterone receptors, absence of aneuploidy, low proliferative rate, little periductal angiogenesis, absence of HER2/*neu* and p53, and normal bcl-2 expression. Intermediate-grade intraductal carcinomas tend to have mixed patterns of biologic marker expression.

Grading has been a component of other classification schemes for assessing the effectiveness of breast conservation therapy in the treatment of intraductal carcinoma. Including those cited earlier, at least six classifications have been proposed (58). These have been based on some or all of the following features: architecture, nuclear grade, presence or absence of necrosis, lesion size, and cell polarity. Most classifications have emphasized nuclear grade, necrosis, and architecture. Generally, three grades have been proposed: high, intermediate, and low grade. There is a significant correlation between the grade of intraductal carcinoma and a corresponding invasive component, if present, regardless of grading system (113). The grading categories also have significant associations with biologic characteristics of intraductal carcinoma, especially lesions classified as high and low grade. High-grade lesions typically exhibit the following features: absence of estrogen and progesterone receptor expression, aneuploidy, high proliferative rate, periductal angiogenesis, membrane reactivity for HER2/*neu*, nuclear reactivity for p53, and abnormal bcl-2 expression. Conversely, low-grade intraductal carcinomas are usually characterized by the following: presence of estrogen and progesterone receptors, absence of aneuploidy, low proliferative rate, little periductal angiogenesis, absence of HER2/*neu* and p53 expression, and normal bcl-2 expression. Intermediate-grade intraductal carcinomas tend to have mixed patterns of biologic marker expression.

No single grading system for intraductal carcinoma has been demonstrated to be notably superior for anticipating successful breast conservation and none has gained universal acceptance. A consensus conference convened in 1997 did not endorse any single system of classification but recommended that a pathology report for intraductal carcinoma provides information about the descriptive characteristics considered to be necessary in most grading schemes (99). The three essential elements noted were: nuclear grade, necrosis, and architectural pattern(s). It was observed that the pathology report should reflect the highest nuclear grade but may indicate the relative proportions of grade when there is heterogeneity. Necrosis was defined as the "presence of ghost cells and karyorrhectic debris." Five architectural patterns were identified: comedo, cribriform, papillary, micropapillary, and solid. It was specified that comedo referred "to solid intraepithelial growth within the basement membrane with central (zonal) necrosis. Such lesions are often but not invariably of high nuclear grade." Other elements recommended for inclusion in the diagnosis were lesion "size (extent, distribution)" and margin status. No particular methods for assessing size or margins were suggested.

Size of Intraductal Carcinoma

Lesion size is difficult to consistently determine in many cases. When intraductal carcinoma is limited to a single tissue block, it may be possible to obtain an accurate measurement of size. Determining size when intraductal carcinoma is distributed in more than one tissue block from a single biopsy sample, or if it is in more than one biopsy specimen, is very imprecise. Kestin et al. (114) were unable to determine tumor size in 58% of the cases they analyzed. For this and other reasons summarized by Schnitt et al. (115), classifications for assessing the prognosis of intraductal carcinoma that depend on and offer precise size categories may be viewed, at best, as general guidelines rather than as a strict criteria for making therapeutic decisions.

It is exceedingly unusual for intraductal carcinoma to be limited to a needle core biopsy sample. This material is not suitable for determining the size of intraductal carcinoma even if the procedure is performed for calcifications alone and calcifications are no longer present in a follow-up mammogram. The needle biopsy specimen only rarely provides a single intact sample of the lesion, and it is not feasible to reassemble the intraductal carcinoma foci from multiple samples to obtain a single measurement.

Intraductal Carcinoma and Microinvasion

The diagnosis of intraductal carcinoma by needle core biopsy cannot be relied upon in all cases to exclude invasive carcinoma in the affected breast. Several studies have reported the frequency of invasive carcinoma detected by excisional biopsy after a needle core biopsy diagnosis of intraductal carcinoma to be in the range of 15% to 27% (7,56,116–118). The diagnosis of intraductal carcinoma was reportedly more reliable with a directional vacuum-assisted biopsy procedure than with an automated needle biopsy system in one study (56).

Ultrastructural studies have detected foci of discontinuity in the basement membranes of ducts with intraductal carcinoma (119), and similar observations have been reported in tissues studied by immunohistochemistry (120). Breaks in the basement membrane are more common when intraductal carcinoma is of the comedo type or has a high nuclear grade. In such regions, the neoplastic epithelium appears to protrude from the duct, coming in contact with the stroma while it remains connected to the intraductal neoplasm (121). This finding often elicits diagnostic uncertainty, reflected in such caveats as "microinvasion suspected" or "microinvasion cannot be ruled out."

When microinvasion is present, carcinoma cells are distributed singly or as small groups that have irregular shapes in the periductal stroma with no particular orientation relative to the intraductal carcinoma (Fig. 8.60). The stroma sometimes appears less dense at sites of microinvasion than in other areas around ducts and lobules containing intraductal carcinoma. Detecting carcinoma cells in the stroma can be difficult when there is a marked periductal reaction. Microinvasion should be suspected at sites where there is a lymphocytic reaction around or near ducts with intraductal carcinoma. A granulomatous reaction may be elicited at foci of microinvasion (122). In this setting, tumor cells can resemble histiocytes, and it may require immunostains for cytokeratin to confirm their presence outside the ducts (see Fig. 8.60). Carcinomatous epithelium displaced by needling procedures should not be misinterpreted as intrinsic invasive carcinoma (Fig. 8.55).

Microinvasion is more often associated with high-grade and comedo intraductal carcinoma, but it may occur in other types (84). There have been several studies that identified features of intraductal carcinoma in core biopsy specimens that were predictive of detecting invasive carcinoma in the subsequent lumpectomy. Renshaw (117) reported that invasive carcinoma in the excisional biopsy specimen was significantly associated with cribriform/papillary architecture and necrosis in the intraductal carcinoma and more than 4 mm of lobular extension. Hou et al. (123) also found lobular extension to be predictive of invasion. Other features of intraductal carcinoma in a needle core biopsy sample that have been cited as predictive of invasion include the presence of a mass lesion on the imaging study (123–125), high nuclear

grade (126–128), extensive calcifications (126,127), and a palpable lesion (128).

In light of the foregoing discussion, it is evident that there are instances in which the presence or absence of microinvasion can be difficult to determine with certainty, even with the immunohistochemical reagents currently

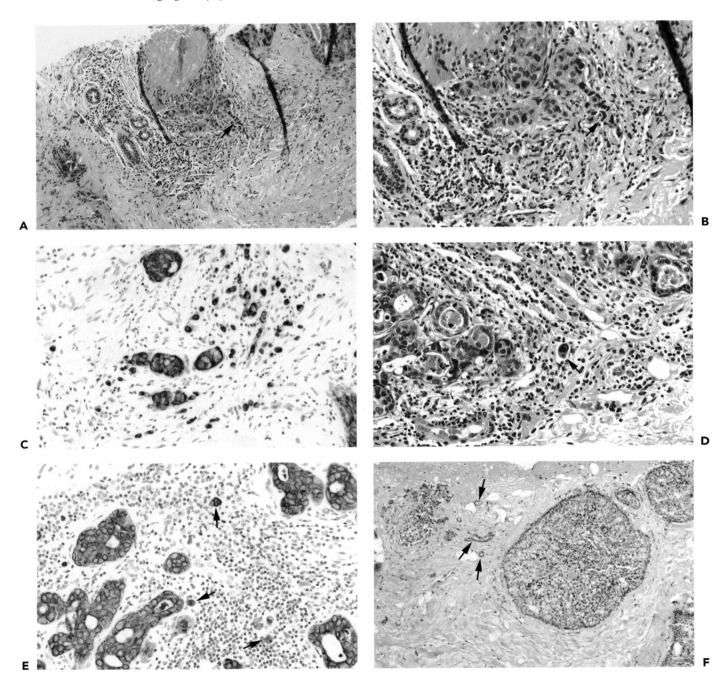

Figure 8.60 Intraductal carcinoma with microinvasion. Three different patterns of microinvasion found in needle core biopsy specimens are shown. **A, B:** Microinvasion here consists of a linear strand of tumor cells *(arrow)* extending into the stroma surrounded by a lymphocytic reaction. **C:** Carcinoma cells in the stroma are highlighted here by the CAM 5.2 cytokeratin immunostain (immunoperoxidase). **D:** Another needle core biopsy specimen in which there is an isolated carcinoma cell *(arrow)* in the perilobular stroma. **E:** Invasive carcinoma cells *(arrows)* are highlighted by an immunostain for CAM 5.2 cytokeratin (immunoperoxidase). **F:** Well-differentiated infiltrating duct carcinoma is present in the stroma *(arrows)* to the left of a large duct with intraductal carcinoma.

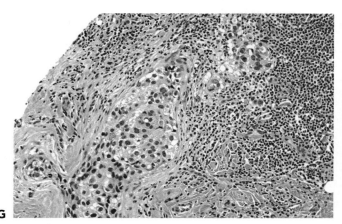 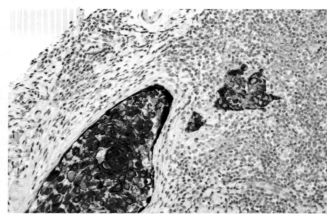

G   H

Figure 8.60 *(continued)* **G, H:** Microinvasive carcinoma surrounded by lymphocytes next to intraductal carcinoma in a needle core biopsy sample. Myoepithelium around the intraductal carcinoma stains brown and the carcinoma cells are red. The microinvasive carcinoma (right) lacks myoepithelium (triple immunostain).

available. Some guidelines can be suggested based on experience examining numerous specimens in which microinvasion was a concern.

1. The presence of myoepithelial cells is the most convincing evidence of intraductal carcinoma, especially if demonstrated with the p63 immunostain. It is essential to use more than one immunostain because reactivity is not equally intense with all reagents (129).
2. Absence of demonstrable reactivity with an appropriate marker usually means that myoepthelial cells are not present, although they can be severely attenuated and difficult to recognize. Loss of the myoepithelial cell layer occurs in some but not all intraductal carcinomas. By itself, absence of myoepithelial cells is not indicative of invasive carcinoma, and the interpretation of this finding depends on the complete histologic appearance of the lesion in the corresponding H&E section.
3. A new consecutive H&E section must be prepared whenever immunostains are performed for suspected microinvasion. This is necessary because the structure of the tissue changes as additional slides are made.
4. Cytokeratin immunostains are essential for the evaluation of any focus suspected to be the site of microinvasion. It is recommended that at least two different stains be used (e.g., CK7, AE1/3) because of the variable reactivity of carcinoma cells. Cytokeratin immunostaining highlights the distribution of epithelial cells and distinguishes epithelial cells from histiocytes.
5. Immunostains for basement membrane components laminin and collagen type IV are sometimes helpful. Absence of reactivity for both components indicates a strong likelihood of invasive carcinoma, especially if coupled with absence of myoepithelial cells.
6. Reactivity for one or both basal lamina components in the absence of myoepithelial cells presents the most difficult diagnostic situation that requires assessment of the entire lesion including multiple H&E levels if possible. The presence of laminin and collagen type IV

favors a diagnosis of in situ carcinoma. However, consideration must given to the possibility that basal lamina may be formed at sites of invasion. With present routine diagnostic techniques, the distinction between basal lamina formed at sites of invasion and basement membranes in in situ carcinoma cannot be resolved with confidence in all cases.

It is essential to use the term *microinvasion* for lesions with no single focus of invasive carcinoma that is 1 mm or larger in diameter. This definition has been adopted by the TNM staging system with the rubric T1mic. When multiple foci of such microinvasion are present, there is no precise method for estimating their aggregate diameter, and these cases qualify as intraductal carcinoma with multifocal microinvasion. Invasive foci larger than 1 mm are diagnosed as invasive duct carcinoma and reported on the basis of measured size (Fig. 8.61).

de Mascarel et al. (130) subclassified microinvasive duct carcinoma into type 1 (single tumor cells) and type 2 (clusters of tumor cells). None of the 59 type 1 patients who had axillary lymph nodes removed had nodal metastases. On the other hand, there were nodal metastases in 14 (10%) of the 139 patients with type 2 microinvasion who had axillary lymph nodes examined. Distant metastases were reported in 2 (3%) of the 72 patients with type 1 microinvasion and in 12 (7%) of 171 with type 2 microinvasion. The survival of patients with type 1 microinvasive carcinoma was similar to that of women with pure intraductal carcinoma and significantly better that of patients with type 2 microinvasion.

SUMMARY OF TREATMENT RECOMMENDATIONS

The treatment recommendation is made on the basis of clinical and pathologic findings in consultation with the patient. Important considerations include the manner of

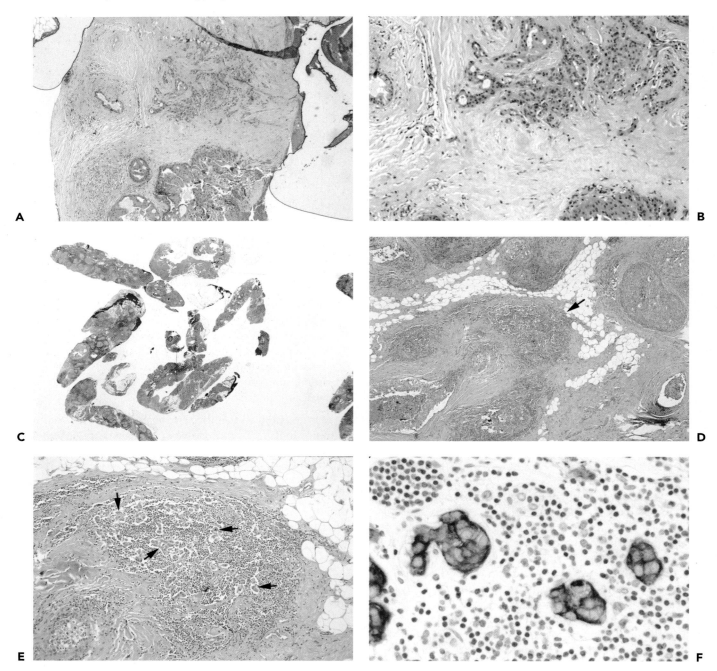

Figure 8.61 **Intraductal carcinoma with invasion. A, B:** A 1-mm focus of orderly invasive apocrine duct carcinoma is present in the upper half of this needle core biopsy specimen. Apocrine intraductal carcinoma is apparent below the invasive area. **C:** Another specimen that consisted of multiple needle core biopsy samples with extensive intraductal carcinoma. **D:** The specimen shown in **(C)** contained these areas of solid high-grade intraductal carcinoma and a 2-mm focus of invasive ductal carcinoma in a marked lymphocytic reaction *(arrow)*. **E:** A magnified view of the invasive ductal carcinoma *(arrows)*. **F:** Groups of invasive carcinoma cells are highlighted by the CAM 5.2 keratin immunostain (immunoperoxidase).

clinical presentation (e.g., palpable, incidental, or mammographic), extent by mammography, size measured grossly or microscopically when possible, margin status of the lumpectomy specimen, and histologic features of the intraductal carcinoma such as nuclear grade, growth pattern (e.g., cribriform, comedo, or solid papillary), and the presence or absence of necrosis. The issue is complicated

by the many different combinations of these and other features that can occur in a given case.

Numerous studies cited indicate that margin status and the biologic characteristics of intraductal carcinoma represented histologically by nuclear grade and the presence or absence of necrosis are the most important predictors of local recurrence in the breast after breast conservation with or without radiotherapy. Tumor size correlates well with the extent of the lesion and thus influences margin status. Biologic characteristics, at least partially reflected in the histologic appearance of intraductal carcinoma, have a complex influence on the success of treatment by affecting the rate of growth (and to some extent the time to detection of clinical recurrences) and radiosensitivity of residual intraductal carcinoma after lumpectomy. Consequently, it is possible for patients with comparable amounts of incompletely excised residual high-grade (comedo) and low-grade (cribriform) intraductal carcinoma who receive the same treatment to have similar absolute risks for breast recurrence, but they may differ in time to clinical detection of recurrence, especially of invasive lesions, and in responsiveness to radiotherapy or antiestrogens.

Retrospective and prospective randomized studies have demonstrated that radiotherapy after excisional surgery reduces the chance of recurrence in the breast by about 50%. The degree to which a reduced frequency of breast recurrence contributes to overall survival remains to be determined for patients with intraductal carcinoma. The possibility that there could be a survival advantage conferred by reducing breast recurrences is suggested by a meta-analysis of randomized studies of radiotherapy and breast conservation in women with invasive breast carcinoma that detected this beneficial effect. The addition of tamoxifen to breast conservation therapy reduces breast recurrences in women with estrogen receptor positive intraductal carcinoma.

Radiotherapy is usually indicated for any of the following circumstances: high-grade intraductal carcinoma, when margins are close (variously described as 10 mm or less), and for patients younger than 50 years. Tamoxifen may be added for hormone receptor positive intraductal carcinoma. Omitting radiotherapy is a consideration for some women older than 50 years with a widely clear margin (variously defined as more than 10 mm) and low-grade histology without necrosis. This type of intraductal carcinoma is very likely to be hormone receptor positive and therefore amenable to adjuvant tamoxifen treatment.

Mammography is an essential component of the clinical follow-up of women treated by breast conserving surgery with or without radiotherapy and/or tamoxifen. Particular attention should be paid to the mammographic follow-up of the contralateral breast in women with atypical hyperplasia or LCIS coexisting with intraductal carcinoma. The role of routine MR screening in the follow-up of women with intraductal carcinoma treated by breast conservation remains to be determined.

Some patients may choose mastectomy even if they are candidates for breast conservation. Mastectomy is preferable for the patient with such widespread intraductal carcinoma that negative margins cannot be achieved with a cosmetically acceptable surgical procedure. Many but not all of these patients have dispersed calcifications on mammography. Lumpectomy with or without radiation will suffice for most women with intraductal carcinoma limited to a single focus on the basis of pathologic and clinical findings, if the margins of excision are negative, if the lesion is not comedotype with necrosis and high nuclear grade, and it is small (variously defined as less than 1.0 cm or less than 2.5 cm). Radiation after lumpectomy is recommended regardless of size if the intraductal carcinoma has high nuclear grade, necrosis or is distinctively of the comedo carcinoma type or the margins are indeterminate or are involved.

Axillary dissection is not indicated in the majority of patients with intraductal carcinoma. Some low axillary lymph nodes may be taken with the axillary tail of the breast in the course of a mastectomy. If the lesion is extensive intraductal carcinoma, especially comedo type with marked duct distortion, it would be prudent to perform sentinel lymph node mapping because of concern for undetected invasion.

Treatment for the majority of patients with microinvasive duct carcinoma previously described in the literature has been mastectomy. The overall outcome was relatively favorable after mastectomy, but the studies were not directly comparable because of differing criteria for defining microinvasion. Patients treated by breast conservation were described in several reports with results indicating that this was equally effective as mastectomy. These and other published reports indicate that the presence of microinvasion, as variously defined in the past or as currently described in the TNM staging system (T1mic), probably has little independent impact on the effectiveness of conservation therapy for local control in the breast. The characteristics of the intraductal carcinoma that are associated with microinvasion, such as high grade, the presence of necrosis, and lesion size are crucial determinants for treatment. The significance of multiple microinvasive foci is yet to be determined. The finding of microinvasion will lead to axillary lymph node staging, often by sentinel lymph node mapping, in many patients prior to consideration of systemic therapy.

REFERENCES

Ductal Hyperplasia-Usual and Atypical

1. Connolly JL, Schnitt SJ. Benign breast disease. Resolved and unresolved issues. *Cancer.* 1993;71:1187–1189.
2. Bodian CA, Perzin KH, Lattes R, Hoffman P. Reproducibility and validity of pathologic classifications of benign breast disease and implications for clinical applications. *Cancer.* 1993;71:3908–3913.
3. Rosai J. Borderline epithelial lesions of the breast. *Am J Surg Pathol.* 1991;15:209–221.
4. Schnitt SJ, Connolly JL, Tavassoli FA, et al. Interobserver reproducibility in the diagnosis of ductal proliferative breast lesions using standardized criteria. *Am J Surg Pathol.* 1992;16:1133–1143.
5. Palli D, Galli M, Bianchi S, et al. Reproducibility of histological diagnosis of breast lesions: results of a panel in Italy. *Eur J Cancer.* 1996;32A:603–607.
6. Helvie MA, Hessler C, Frank TS, Ikeda DM. Atypical hyperplasia of the breast: mammographic appearance and histologic correlation. *Radiology.* 1991;179:759–764.
7. Jackman RJ, Nowels KW, Shepard MJ, et al. Stereotaxic large-core needle biopsy of 450 nonpalpable breast lesions with surgical correlation in lesions with cancer or atypical hyperplasia. *Radiology.* 1994;193:91–95.
8. Liberman L, Cohen MA, Abramson AF, et al. Atypical ductal hyperplasia diagnosed at stereotaxic core biopsy of breast lesions: an indication for surgical biopsy. *Am J Roentgenol.* 1995;164:1111–1113.
9. Bodian CA, Perzin KH, Lattes R, et al. Prognostic significance of benign proliferative breast disease. *Cancer.* 1993;71:3896–3907.
10. Page DL, Rogers LW. Combined histologic and cytologic criteria for the diagnosis of mammary atypical ductal hyperplasia. *Hum Pathol.* 1992;23:1095–1097.

11. Rubin E, Visscher DW, Alexander RW, et al. Proliferative disease and atypia in biopsies performed for nonpalpable lesions detected mammographically. *Cancer.* 1988;61:2077–2082.

12. Stomper PC, Cholewinski SP, Penetrante RB, et al. Atypical hyperplasia, frequency and mammographic and pathologic relationships in excisional biopsies guided by mammography and clinical examination. *Radiology.* 1993;189:667–671.

13. Orel SG, Rosen M, Miles C, Schnall MD. MR imaging guided 9-gauge vacuum assisted core needle breast biopsy: initial experience. *Radiology.* 2006; 238:54–61.

14. Perlet C, Heywang-Kobrunner SH, Heinig A, et al. Magnetic resonance-guided, vacuum-assisted breast biopsy: results from a European multicentre study of 538 lesions. *Cancer.* 2006;106:982–990.

15. Liberman L, Holland AE, Marjan D, et al. Underestimation of atypical ductal hyperpasia at MRI-guided 9-gauge vacuum-assisted breast biopsy. *Am J Roentgenol.* 2007;188:684–690.

16. Rosen PP, Cantrell B, Mullen DL, DePalo A. Juvenile papillomatosis (Swiss cheese disease) of the breast. *Am J Surg Pathol.* 1980;4:3–12.

17. Wilson M, Cranor ML, Rosen PP. Papillary duct hyperplasia of the breast in children and young women. *Mod Pathol.* 1993;6:570–574.

18. Arapantoni-Dadioti P, Panayiotides J, Georgakila H, Lekka J. Significance of intracytoplasmic lumina in the differential diagnosis between epithelial hyperplasia and carcinoma in situ of the breast. *Breast Dis.* 1996;9: 277–282.

19. Ozaki D, Kondo Y. Comparative morphometric studies of benign and malignant intraductal proliferative lesions of the breast by computerized image analysis. *Hum Pathol.* 1995;26:1109–1113.

20. Ohuchi N, Abe R, Takahashi T, et al. Three-dimensional atypical structure in intraductal carcinoma differentiating from papilloma and papillomatosis of the breast. *Breast Cancer Res Treat.* 1985;5:57–65.

21. Barbareschi M, Pecciarini L, Gangi MG, et al. p63, a p53 homologue, is a selective nuclear marker of myoepithelial cells of the human breast. *Am J Surg Pathol.* 2001;25:1054–1060.

22. Kalof AN, Tam D, Beatty B, Cooper K. Immunostaining patterns of myoepithelial cells in breast lesions: a comparison of CD10 and smooth muscle myosin heavy chain. *J Clin Pathol.* 2004;57:625–629.

23. Moritani S, Kushima R, Sugihara H, et al. Availability of CD10 immunohistochemistry as a marker of breast myoepithelial cells on paraffin sections. *Mod Pathol.* 2002;15:397–405.

24. Lerwill M. Current practical applications of diagnostic immunohistochemistry in breast pathology. *Am J Surg Pathol.* 2004;28:1076–1091.

25. Tavassoli FA, Norris HJ. A comparison of the results of long-term follow-up for atypical intraductal carcinoma of the breast. *Cancer.* 1990;65:518–529.

26. Tavassoli FA. Intraductal hyperplasias, ordinary and atypical. In: Tavassoli FA, ed. *Pathology of the Breast.* New York: Elsevier Science Publishing Co.; 1992:155–191.

27. Fisher ER, Costantino J, Fisher B, et al. Pathologic findings from the National Surgical Adjuvant Breast Project (NSABP) Protocol B-17. Intraductal carcinoma (ductal carcinoma in situ). *Cancer.* 1995;75:1310–1319.

28. Lubelsky SM, Bane AL, Shin V, et al. Columnar cell lesions and flat epithelial atypia: incidence and significance in a mammographically screened population. *Mod Pathol.* 2005;18(suppl):41A.

29. Rosen PP. Columnar cell hyperplasia is associated with lobular carcinoma in situ and tubular carcinoma. *Am J Surg Pathol.* 1999;23:1561.

30. Rosen PP. Ductal hyperplasia. Ordinary and atypical. In: Rosen PP, ed. *Breast Pathology.* 2nd ed. Philadelphia, PA: Lippincott, Williams & Wilkins; 2001:215–223.

31. Tavassoli FA, Hoefler H, Rosai J, et al. Intraductal proliferative lesions. In: Tavassoli FA, Devilee P, eds. *Pathology and Genetics of Tumours of the Breast and Female Genital Organs.* Lyon: IARC Press; 2003:63–67.

32. Oyama T, Maluf H, Koerner F. Atypical cystic lobules: an early stage in the formation of low-grade ductal carcinoma in situ. *Virchows Arch.* 1999;435: 413–421.

33. Goldstein NS, Lacerna M, Vicini F. Cancerization of lobules and atypical ductal hyperplasia adjacent to ductal carcinoma *in situ* of the breast. *Am J Clin Pathol.* 1998;110:357–367.

34. Fraser JL, Raza S, Chorny K, et al. Columnar alteration with prominent apical snouts and secretions: a spectrum of changes frequently present in breast biopsies performed for microcalcifications. *Am J Surg Pathol.* 1998; 22:1521–1527.

35. Fraser JL, Pliss N, Connolly JL, Schnitt SJ. Immunophenotype of columnar alteration with prominent apical snouts and secretions (CAPSS). *Mod Pathol.* 2000;13:21A.

36. Noel J-C, Fayt I, Fernandes-Aguillar S, et al. Proliferating activity in columnar cell lesions of the breast. *Virchows Arch.* 2006;449:617–621.

37. Dabbs DJ, Carter G, Fudge M, et al. Molecular alterations in columnar cell lesions of the breast. *Mod Pathol.* 2006;19:344–349.

38. Kaneko M, Arihiro K, Takeshima Y, et al. Loss of heterozygosity and microsatellite instability in epithelial hyperplasia of the breast. *J Exp Ther Oncol.* 2002;2:9–18.

39. Schnitt SJ, Vincent-Salomon A. Columnar cell lesions of the breast. *Adv Anat Pathol.* 2003;10:113–124.

40. Guerra-Wallace MM, Christensen WN, White RL. A retrospective study of columnar alteration with prominent apical snouts and secretions and the association with cancer. *Am J Surg.* 2004;188:395–398.

41. Chivukula M, Bhargava R, Tseng G, Dabbs DJ. Clinico-pathologic implications of "flat epithelial atypia" in core needle biopsy specimens of the breast. *Am J Clin Pathol.* 2009;131:802–808.

42. Piubello Q, Parisi A, Eccher A, et al. Flat epithelial atypia on core needle biopsy. Which is the right management? *Am J Surg Pathol.* 2009;33: 1078–1084.

43. Senetta R, Campanino PP, Mariscotti G, et al. Columnar cell lesions associated with breast calcifications on vacuum-assisted core biopsies: clinical, radiographic, and histological correlations. *Mod Pathol.* 2009;22: 762–769.

44. Collins LC, Achacoso NA, Nekhlyudov L, et al. Clinical and pathologic features of ductal carcinoma in situ associated with the presence of flat epithelial atypia: an analysis of 543 patients. *Mod Pathol.* 2007;20: 1149–1155.

45. Abdel-fatah TM, Powe DG, Hodi Z, et al. High frequency of coexistence of columnar cell lesions, lobular neoplasia, and low grade ductal carcinoma in situ with invasive tubular carcinoma and invasive lobular carcinoma. *Am J Surg Pathol.* 2007;31:416–426.

46. Sahoo S, Recant WM. Triad of columnar cell alteration, lobular carcinoma in situ, and tubular carcinoma of the breast. *Breast J.* 2005;11:140–142.

47. Turashvili G, Hayes M, Gilks B, et al. Are columnar cell lesions the earliest histologically detectable non-obligate precursor of breast cancer? *Virchows Arch.* 2008;452:589–598.

48. Boulos FI, Dupont WD, Simpson JF, et al. Histologic associations and long-term cancer risk in columnar cell lesions of the breast. A retrospective cohort and a nested core-control study. *Cancer.* 2008;75:2415–2421.

49. Tocino I, Garcia BM, Carter D. Surgical biopsy findings in patients with atypical hyperplasia diagnosed by stereotaxic core needle biopsy. *Ann Surg Oncol.* 1996;3:483–488.

50. Jackman RJ, Birdwell RL, Ikeda DM. Atypical ductal hyperplasia: can some lesions be defined as probably benign after stereotactic 11-gauge vacuum-assisted biopsy, eliminating the recommendation for surgical excision? *Radiology.* 2002;224:548–554.

51. Maganini RO, Klem DA, Huston BJ, et al. Upgrade rate of core biopsy-determined atypical ductal hyperplasia by open excisional biopsy. *Am J Surg.* 2001;182:355–358.

52. Winchester DJ, Bernstein JR, Jeske JM, et al. Upstaging of atypical ductal hyperplasia after vacuum-assisted 11-gauge stereotactic core needle biopsy. *Arch Surg.* 2003;138:619–623.

53. Brem RF, Behrndt VS, Sanow L, Gatewood OM. Atypical ductal hyperplasia: histologic underestimation of carcinoma in tissue harvested from impalpable breast lesions using 11-gauge stereotactically guided directional vacuum-assisted biopsy. *Am J Roentgenol.* 1999;172:1405–1407.

54. Moore MM, Hargett CW, Hanks JB, et al. Association of breast cancer with the finding of atypical ductal hyperplasia at core breast biopsy. *Ann Surg.* 1997;225:726–731.

55. Gadzala DE, Cederbom GJ, Bolton JS, et al. Appropriate management of atypical ductal hyperplasia diagnosed by stereotactic core needle breast biopsy. *Ann Surg Oncol.* 1977;4:283–286.

56. Burbank F. Stereotactic breast biopsy of atypical ductal hyperplasia and ductal carcinoma in situ lesions: improved accuracy with directional, vacuum-assisted biopsy. *Radiology.* 1997;202:843–847.

57. Renshaw AA, Cartagena N, Schenkman RH, et al. Atypical ductal hyperplasia in breast core needle biopsies. *Am J Clin Pathol.* 2001;116:92–96.

58. Wagoner MJ, Laronga C, Acs G. Extent and histologic pattern of atypical ductal hyperplasia present on needle core biopsy specimens of the breast can predict ductal carcinoma in situ in subsequent excision. *Am J Clin Pathol.* 2009;131:112–121.

59. Kodlin D, Winger EE, Morgenstern NL, Chen V. Chronic mastopathy and breast cancer: a follow-up study. *Cancer.* 1977;39:2603–2607.

60. Dupont WD, Page DL. Breast cancer risk associated with proliferative disease, age at first birth, and family history of breast cancer. *Am J Epidemiol.* 1987;1225:769–779.

61. Krieger N, Hiatt RA. Risk of breast cancer after benign breast diseases. Variation by histologic type, degree of atypia, age at biopsy, and length of follow-up. *Am J Epidemiol.* 1992;135:619–631.

62. Davis HH, Simons M, Davis JB. Cystic disease of the breast: relationship to carcinoma. *Cancer.* 1964;17:957–978.

63. Page DL, DuPont WD, Rogers LW, Rados MS. Atypical hyperplastic lesions of the female breast. A long-term follow-up study. *Cancer.* 1985;55: 2698–2708.

64. Connolly J, Schnitt S, London S, et al. Both atypical lobular hyperplasia (ALH) and atypical ductal hyperplasia (ADH) predict for bilateral breast cancer risk. *Lab Invest.* 1992;66:13A.

65. Carter CL, Corle DK, Micozzi MS, et al. A prospective study of the development of breast cancer in 16,692 women with benign breast disease. *Am J Epidemiol.* 1988;128:467–477.

66. London SJ, Connolly JL, Schnitt SJ, Colditz GA. A prospective study of benign breast disease and the risk of breast cancer. *JAMA.* 1992;267:941–944.

67. Dupont WD, Page DL. Risk factors for breast cancer in women with proliferative breast disease. *N Engl J Med.* 1985;312:146–151.

68. Ma L, Boyd NF. Atypical hyperplasia and breast cancer risk: a critique. *Cancer Causes Control.* 1992;3:517–525.

69. Jensen RA, Page DL, Dupont WD, Rogers LW. Invasive breast cancer risk in women with sclerosing adenosis. *Cancer.* 1989;64:1977–1983.

Intraductal Carcinoma

70. Ernster VL, Barclay J, Kerlikowske K, et al. Incidence of and treatment for ductal carcinoma in situ of the breast. *JAMA.* 1996;275:913–918.
71. Ernster VL, Barclay J. Increases in ductal carcinoma in situ (DCIS) of the breast in relation to mammography: a dilemma. *J Natl Cancer Inst Monograph.* 1997;22:151–156.
72. Ward BA, McKhann CF, Ravikumar TS. Ten-year follow-up of breast carcinoma in situ in Connecticut. *Arch Surg.* 1992;127:1392–1395.
73. Chu KC, Tarone RE, Kessler LG, et al. Recent trends in U.S. breast cancer incidence, survival, and mortality rates. *JNCI.* 1996;88:1571–1579.
74. Verbeek ALM, Hendriks JHCL, Holland R, et al. Reduction of breast cancer mortality through mass screening with modern mammography: first results of the Nijmegen Project 1975–1981. *Lancet.* 1984;1:1222–1224.
75. Ciatto S, Cataliotti L, Distante V. Nonpalpable lesions detected with mammography: review of 512 consecutive cases. *Radiology.* 1987;165: 99–102.
76. Dershaw DD, Abramson A, Kinne DW. Ductal carcinoma in situ: mammographic findings and clinical implications. *Radiology.* 1989;170:411–415.
77. Stomper PC, Connolly JL, Meyer JE, Harris JR. Clinically occult ductal carcinoma in situ detected with mammography: analysis of 100 cases with radiologic-pathologic correlation. *Radiology.* 1989;172:235–241.
78. Holland R, Hendriks JHCL, Verbeek ALM, et al. Extent, distribution, and mammographic/histological correlations of breast ductal carcinoma in situ. *Lancet.* 1990;335:519–522.
79. Lagios MD. Multicentricity of breast carcinoma demonstrated by routine correlated subgross and radiographic examination. *Cancer.* 1977;40: 1726–1734.
80. Stomper PC, Connolly JL. Ductal carcinoma in situ of the breast: correlation between mammographic calcification and tumor subtype. *Am J Roentgenol.* 1992;159:483–485.
81. Zunzunegui R, Chung MA, Oruwari J, et al. Casting-type calcifications with invasion and high-grade ductal carcinoma in situ. A more aggressive disease? *Arch Surg.* 2003;138:537–540.
82. Evans A, Pinder S, Wilson R, et al. Ductal carcinoma in situ of the breast: correlation between mammographic and pathologic findings. *Am J Roentgenol.* 1994;162:1307–1311.
83. Evans AJ, Pinder SE, Ellis IO, et al. Correlations between the mammographic features of ductal carcinoma in situ (DCIS) and c-erb-s oncogene expression. *Clin Radiol.* 1994;49:559–562.
84. Patchefsky AS, Schwartz GF, Finkelstein SD, et al. Heterogeneity of intraductal carcinoma of the breast. *Cancer.* 1989;63:731–741.
85. Menell JH, Morris EA, Dershaw DD, et al. Determination of the presence and extent of pure ductal carcinoma in situ by mammography and magnetic resonance imaging. *Breast J.* 2005;11:382–390.
86. Gilles R, Zafrani B, Guinebretiere J-M, et al. Ductal carcinoma in situ: MR Imaging-histopathologic correlation. *Radiology.* 1995:196:415–419.
87. Orel S, Schnall M, Livolsi V, Troupin R. Suspicious breast lesions: MR imaging with radiologic-pathologic correlation. *Radiology.* 1994;190: 485–493.
88. Heywang-Köbrunner S. Contrast-enhanced magnetic resonance imaging of the breast. *Invest Radiol.* 1994;29:94–104.
89. Orel SG, Mendonca MH, Reynolds C, et al. MR imaging of ductal carcinoma in situ. *Radiology.* 1997;202:413–420.
90. Pediconi F, Catalano C, Roselli A, et al. Contrast-enhanced MR mammography for evaluation of the contralateral breast in patients with diagnosed unilateral breast cancer or high risk lesions. *Radiology.* 2007;243:670–680.
91. Cheng L, Al-Kaisi NK, Liu AY, Gordon NH. The results of intraoperative consultations in 181 ductal carcinomas in situ of the breast. *Cancer.* 1997; 80:75–79.
92. Rosen PP. Frozen section diagnosis of breast lesions. Recent experience with 556 consecutive biopsies. *Ann Surg.* 1978;187:17–19.
93. Rosen PP, Senie R, Schottenfeld D, Ashikari R. Noninvasive breast carcinoma: frequency of unsuspected invasion and implication for treatment. *Ann Surg.* 1979;189:98–103.
94. Wellings SR, Jensen HM, Marcum RG. An atlas of subgross pathology of the human breast with special reference to possible precancerous lesions. *JNCI.* 1975;55:231–273.
95. Barsky SH, Siegal GP, Jannotta F, Liotta LA. Loss of basement membrane components by invasive tumors but not by their benign counterparts. *Lab Invest.* 1983;49:140–147.
96. Farshid G, Moinfar F, Meredith DJ, et al. Spindle cell ductal carcinoma in situ. An unusual variant of ductal intra-epithelial neoplasia that stimulates ductal hyperplasia or a myoepithelial proliferation. *Virchows Arch.* 2001; 439:70–77.
97. Kawasaki, T, Nakamura S, Sakamoto G, et al. Neuroendocrine ductal carcinoma in situ (NE-DCIS) of the breast-comparative clinicopathologic study of 20 NE-DCIS cases and 274 non-NE-DCIS cases. *Histopathology.* 2008;53: 288–298.
98. Lennington WJ, Jensen RA, Dalton LW, Page DL. Ductal carcinoma in situ of the breast. Heterogeneity of individual lesions. *Cancer.* 1994;73:118–124.
99. Consensus Conference Committee. Consensus conference on the classification of ductal carcinoma in situ. *Cancer.* 1997;80:1798–1802.
100. Wen P, Marsh WL. SMMHC-p63 cocktail improves detection of myoepithelial layer in high-grade ductal carcinoma in-situ. *Mod Pathol.* 2005;18(suppl): 54a–55a.
101. Bose S, Lesser ML, Norton L, Rosen PP. Immunophenotype of intraductal carcinoma. *Arch Pathol Lab Med.* 1996;100:81–85.
102. Muir R, Aitkenhead AC. The healing of intraduct carcinoma of the mamma. *J Pathol Bacteriol.* 1934;38:117–127.
103. Davies JD. Hyperelastosis, obliteration and fibrous plaques in major ducts of the human breast. *J Pathol.* 1973;110:13–26.
104. Bryan BA, Schnitt SJ, Collins LC. Ductal carcinoma in situ with basal-like phenotype: a possible precursor to invasive basal-like breast cancer. *Mod Pathol.* 2006;19:617–621.
105. Dabbs DJ, Chivukula M, Carter G, Bhargava R. Basal phenotype of ductal carcinoma in situ: recognition and immunohistologic profile. *Mod Pathol.* 2006;19:1506–1511.
106. Chan JKC, Ng WF. Sclerosing adenosis cancerized by intraductal carcinoma. *Pathology.* 1987;19:425–428.
107. Eusebi V, Collina G, Bussolati G. Carinoma in situ in sclerosing adenosis of the breast: an immunocytochemical study. *Semin Diagn Pathol.* 1989;6: 146–152.
108. Oberman HA, Markey BA. Non-invasive carcinoma of the breast presenting in adenosis. *Mod Pathol.* 1991;4:31–35.
109. Taylor HB, Norris HJ. Epithelial invasion of nerves in benign diseases of the breast. *Cancer.* 1967;20:2245–2249.
110. Tsang WYW, Chan JKC. Neural invasion in intraductal carcinoma of the breast. *Hum Pathol.* 1992;23:202–204.
111. Rosen PP. Coexistant lobular carcinoma in situ and intraductal carcinoma in a single lobular-duct unit. *Am J Surg Pathol.* 1980;4:241–246.
112. Goldstein NS, Murphy T. Intraductal carcinoma associated with invasive carcinoma of the breast. A comparison of the two lesions with implications for intraductal carcinoma classification systems. *Am J Clin Pathol.* 1996;106:312–318.
113. Douglas-Jones AG, Gupta SK, Attanoos RL, et al. A critical appraisal of six modern classifications of ductal carcinoma in situ of the breast (DCIS): correlation with grade of associated invasive carcinoma. *Histopathology.* 1996;29:397–409.
114. Kestin I, Goldstein NS, Lacerna MD, et al. Factors associated with local recurrence of mammographically detected ductal carcinoma in situ in patients given breast conserving therapy. *Cancer.* 2000;88:596–607.
115. Schnitt SJ, Connolly JL. Classification of ductal carcinoma in situ: striving for clinical relevance in the era of breast conserving therapy. *Hum Pathol.* 1997;28:887–880.
116. Liberman L, Dershaw DD, Rosen PP, et al. Stereotaxic core biopsy of breast carcinoma: accuracy at predicting invasion. *Radiology.* 1995;194:379–381.
117. Renshaw AA. Predicting invasion in the excision specimen from breast core needle biopsy specimens with only ductal carcinoma in situ. *Arch Pathol Lab Med.* 2002;126:39–41.
118. Mendez I, Andreu FJ, Saez E, et al. Ductal carcinoma in situ and atypical ductal hyperplasia of the breast diagnosed at stereotactic core biopsy. *Breast J.* 2001;7:14–18.
119. Ozzello L. Ultrastructure of intra-epithelial carcinomas of the breast. *Cancer.* 1971;28:1508–1515.
120. Rajan PB, Perry RH. A quantitative study of patterns of basement membrane in ductal carcinoma in situ (DCIS) of the breast. *Breast J.* 1995;1: 315–321.
121. Ozzello L. The behaviour of basement membranes in intraductal carcinoma of the breast. *Am J Pathol.* 1959;35:887–899.
122. Coyne J, Haboubi NY. Micro-invasive breast carcinoma with granulomatous stromal response. *Histopathology.* 1992;20:184–185.
123. Hou L, Sneige N, Hunt KK, et al. Predictors of invasion in patients with core-needle biopsy-diagnosed ductal carcinoma in situ and recommendations for a selective approach to sentinel lymph node biopsy in ductal carcinoma in situ. *Cancer.* 2006;107:1760–1768.
124. Jackman RJ, Burbank F, Parker SH, et al. Stereotactic breast biopsy of nonpalpable lesions: determinants of ductal carcinoma in situ underestimation rates. *Radiology.* 2001;218:497–502.
125. King TA, Farr Jr GH, Cederblom GI, et al. A mass on breast imaging predicts coexisting invasive carcinoma in patients with a core biopsy diagnosis of ductal carcinoma in situ. *Am Surg.* 2001;67:907–912.
126. Bagnall MJ, Evans AJ, Wilson AR, et al. Predicting invasion in mammographically detected microcalcification. *Clin Radiol.* 2001;56:828–832.
127. Hoorntje LE, Schipper ME, Peeters PH, et al. The finding of invasive cancer after a preoperative diagnosis of ductal carcinoma in situ: causes of ductal carcinoma in situ underestimates with stereotactic 14-gauge needle biopsy. *Ann Surg Oncol.* 2003;10:748–753.
128. Yen TW, Hunt KK, Rose MI, et al. Predictors of invasive breast cancer in patients with an initial diagnosis of ductal carcinoma in situ: a guide to selective use of sentinel lymph node biopsy in management of ductal carcinoma in situ. *J Am Coll Surg.* 2005;200:516–526.
129. Hilson JB, Schnitt SJ, Collins LC. Phenotypic alterations in ductal carcinoma in situ-associated myoepithelial cells. Biologic and diagnostic implication. *Am J Surg Pathol.* 2009;33:227–232.
130. de Mascarel I, MacGrogan G, Mathoulin-Pelissier S, et al. Breast ductal carcinoma in situ with microinvasion. A definition supported by a long-term study of 1248 serially sectioned ductal carcinomas. *Cancer.* 2002; 94:2134–2142.

Invasive Duct Carcinoma

9

This is the largest group of malignant mammary tumors constituting 75% to 80% of mammary carcinomas. A generic term sometimes employed is *invasive duct carcinoma, not otherwise specified* (NOS). This is a useful designation that recognizes the distinction between the majority of invasive duct carcinomas and other, specific forms of duct carcinoma, such as tubular, medullary, metaplastic, colloid, and adenoid cystic carcinoma.

Invasive duct carcinoma NOS includes a subset of tumors that express in part characteristics of one of the specific types of breast carcinoma but do not constitute pure examples of the individual tumors. One example of this phenomenon is invasive duct carcinoma with lobular carcinoma features (Fig. 9.1). Foci of tubular, mucinous, or papillary differentiation can be found in invasive duct carcinomas. When evidence of a mixed growth pattern is present in a needle core biopsy, the findings should be reported descriptively, with final classification reserved for the excisional biopsy specimen. The relatively favorable prognosis associated with some specific histologic types has been found to apply only to those tumors composed entirely or in very large part of the designated pattern. Invasive duct carcinoma with a minor portion of a specific subtype is likely to have the prognosis of the dominant invasive duct carcinoma component.

The specimens obtained in a needle core biopsy procedure often include multiple samples of tumor tissue (Fig. 9.2). On occasion only a small fragment of the lesion may be present (Fig. 9.3). All tissue on a slide must be carefully examined to ensure that this very limited material is not overlooked. In the most extreme circumstance, the evidence is so scant that a diagnosis of carcinoma cannot be made with confidence, and an excisional biopsy is necessary to determine if carcinoma is present.

Although it is technically possible to examine needle core biopsy specimens by frozen section, this is not a standard practice and should only rarely be done in exceptional situations when there is strong clinical evidence that carcinoma is present, and there are compelling clinical circumstances that warrant immediate intervention after the diagnosis has been rendered (Fig. 9.4). Major reasons for avoiding frozen section diagnosis of needle core biopsy samples are the loss of tissue from these small specimens during slide preparation and the potential for misdiagnosis of a number of benign lesions that mimic carcinoma. The concern over interpretive issues that apply to these lesions when they are excised intact and examined by frozen section is enhanced in the disrupted form presented by needle core biopsy samples.

CLINICAL PRESENTATION

There are no specific clinical features that distinguish invasive duct carcinoma from other types of invasive carcinoma and some benign tumors. The lesions occur throughout the age range of breast carcinoma. Invasive duct carcinoma typically forms a solid tumor. Cystic change in this group of lesions is extremely uncommon but may be a manifestation of necrosis.

Size

The measured gross *size* of a mammary carcinoma is one of the most significant prognostic variables. Survival decreases with increasing tumor size of invasive duct carcinoma and most of the subtypes of breast carcinoma, and there is a coincidental rise in the frequency of axillary nodal metastases (1,2). This phenomenon applies not only to the overall spectrum of primary tumor size, but also within subsets such as those defined by TNM (tumor–node–metastasis) staging. For example, among T_1 breast carcinomas (less than or equal to 2 cm in diameter), there is a significant relationship between size, the frequency of nodal metastases, and prognosis when the tumors are stratified in 5-mm groups (3,4).

Roger et al. (5) reported the following significant ($P < 0.0001$) distribution of the frequency of axillary nodal involvement in relation to tumor size in a series of 534 patients: T_1a (0–0.5 cm) (3%); T_1b (0.6–1.0 cm) (10%); 1.1 to 15 cm (21%); 1.6 to 2.0 cm (35%). Data from the Breast Cancer Surveillance Consortium for 786,846 women aged 40 to 89 years with breast carcinomas diagnosed by screening mammography revealed negative axillary lymph nodes

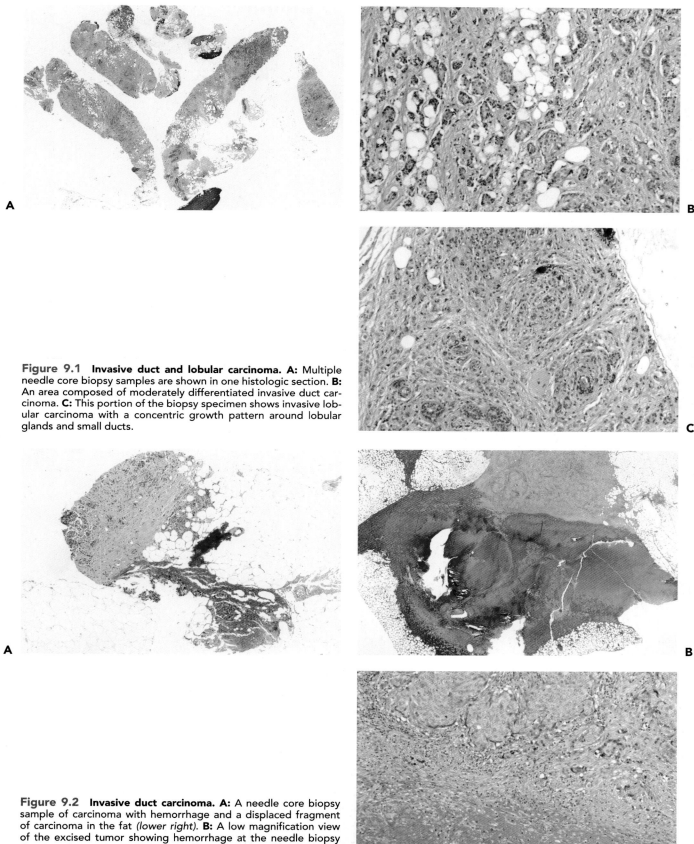

Figure 9.1 Invasive duct and lobular carcinoma. A: Multiple needle core biopsy samples are shown in one histologic section. **B:** An area composed of moderately differentiated invasive duct carcinoma. **C:** This portion of the biopsy specimen shows invasive lobular carcinoma with a concentric growth pattern around lobular glands and small ducts.

Figure 9.2 Invasive duct carcinoma. A: A needle core biopsy sample of carcinoma with hemorrhage and a displaced fragment of carcinoma in the fat *(lower right)*. **B:** A low magnification view of the excised tumor showing hemorrhage at the needle biopsy site. Invasive carcinoma is present above the area of hemorrhage. **C:** Granulation tissue is present between the poorly differentiated invasive duct carcinoma above and the blood clot.

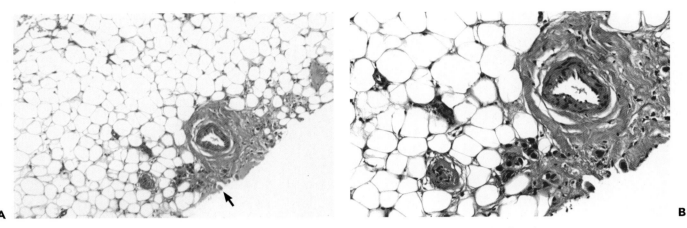

Figure 9.3 Invasive duct carcinoma. A, B: A small group of atypical epithelial cells in fat *(arrow)* around a blood vessel in this needle core biopsy specimen was the only evidence of carcinoma. The material was not considered diagnostic. Excisional biopsy of an 8-mm circumscribed tumor revealed invasive poorly differentiated duct carcinoma.

in 91.8%, 78.2%, and 57.9% of patients with tumors that measured 0 to 10 mm, 11 to 20 mm, and 21 to 50 mm, respectively (6).

Analysis of the tumor size of primary breast carcinomas recorded in SEER registry data revealed a progressive increase in the proportion of smaller tumors between 1975 and 1999 (7). The proportion of carcinomas that measured less than 1 cm rose from less than 10% in the period

1975 to 1979 to about 25% in 1995 to 1999 among node-negative patients. Among node-positive patients the proportion with tumors less than 2 cm rose from about 20% to 33% between the same time periods. In both groups, the trends toward smaller tumors were statistically significant. These trends in tumor size distribution were matched by increased relative survival rates in the node-negative and node-positive groups.

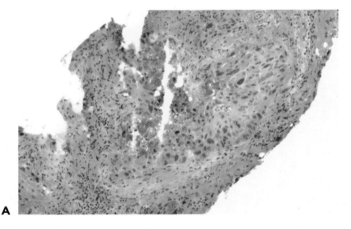

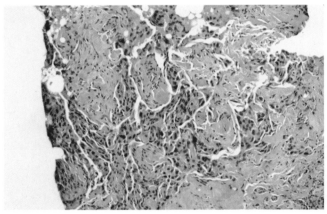

Figure 9.4 Invasive duct carcinoma, frozen section. A: This frozen section preparation from a needle core biopsy specimen shows duct carcinoma with necrosis and poorly differentiated nuclear grade. The presence of invasion could not be established from this sample. **B:** Invasive poorly differentiated duct carcinoma was evident in the paraffin section from the frozen tissue sample. The tissue is distorted by frozen section artefact. **C:** The appearance of the tumor without frozen section artefact is shown here in the excisional biopsy specimen.

Size and Prognosis

Long-term follow-up is necessary to fully assess the prognosis of patients who had invasive carcinoma with a favorable stage such as $T_1N_0M_0$. The 20-year overall survival in a Finish Cancer Registry study was 54% (95% CI: 48–60%), and the survival rate corrected for non-breast carcinoma deaths was 81% (95% CI: 75–87%) (8). In patients with T_1a–b tumors, the corrected 20-year survival rate was 92% (95% CI: 86–96%), and in the T_1c group corrected 20-year survival was 75% (95% CI: 64–86%). During the first 15 years of follow-up, the risk of death due to breast carcinoma was 0.70% per year of follow-up, rising to 0.80%, 1.51%, and 1.19% per year in each of the subsequent 5-year intervals. During the same period, the risk of death due to nonmammary carcinoma was 0.23%, 0.45%, 0.88%, and 0.71% per year in each 5-year period.

The interaction of the number of involved lymph nodes and tumor size is important prognostically in stage II patients. Quiet et al. (9) found that the long-term disease-free survival after mastectomy was 81% in patients, with one lymph node metastasis and a tumor 2 cm or smaller, compared with 59% if the tumor was larger than 2 cm.

Because many carcinomas have asymmetric shapes, the measurement of size is generally reported in terms of the greatest diameter. The gross measurement of the size of a carcinoma is only an approximation of the actual amount of invasive tumor present (10,11). In some tumors, a considerable part of the mass is composed of invasive carcinoma, whereas other lesions of comparable size may have a substantial component of intraductal carcinoma, resulting in a lesser volume of invasive carcinoma. Measurement of the invasive component exclusive of peripheral extensions of intraductal carcinoma is recommended when it is practical on the basis of histologic sections.

Size and Needle Core Biopsy Samples

It is rarely possible to accurately measure the size of an invasive carcinoma in a needle core biopsy specimen because it is difficult to ensure that the sample represents a complete diameter in the largest dimension. When microinvasive ductal carcinoma is found in a needle core biopsy specimen, it is possible that a larger invasive lesion will be found when an excisional biopsy is performed. A small invasive focus may be limited to one of multiple levels prepared from a paraffin block (12). Correlation of the needle core biopsy specimen with the dimensions of a small lesion seen on a mammogram can be useful in some circumstances to confirm the size of a carcinoma and to assess the contour of the tumor.

A review of tumor sizes determined in mammograms and excised specimens found no evidence that a prior needle core biopsy influenced the measurement of the tumors (13). The study evaluated 138 mammographically detected T_1 invasive carcinomas, including 61 sampled by core biopsy before excision and 77 excised without a core biopsy. The mean differences between mammographic and pathologic sizes in the two groups were not significantly different (2.3 mm and 1.96 mm, respectively). However, there are circumstances in which needle core biopsy sampling removes a substantial portion of a small invasive carcinoma to the extent that the remaining tumor in the excised specimen no longer accurately reflects the pre-biopsy size. In such situations, size based on imaging studies may be more accurate than pathologic measurements.

Size and Multifocal Carcinoma

A minority of patients have clinically or grossly identifiable multifocal tumor in the same breast quadrant, or multicentric tumors in more than one quadrant. When clinically apparent, multiple nodules may be sampled by needle core biopsies to confirm this impression. The sixth edition of the American Joint Committee on Cancer Staging Manual (AJCC) (14) refers to tumor size as the diameter of the largest invasive lesion when multiple separate invasive tumors are present. There are no AJCC guidelines for distinguishing between discontinuous portions of a single focus and separate tumors. It is reasonable to conclude that separate primary tumors are present if each focus includes intraductal carcinoma and there is nonneoplastic breast tissue between the foci. Connolly (15) observed that based on AJCC guidelines, "If the foci are clearly separate, measure the largest for pT. This area requires a lot of judgement."

Jain et al. (16) described a study of 139 patients with synchronous, multifocal invasive breast carcinomas. The mean tumor diameter of the largest focus in multifocal cases was 2.1 cm, whereas the mean aggregate diameter of multifocal tumors was 3.6 cm. When staging was based on the single largest invasive tumor, patients with multifocal carcinoma were more likely to have axillary nodal metastases than those with a single tumor of equivalent size. Data obtained by Andea et al. (17) also suggest that the aggregate diameter of grossly measurable nodules should be used to determine tumor size or T stage rather than the current convention of staging on the basis of the largest nodule. When aggregate tumor diameter was calculated, multifocal and unifocal carcinomas of similar size did not differ significantly with respect to nodal status (18). Coombs and Boyages (19) obtained a similar result in an analysis of 94 (11.1%) patients with multifocal carcinoma in a series of 848 women with breast carcinoma. Axillary nodal metastases were present in 52.1% of patients with multifocal carcinoma and in 37.5% of those with unifocal tumors. When tumor size among those with multifocal carcinoma was based only on the largest lesion, patients with multifocal tumors had more frequent nodal metastases than women with unifocal tumors of equivalent diameter. This difference was substantially diminished when aggregate tumor size was taken into consideration for multifocal tumor cases.

For staging on the basis of the standards set forth by the AJCC, tumor size in patients with multifocal carcinoma will be reported as the largest tumor diameter until these rules are adjusted. In clinical practice it should be appreciated that this rule leads to understaging of tumor size in some cases. It would be prudent for the individual pathology report to provide the size (diameter) of the single largest invasive tumor focus and the aggregate size on the basis of largest diameters of all measurable invasive tumor foci. This information can be provided separately for multiple grossly evident invasive lesions and for foci that are histologically identified.

As noted previously, needle core biopsy samples are not a reliable basis for measuring tumor diameter in many cases, and these samples cannot be relied upon to determine whether multifocal invasive carcinoma is present. Problems also arise in the determination of tumor size that takes into account the span of invasive carcinoma in the core biopsy sample and tumor remaining at the biopsy site in the excisional specimen.

Size and Magnetic Resonance Imaging

Magnetic resonance (MR) imaging offers a clinical, objective method for determining tumor volume without the necessity for calculations based on pathologic tumor measurements. MR measurements of tumor diameter correlate more closely with pathologic tumor size than do measurements by mammography, ultrasound or clinical examination (20). MR has also proven to be the most accurate method for measuring tumor size during neoadjuvant chemotherapy (21).

Grading

Histologic grading of invasive duct carcinomas is an estimate of structural differentiation, limited to the invasive portion of the tumor (Fig. 9.5). The most widely used histologic grading system is based on criteria established by Bloom and Richardson (22) and Elston and Ellis (23). The parameters measured are the extent of tubule formation, nuclear size, and mitotic rate. Each of the three elements is assigned a score on a scale of 1 to 3, and the final grade is determined by the sum of the scores. Histologic grade is usually expressed in three categories: scores 3 to 5, well differentiated or grade 1; scores 6 to 7, intermediate or grade 2; scores 8 to 9, poorly differentiated or grade 3. A modified Scarff–Bloom–Richardson system presented by Robbins et al. (24) is outlined in Table 9.1.

Nuclear grading is the cytologic evaluation of tumor nuclei in comparison with the nuclei of normal mammary epithelial cells (Fig. 9.6). Because nuclear grading does not involve an assessment of the growth pattern of the tumor, this procedure is applicable not only to invasive duct carcinoma but also other subtypes of mammary carcinoma. The most widely employed system for nuclear grading, introduced by Black et al. (25) and Cutler et al. (26) is usually reported in terms of three categories: well differentiated, intermediate, and poorly differentiated. By convention, the sequence of numerical designations originally used for nuclear grading was the reverse of histologic grading, but more recently, there has been a trend to employ a numbering system that conforms to histologic grading (grade 1, well differentiated; grade 2, moderately differentiated;

grade 3, poorly differentiated). Because of the potential for confusion on this issue, it is preferable to employ descriptive terms for nuclear grading rather than numerals.

Several studies have investigated the accuracy of histologic grading based on needle core biopsy specimens when compared with the final grade determined from the excised tumor. The reported concordance rates ranged from 59% to 75% (27–29). In the same studies, concordance with respect to tumor type ranged from 66.6% to 81.0%. These data suggest that classification and grading of invasive carcinomas based on the needle core biopsy sample should be regarded as provisional. This consideration should be borne in mind when neoadjuvant therapy is administered on the basis of a diagnosis made with a needle core biopsy sample. Tumor heterogeneity is the most common source of discordant classification and grading but interobserver and intraobserver variation are also factors.

The histologic and nuclear grades of a given tumor coincide in many but not all invasive duct carcinomas (30). Nuclear and histologic grade have been shown to be useful predictors of prognosis for patients stratified by stage of disease, especially those without axillary lymph node metastases (31,32). Increasing tumor grade has been associated with several factors that are related to an increased risk for breast recurrence after conservation therapy, including greater tumor size, diagnosis at the relatively young age, and absence of estrogen receptor expression. Although some investigators found a significant relationship between grade and local recurrence (33), others concluded that grade was not a significant predictor of local recurrence (34). In patients with relatively favorable stage I carcinomas treated by lumpectomy without radiotherapy, the tumor recurred sooner and with greater frequency after a median follow-up of 58 months in patients with high-grade carcinomas (35).

Women with *BRCA1* mutations have a significantly higher frequency of poorly differentiated carcinomas when compared with individuals not carrying this mutation. *BRCA1* mutations occurring in sporadic and familial breast carcinomas have been associated with similar patterns of poorly differentiated growth (36). This is manifested by a nuclear grade denoting poor differentiation (36), low frequency of estrogen receptor positivity (36), and a high histologic grade (37). Mammography did not detect a significant difference in the radiographic appearance of carcinomas in *BRCA1* carriers (38).

Stromal Inflammatory Cell Infiltrate

The stromal inflammatory cell infiltrate within and around invasive duct carcinomas usually consists of mature lymphocytes with a variable admixture of plasma cells, neutrophils, mast cells, and macrophages (Fig. 9.7). Rarely neutrophils or eosinophils are prominent. Nonmedullary duct carcinomas with a prominent lymphocytic reaction tend to be poorly differentiated, and they are almost always negative for estrogen and progesterone receptors. Studies of the lymphocyte subgroups infiltrating mammary carcinomas

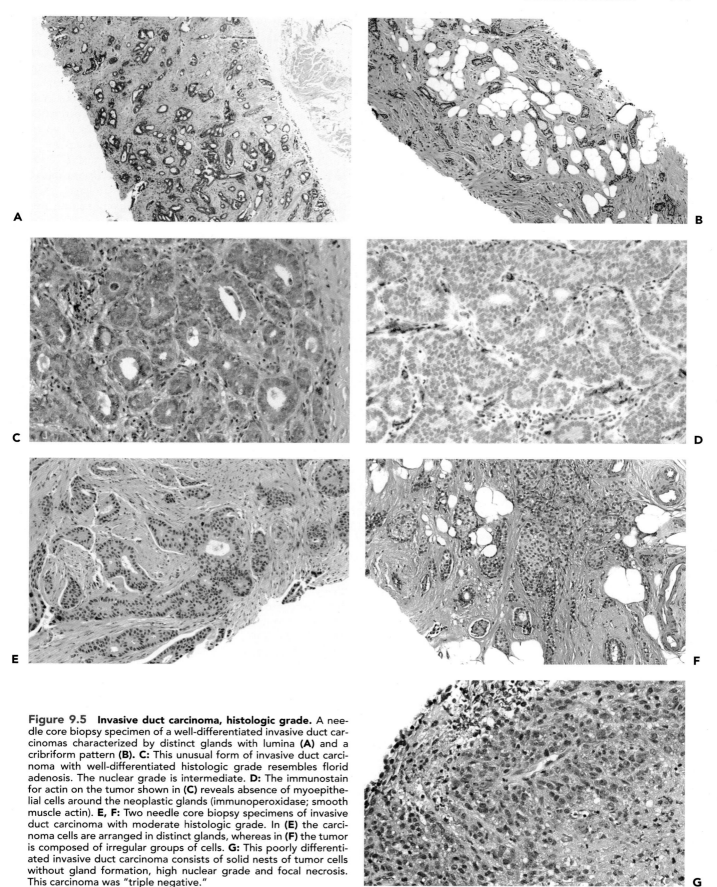

Figure 9.5 Invasive duct carcinoma, histologic grade. A needle core biopsy specimen of a well-differentiated invasive duct carcinomas characterized by distinct glands with lumina **(A)** and a cribriform pattern **(B). C:** This unusual form of invasive duct carcinoma with well-differentiated histologic grade resembles florid adenosis. The nuclear grade is intermediate. **D:** The immunostain for actin on the tumor shown in **(C)** reveals absence of myoepithelial cells around the neoplastic glands (immunoperoxidase; smooth muscle actin). **E, F:** Two needle core biopsy specimens of invasive duct carcinoma with moderate histologic grade. In **(E)** the carcinoma cells are arranged in distinct glands, whereas in **(F)** the tumor is composed of irregular groups of cells. **G:** This poorly differentiated invasive duct carcinoma consists of solid nests of tumor cells without gland formation, high nuclear grade and focal necrosis. This carcinoma was "triple negative."

TABLE 9.1
A MODIFIED SCARFF–BLOOM–RICHARDSON GRADING

Tubule/Formation

Score 1: >75% of tumor has tubules
Score 2: 10–75% of tumor has tubules
Score 3: <10% tubule formation

Nuclear Size

Score 1: tumor nuclei similar to normal duct cell nuclei
(2–3× rbc)
Score 2: intermediate-size nuclei
Score 3: very large nuclei, usually vesicular with
prominent nucleoli

Mitotic Count

On the basis of 10 HPF from edge of tumor (40× objective,
400× magnification, field area 0.196 mm^2)
Score 1: 0–7 mitoses
Score 2: 8–14 mitoses
Score 3: ≥15 mitoses

From Robbins P, Pinder S, de Klerk N, et al. Histological grading of
breast carcinomas: a study of interobserver agreement. *Hum Pathol.*
1995;26:873–879, with permission.

indicate that they are largely T lymphocytes (39) consisting mainly of T4 (CD4+) helper and T8 (CD8+) cytotoxic suppressor cells (40).

Mast cells can be detected in the tumor stroma by immunostaining for c-Kit (CD117). The presence of mast cells in stroma associated with breast carcinoma was reported to be a marker of favorable prognosis, especially in node-negative women (41). Studies of the prognostic significance of mast cells have been done on excised tumors. It remains to be determined whether needle core biopsies provide adequate samples for reliably evaluating mast cell infiltration in breast carcinomas.

Lymphovascular Invasion

The presence of lymphatic tumor emboli (Fig. 9.8) in the breast is an unfavorable prognostic finding. For this purpose, lymphatics are defined as vascular channels lined by endothelium without supporting smooth muscle or elastica. Most lymphatics do not contain red blood cells, but undoubtedly some blood capillaries are included in this definition. Nonvascular spaces can be formed around nests of tumor cells within an invasive carcinoma as a result of tissue retraction during processing, so-called *shrinkage* or *retraction* artefact (Fig. 9.9). It can be difficult to distinguish retraction artefact from true lymphatic spaces (42). Assessment for lymphatic invasion (LI) is more reliably accomplished in breast parenchyma adjacent to or well beyond the invasive tumor margin, where these artefacts are less often present (43). An unusual pattern of necrosis in carci-

noma that involves pseudoangiomatous stromal hyperplasia can simulate LI by carcinoma (Fig. 9.10).

Retraction artefact is more commonly found in ductal than in lobular carcinomas or in carcinomas with ductal and lobular features. Carcinomas with retraction artefact tend to exhibit high histologic and nuclear grade. Acs et al. (44) found that there was a significant direct correlation between the presence of retraction artefact and the presence of lymphatic tumor emboli in node-negative patients. Furthermore, node-negative patients with retraction artefact had a significantly higher frequency of distant metastases than patients without retraction artefact. These findings led the investigators to suggest that retraction artefact may reflect significant aspects of tumoral–stromal interaction, possibly related to the formation of lymphatic channels and not simply a passive phenomenon due to incomplete tissue fixation. The presence of micropapillary features, which may represent a special type of retraction artefact, in invasive duct carcinomas also appears to predispose to axillary nodal metastases (45). Immunostains are useful for distinguishing between retraction artifact and LI.

Controversy exists over the presence of intratumoral vascular channels and whether lymphangiogenesis occurs in carcinomas. The availability of antibodies with a high degree of specificity for lymphatic endothelium has facilitated investigation of these issues. In general, it has been observed that lymphangiogenesis is limited or absent within breast carcinomas and that lymphatic vessel density is substantially greater in peritumoral than in intratumoral stroma (46–48).

Before the availability of lymphatic endothelial markers, efforts to identify lymphatic spaces by using immunoperoxidase reagents associated with blood vessel endothelial cells (factor VIII, CD34 or CD31, and blood group antigens) met with limited success (49–51). Reactivity is strongest in blood vessel endothelium and weakest or absent in lymphatic endothelium. D2-40 is a monoclonal antibody directed at podoplanin with a high degree of specificity for the endothelium of lymphatic vessels in normal tissues and lymphatics in the stroma associated with carcinomas (52,53). A nonneoplastic vascular channel that is D2-40(+) and CD31(−) and/or CD34(−) is very likely to be a lymphatic space whereas the reverse immunophenotype [D2-40(−), CD31(+), and/or CD34(+)] is highly associated with a blood vessel channel. In a study using the CD34 and D2-40 antibodies, Van den Eynden et al. (54) were able to localize blood vessel [D2-40(−), CD34(+) and lymphatic D2-40(+), CD34(−) or (+)] tumor emboli. Intratumoral and peritumoral sites of lymphovascular invasion were tabulated separately. The presence of axillary nodal metastases was associated with peritumoral but not with intratumoral lymphatic tumor emboli detected by the D2-40 immunostain in studies by Van den Eynden et al. (54) and de Mascarel et al. (55). The observation that periductal myoepithelial cells are sometimes reactive D2-40 (56) indicates a potential source of misdiagnosis of lymphatic tumor emboli when intraductal carcinoma becomes detached from the myoepithelial layer and is displaced into a duct lumen. This phenomenon is found most commonly in

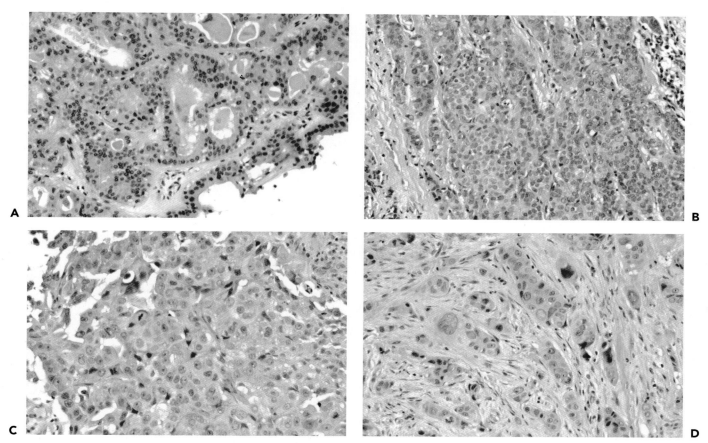

Figure 9.6 **Invasive duct carcinoma, nuclear grade. A:** Well-differentiated nuclear grade is characterized by cells having small, regular, round nuclei with even chromatin, lacking nucleoli and mitoses. **B, C:** Moderately differentiated nuclear grade is characterized by modest nuclear pleomorphism and enlargement, with nucleoli in some nuclei. The nuclei are slightly hyperchromatic. **D:** Poorly differentiated nuclear grade features marked nuclear pleomorphism and enlargement with hyperchromasia.

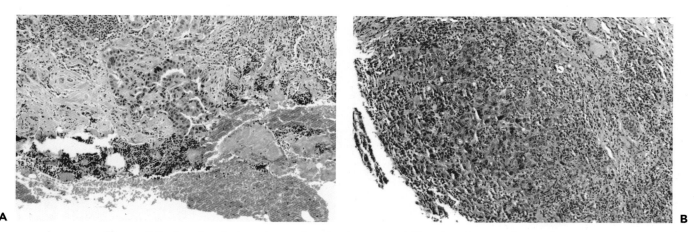

Figure 9.7 **Invasive duct carcinoma, lymphoplasmacytic infiltration. A:** A needle core biopsy specimen showing modest lymphocytic reaction associated with invasive duct carcinoma. **B:** Extreme lymphoplasmacytic infiltration in a needle core biopsy sample from a poorly differentiated invasive duct carcinoma. Medullary carcinoma would be considered in the differential diagnosis of such a specimen. In this instance, the excised tumor was not classified as medullary carcinoma because it had areas of invasive growth.

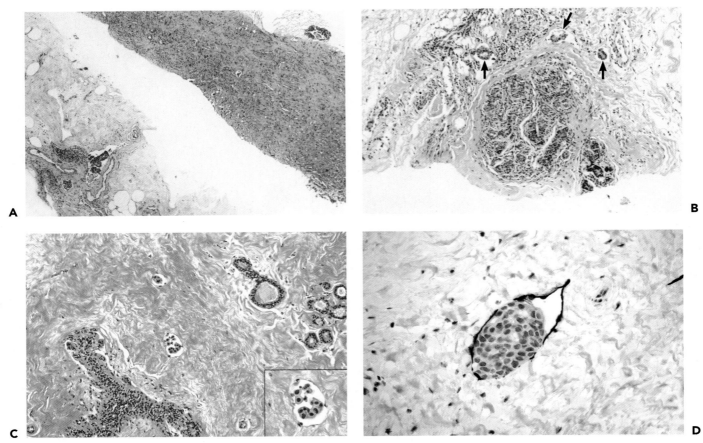

Figure 9.8 **Invasive duct carcinoma with lymphatic tumor emboli. A:** This needle core biopsy specimen shows clusters of carcinoma cells in dilated lymphatic spaces among small blood vessels *(left)* adjacent to a sample of invasive poorly differentiated duct carcinoma *(right)*. **B:** Lymphatic tumor emboli *(arrows)* are located in the stroma around a lobule in a needle core biopsy specimen. **C:** Carcinoma cells in lymphatic channels. **D:** A lymphatic channel containing carcinoma cells is immunoreactive for D2-40 (immunoperoxidase).

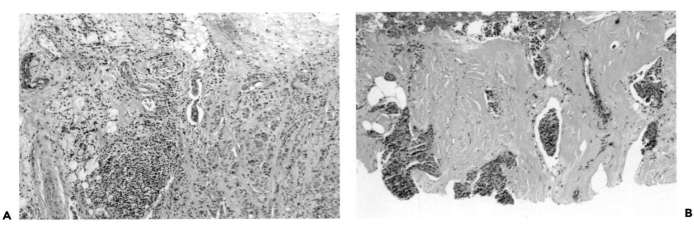

Figure 9.9 **Invasive duct carcinoma with retraction artefact. A:** Two clusters of carcinoma cells are present in a bilobed space in the midst of this needle core biopsy specimen. The contour of the space closely duplicates the shape of the carcinoma that it contains. This is hallmark of retraction artefact. **B:** Retraction artefact in a needle core biopsy specimen from an invasive duct carcinoma.

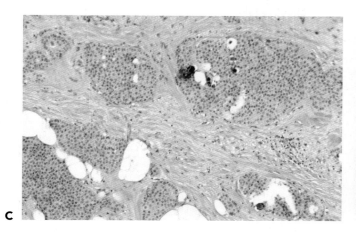

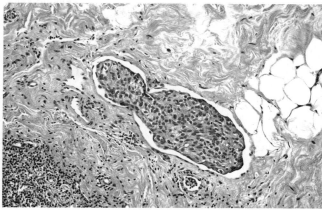

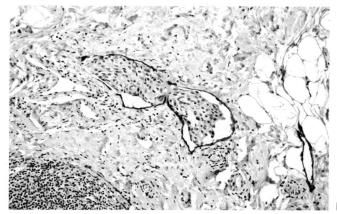

Figure 9.9 *(continued)* **C:** No retraction artefact was present in the excisional biopsy of the tumor shown in **(B). D, E:** A bilobed focus of invasive duct carcinoma in a space with the appearance of retraction artefact. Immunoreactivity for D2-40 **(E)** demonstrates that this is intralymphatic carcinoma.

excisional biopsy specimens at sites of prior vacuum-assisted needle core biopsy procedures.

Monoclonal and polyclonal antibodies directed at the endothelial hyaluronan receptor-1 (LYVE-1) have also proven to be useful for detecting lymphatic tumor emboli associated with breast carcinomas (57,58). In studies with smaller number of cases, the presence of lymphatic tumor emboli detected with the LYVE-1 antibody proved to be associated with the presence of axillary nodal metastases and a poor prognosis (57,58).

Presently, antibodies to D2-40, LYVE-1, and other endothelial markers can be employed in individual cases where there may be uncertainty about the presence of lymphovascular invasion at a particular site in the tissues. Whenever such an investigation is undertaken, a contemporaneous hematoxylin and eosin (H&E)-stained section must always be made to ensure correlation of the immunostained sections with the histologic appearance of the tissue. Screening of breast carcinoma specimens with markers for lymphatic endothelium is presently an investigational

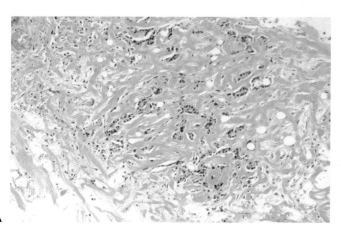

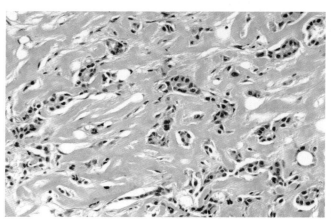

Figure 9.10   Invasive duct carcinoma with necrosis. A, B: The invasive duct carcinoma in this needle core biopsy specimen is growing in stroma that has a pseudoangiomatous architecture.

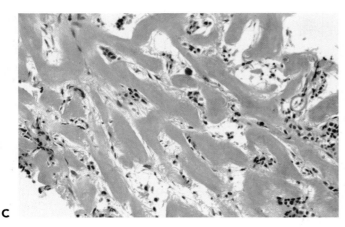
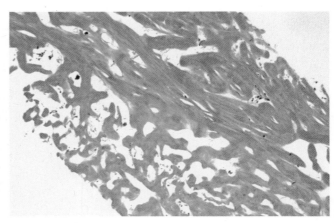

C   D

Figure 9.10 *(continued)* **C, D:** The pseudoangiomatous pattern is accentuated in areas of necrosis.

procedure, the results of which have yet to be correlated with long-term follow-up results.

Extratumoral lymphatic tumor emboli in the breast are found associated with approximately 15% of invasive duct carcinomas that have been examined in excisional biopsy specimens. The majority of these patients also have axillary lymph node metastases, but lymphatic tumor emboli are found in the breast surrounding invasive duct carcinomas in 5% to 10% of patients who have pathologically negative lymph nodes in routine H&E slides. Several studies have shown that lymphatic emboli are prognostically unfavorable in node-negative patients treated by mastectomy (9,59–61) and by breast conservation therapy (62).

Lymphatic tumor emboli do not predispose to local recurrence in patients treated by mastectomy (60), but they have been associated with an increased risk for recurrence in the breast after breast conservation therapy (62). Liljegren et al. (63) reported that the relative risk for recurrence in the breast after conservation therapy was 1.9% (95% CI, 1.1–3.5) in a comparison of women with or without peritumoral lymphatic tumor emboli.

Lymphatic tumor emboli detected with the D2-40 immunostain in node-negative patients are also associated with a significant risk for distant but not for local recurrence. Aranaout-Alkarain et al. (64) used D2-40 to detect lymphatic tumor emboli in 303 invasive carcinomas from node-negative women with a median follow-up of 7.6 years. LI was found in 27%, mainly at the perimeter of the carcinomas. Patients with lymphatic tumor emboli detected by this method had a significantly higher frequency of distant recurrence and shorter survival than those without this finding.

The deleterious effect of lymphatic tumor emboli is most pronounced in women with $T_1N_0M_0$ disease. In a 10-year follow-up study of 378 patients treated for $T_1N_0M_0$ carcinoma, 33% of 30 women with lymphatic emboli died of the disease. Death due to breast carcinoma was observed in 20% of the 348 women who did not have lymphatic emboli (3). Another study comparing similar subsets of $T_1N_0M_0$ patients found recurrences in 32% of those with lymphatic emboli and in 10% of controls (65). In stage I patients with tumors larger than 2 cm ($T_2N_0M_0$), those with lymphatic

emboli also experienced a higher metastatic rate (61). Metastases that develop in node-negative patients who have peritumoral lymphatic emboli tend to occur more than 5 years after diagnosis, and they are almost always systemic.

Blood vessel invasion is defined as penetration by tumor into the lumen of an artery or vein. These vascular structures can be identified by the presence of a smooth muscle wall supported by elastic fibers. It is usually necessary to employ special histochemical procedures (e.g., orcein or Verhoeff-van Gieson stains) that selectively highlight elastic tissue in order to detect this component of the vascular wall. Elastic fibers are often deposited around ducts that contain intraductal carcinoma within an invasive tumor, and the resulting appearance in an elastic tissue stain may be difficult to distinguish from vascular invasion. Because larger vascular components in the breast usually consist of a paired artery and vein, vascular invasion should only be diagnosed with confidence when tumor is demonstrated within one or both of a pair of vessels demonstrated by an elastic tissue stain. The independent prognostic significance of true blood vessel invasion has not been definitively determined.

Angiogenesis

Angiogenesis associated with breast carcinomas reflects the capacity of neoplastic tissue to induce vascular proliferation (66). Tumor growth is enhanced not only by increased perfusion associated with neovascularization, but also by the paracrine mitogenic effects of growth factors produced by endothelial cells (65). Pathologic studies of angiogenesis in breast carcinoma have examined the relevance of tumor vascularity to known prognostic markers and to prognosis. To perform such studies, histologic sections of paraffin embedded tissue are stained with an immunohistochemical marker for endothelial cells (67) (Fig. 9.11). Vessel counts are recorded in foci of greatest vascular density, so-called *hot spots*, by counting the number of immunostained structures in a predetermined number of fields at a fixed magnification (68). A significant problem in the method of assessment based on detecting hot spots is the heterogeneity of vascularity with breast carcinomas. A study of angiogenesis

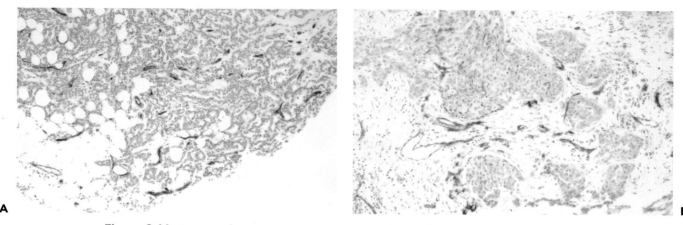

Figure 9.11   Invasive duct carcinoma with angiogenesis. A, B: Vascularity is demonstrated in the needle core biopsy specimens of two invasive duct carcinomas with the immunostain for CD34 (immunoperoxidase). The tumor invades fat in **(A)** and fibrous stroma in **(B)**.

in multiple blocks from individual carcinomas revealed an average coefficient of variation (CV) of 11.1% for vessel counts in hot spots in different sections from a single paraffin block and a CV of 24.4% when hot spots in sections from different blocks from the same tumor were compared (69). The authors concluded that "one must carefully scan all the available tumor material in each case for the best spot." Counts based on limited samples, such as needle core biopsies or one section of a tumor could be highly misleading. Consequently conventional needle core biopsy specimens are not suitable for estimating angiogenesis by current methods.

Perineural Invasion

Perineural invasion can be found in approximately 10% of invasive duct carcinomas (Fig. 9.12). It tends to occur in high-grade tumors, frequently in association with lymphatic tumor emboli, but it has not been proven to have independent prognostic significance.

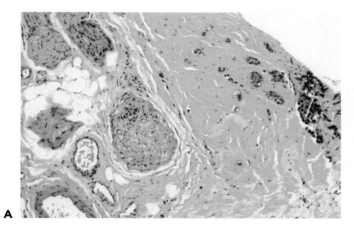

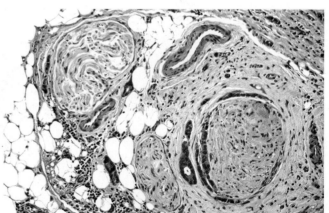

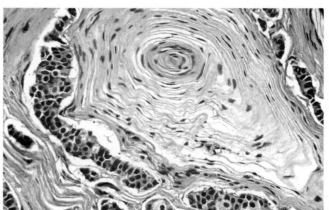

Figure 9.12   Invasive duct carcinoma with perineural infiltration. A, B: Carcinoma cells are shown invading in and around nerves in needle core biopsy specimens from two patients. **C:** Carcinoma surrounding a pacinian corpuscle resembles perineural infiltration.

Stromal Elastosis

Abundant elastosis in the stroma of an invasive duct carcinoma is significantly associated with estrogen receptor positivity (Fig. 9.13). The significance of elastosis as an independent prognostic variable remains controversial (70,71).

Absence of Myoepithelium

Invasive duct carcinoma lacks myoepithelium, a characteristic that helps to distinguish it from benign proliferative lesions, with the exception of microglandular adenosis. Because loss of myoepithelium occurs in some, but not all in situ carcinomas, failure to detect myoepithelium is not by itself diagnostic of invasive carcinoma. Cross-reactivity of stromal cells with myoepithelial markers can be a confounding factor by creating the false impression that myoepithelium is present (Fig. 9.14). For this reason, the p63 immunostain is preferable because reactivity is limited to myoepithelial cell nuclei. It is often also useful to employ a cytokeratin stain to highlight the growth pattern of the

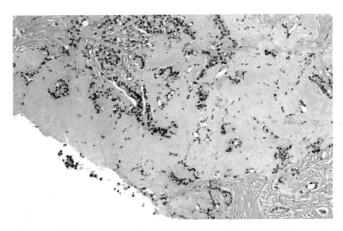

Figure 9.13 Invasive duct carcinoma with stromal elastosis. The stroma in this needle core biopsy specimen contains homogeneous masses of amphophilic elastin in invasive duct carcinoma.

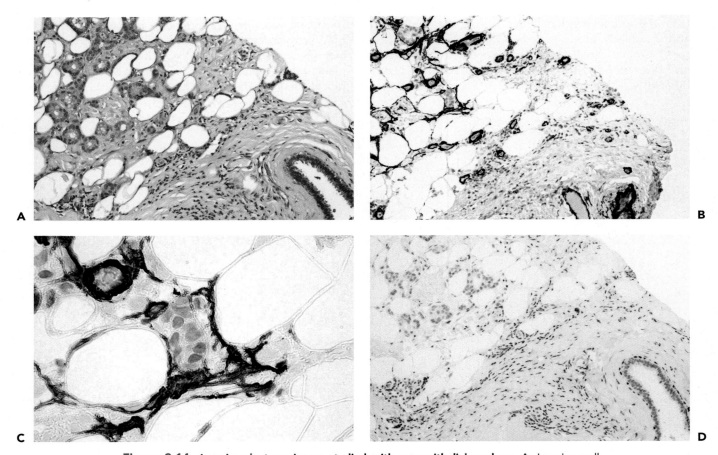

A   **B**   **C**   **D**

Figure 9.14 Invasive duct carcinoma studied with myoepithelial markers. A: Invasive well-differentiated duct carcinoma in a needle core biopsy specimen. **B, C:** The smooth muscle actin stain on the tumor in **(A)** is reactive with vascular structures and stromal cells. The stromal background staining encircles carcinoma glands in a manner that simulates myoepithelium (immunoperoxidase). **D:** No nuclear reactivity is present around the invasive carcinoma with the p63 immunostain. This confirms that myoepithelium is absent. p63-positive myoepithelial cells encircle a duct in the lower right corner (immunoperoxidase).

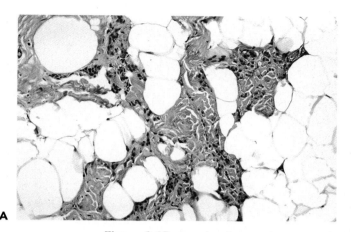
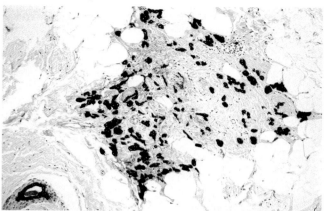

Figure 9.15 **Invasive duct carcinoma, cytokeratin stain. A:** This glandular proliferation in fibrofatty tissue is very suggestive of invasive carcinoma in a needle core biopsy specimen. **B:** The AE1/AE3 cytokeratin stain highlights the structure of the lesion that is typical for invasive carcinoma (immunoperoxidase).

lesion when seeking to identify small foci of invasive carcinoma (Fig. 9.15).

Intraductal Carcinoma

Invasive duct carcinoma arises from intraductal carcinoma and the two components usually have similar structural and cytologic features. Molecular analysis of microdissected paired samples of intraductal and invasive components of single tumors found that they had undergone similar chromosomal changes (72). Attention has been directed to the pattern and distribution of intraductal carcinoma as a prognostic variable in patients with invasive duct carcinoma. The presence of intraductal carcinoma in a needle core biopsy specimen coexisting with invasive duct carcinoma should be noted. Included in the diagnostic report should be a description of the structural pattern, nuclear grade, and the presence or absence of necrosis and calcifications.

Invasive duct carcinomas vary in the relative proportions of intraductal and invasive components. As the proportion of intraductal carcinoma increases for any gross tumor size, there is a trend to decreased nodal metastases and a more favorable prognosis. Lesions with a prominent intratumoral intraductal component tend to have intraductal carcinoma outside the main tumor and multicentric foci of carcinoma in other quadrants of the breast. The distribution of intraductal carcinoma in and around the primary tumor appears to correlate with the risk for recurrence in the breast after lumpectomy and radiation therapy (73) but has no bearing on the risk for systemic recurrence in women treated by breast conservation or mastectomy (74). Recurrence occurs more often in the breast after lumpectomy and radiation therapy in women who have comedocarcinoma or extensive intraductal carcinoma, defined as intraductal carcinoma within and around an invasive tumor that comprises at least 25% of the neoplasm. The increased risk for local recurrence after breast conservation attributable to an extensive intraductal component is probably a manifestation of a greater

probability of there being carcinoma at the margin of excision and remains in the breast. In patients with negative margins, the presence of extensive intraductal carcinoma does not increase the risk for local recurrence in the breast after breast conservation therapy (75,76). A reliable estimate of the proportion of intraductal carcinoma in the lesion and its extent beyond the invasive area cannot be determined from conventional needle core biopsy samples.

Basal-like Phenotype

A subset of invasive mammary carcinomas expresses high molecular weight cytokeratins that have been associated mainly, but not exclusively, with the cells that comprise the myoepithelial or "basal" layer of the mammary gland epithelium (77). In particular, attention has centered on CK5, CK5/6, CK14, and CK17 that have been referred to as "basal keratins" because of their predominant localization in the basal (myopepithelial) region. Invasive carcinomas of the breast that express one or more of these cytokeratins are described as having a "basal-like phenotype." Since cells that express basal cytokeratins occur in the glandular as well as the myoepithelial layers of the mammary epithelium it cannot be inferred that a particular invasive carcinoma with the basal immunophenotype arose specifically from the myoepithelium. Hence terms such as *basal phenotype* or *basal-like* refer to cytokeratin expression and other features rather than histogenesis. Basal-like carcinomas that do not express estrogen receptor, progesterone receptor, or HER2/*neu* and are referred to as "triple negative" (Fig. 9.16). Almost all basal-like carcinomas fall within the category of the invasive ductal carcinomas, NOS.

El-Rehim et al. (78) studied cytokeratin expression in invasive breast carcinomas nearly 75% of which were conventional ductal type. The samples were analyzed for cytokeratins associated with luminal epithelium (CK7/8, 18, 19) and basal cells (CK5/6, CK14). Four patterns of immunoreactivity were found: luminal phenotype represented

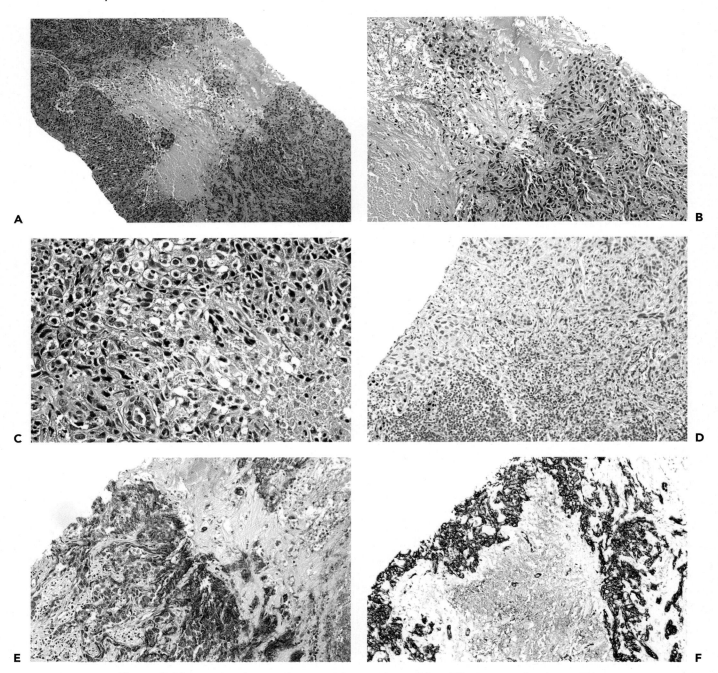

Figure 9.16 **Invasive duct carcinoma, triple negative and basal-like immunophenotype.** This needle core biopsy sample is from a 30-year-old woman. **A–C:** Invasive duct carcinoma, poorly differentiated, with prominent lymphocytic infiltration and focal necrosis, features commonly found in triple negative and basal-like carcinomas. **D:** The carcinoma did not express hormone receptors or HER2/neu. Estrogen receptor reactivity is evident in the nuclei of nonneoplastic lobular cells (lower left) (immunoperoxidase). **E, F:** The carcinoma was immunoreactive for CK5/6 **(E)** and EGFR **(F)**, markers of basal-like immunophenotype.

by one or more luminal cytokeratins only (71.4%); combined phenotype with luminal and basal markers expressed 27.4%); basal phenotype in which only a basal cytokeratin was expressed (0.8%); and a null phenotype that was not reactive for either cytokeratin type (0.4%). These results indicate that breast carcinomas with a pure basal immunophenotype are uncommon. Luck et al. (79) found that 41 of 350 (12%) screen-detected breast carcinomas were characterized

as basal-like because 10% or more of the tumor cells expressed CK5/6 or CK14. Basal-like carcinomas were more likely to form an ill-defined, nonspiculated mass than non-basal-like carcinomas.

Fulford et al. (80) described histologic features that were associated with the basal-like phenotype among high-grade invasive duct carcinomas. In this study, the basal-like phenotype was based on the presence of CK14 expression that was found in 88 of 453 (19.4%) of the tumors examined. The basal-like phenotype was significantly associated with a high mitotic count. Mitosis counts exceeding 40 per 10 high power fields (10 HPF) occurred in 59% of basal-like phenotype carcinomas and in 30% of non-basal-like phenotype carcinomas. Structural features found with significantly greater frequency in carcinomas with the basal-like phenotype included a partly or completely pushing rather than infiltrative external border, a central scar, necrosis and a more prominent lymphoid infiltrate.

A carcinoma cannot be identified as having the basal-like phenotype solely on the basis of the triple-negative marker status. Not all triple-negative tumors express basal cytokeratins and a subset of basal-like carcinomas are not triple negative (81,82). Invasive duct carcinomas with the basal-like phenotype display increased expression of p53 and epidermal growth factor receptor (EGFR) (83). The combination of ER(−), HER2/*neu*(−), and CK5/6(+) has a 76% sensitivity and 100% specificity for the identification of basal-like carcinomas (84).

Attention has focused on the relationship of the basal-like phenotype to prognosis. In 1987 Dairkee et al. (85) reported that the expression of CK5 and CK17 was associated with early recurrence and reduced survival. Subsequently, Banerjee et al. (86) compared patients with basal-like carcinomas to a group with nonbasal-like carcinomas who were matched for age, nodal status, and tumor grade. The basal-like phenotype was based on the expression of at least one of several cytokeratins (CK5/6, CK14, CK17). Patients with basal-like carcinomas had significantly higher recurrence rates locally and systemically, as well as significantly shorter disease-free and lower overall survival rates. The relationship of the basal-like phenotype to chemotherapy response remains to be determined. Banerjee et al. (86) reported that anthracycline-based chemotherapy was less effective in patients with basal-like tumors when compared to matched controls. Others have reported greater success with neoadjuvant therapy in women with basal-like carcinomas (87,88). Haffty et al. (89) reported that the basal-like phenotype was associated with a significantly reduced disease-free survival, poorer overall survival but that the basal-like phenotype did not predispose to local breast recurrence after conservative surgery and radiotherapy.

In considering these and other studies, it should be noted that diverse criteria used to define the basal-like phenotype in clinical studies include EGFR and cytokeratin expression, triple negative status, and other molecular characteristics. A standardized definition for the basal-like phenotype as applied in clinical practice has yet to be agreed upon. The absence of a universally accepted definition was highlighted by Tang et al. (90) who analyzed "4 major molecular classification in the literature that divide breast carcinoma into basal and nonbasal subtypes, with basal subtypes associated with poor prognosis." They applied the four classifications to 195 carcinomas. The rates of basal subtype for invasive carcinomas ranged from 14% to 40% overall and from 19% to 76% in high-grade carcinomas. The different classifications based on patterns of cytokeratin, EGFR, and triple-negative status not only produced different frequencies of basal-like subtype, but they were also found not to be "interchangeable."

REFERENCES

1. Say CC, Donegan WL. Invasive carcinoma of the breast: prognostic significance of tumor size and involved axillary lymph nodes. *Cancer.* 1974;34: 468–471.
2. Smart CR, Myers MH, Gloecker LA. Implications for SEER data on breast cancer management. *Cancer.* 1978;41:787–789.
3. Rosen PP, Saigo PE, Braun Jr DW, et al. Predictors of recurrence in Stage I (T$_1$N$_0$M$_0$) breast carcinoma. *Ann Surg.* 1981;193:15–25.
4. Rosen PP, Saigo PE, Braun Jr DW, et al. Prognosis in Stage II (T$_1$N$_1$M$_0$) breast cancer. *Ann Surg.* 1981;194:576–584.
5. Roger V, Beito G, Jolly PC. Factors affecting the incidence of lymph node metastases in small cancers of the breast. *Am J Surg.* 1989;157:501–502.
6. Weaver DL, Rosenberg RD, Barlow WE. Pathologic findings from the breast cancer surveillance consortium. Population-based outcomes in women undergoing biopsy after screening mammography. *Cancer.* 2006;106:732–742.
7. Elkin EB, Hudis C, Begg CB, Schrag D. The effect of changes in tumor size on breast cancer survival in the U.S.: 1975–1999. *Cancer.* 2005;104; 1149–1157.
8. Joenusu H, Pylkkanen L, Toikkanen S. Late mortality from pT1N0M0 breast carcinoma. *Cancer.* 1999;85:2183–2189.
9. Quiet CA, Ferguson DJ, Weichselbaum RR, Hellman S. Natural history of node-positive breast cancer: the curability of small cancers with a limited number of positive nodes. *J Clin Oncol.* 1996;14:3105–3111.
10. Seidman JD, Schnaper LA, Aisner SC. Relationship of the size of the invasive component of the primary breast carcinoma to axillary lymph node metastasis. *Cancer.* 1995;75:65–71.
11. Silverberg SG, Chitale AR. Assessment of significance of proportions of intraductal and infiltrating tumor growth in ductal carcinoma of the breast. *Cancer.* 1978;32:830–837.
12. Renshaw AA. Minimal(<0.1 cm) invasive carcinoma in breast core needle biopsies. *Arch Pathol Lab Med.* 2004;128:996–999.
13. Charles M, Edge SB, Winston JS, et al. Effect of stereotactic core needle biopsy on pathologic measurement of tumor size of T1 invasive breast carcinomas presenting as mammographic masses. *Cancer.* 2003;97:2137–2141.
14. Greene FL, Page DL, Fleming ID, et al., eds. *For the American Joint Committee on Cancer. AJCC Cancer Staging Manual.* 6th ed. New York: Springer-Verlag; 2002.
15. Connolly J. Changes and problematic areas in interpretation of the AJCC Cancer Staging Manual, 6th ed., for breast cancer. *Arch Pathol Lab Med.* 2006;130:287–291.
16. Jain S, Rezo A, Shadbolt B, Dahlstrom JE. Synchronous multiple ipsilateral breast cancers: implications for patient management. *Pathology.* 2009;41:57–67.
17. Andea AA, Bouwman D, Wallis T, Visscher DW. Correlation of tumor volume and surface area with lymph node status in patients with multifocal/multicentric breast carcinoma. *Cancer.* 2004;100:20–27.
18. Andea AA, Wallis T, Newman LA, et al. Pathologic analysis of tumor size and lymph node status in multifocal/multicentric breast carcinoma. *Cancer.* 2002;94:1383–1390.
19. Coombs NJ, Boyages J. Multifocal and multicentric breast cancer: does each focus matter? *J Clin Oncol.* 2005;23:7497–7502.
20. Berg WA, Gutierrez L, Ness-Aiver MS, et al. Diagnostic accuracy of mammography, clinical examination, US, and MR imaging in preoperative assessment of breast cancer. *Radiology.* 2004;233:830–849.
21. Yeh E, Slantez P, Kopans SB, et al. Prospective comparison of mammography, sonography, and MRI in patients undergoing neoadjuvant chemotherapy for palpable breast cancer. *Am J Roentgenol.* 2005;184:868–877.
22. Bloom HJG, Richardson WW. Histological grading and prognosis in breast cancer. A study of 1049 cases, of which 359 have been followed 15 years. *Br J Cancer.* 1957;11:359–377.
23. Elston CW, Ellis IO. Pathological prognostic factors in breast cancer. I. The value of histological grade in breast cancer: experience from a large study with long-term follow-up. *Histopathology.* 1991;19:403–410.
24. Robbins P, Pinder S, de Klerk N, et al. Histological grading of breast carcinomas: a study of interobserver agreement. *Hum Pathol.* 1995;26:873–879.
25. Black MM, Speer FD. Nuclear structure in cancer tissues. *Surg Gynecol Obstet.* 1957;105:97–105.
26. Cutler SJ, Black MM, Mork T, et al. Further observations on prognostic factors in cancer of the female breast. *Cancer.* 1969;24:653–667.
27. Harris GC, Denley HE, Pinder SE, et al. Correlation of histologic prognostic factors in core biopsies and therapeutic excisions of invasive breast carcinoma. *Am J Surg Pathol.* 2003;27:11–15.
28. Sharifi S, Peterson MK, Baum JK, et al. Assessment of pathologic prognostic factors in breast core needle biopsies. *Mod Pathol.* 1999;12:941–945.
29. Andrade VP, Gobbi H. Accuracy of typing and grading invasive mammary carcinomas on core needle biopsy compared with the excisional specimen. *Virchows Arch.* 2004;445:597–602.
30. Goldstein NS, Murphy T. Intraductal carcinoma associated with invasive carcinoma of the breast. A comparison of the two lesions with implications for intraductal carcinoma classification systems. *Am J Clin Pathol.* 1996;106:312–318.
31. Dawson PJ, Ferguson DJ, Karrison T. The pathologic findings of breast cancer in patients surviving 25 years after radical mastectomy. *Cancer.* 1982;50: 2131–2138.

32. LeDoussal V, Tubiana-Hulin M, Friedman S, et al. Prognostic value of histologic grade/nuclear components of Scarff–Bloom–Richardson (SBR). An improved score modification based on a multivariate analysis of 1262 invasive ductal carcinomas. *Cancer.* 1989;64:1914–1921.

33. Locker A, Ellis IO, Morgan DA, et al. Factors influencing local recurrence after excision and radiotherapy for primary breast cancer. *Br J Surg.* 1989;76:890–894.

34. Nixon AJ, Schnitt SJ, Gelman R, et al. Relationship of tumor grade to other pathologic features and to treatment outcome of patients with early stage breast carcinoma treated with breast-conserving therapy. *Cancer.* 1996;78:426–431.

35. Schnitt SJ, Hayman J, Gelman R, et al. A prospective study of conservative surgery alone in the treatment of selected patients with stage I breast cancer. *Cancer.* 1996;77:1094–1100.

36. Karp SE, Tonin PN, Begin LR, et al. Influence of BRCA1 mutations on nuclear grade and estrogen receptor status of breast carcinoma in Ashkenazi Jewish women. *Cancer.* 1997;80:435–441.

37. Breast Cancer Linkage Consortium. Pathology of familial breast cancer: differences between breast cancers in carriers of BRCA1 and BRCA2 mutations and sporadic cases. *Lancet.* 1997;349:1505–1510.

38. Helvie MA, Roubidoux MA, Weber BL, Merajver SD. Mammography of breast carcinoma in women who have mutations of the breast cancer gene BRCA1: initial experience. *Am J Roentgenol.* 1997;168:1599–1602.

39. Bilik R, Mor C, Haraz B, Moroz C. Characterization of T-lymphocyte subpopulations infiltrating breast cancer. *Cancer Immunol Immunother.* 1989;28:143–147.

40. Whiteside TL, Miescher S, Hurlimann J, et al. Clonal analysis and in situ characterization of lymphocytes infiltrating human breast carcinomas. *Cancer Immunol Immunother.* 1986;23:169–173.

41. Dabiri S, Huntsman D, Makretsov N, et al. The presence of stromal mast cells identifies a subset of invasive breast cancers with a favorable prognosis. *Mod Pathol.* 2004;17:690–695.

42. Gilchrist KW, Gould VE, Hirschl S, et al. Interobserver variation in the identification of breast carcinoma in intramammary lymphatics. *Hum Pathol.* 1982;13:170–172.

43. Rosen PP. Tumor emboli in intramammary lymphatics in breast carcinoma: pathologic criteria for diagnosis and clinical significance. *Pathol Annu.* 1983;18(pt 2):215–232.

44. Acs G, Dumoff KL, Solin LJ, et al. Extensive retraction artefact correlates with lymphatic invasion and nodal metastasis and predicts poor outcome in early stage breast carcinoma. *Am J Surg Pathol.* 2007;31:129–140.

45. Acs G, Paragh G, Chuang S-T, et al. The presence of micropapillary features and retraction artefact in needle core biopsy material predicts lymph node metastasis in breast carcinoma. *Am J Surg Pathol.* 2009;33:202–210.

46. Agarwal B, Saxena R, Morimiya A, et al. Lymphangiogenesis does not occur in breast cancer. *Am J Surg Pathol.* 2005;29:1449–2455.

47. Williams CS, Leek RD, Robson AM, et al. Absence of lymphangiogenesis and intratumoral lymph vessels in human metastatic breast cancer. *J Pathol.* 2003;200:195–206.

48. Vlengel MM, Bos R, van der Groep P, et al. Lack of lymphangiogenesis during breast carcinogenesis. *J Clin Pathol.* 2004;57:746–751.

49. Hanau CA, Machera H, Miettinen M. Immunohistochemical evaluation of vascular invasion in carcinomas with five different markers. *Appl Immunohistochem.* 1993;1:46–50.

50. Lee AKC, DeLellis RA, Wolfe HJ. Intramammary lymphatic invasion in breast carcinoma. Evaluation using ABH isoantigens as endothelial markers. *Am J Surg Pathol.* 1986;10:589–594.

51. Saigo PE, Rosen PP. The application of immunohistochemical stains to identify endothelial-lined channels in mammary carcinoma. *Cancer.* 1987;59:51–54.

52. Kahn HJ, Marks A. A new monoclonal antibody, D2-40, for detection of lymphatic invasion in primary tumors. *Lab Invest.* 2002;82:1255–1257.

53. Fukunaga M. Expression of D2-40 in lymphatic endothelium of normal tissues and in vascular tumors. *Histopathology.* 2005;46:396–402.

54. Van den Eynden GG, van der Auwera I, van Laere SJ, et al. Distinguishing blood and lymph vessel invasion in breast cancer: a prospective immunohistochemical study. *Br J Cancer.* 2006;94:1643–1649.

55. de Mascarel I, MacGrogan G, Debled M, et al. D2-40 in breast cancer: should we detect more vascular emboli? *Mod Pathol.* 2009;22:216–222.

56. Rabban JT, Chen Y-Y. D2-40 expression in breast myoepithelium: potential pitfalls in distinguishing intralymphatic carcinoma from in situ carcinoma. *Hum Pathol.* 2008;39:175–183.

57. Kato T, Prevo R, Steers G, et al. A quantitative analysis of lymphatic vessels in human breast cancer based on LYVE-I immunoreactivity. *Br J Cancer.* 2005;93:1168–1174.

58. Bono P, Wasenius V-M, Lundin J, et al. High LYVE-I positive lymphatic vessel numbers are associated with poor outcome in breast cancer. *Clin Cancer Res.* 2004;10:7144–7149.

59. Bettelheim R, Penman HG, Thornton-Jones H, Neville AM. Prognostic significance of peritumoral vascular invasion in breast cancer. *Br J Cancer.* 1984;50:771–777.

60. Nime F, Rosen PP, Thaler H, et al. Prognostic significance of tumor emboli in intramammary lymphatics in patients with mammary carcinoma. *Am J Surg Pathol.* 1977;1:25–30.

61. Lauria R, Perrone F, Carlomagno C, et al. The prognostic value of lymphatic and blood vessel invasion in operable breast cancer. *Cancer.* 1995;76:1772–1778.

62. Clemente CG, Boracchi P, Andreola S, et al. Peritumoral lymphatic invasion in patients with node-negative mammary duct carcinoma. *Cancer.* 1992;69:1396–1403.

63. Liljegren G, Holmberg I, Bergh J, et al. 20-year results after sector resection with or without postoperative radiotherapy for Stage I breast cancer: a randomized trial. *J Clin Oncol.* 1999;17:2326–2333.

64. Aranaout-Alkarain A, Kahn HJ, Narod SA, et al. Significance of lymph vessel invasion identified by the endothelial lymphatic marker D2-40 in node negative breast cancer. *Mod Pathol.* 2007;20:183–191.

65. Roses DF, Bell DA, Flotte TJ, et al. Pathologic predictors of recurrence in Stage 1 ($T_1N_0M_0$) breast cancer. *Am J Clin Pathol.* 1982;78:817–820.

66. Rak JW, St Croix BD, Kerbel RS. Consequences of angiogenesis for tumor progression, metastasis and cancer therapy. *Anti-Cancer Drugs.* 1995;6:3–18.

67. Horak ER, Leek R, Klenk N, et al. Angiogenesis, assessed by platelet/endothelial cell adhesion molecule antibodies, as indicator of node metastases and survival in breast cancer. *Lancet.* 1992;340:1120–1124.

68. Weidner N, Gasparini G. Determination of epidermal growth factor receptor provides additional prognostic information to measuring tumor angiogenesis in breast carcinoma patients. *Breast Cancer Res Treat.* 1994;29:97–107.

69. de Jong JS, van Diest PJ, Baak JPA. Methods in laboratory investigation. Heterogeneity and reproducibility of microvessel counts in breast cancer. *Lab Invest.* 1995;73:922–926.

70. Tamura S, Enjoji M. Elastosis in neoplastic and non-neoplastic tissues from patients with mammary carcinoma. *Acta Pathol Jpn.* 1988;38:1537–1546.

71. Glaubitz LC, Bowen JH, Cox ED, McCarty KS. Elastosis in human breast cancer. Correlation with sex steroid receptors and comparison with clinical outcome. *Arch Pathol Lab Med.* 1984;108:27–30.

72. Aubele M, Mattis A, Zitzelsberger H, et al. Extensive ductal carcinoma *in situ* with small foci of invasive ductal carcinoma: evidence of genetic resemblance by CGH. *Int J Cancer.* 2000;85:82–86.

73. Schnitt SJ, Connolly JL, Harris JR, et al. Pathologic predictors of early local recurrences in Stage I and II breast cancer treated by primary radiation therapy. *Cancer.* 1984;53:1049–1057.

74. Rosen PP, Kinne DW, Lesser ML, Hellman S. Are prognostic factors for local control of breast cancer treated by primary radiotherapy significant for patients treated by mastectomy? *Cancer.* 1986;57:1415–1420.

75. Hurd TC, Sneige N, Allen PK, et al. Impact of extensive intraductal component on recurrence and survival in patients with stage I and II breast cancer treated with breast conservation therapy. *Ann Surg Oncol.* 1997;4:119–124.

76. Schnitt SJ, Abner A, Gelman R, et al. The relationship between microscopic margins of resection and the risk of local recurrence in patients with breast cancer treated with breast-conserving surgery and radiation therapy. *Cancer.* 1994;74:1746–1751.

77. Gusterson BA, Ross DT, Heath VJ, Stein T. Basal cytokeratins and their relationship to the cellular origin and functional classification of breast cancer. *Breast Cancer Res.* 2005;7:143–148.

78. El-Rehim DMA, Pinder SE, Paish CE, et al. Expression of luminal and basal cytokeratins in human breast carcinoma. *J Pathol.* 2004;203:661–671.

79. Luck AA, Evans AJ, James JJ, et al. Breast carcinoma with basal phenotype: mammographic findings. *Am J Roentgenol.* 2008;191:346–351.

80. Fulford LG, Easton DF, Reis-Filho JS, et al. Specific morphological features predictive for the basal phenotype in grade 3 invasive ductal carcinoma of breast. *Histopathology.* 2006;49:22–34.

81. Reis-Filho JS, Tutt ANJ. Triple negative tumours: a critical review. *Histopathology.* 2008;52:108–118.

82. Rakha EA, Ellis IO. Triple negative/basal-like breast cancer: a review. *Pathology.* 2009;41:40–47.

83. Korsching E, Packeisen J, Agelopoulos K, et al. Cytogenetic alterations and cytokeratin expression patterns in breast cancer: integrating a new model of breast differentiation into cytogenetic pathways of breast carcinogenesis. *Lab Invest.* 2002;82:1525–1533.

84. Nielsen TO, Hsu FD, Jensen K, et al. Immunohistochemical and clinical characterization of the basal-like subtype of invasive breast carcinoma. *Clin Cancer Res.* 2004;10:5367–5374.

85. Dairkee SH, Mayall BH, Smith HS, Hackett AJ. Monoclonal marker that predicts early recurrence of breast cancer. *Lancet.* 1987;1:514.

86. Banerjee S, Reis-Filho JS, Ashley S, et al. Basal-like breast carcinomas: clinical outcome and response to chemotherapy. *J Clin Pathol.* 2006;59:729–735.

87. Carey LA, Dees EC, Sawyer LR, et al. The triple negative paradox: primary tumor chemosensitivity of the basal-like breast cancer phenotype. *Breast Cancer Res Treat.* 2004;88:S48.

88. Rouzier R, Perou CM, Symmons WF, et al. Breast cancer molecular subtypes respond differently to perioperative chemotherapy. *Clin Cancer Res.* 2005;11:5678–5685.

89. Haffty BG, Yang Q, Reiss M, et al. Locoregional relapse and distant metastasis in conservatively managed triple negative early stage breast cancer. *J Clin Oncol.* 2006;24:5652–5657.

90. Tang P, Wang J, Bourne P. Molecular classifications of breast carcinoma with similar terminology and different definitions: are they the same? *Hum Pathol.* 2008;39:506–513.

Tubular Carcinoma 10

Tubular carcinoma is "a highly differentiated invasive carcinoma whose cells are regular and arranged in well-defined tubules typically one-cell layer thick and surrounded by an abundant fibrous stroma" (1) (Fig. 10.1). The term "tubular" refers to the presence of neoplastic glands that resemble breast ductules. This characteristic is the main source of difficulty in recognizing the lesion, especially in the limited sample of a needle core biopsy (Fig. 10.2).

The development of laser microdissection has made it possible to obtain relatively pure microscopic samples of neoplastic glandular tissue for molecular analysis. In a study of 18 pure tubular carcinomas, sampled by laser microdissection and investigated by comparative genomic hybridization, Waldman et al. detected an average of 3.6 chromosomal alterations per tumor (2). Tubular carcinomas had significantly fewer chromosomal alterations overall and significantly more frequent 16q gains when compared with a group of nontubular invasive duct carcinomas. The authors concluded that pure tubular carcinomas are a distinct form of mammary carcinoma that may not evolve into less well-differentiated tumors.

The diagnosis of tubular carcinoma does not apply to carcinomas in which tubular structures are formed by less well-differentiated cells or have a more complex growth pattern (Fig. 10.3). The pattern of glandular growth in nontubular well-differentiated duct carcinoma is partly tubular but in areas the proliferation is more florid and the epithelium of the glands may be more than one-cell thick. Some glands develop micropapillae, cribriform transluminal bridging, or microgland structures. In pure tubular carcinoma an occasional mitotic figure may be encountered but there is little cytological pleomorphism. When present, the intraductal carcinoma or ductal carcinoma in situ (DCIS) has cribriform or micropapillary structure. Often the intraductal proliferation at the site of tubular carcinoma is so orderly that it is indistinguishable from atypical duct hyperplasia, although it probably is the DCIS that gave rise to the invasive lesion.

Pure tubular carcinomas constitute less than 2% of all female breast carcinomas. The incidence of this lesion is influenced by the nature of the population under investigation. Before the widespread use of mammography, 5% of 382 $T_1N_0M_0$ breast carcinomas in one series were classified as tubular (3). When stratified by size, 9% of carcinomas 1.0 cm or smaller were tubular, a substantially higher proportion than the 2% of tubular carcinomas among tumors that measured 1.1 to 2.0 cm. Tubular carcinoma was less frequent among women with $T_1N_1M_0$ disease (1.5% of 142 patients), reflecting the relatively low frequency of axillary metastases from these tumors (4). In the Breast Cancer Detection Demonstration Projects, 8% of invasive carcinomas 1.0 cm or less in diameter were of the tubular variety (5).

Tubular carcinomas have structural features that render the lesions detectable by mammography. Most tubular carcinomas are spiculated and calcifications are often present (6). Leibman et al. (7) reported that the average radiographic size of tubular carcinomas was 0.8 cm in patients with nonpalpable lesions and 1.2 cm when the lesions were palpable. It may be difficult to distinguish tubular carcinoma from radial scar in mammograms, a problem compounded by the fact that tubular carcinoma can arise in a radial scar (8,9) (Fig. 10.4). Ultrasonography may detect tubular carcinomas that are inapparent on mammography. Because the majority of tubular carcinomas are detected by imaging studies, they are often the target of needle core biopsy sampling (10).

The median age at diagnosis is in the mid to late 40s with a range from 24 to 92 years (11–13). Superficial tumors are fixed to the skin, producing retraction in a small number of cases. When a tubular carcinoma arises from the major lactiferous ducts in the nipple or slightly lower in the subareolar region, it is difficult to distinguish clinically and pathologically from florid papillomatosis of the nipple. The finding of Paget disease in the nipple epidermis supports the diagnosis of tubular carcinoma in this setting. Almost all tubular carcinomas have been positive for estrogen and progesterone receptors (14,15) (Fig. 10.5). Fewer than 5% of tubular carcinomas are positive for the HER2/*neu* by immunohistochemistry (16) and none of 55 tubular carcinomas studied by fluorescence in situ hybridization (FISH) exhibited HER2/*neu* gene amplification (17).

The distribution of the small neoplastic glands or tubules in histological sections of tubular carcinoma is

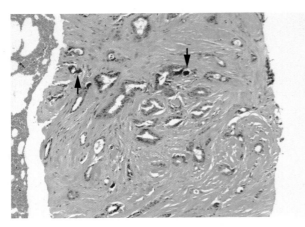

Figure 10.1 Tubular carcinoma. This needle core biopsy specimen shows small, evenly distributed glands. Calcifications are visible *(arrows).*

largely haphazard, but they tend to be relatively evenly spaced throughout the lesion. An important clue to the diagnosis of tubular carcinoma that should be searched for in a needle core biopsy specimen is evidence of lesional glands invading fat beyond fibrous stroma (see Fig. 10.4C).

Although this distribution can occur in adenosis or a radial sclerosing lesion, it is more likely to be found in tubular carcinoma.

The glands may have virtually any shape but the majority of the glands have irregular, angular contours (see Fig. 10.2). In exceptionally well-differentiated tubular carcinomas, especially tumors smaller than 1 cm, it is possible to find round or oval glands of relatively uniform caliber which resemble microglandular adenosis (18,19) (see Fig. 10.2B). If cribriform and papillary growth are present in the neoplastic glands, the tumor is best classified as invasive well-differentiated duct carcinoma rather than as pure tubular carcinoma (see Fig. 10.3).

The glands of tubular carcinoma are composed only of neoplastic epithelial cells, typically distributed in a single layer (Fig. 10.6). The cells are cuboidal or columnar with round or oval hyperchromatic nuclei that tend to be basally oriented. Nucleoli are inapparent and mitoses are very rarely present. Apocrine-type cytoplasmic "snouts" are often evident at the luminal cell border. The cytoplasm is usually amphophilic. Eosinophilic or nearly clear apocrine cytoplasm rarely occurs in a pure tubular carcinoma. An uncommon type of tubular carcinoma is composed of tumor cells

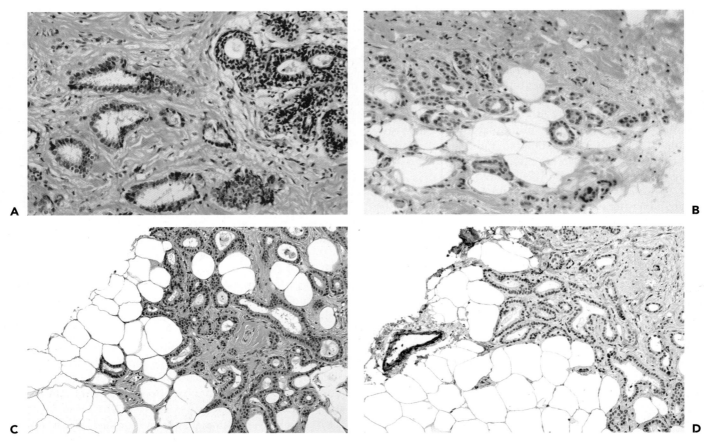

Figure 10.2 Tubular carcinoma. The carcinomatous ductules are formed by a single layer of uniform cuboidal cells. **A:** A normal terminal duct is shown on the right for contrast with the angular carcinomatous structures. **B:** This carcinoma is composed partly of glands with rounded shapes. **C, D:** Tubular carcinoma composed of glands with various shapes invades fat. Absence of myoepithelium is demonstrated in **(D)** by the myosin immunostain. A blood vessel is myosin positive (immunoperoxidase).

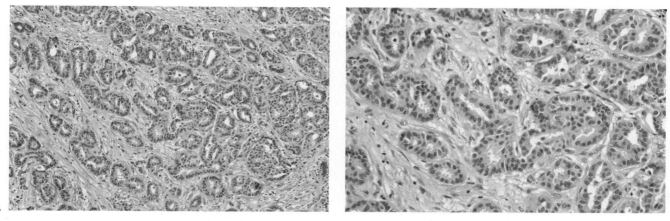

Figure 10.3 Well-differentiated invasive duct carcinoma. A, B: The glandular pattern is more complex than in tubular carcinoma. Intraglandular proliferation is evident.

with intracytoplasmic mucin and mucin in the neoplastic gland lumens (Fig. 10.7).

The primary considerations in the differential diagnosis of tubular carcinoma are sclerosing adenosis and radial sclerosing lesions. Sclerosing adenosis is composed in varying proportions of compact whorled, elongated, and largely compressed and open glands with interlacing spindly myoepithelial cells. The lobulocentric distribution of sclerosing adenosis is absent from tubular carcinoma. Because proliferation of myoepithelial cells is an integral part of sclerosing

adenosis and these cells are not present in tubular carcinoma, it is helpful to employ immunohistochemical stains for myoepithelial cells when dealing with a difficult problem (20). The preferred stain for myoepithelium is the nuclear marker p63 since it does not cross-react with stromal myofibroblasts (Fig. 10.8). Other relatively specific immunostains are CD10, myosin, and calponin. Immunoreactivity for myoepithelial markers may vary from case to case, and it is therefore prudent to employ p63 and at least one other stain at the outset. A contemporaneous hematoxylin

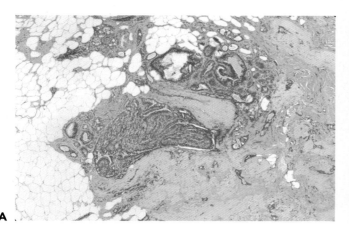

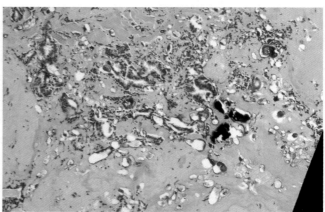

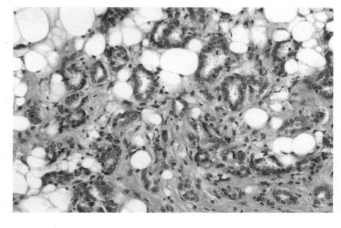

Figure 10.4 Tubular carcinoma arising in a radial scar. This nonpalpable lesion was detected on mammography as a mass with calcifications. **A:** This portion consists of sclerosing adenosis and papillary duct hyperplasia surrounded by tubular carcinoma. The scleroelastotic core is seen on the right. **B:** Glandular proliferation in the sclerotic core with numerous calcifications is shown. This area was not diagnostic of carcinoma in the H&E section alone but proved to be part of the tubular carcinoma when the actin immunostains revealed absence of myoepithelium. **C:** Tubular carcinoma invading fat at the periphery of the tumor.

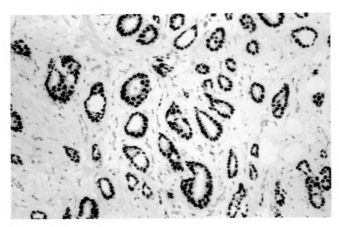

Figure 10.5 **Tubular carcinoma.** Nuclei in the carcinomatous glands are immunoreactive for estrogen receptor (immunoperoxidase).

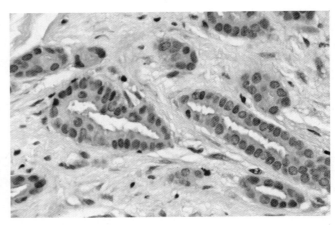

Figure 10.6 **Tubular carcinoma.** A needle core biopsy specimen with uniformly distributed tubular carcinoma glands.

and eosin (H&E) recut should be prepared whenever immunostains are performed. Intact and largely continuous basement membranes are present around the glands of sclerosing adenosis whereas these structures are absent or poorly formed in tubular carcinomas when studied with reagents to detect laminin, type IV collagen, and basement membrane proteoglycan (20,21) (Fig. 10.8) or with the reticulin stain. Elastosis found in many tubular carcinomas, is absent from or minimally present in sclerosing adenosis (Fig. 10.9).

Radial sclerosing lesions are composed of adenosis and duct hyperplasia or papilloma, often accompanied by cysts. Varying proportions of these components are found in individual lesions and some consist entirely of adenosis or of papilloma. Stromal elastosis is a feature of many radial sclerosing lesions, especially when adenosis is not a prominent component. Immunostains will usually detect myoepithelial cells in portions of a radial sclerosing lesion with adenosis, but sometimes these cells are noticeably attenuated and difficult to detect or focally inapparent in

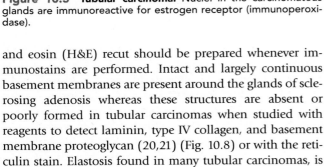

A

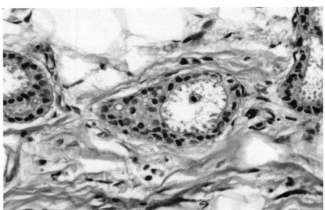

B

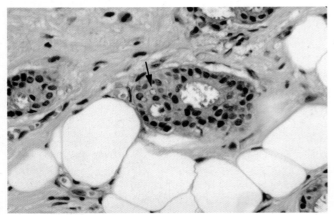

C

Figure 10.7 **Tubular carcinoma with intracytoplasmic mucin.** **A, B:** The carcinoma is composed mainly of glands formed by cuboidal cells. Some cells have intracytoplasmic lumina. **C:** The lumina in some intracytoplasmic vacuoles are outlined in red with the mucicarmine stain *(arrow)*.

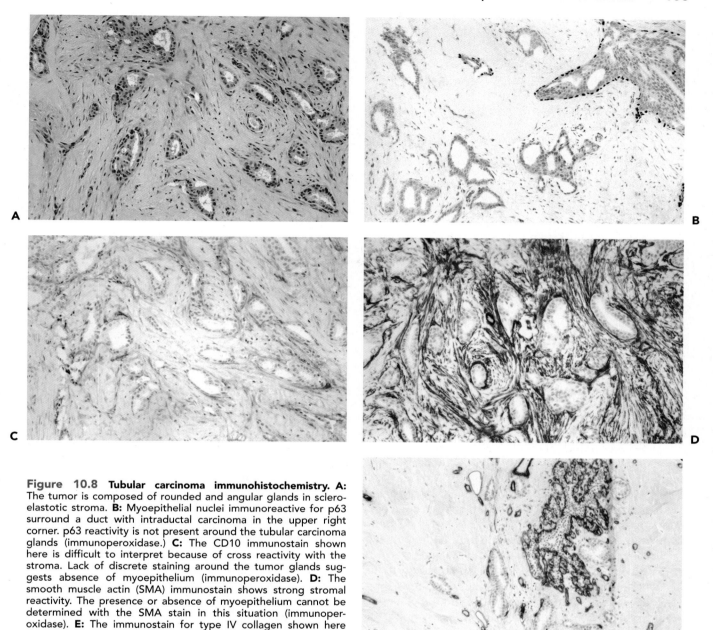

Figure 10.8 Tubular carcinoma immunohistochemistry. A: The tumor is composed of rounded and angular glands in scleroelastotic stroma. **B:** Myoepithelial nuclei immunoreactive for p63 surround a duct with intraductal carcinoma in the upper right corner. p63 reactivity is not present around the tubular carcinoma glands (immunoperoxidase.) **C:** The CD10 immunostain shown here is difficult to interpret because of cross reactivity with the stroma. Lack of discrete staining around the tumor glands suggests absence of myoepithelium (immunoperoxidase). **D:** The smooth muscle actin (SMA) immunostain shows strong stromal reactivity. The presence or absence of myoepithelium cannot be determined with the SMA stain in this situation (immunoperoxidase). **E:** The immunostain for type IV collagen shown here highlights basement membranes of a duct and small blood vessels. Immunoreactivity is absent around tubular carcinoma glands in this needle core biopsy specimen (immunoperoxidase).

areas of densely sclerotic papilloma. The latter characteristic can result in misleading results when immunostains for myoepithelium are done on needle core biopsy samples where contextual information from the surrounding tissue is not available. A sclerosing lesion in which there is distinct apocrine metaplasia is unlikely to be tubular carcinoma, even when myoepithelium appears to be absent in a needle core biopsy sample.

Because of the limited sampling provided by a needle core biopsy, the diagnosis of pure tubular carcinoma is sometimes uncertain in this material. Difficulty arises especially when only a small portion of the lesion is present in the specimen. Greater confidence in a diagnosis of "pure"

tubular carcinoma by needle core biopsy can be obtained by correlating the pathological and radiological findings, especially if it is determined that the lesion seen mammographically has been completely or nearly completely removed by the biopsy procedure. Nonetheless, it is prudent practice in many cases to indicate in the needle core biopsy report that the final classification of the carcinoma will depend on the findings in an excisional biopsy specimen.

A tumor with areas of invasive lobular and tubular carcinoma is referred to as *tubulolobular carcinoma* (22) (Fig. 10.10). The precise position of tubulolobular carcinoma in the classification of breast carcinomas is uncertain because it has been regarded as a variant of tubular

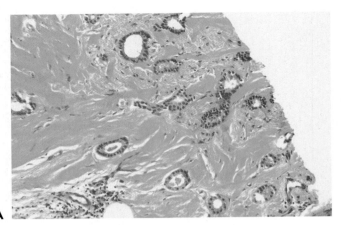

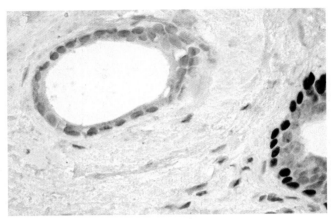

Figure 10.9 **Tubular carcinoma with elastosis. A:** This needle core biopsy specimen from a non-palpable tumor shows basophilic elastic tissue in the stroma of a tubular carcinoma. **B:** The carcinoma on the left is devoid of p63 positive myoepithelial cells. To the right there is a lobular gland with p63 positive nuclei (immunoperoxidase).

carcinoma by some authors, and as a form of invasive lobular carcinoma by others. Tubulolobular carcinomas range in size from 0.3 cm to 2.5 cm with a mean size of about 1.3 cm (22–24). When present, in situ carcinoma may be lobular carcinoma in situ (LCIS), DCIS, or LCIS and DCIS (22–24). DCIS alone is found more often in pure tubular carcinoma than in tubulolobular carcinoma, whereas tubulolobular carcinomas are more likely to be accompanied by LCIS only (22,23).

Varying proportions of tubular and invasive lobular carcinoma are found in tubulolobular carcinomas. In one study of 11 cases, tubular and lobular carcinoma were nearly equally present in 3 (27%), lobular carcinoma was predominant in 5 (46%), and the tubular pattern was more pronounced in 3 (27%) (24). Multifocality is more frequent in tubulolobular carcinoma than in pure tubular carcinoma, having been found in 19% (24) and 29% (22) of tubulolobular cases in two studies. By comparison, the frequency of multifocality in pure tubular carcinomas was 10% (24) and 20% (22). Patients with tubulolobular carcinoma are slightly more likely to have axillary lymph node

metastases than women with pure tubular carcinoma (22–24), but a prognosis closer to that of pure tubular carcinoma than that of invasive lobular carcinoma (22,23).

The observation that almost all tubulolobular carcinomas in three studies were E-cadherin positive supports ductal histogenesis since loss of E-cadherin reactivity is associated with invasive lobular carcinoma (22,24,25). E-cadherin immunoreactivity was found in invasive tubular and invasive lobular components, even in tumors where the invasive lobular pattern was more prominent. In one study α-catenin and β-catenin were expressed in 50% and 62.5%, respectively, of tubulolobular carcinomas (25). Esposito et al. (24) detected membranous reactivity for α, β, and γ catenin, in all tubulolobular and tubular carcinomas they studied. Infiltrating lobular carcinomas displayed cytoplasmic staining for β and γ-catenin but no reactivity for α-catenin. In this study all tubular and tubulolobular carcinomas had membranous reactivity for E-cadherin. Membranous E-cadherin reactivity was absent from lobular carcinomas. Immunoreactivity for the high-molecular weight cytokeratin 34βE12 (K903) was observed in about

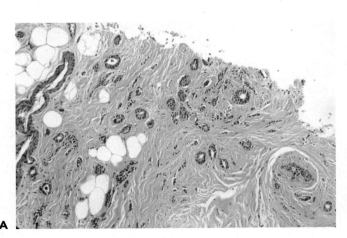

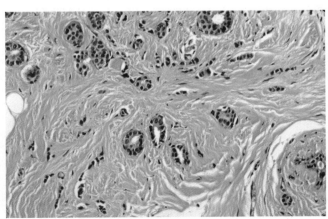

Figure 10.10 **Tubulolobular carcinoma. A, B:** This needle core biopsy specimen has elements of invasive lobular and tubular carcinoma.

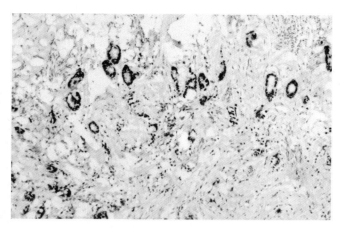

Figure 10.11 Tubulolobular carcinoma. Nuclear immunoreactivity for estrogen receptors is present in the tubular and invasive lobular components (immunoperoxidase).

50% of tubular, tubulolobular, and invasive lobular carcinomas. Wheeler et al. (23) found that 25 of 27 tubulolobular carcinomas were immunoreactive for cytokeratin K903, a marker that has been associated with lobular differentiation (26,27). Three-dimensional modeling of tubular and tubulolobular carcinomas revealed a growth pattern in which cavitary glandular structures were connected by network of slender, solid cords of single cells (28). In tubulolobular carcinomas the connecting network of single cells appeared to consist of longer strands that might account for the histological pattern suggestive of invasive lobular carcinoma. Overall the mixed immunophenotype of tubulolobular carcinomas reflects the ductal and lobular histological components of these tumors, with the preponderance of evidence supporting ductal histogenesis. Almost all tubulolobular carcinomas are immunoreactive for estrogen and progesterone receptors (22,23) (Fig. 10.11).

As greater experience with tubulolobular carcinoma is obtained, it is likely to emerge as a separate subtype of mammary carcinoma, distinct from tubular and invasive lobular carcinoma. Presently, patients with tubulolobular carcinoma should be viewed as having a good prognosis. It remains to be seen if the prognosis equals the exceptionally favorable outcome of pure tubular carcinoma.

Tissue between the glands in tubular carcinomas often appears different from stroma in the surrounding breast, sometimes as a result of abundant elastic tissue (29). However, elastosis can be a prominent feature of nontubular carcinomas and some benign lesions, particularly those with the "radial scar" pattern. Other stromal alterations that may be seen include dense collagenization or loosening of the stroma caused by the accumulation of metachromatic ground substances. If present at all, there is at most a mild lymphocytic reaction. Blood vessel invasion and lymphatic tumor emboli are virtually never seen in tubular carcinoma. Calcifications are found in many tubular carcinomas, distributed in the neoplastic glands, in the stroma or in the DCIS component. DCIS can be found in at least two-thirds of tubular carcinomas. It typically has papillary or cribriform patterns or a mixture of the two (12) (Fig. 10.12). Micropapillary DCIS is especially common and the growth pattern is frequently so orderly that it is not distinguishable from atypical duct hyperplasia.

Tubular and tubulolobular carcinoma frequently arise in breast tissue that is the site of a multifocal, distinctive proliferation in terminal duct–lobular units and ducts now referred to as columnar cell lesions. The spectrum of columnar cell proliferation ranges from columnar cell change and simple columnar cell hyperplasia (CCH), through CCH with atypia to DCIS. Cystic dilatation often accompanies these epithelial alterations, especially in terminal duct–lobular units where the condition seems to arise. Goldstein and O'Malley (30) referred to carcinoma in this setting as "cancerization of small ectatic ducts of the breast by DCIS cells with apocrine snouts." Features common to columnar cell lesions are nuclear hyperchromasia, a high nuclear-to-cytoplasmic ratio, and apocrine snouts at the luminal borders of ducts and ductules. The lesions are prone to develop distinctive, ossifying calcifications. The most subtle expression of this condition is formed by cuboidal or low

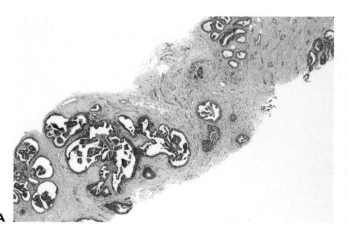

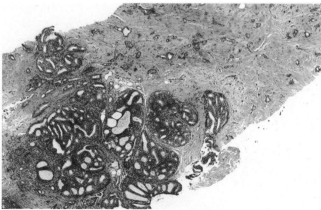

A **B**

Figure 10.12 Tubular carcinoma with intraductal carcinoma. Two needle core biopsy specimens of tubular carcinoma *(upper right)* are shown. **A:** Papillary intraductal carcinoma. **B:** Cribriform intraductal carcinoma.

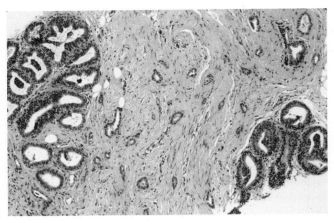

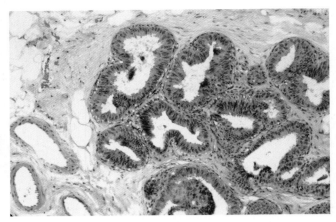

Figure 10.13 Columnar cell hyperplasia. A: Atypical columnar cell hyperplasia is present in ductules on the right and left borders of this needle core biopsy specimen showing tubular carcinoma in the center. The hyperplastic change consists of crowded cuboidal and low columnar cells. **B:** Atypical columnar cell hyperplasia in which focal cell crowding results in the formation of small mounds of columnar cells. One papillary structure is present at the lower border. Myoepithelial cells with vacuolated cytoplasm are present at the outer border of the epithelium in many glands.

columnar cells with the foregoing cytologic features distributed in a single layer (Fig. 10.13). Progressive hyperplasia is marked by crowding of cells that become increasingly compressed, columnar, and come to have nuclei distributed in a haphazard pattern with respect to the basement membrane (Fig. 10.14). The presence of blunt micropapillae or cribriform growth composed of the same proliferative cells with

"streaming" or condensation of cells toward the lumen is indicative of atypical CCH (Fig. 10.15).

Columnar cell lesions are associated with LCIS as well as tubular carcinoma (31,32) (Fig. 10.16). Because CCH is prone to develop calcifications, often at multiple sites, it is a relatively common finding in needle core biopsy samples from women with nonpalpable mamographically detected

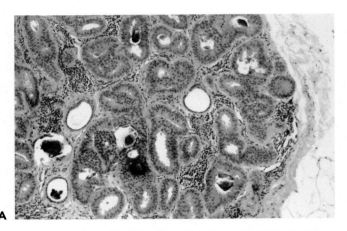

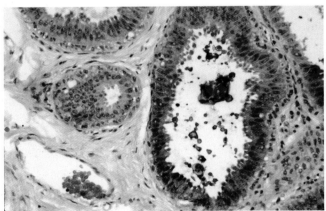

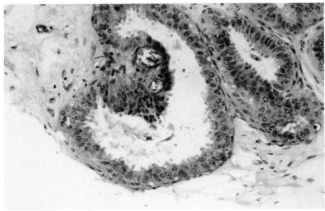

Figure 10.14 Columnar cell hyperplasia. A: The complex intraglandular proliferation with calcifications represents columnar cell duct hyperplasia with an adenosis pattern. **B:** The larger gland on the right shows cytologic atypia with a disorderly distribution of hyperchromatic nuclei. Apical cytoplasmic blebs are prominent at the luminal borders and the larger gland contains calcification. Hyperplastic myoepithelial cells are visible around the glands. **C:** An epithelial mound with ossifying calcification.

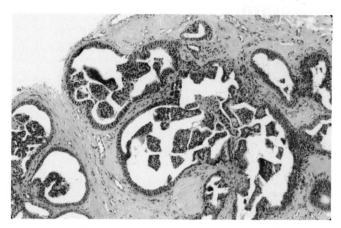

Figure 10.15 Tubular carcinoma with papillary intraductal carcinoma. A magnified view of intraductal carcinoma from the tumor shown in Fig. 10.16.

calcifications. The distinctive "ossifying" calcifications have a characteristic outer band of eosinophilic material that resembles ostoid and central basophilic calcific deposits. Excisional biopsy should be performed after a needle core biopsy diagnosis of CCH with atypia. Additional information about columnar cell lesions can be found in Chapter 8.

Most patients with tubular or tubulolobular carcinoma have a single mass detected by palpation or an imaging procedure. However, sampling of surgical biopsy speci-

mens reveals multifocal tubular carcinoma lesions growing as seemingly separate foci in up to 20% of patients with tubular carcinoma and in nearly 30% of patients with tubulolobular carcinoma (22). DCIS may be found in the individual carcinomatous areas.

It is difficult to distinguish between unifocal and multifocal tubular or tubulolobular carcinomas in needle core biopsy specimens unless carcinoma is found in samples from anatomically different sites.

Tubular carcinoma has a very favorable prognosis when the diagnosis is restricted to "pure" tubular carcinomas (11,12). In a series of patients with $T_1N_0M_0$ breast carcinomas treated by modified or radical mastectomy and followed for a median of 18 years there were no recurrences among patients with tubular carcinoma (33). The frequency of axillary lymph node metastases resulting from pure tubular carcinoma is about 10% (2,3,9–11). Based on a literature review of 680 patients with pure tubular carcinomas, Papadatos et al. (34) reported that nodal metastases were found in 16 of 244 cases (6.6%; 95% CI 1.7–11.4). Affected lymph nodes are usually in the low axilla (level I) and only rarely are more than three lymph nodes involved (12). Metastases in lymph nodes tend to reproduce the tubular growth pattern of the primary tumor but less well-differentiated or solid metastases may be encountered. Axillary lymph node metastases were encountered in about 30% of patients with tubulolobular carcinoma who had an axillary dissection (22).

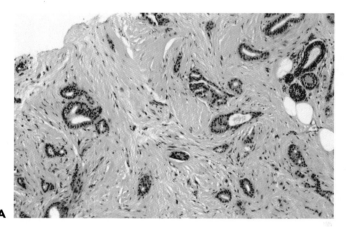

A

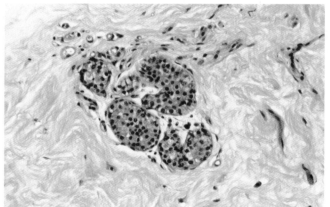

B

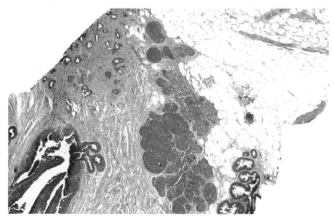

C

Figure 10.16 Tubular carcinoma and lobular carcinoma in situ. Needle core biopsy samples from a radiographically detected lesion. **A:** Pure tubular carcinoma. **B:** A separate focus of lobular carcinoma in situ. **C:** The triad of tubular carcinoma (upper left), lobular carcinoma in situ (center), and atypical columnar cell duct hyperplasia (lower left and lower right).

Patients with unifocal pure tubular carcinoma are considered to be excellent candidates for breast conservation therapy. If a unifocal pure tubular carcinoma is excised with an adequate negative margin and there is not extensive DCIS in the surrounding breast, postoperative radiotherapy has been omitted in selected cases. In one series, there were no breast recurrences among 21 patients with tubular carcinoma treated by lumpectomy and radiotherapy (35). Bradford et al. (36) reported no breast or systemic recurrences in 38 women treated by excision, including 17 who did not have breast irradiation.

Patients with multifocal tubular carcinoma, coexistent extensive DCIS, or evidence of other invasive lesions in the breast usually have radiotherapy after excision, or they may require mastectomy. Sentinel lymph node mapping should be performed in patients with a tubular or tubulolobular carcinoma larger than 1 cm, when there are multifocal invasive lesions, or if there are other indications that suggest axillary nodal metastases. In view of the extremely favorable prognosis of tubular carcinoma, there is no evidence that systemic adjuvant therapy would prove beneficial, except for women with tumors larger than 3 cm, if there are axillary metastases or if there is also a less well-differentiated carcinoma in the ipsilateral or contralateral breast.

Patients with mixed tubular carcinomas should receive treatment appropriate for an infiltrating duct carcinoma of the grade of the nontubular component as determined by tumor size and stage. This is likely to include postoperative radiotherapy and systemic adjuvant therapy if the tumor is larger than 1 cm.

The presence of multifocal carcinoma at the primary site appears to predispose patients with tubular and tubulolobular carcinoma to develop axillary lymph node metastases, perhaps because of the greater tumor volume associated with multifocality (22).

REFERENCES

1. World Health Organization. *Histological Typing of Breast Tumours.* 2nd ed. *International Histological Classification of Tumours #2.* Geneva: World Health Organization; 1981:19.
2. Waldman FM, Hwang ES, Etsell J, et al. Genomic alterations in tubular breast carcinomas. *Hum Pathol.* 2001;32:222–226.
3. Rosen PP, Saigo PE, Braun Jr DW, et al. Predictors of recurrence in Stage I ($T_1N_0M_0$) breast carcinoma. *Ann Surg.* 1981;193:15–25.
4. Rosen PP, Saigo PE, Braun Jr DW, et al. Prognosis in Stage II ($T_1N_1M_0$) breast cancer. *Ann Surg.* 1981;194:576–584.
5. Beahrs O, Shapiro S, Smart C. Report of the working group to review the National Cancer Institute-American Cancer Society Breast Cancer Detection Demonstration Projects. *J Natl Cancer Inst.* 1979;62:640–709.
6. Elson BC, Helvie MA, Frank TS, et al. Tubular carcinoma of the breast: mode of presentation, mammographic appearance, and frequency of nodal metastases. *Am J Roentgenol.* 1993;161:1173–1176.
7. Leibman AJ, Lewis M, Kruse B. Tubular carcinoma of the breast: mammographic appearance. *Am J Roentgenol.* 1993;160:263–265.
8. Vega A, Garijo. Radial scar and tubular carcinoma. Mammographic and sonographic findings. *Acta Radiologica.* 1993;34:43–47.
9. Frouge C, Tristant H, Guinebretière J-M, et al. Mammographic lesions suggestive of radial scars: microscopic findings in 40 cases. *Radiology.* 1995;195:623–625.
10. Mitnick JS, Gianutsos R, Pollack AH, et al. Tubular carcinomas of the breast: sensitivity of diagnostic techniques and correlation with histopathology. *Am J Roentgenol.* 1999;172:319–323.
11. Peters GN, Wolff M, Haagensen CD. Tubular carcinoma of the breast. Clinical pathologic correlations based on 100 cases. *Ann Surg.* 1981;193:138–149.
12. McDivitt RW, Boyce W, Gersell D. Tubular carcinoma of the breast. Clinical and pathological observations concerning 135 cases. *Am J Surg Pathol.* 1982;6:401–410.
13. Deos PH, Norris HJ. Well differentiated (tubular) carcinoma of the breast. *Am J Clin Pathol.* 1982;78:1–7.
14. Winchester DJ, Sahin AA, Tucker SL, Singletary SE. Tubular carcinoma of the breast. Predicting axillary nodal metastases and recurrence. *Ann Surg.* 1996;223:342–347.
15. Masood S, Barwick KW. Estrogen receptor expression of the less common breast carcinomas. *Am J Clin Pathol.* 1990;93:437–442.
16. Fasano M, Vamvakos E, Delgado Y, et al. Tubular carcinoma of the breast: immunohistochemical and DNA flow cytometric profile. *The Breast J.* 1999;5:252–255.
17. Oakley GJ, Tubbs RR, Crowe J, et al. HER-2 amplification in tubular carcinoma of the breast. *Am J Clin Pathol.* 2006;126:55–59.
18. Rosen PP. Microglandular adenosis. A benign lesion simulating invasive mammary carcinoma. *Am J Surg Pathol.* 1983;7:137–144.
19. Shen SS, Sahin AA. Invasive ductal carcinoma of the breast with a microglandular adenosis pattern. *Ann Diagn Pathol.* 2004;8:39–42.
20. Joshi MG, Lee AKC, Pedersen CA, et al. The role of immunocytochemical markers in the differential diagnosis of proliferative and neoplastic lesions of the breast. *Mod Pathol.* 1996;9:57–62.
21. Ekblom P, Miettinen M, Forsman L, Andersson LC. Basement membrane and apocrine epithelial antigens in differential diagnosis between tubular carcinoma and sclerosing adenosis of the breast. *J Clin Pathol.* 1984;37:357–363.
22. Green I, McCormick B, Cranor M, Rosen PP. A comparative study of pure tubular and tubulolobular carcinoma of the breast. *Am J Surg Pathol.* 1997;21:653–657.
23. Wheeler DT, Tai LH, Bratthauer GL, et al. Tubulolobular carcinoma of the breast. An analysis of 27 cases of a tumor with a hybrid morphology and immunoprofile. *Am J Surg Pathol.* 2004;28:1587–1593.
24. Esposito NN, Chivukula M, Dabbs DJ. The ductal phenotypic expression of the E-cadherin/catenin complex in tubulolobular carcinoma of the breast: an immunohistochemical and clinicopathologic study. *Mod Pathol.* 2007;20:130–138.
25. Kuroda H, Tamaru J, Takeuchi I, et al. Expression of E-cadherin, alpha-catenin, and beta-catenin in tubulolobular carcinoma of the breast. *Virchows Arch.* 2006;448:500–505.
26. Bratthauer GL, Miettinen M, Tavassoli FA. Cytokeratin immunoreactivity in lobular intraepithelial neoplasia. *J Histochem Cytochem.* 2003;51:1527–1531.
27. Bratthauer GL, Monifar F. Stamatakos MD, et al. Combined E-cadherin and high molecular weight cytokeratin immunoprofile differentiates lobular, ductal, and hybrid mammary intraepithelial neoplasias. *Hum Pathol.* 2002;33:620–627.
28. Marchio C, Sapino A, Arisio R, Bussolati G. A new vision of tubular and tubulolobular carcinomas of the breast, as revealed by 3-D modeling. *Histopathology.* 2006;48:556–562.
29. Tremblay G. Elastosis in tubular carcinoma of the breast. *Arch Pathol.* 1974;98:302–307.
30. Goldstein NS, O'Malley BA. Cancerization of small ectatic ducts of the breast by ductal carcinoma in situ cells with apocrine snouts. A lesion associated with tubular carcinoma. *Am J Clin Pathol.* 1997;107:561–566.
31. Rosen PP. Columnar cell hyperpasia is associated with lobular carcinoma *in situ* and tubular carcinoma. *Am J Surg Pathol.* 1999;23:1561.
32. Abdel-Fatah TMA, Powe DG, Hodi Z, et al. High frequency of coexistence of columnar cell lesions, lobular neoplasia, and low grade ductal carcinoma in situ with invasive tubular carcinoma and invasive lobular carcinoma. *Am J Surg Pathol.* 2007;31:417–426.
33. Rosen PP, Groshen S, Saigo PE, et al. A long-term follow-up study of survival in Stage I ($T_1N_0M_0$) and Stage II ($T_1N_1M_0$) breast carcinoma. *J Clin Oncol.* 1989;7:355–366.
34. Papadatos G, Rangan AM, Psarianos T, et al. Probability of axillary node involvement in patients with tubular carcinoma of the breast. *Br J Surg.* 2001;88:860–864.
35. Haffty BG, Perotta PL, Ward B, et al. Conservatively treated breast cancer: outcome by histologic subtype. *The Breast J.* 1997;3:7–14.
36. Bradford WZ, Christensen WN, Fraser H Cloninger TE. Treatment of pure tubular carcinoma of the breast. *The Breast J.* 1998;4:437–440.

Papillary Carcinoma

11

About 1% to 2% of breast carcinomas can be classified as papillary in women, and a slightly greater percentage of male breast carcinomas are papillary. A distinction should be made between invasive and noninvasive papillary carcinoma (1). Intracystic carcinoma is a variant of in situ papillary carcinoma that may also have an invasive component (1–3).

Women with solid or cystic papillary carcinoma of the breast are reportedly older than patients with other types of carcinoma, with a mean age ranging from 63 to 71 years. Nearly 50% of papillary carcinomas arise in the central part of the breast, and as a consequence, nipple discharge has been described in up to one-third of patients. Bleeding from the nipple occurs in a higher percentage of patients with papillary carcinoma than in those with a papilloma. The average size of papillary carcinoma clinically is 2 to 3 cm. Papillary carcinomas are usually rich in estrogen and progesterone receptors (4), and they tend to have a low growth rate when measured by thymidine labeling (5).

Papillary carcinomas often appear as rounded, circumscribed mass lesions on mammography (6,7). If part of the contour lacks circumscription on mammography, an invasive component may be present (7–9). Examination by ultrasound can suggest a papillary tumor when a solid area is detected in a hypoechoic cystic lesion (7–10). When present, calcifications tend to be punctated and associated with intraductal papillary carcinoma (10). Coarse, pleomorphic calcifications may develop in areas of sclerosis or resolved hemorrhage. Needle core biopsy can be used effectively for the diagnosis of papillary carcinoma. A series of 26 papillary lesions diagnosed by needle core biopsy included seven classified as papillary carcinoma in situ (11). Invasive carcinoma was found in three (43%) of subsequent excisional biopsy specimens.

The term *papillary* applies to carcinomas in which the underlying microscopic pattern is predominantly frond forming. Many papillary carcinomas have cystic areas, but this is not necessary for the diagnosis. When cyst formation is minimal or absent, separate fronds may be inconspicuous, and the papillary character is appreciated because the epithelium is supported by a network of fibrovascular stroma. Papillary carcinomas that do not form fronds are referred to as *solid papillary carcinomas*.

The epithelium on the papillae in papillary carcinomas is composed of cells arranged in the patterns typically found in intraductal carcinoma, that include papillary, micropapillary, cribriform, reticular, and solid appearances (Fig. 11.1). In most cases, the epithelial proliferation fills part or all of the space between neighboring fibrovascular stromal cores and contributes to the formation of complex patterns of papillae, glandular spaces, and solid areas within the lesion.

Fibrovascular stroma is present to some extent in all papillary carcinomas, but it tends to be less evenly distributed in carcinomas than in benign papillary lesions (Figs. 11.1 and 11.2). Rarely, a low-grade papillary carcinoma has a very orderly frond-forming structure with epithelium limited to the surfaces of the fibrovascular stroma. These lesions are very difficult to distinguish from papillomas in hematoxylin and eosin (H&E)-stained sections, especially in needle core biopsy samples, but they are devoid of myoepithelium when studied with immunostains (Fig. 11.2). Some papillary carcinomas have areas in which there are relatively broad fibrous stalks with extensive sclerosis (Fig. 11.3).

The epithelial cells in papillary carcinomas grow in a less orderly fashion than in papillomas. This is manifested by uneven stratification and loss of epithelial cell polarity with respect to the basement membrane (Fig. 11.4). Epithelial cell nuclei are characteristically hyperchromatic regardless of cytologic grade, and there is usually a high nuclear-to-cytoplasmic ratio. Mitotic figures are variably present and usually more numerous in lesions that exhibit the most severe cytologic atypia. The tumor cells sometimes have secretory "snouts" at the luminal surface (Fig. 11.5). Intracytoplasmic mucin vacuoles may be conspicuous (Fig. 11.6). Mucin may accumulate between papillary fronds (Fig. 11.7). Apocrine areas in a papillary carcinoma exhibit cytologic atypia consistent with the rest of the tumor and therefore differ from the bland foci of apocrine metaplasia sometimes encountered in papillomas. The presence of histologically benign apocrine

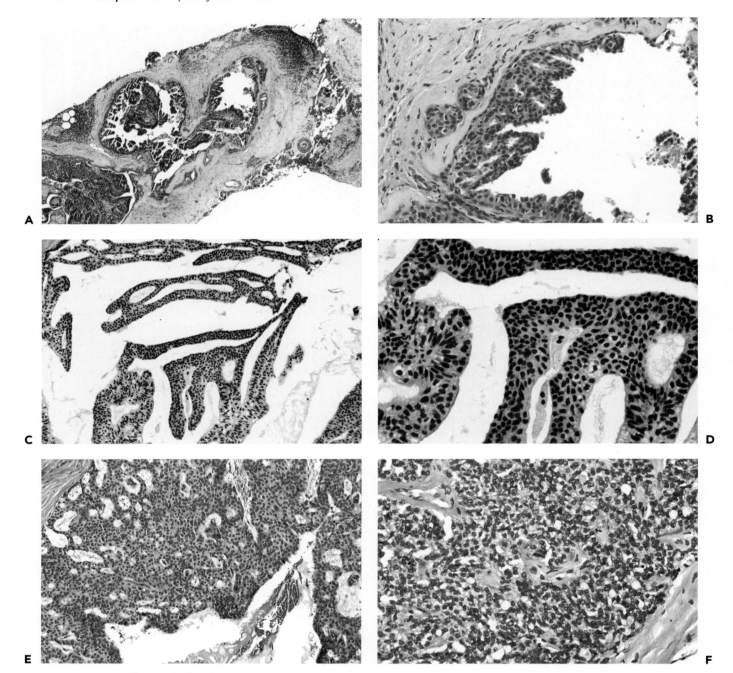

Figure 11.1 **Papillary carcinoma.** Various growth patterns are represented in these needle core biopsy specimens. **A, B:** Papillary and micropapillary intraductal carcinoma. Myoepithelial cells represented by oval nuclei arranged parallel to the basement membrane are seen beneath the micropapillary carcinoma in **(B). C, D:** Arborizing cribriform and micropapillary intraductal carcinoma with well-differentiated nuclear grade. **E:** Cribriform structure. **F:** Solid architecture.

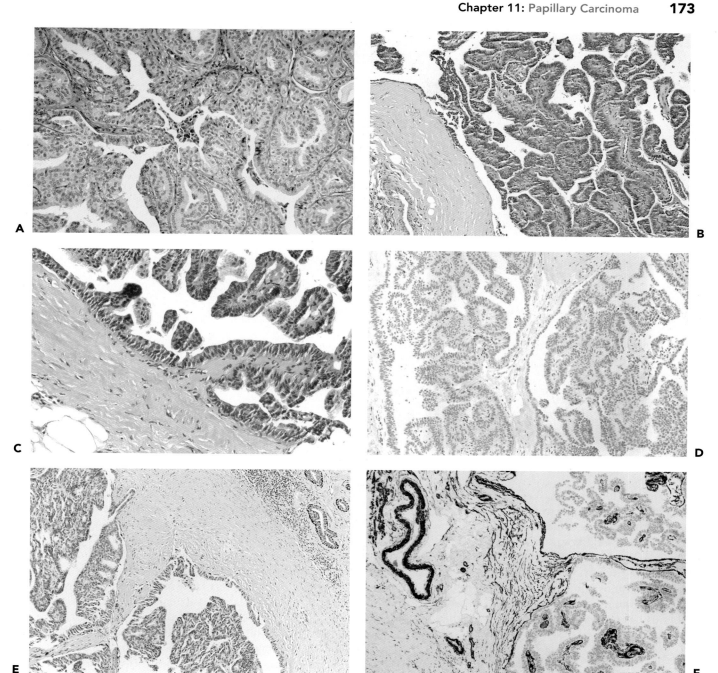

Figure 11.2 Papillary carcinoma, low grade. A: The fibrovascular stroma forms slender, branching strands in this orderly lesion with foci of residual papilloma represented by regular columnar epithelium, seen mainly near the lower right corner. **B, C:** Very orderly frond-forming papillary carcinoma that resembles a papilloma. **D:** Absence of myoepithelium in the lesion shown in **(B, C)** is demonstrated by the negative CD10 immunostain (immunoperoxidase). **E:** The p63 immunostain was also negative. Note p63 reactivity around normal ducts **(upper right)** (immunoperoxidase). **F:** The SMA immunostain highlights stromal cells and vascular structures. No myoepithelial reactivity is evident (immunoperoxidase).

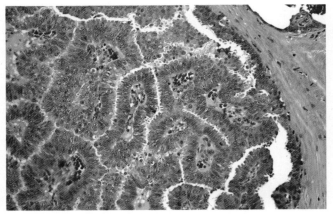

G

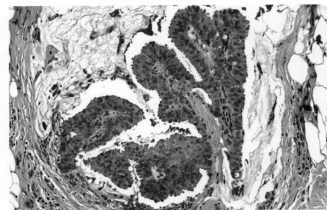

H

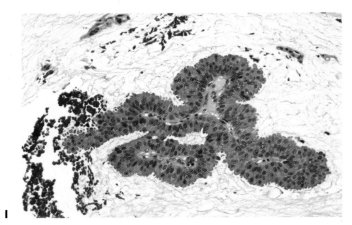

I

Figure 11.2 *(continued)* **G–I:.** Needle core biopsy samples from an orderly invasive papillary carcinoma. Intraductal papillary carcinoma is shown in **(G).** Frond-forming invasive papillary carcinoma with mucin formation. Note the stroma in the invasive papillary fronds **(H, I).**

elements is almost always associated with a papilloma rather than a papillary carcinoma. When present, microcalcifications are more often found in glandular portions of the lesion than in the stroma (Fig. 11.8).

Myoepithelial cells, which are distributed relatively uniformly and proportionately with the epithelium of benign papillary lesions, are characteristically absent from papillary carcinoma. Less often they are present as a discontinuous layer or even hyperplastic in carcinomatous areas

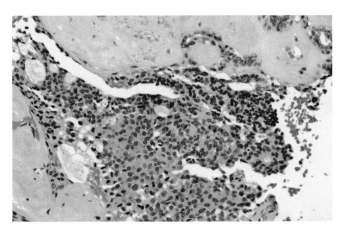

Figure 11.3   Papillary carcinoma. Dense collagenization with finely granular basophilic calcification **(upper center)** is present in this lesion.

(12,13) (Figs. 11.1, 11.2, 11.5, and 11.9). Although myoepithelial cells can sometimes be visualized in H&E sections of a papillary carcinoma the most reliable method for detecting them is with immunohistochemistry. Cytoplasmic markers associated with myoepithelium include CD10, smooth muscle actin (SMA), calponin, myosin, and CK5/6. The cytoplasmic markers are sometimes cross-reactive with stromal myofibroblasts or vascular structures. The degree to which this cross-reactivity will occur is unpredictable, and quite variable with respect to individual markers. Thus, there may be considerable stromal reactivity for SMA in a given case and greater myoepithelial specificity for CD10 in the same tissue. The nuclear marker p63 is present in myoepithelial cells and it exhibits no cross-reactivity for stroma. However, p63 can be expressed in the nuclei of epithelial cells in a papillary lesion (14). p63-positive epithelial cells can be readily distinguished from myoepithelium by their position in the epithelium. Whenever possible, it is prudent to employ a panel of several markers when evaluating myoepithelium in a papillary tumor in order to compensate for issues of variable and cross-reactivity (15–17). Such a panel should always include p63 and representative cytoplasmic markers such as CD10, calponin, and SMA. A contemporary H&E recut should be prepared at the same time as the immunostains. Cytokeratin immunostains are very helpful when investigating the possibility of invasion in a papillary carcinoma.

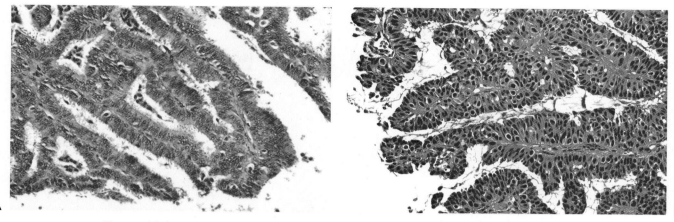

Figure 11.4 Papillary carcinoma. A: The columnar carcinoma cells in this orderly tumor are closely arrayed along the basement membrane. There is a high nuclear-to-cytoplasmic ratio and loss of nuclear polarity with respect to the basement membrane. **B:** Orderly papillary carcinoma with mucin between fronds in a needle core biopsy sample from a 55-year-old woman.

Figure 11.5 Papillary carcinoma. Papillary intraductal carcinoma is present in this needle core biopsy specimen from a circumscribed, nonpalpable tumor detected by mammography. A myoepithelial cell layer is present at the periphery of the lesion.

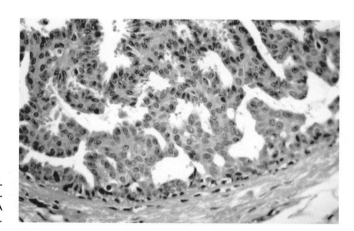

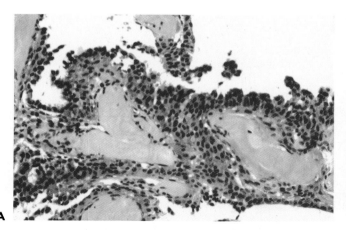
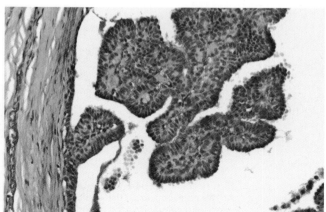

Figure 11.6 Papillary carcinoma with intracytoplasmic mucin. A: Intracytoplasmic mucin is represented by discrete, pale blue vacuoles. **B:** The mucin is stained magenta by the mucicarmine stain.

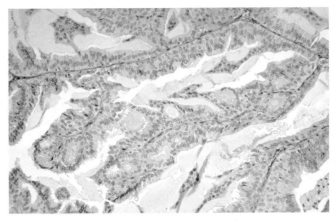

Figure 11.7 **Papillary carcinoma with extracellular mucin.** This papillary carcinoma with apocrine differentiation has a micropapillary structure and unusually abundant mucin secretion between papillary fronds.

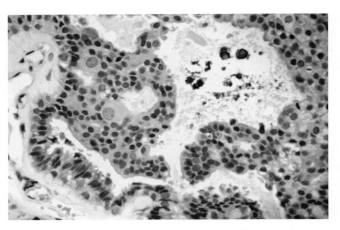

Figure 11.8 **Papillary carcinoma with calcification.** Granular calcifications are present in a glandular lumen in this needle core biopsy specimen. The picture shows papillary carcinoma with a micropapillary pattern.

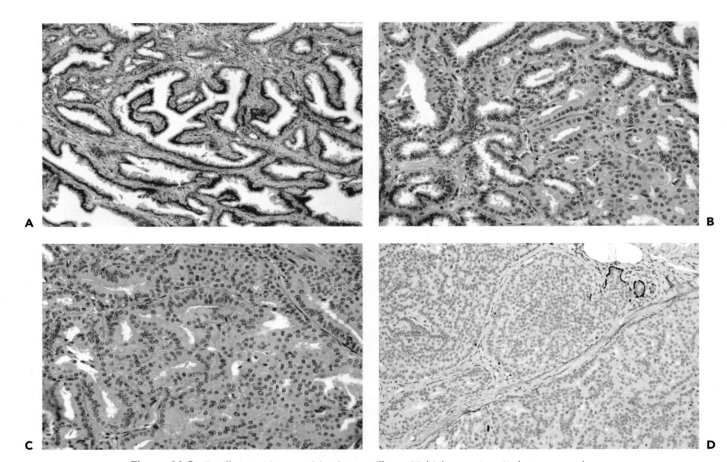

Figure 11.9 **Papillary carcinoma arising in a papilloma.** Multiple areas in a single tumor are shown. **A:** This papilloma has a thin, uniform layer of cuboidal and low columnar cells overlying prominent myoepithelial cells and broad strands of stroma. **B:** An enlarged view from another region shows hyperplastic epithelium on the left merging with atypical glandular hyperplasia on the right composed of cells with eosinophilic cytoplasm. Note the loss of myoepithelial cells and more slender stromal strands on the right. **C:** Carcinoma with a cribriform structure. Note the persisting inconspicuous arborizing stroma and virtual absence of myoepithelial cells. **D:** Residual myoepithelial cells are highlighted by the p63 immunostain (upper right) in the solid papillary intraductal carcinoma (immunoperoxidase).

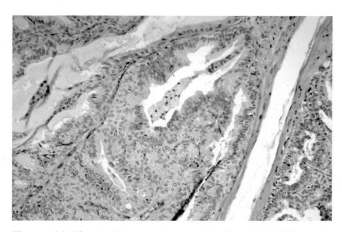

Figure 11.10 Papillary carcinoma with dimorphic differentiation. Polygonal cells are shown surmounted by columnar cells.

Lefkowitz et al. (3) drew attention to papillary carcinomas containing cuboidal cells with abundant clear or faintly eosinophilic cytoplasm located mainly near the basement membrane, either singly, in small clusters, or in broad sheets. In some instances, the polygonal cells with pale cytoplasm become quite numerous, creating solid and cribriform regions beneath a superficial layer of columnar epithelium (Fig. 11.10). Despite the difference in cytoplasmic features between the clear cells and the columnar carcinomatous cells, the nuclei of the two cell types are similar, and both cell types are immunoreactive for cytokeratin. There is no reactivity for SMA or p63 in the polygonal cells. Both cell types are of epithelial origin, and this pattern is referred to as dimorphic papillary carcinoma.

Although myoepithelial cells can sometimes be visualized in H&E sections of a papillary carcinoma, the most reliable method for detecting them is with immunohistochemistry. Cytoplasmic markers associated with myoepithelium include S-100 CK14, 34BE12, CD10, SMA, calponin, CK5/6, and myosin. The cytoplasmic markers are sometimes cross-reactive with stromal myofibroblasts or vascular structures. The degree to which this cross-reactivity will occur is unpredictable, and quite variable with respect to individual markers. Thus, there may be considerable stromal reactivity for SMA in a given case and greater myoepithelial specificity for CD10 in the same tissue.

The term *encapsulated papillary carcinoma* has arisen from immunohistochemical studies of myoepithelial markers in solid papillary carcinomas. Hill and Yeh (15) investigated a series of papillary carcinomas and found five with "no or only focal staining of the basal" myoepithelial cell layer for calponin, smooth muscle myosin-heavy chain, and p63. Absence of myoepithelial reactivity led these authors to suggest that such carcinomas are "part of a spectrum of progression intermediate between in situ and invasive disease" and to "consider these lesions to be an encapsulated variant of breast carcinoma," termed *encapsulated papillary carcinoma*.

In a report on five immunostain myoepithelial markers (calponin, p63, CD10, CK5/6, and smooth muscle myosin-heavy chain), Collins et al. (16) investigated the distribution of myoepithelial cells in 22 tumors that had been classified as "intracystic papillary carcinomas." On the basis of the illustrations provided and gross descriptions which referred to "circumscribed," "soft," and "focally hemorrhagic" "nodules," with no mention of a cystic component, these appear to have been solid rather than "intracystic" papillary carcinomas. All of the 22 tumors were devoid of myoepithelial reactivity with the five immunostain markers. The authors observed that absence of myoepithelium created uncertainty about the possible presence of an invasive component in these lesions. However, they recommended treatment "similar to patients with DCIS" (intraductal carcinoma) and suggested that these tumors be called encapsulated papillary carcinoma.

As reported by Hill and Yeh (15), Collins et al. (16), and many other investigators, absence of myoepithelium characterizes the invasive component of papillary carcinoma, whether solid or cystic, and myoepithelium is not detectable in some but not all in situ cystic and solid papillary intraductal carcinomas. Loss of myoepithelium can be used to distinguish some in situ papillary carcinomas from papillomas, but by itself the absence of myoepithelium is not a basis for separating in situ from invasive papillary carcinomas. In the case of solid papillary carcinoma, the presence of myoepithelium around the entire circumference of the lesion supports the diagnosis of solid papillary intraductal carcinoma. Focal or even complete absence of peripheral myoepithelium in a solid papillary carcinoma renders the tumor "indeterminate for invasion" (17). However, the actual structure of the tumor must also be considered, with the best evidence for invasion being localized change in the growth pattern, such as focal cribriform, tubular, or mucinous carcinoma, which extends beyond the perimeter of the tumor. Absence of myoepithelium around a solid papillary carcinoma that retains a smooth peripheral contour is not definitive evidence of invasion. It is sometimes helpful to use one or more cytokeratin immunostains to detect individual invasive carcinoma cells that may have extended beyond the perimeter of an apparently circumscribed papillary carcinoma.

Encapsulated papillary carcinoma is an alternative term sometimes used for cystic and solid papillary carcinoma. The word *encapsulated* is used by proponents of this term to take cognizance of their uncertainty about the presence of invasion in these lesions. Although it is true that there are examples of cystic and solid types of papillary carcinoma that elicit uncertainty as to the presence of an invasive component, it has not yet been demonstrated that among these uncertain tumors there is an identifiable subset with a propensity to cause metastases in the absence of an evident invasive component. In this circumstance, the advocates of the term *encapsulated* have not clearly indicated whether the diagnosis "encapsulated papillary carcinoma" should apply to all papillary carcinomas that are entirely myoepithelial deficient or only to those where invasion is suspected. Furthermore, no mention is made of lesions that partially lack myoepithelium or of papillary carcinomas endowed with myoepithelium that have foci suspicious for invasion. Additionally, the adjective *encapsulated* suggests encasement, just reverse of suspected microinvasion. Our inability to confidently detect the presence of invasion in some papillary carcinomas reflects the limitations of existing knowledge and technology. This conundrum will probably not be resolved until future research discovers one or more markers that specifically distinguish between in situ and invasion carcinoma cells, an advance that would focus attention on the tumor cells themselves rather on their pattern of growth by which invasion is presently determined. It is preferable to simply describe a papillary carcinoma as cystic, solid, or a combination of cystic and solid and to state that invasion is present, absent, or indeterminate (e.g., "suspected," "cannot be ruled out").

There has been considerable interest in the cytokeratin staining patterns in benign, hyperplasic, and carcinomatous mammary epithelium. Attention has focused on high molecular weight or basal-type cytokeratins. These cytokeratins are identified with immunostains for CK5/6, CK14, and 34BE12 that are reactive with myoepithelial and epithelial cells in duct hyperplasia but show decreased or absent reactivity in conventional intraductal carcinomas. Rabban et al. (18) reported that there was no reactivity for CK5/6 in the neoplastic epithelium of 14 solid papillary carcinomas. However, CK5/6 stained residual nonneoplastic epithelial cells and myoepithelial cells in the carcinomas and was strongly reactive in the epithelium of duct hyperplasia. Tan et al. (19) reported that immunostaining for CK5/6 had higher sensitivity and specificity for distinguishing papillomas from papillary carcinomas than CK14 and 34BE12. The authors developed an immunoscore based on the percentage of cells stained multiplied by staining intensity. The mean immunoscores for CK5/6, CK14, and 34BE12, respectively, in papillomas (107.6, 186.6, 113.1) and papillary carcinomas (12, 29.6, 34.5) were significantly different. It is evident from these results that the expression of these markers, especially CK5/6, is greatly diminished or absent in most papillary carcinomas but that their focal, weak presence does not exclude the diagnosis of papillary carcinoma. If a diagnosis of papillary carcinoma is being contemplated for a papillary tumor in which there is strong epithelial expression of CK5/6, CK14, or 34BE12, the diagnosis should be reconsidered. At present the extent and intensity of staining for these markers have not been shown to correlate with atypical hyperplasia in papillomas.

The solid variant of intraductal papillary carcinoma is not widely recognized (20). Solid papillary intraductal carcinomas are usually well circumscribed and often multinodular. These tumors are composed of ducts nearly or completely filled by a neoplastic epithelial proliferation supported by arborizing fibrovascular stroma (Fig. 11.11). The epithelium has a solid, non-frond-forming structure with variably distributed fibrovascular stromal cords and a

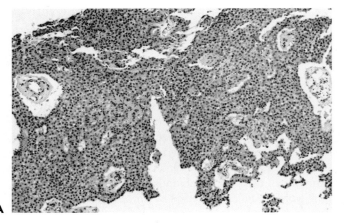

A

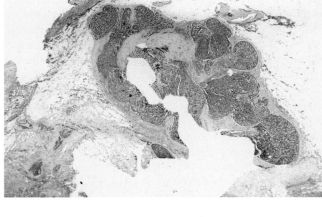

B

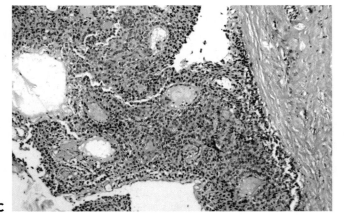

C

Figure 11.11 Solid papillary carcinoma. A: A needle core biopsy specimen shows solid areas of in situ carcinoma arranged around fibrovascular stromal cores. The tumor cells have vacuolated amphophilic cytoplasm and well-differentiated, round nuclei. This specimen could be mistaken for invasive carcinoma if the basic papillary structure were not appreciated. **B:** A low-magnification view of the tumor in the excisional biopsy specimen. **C:** An area at the periphery of the excised tumor duplicating the appearance of the needle core biopsy specimen.

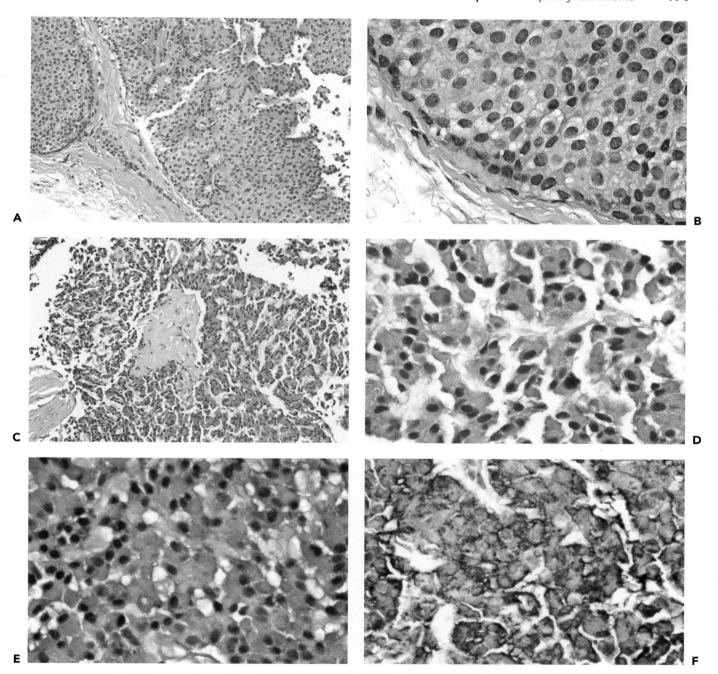

Figure 11.12   Solid papillary carcinoma. A: In this needle core biopsy specimen, the in situ carcinoma contains small cords of fibrovascular stroma that make it possible to recognize the papillary character of the tumor. The circumscribed border is a typical feature of intraductal solid papillary carcinoma. **B:** Magnified view to demonstrate uniform cells with mosaic-like distinct borders. **C:** Needle core biopsy samples from solid papillary carcinoma are often fragmented as shown here. Note the collagenized stroma. Images **(D), (E),** and **(F)** are from the tumor shown in **(C). D:** Plasmacytoid cytology with eccentric nuclei typically found in some solid papillary carcinomas. **E:** Intra- and extracellular mucin are demonstrated with the mucicarmine stain. **F:** Cytoplasmic chromogranin reactivity (immunoperoxidase).

circumscribed border (Fig. 11.12). When cribriform and papillary patterns are present, the stroma is more apparent. Solid areas may be divided into ribbons or trabeculae of neoplastic cells by prominent fibrovascular stroma (Fig. 11.13). Comedo necrosis is infrequent. Collagenization of stroma around and among the ducts occurs to a variable degree, in some cases producing the appearance of a radial sclerosing lesion. Intraductal carcinoma in ducts surrounding a solid papillary carcinoma usually reflects the structure and cytology of the main papillary neoplasm.

The diagnosis of a papillary carcinoma that has arisen in a papilloma can be a problem even with sections of the entire

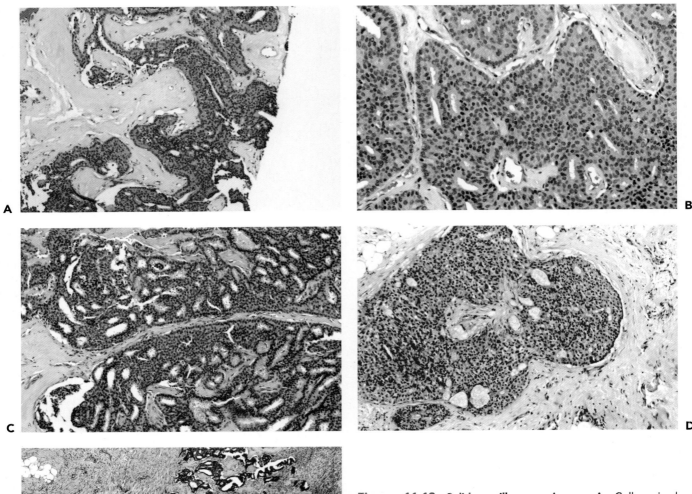

Figure 11.13 Solid papillary carcinoma. A: Collagenized stroma in this needle core biopsy specimen has distorted the structure of an in situ solid papillary carcinoma. This pattern might be mistaken for invasive carcinoma with a trabecular pattern if the papillary character of the lesion were not appreciated. Spaces formed by separation of the epithelium from the strorna are not uncommon in solid papillary carcinoma. **B:** This part of the lesion has a cribriform structure. **C:** Cribriform intraductal carcinoma is apparent in the excisional biopsy specimen of the papillary tumor. **D:** Solid papillary carcinoma is present in a duct at the periphery of the excised tumor. **E:** An area in the center of the excised tumor with reactive stromal proliferation resulting from the prior needle core biopsy. The disrupted glands in granulation tissue are difficult to distinguish from invasive carcinoma.

lesion in hand, a difficulty compounded by the limited and noncontiguous samples in needle core biopsy specimens. Foci of papilloma in such lesions should not impede recognition of the carcinomatous element (see Fig. 11.9). Papillary lesions that have been characterized as "borderline" have modest or substantial areas of benign papillary proliferation as well as more cellular and atypical components. To make a diagnosis of carcinoma in this setting, it is necessary to find low-power microscopic fields where the growth pattern and cytologic appearance of the epithelium between neighboring fibrovascular cores have the pattern of one of the established forms of intraductal carcinoma. Some authors have illustrated focal intraductal carcinoma in papillomas but

classified these lesions as "papillomas with atypical ductal hyperplasia" (21,22). In one of these studies, the relative risk for subsequent carcinoma in women with such papillomas was more than four times that of women with papillomas which lacked atypical hyperplasia or intraductal carcinoma (22). Underdiagnosis of such lesions is likely to result in inadequate treatment that is reflected in the outcome of patients in the aforementioned reports.

Cytoplasmic histochemical and immunohistochemical studies can be helpful for evaluating difficult papillary lesions. Intracytoplasmic mucin indicative of carcinoma is demonstrable with the mucicarmine, alcian blue, and periodic acid–Schiff stains (see Fig. 11.6). In the majority of papillary carcinomas, intracytoplasmic mucin secretion is not prominent, and therefore a negative stain result does not rule out carcinoma. A small number of papillary carcinomas exhibit abundant, diffuse intracellular mucin secretion that can be manifested by signet ring cell formation and the accumulation of extracellular mucin. The cells in a minority of papillary carcinomas contain Grimelius-positive and chromogranin-positive cytoplasmic granules, which have not been demonstrated in the cells of papillomas. These tumors typically have a solid papillary growth pattern with mucinous differentiation. They are usually immunoreactive for synaptophysin, neuron-specific enolase, have mucin-positive cells, and are typically estrogen receptor positive (23) (Fig. 11.14). The accumulation of abundant extracellular mucin creates a pattern that resembles invasive mucinous carcinoma but does not represent invasion if confined within the tumor.

Papillary tumors can undergo complete infarction spontaneously or after a needling procedure. This phenomenon occurs in papillomas (see Chapter 4) and in papillary carcinomas. In many cases, the structure of the lesion is so altered by this phenomenon that is not possible to distinguish between a papilloma and a papillary carcinoma in H&E sections. Immunostains can be helpful in this situation. When reactivity for cytokeratin is preserved, it may be possible to visualize the structure of the tumor (Fig. 11.15) and myoepithelium may be evident if nuclear p63 reactivity is preserved.

The microscopic diagnosis of invasive papillary carcinoma may be difficult. Many papillary carcinomas are bounded by zones of fibrosis, recent or resolved hemorrhage, and chronic inflammation. Similar alterations may also occur within the lesion. Papillary or glandular clusters of epithelial cells within these areas are difficult to interpret. Groups of neoplastic cells distributed parallel to layers of reactive stroma at the border of a papillary carcinoma usually represent entrapped in situ epithelium rather than invasive carcinoma. An actin immunostain is sometimes helpful in this situation, although proliferating myofibroblasts can complicate interpretation. Myofibroblastic staining is avoided if the p63 immunostain is used but this procedure is only useful if the p63 stain reveals myoepithelium throughout the papillary tumor. When myoepithelium is absent from the in situ portion of a papillary carcinoma, myoepithelial immunostains are not helpful for identifying invasive carcinoma. Isolated invasive carcinoma cells can be identified with a cytokeratin immunostain. In general, the most reliable histologic evidence of frank invasion is extension of tumor beyond the zone of reactive changes into the mammary parenchyma and fat.

Papillary lesions that have been subjected to fine needle aspiration or needle core biopsy before excision exhibit alterations that complicate the issue of determining whether there is invasion. Hemorrhage is commonly found in and around the tumor grossly. The best microscopic clues to such manipulation of the tumor are the presence of fresh hemorrhage and acute inflammation associated with "unnatural" fragmentation of the lesion. Tumor cells can be found singly or in clusters deposited in areas of hemorrhage and along the course of the needle. As long as it is known that the lesion was recently "needled," these detached cells are best regarded as the result of trauma rather than as evidence of invasion. Sometimes epithelial cells are also seen in capillary or lymphatic channels after a needle aspiration or needle biopsy procedure. This uncommon finding should be described in the pathology report and may be regarded as a manifestation of invasive carcinoma in some instances (24). Epithelial displacement associated with needling procedures is discussed more extensively in Chapter 28.

It is not possible to rule out invasion from a papillary carcinoma with a needle core biopsy specimen because the sample may not include this aspect of the lesion (Figs. 11.16 and 11.17). The most reliable evidence of invasion is extension of carcinoma beyond the border of the tumor and the adjacent stromal reaction. Cytologically, the invasive component tends to resemble the in situ portion of the lesion. There is usually also an appreciable change in growth pattern between the in situ and invasive components (see Fig. 11.17). Invasive carcinoma arising in solid papillary carcinoma with mucinous differentiation is often mucinous carcinoma (see Fig. 11.14). Invasive tubular, cribriform, solid, and papillary carcinoma can be encountered.

An unusual pattern of true invasion observed in solid papillary carcinomas simulates epithelial displacement associated with needling procedures. This type of invasion is characterized by the presence of one or more irregularly shaped cohesive sheets of carcinoma cells surrounding fat or stroma without the reactive stromal changes that ordinarily accompany invasive carcinoma. These invasive carcinomatous foci abut sharply on normal fat cells, or less often on collagenous stroma, in a fashion suggesting on superficial inspection that they were "pushed" or artifactually displaced to this location (see Fig. 11.17). Features that favor true invasion include the absence at this site of evidence of needling, such as fat necrosis, a distinct needle track, hemorrhage, or tissue disruption. Intimate mingling of carcinoma and normal tissue occurs in these foci, especially in fat, where individual adipose cells are found in the sheet of carcinoma cells. Carcinoma cells appear to be "molded" around fat cells within or at the border of such foci.

Breast conserving surgical treatment by lumpectomy yields excellent clinical control locally in women with noninvasive or invasive papillary carcinoma. Because these lesions are likely to involve ducts in the surrounding breast the excision should include adequate tissue to sample the margins. The risk of local recurrence is greater if the lesion is multifocal. Sentinel lymph node staging should be performed if invasive carcinoma is identified and should be considered when invasion is suspected. Rare instances of axillary nodal metastases have been reported in cases where invasion was not detected (25–27).

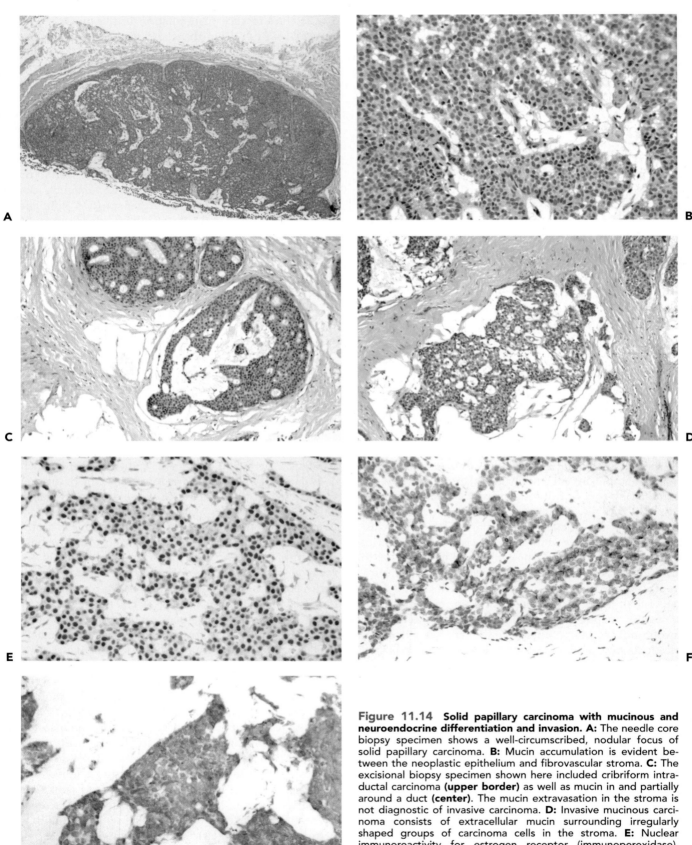

Figure 11.14 Solid papillary carcinoma with mucinous and neuroendocrine differentiation and invasion. A: The needle core biopsy specimen shows a well-circumscribed, nodular focus of solid papillary carcinoma. **B:** Mucin accumulation is evident between the neoplastic epithelium and fibrovascular stroma. **C:** The excisional biopsy specimen shown here included cribriform intraductal carcinoma **(upper border)** as well as mucin in and partially around a duct **(center)**. The mucin extravasation in the stroma is not diagnostic of invasive carcinoma. **D:** Invasive mucinous carcinoma consists of extracellular mucin surrounding irregularly shaped groups of carcinoma cells in the stroma. **E:** Nuclear immunoreactivity for estrogen receptor (immunoperoxidase). **F:** Cytoplasmic immunoreactivity for chromogranin (immunoperoxidase). **G:** Cytoplasmic immunoreactivity for synaptophysin (immunoperoxidase).

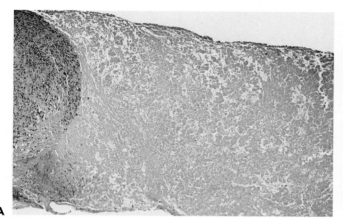

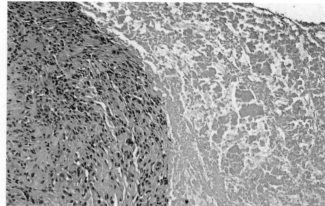

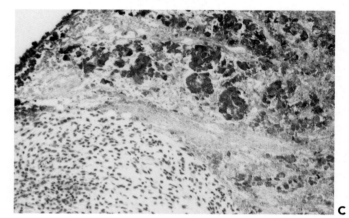

Figure 11.15 Infarcted papillary tumor, probably carcinoma. A, B: The needle core biopsy sample consists of infarcted tumor. Stroma with inflammatory cells is shown on the left. **C:** Papillary clusters of epithelial cells are highlighted in the infarcted tissue by the CK7 immunostain (immunoperoxidase).

Solorzano et al. (25) identified 40 patients with cystic papillary carcinoma who were treated at a single institution between 1985 and 2001. Invasive carcinoma was present in 13 cases, 13 had in situ cystic papillary carcinoma accompanied by intraductal carcinoma, and 14 had intraductal carcinoma confined to the cystic lesion. Metastatic carcinoma was found in axillary lymph nodes from 3 of 10 (30%) women with invasive carcinoma who had lymph nodes examined. No axillary metastases were found in 18 women with noninvasive papillary carcinoma.

By reviewing the records of the California Cancer Registry, Grabowski et al. (28) identified 917 examples of cystic papillary carcinoma of which 47% were intraductal and 53% had an invasive component. The cumulative survivals for intraductal and invasive cases were not significantly different 10 years after diagnosis (96.8% and 94.4%).

Fifty-eight patients with solid papillary carcinoma were identified in the records of two institutions by Nassar et al. (29). Three categories of tumor were described: pure solid papillary carcinomas (SPC, 32.7%), solid papillary carcinomas with extravasated mucin (SPC+M, 8.6%), and solid papillary carcinoma with invasion (SPC+INV, 58.7%). Invasive components were described as neuroendocrine-like (29.5%), mucinous (23.5%), ductal (14.5%),

lobular (3%), tubular (3%), or mixed (26.5%). The mean age at diagnosis was 72 years. Tumor size ranged from less than 1 to 15 cm. All tumors were positive for estrogen receptor and only two were negative for progesterone receptor. The 77 tumors tested were HER2/*neu* negative. All patients were treated surgically by excisional biopsy, supplemented by radiotherapy in nine cases. Among those with invasive carcinoma, 13 had adjuvant hormonal therapy and 3 also received chemotherapy. Axillary lymph nodes were examined in 30 (88.2%) cases, consisting of lymph nodes alone in 4 and axillary dissection in 26. Six of the 30 (20%) had positive axillary lymph nodes ranging from 1 to 10 (mean 4). The primary tumor in each of the patients with axillary nodal metastases had an invasive component that measured 1.5 cm or less. Axillary nodal metastases were observed with various histologic types of primary invasive carcinoma which the metastatic foci usually duplicated. Follow-up for a mean of 9.4 years was obtained for 28 patients. Five patients developed "chest wall" recurrences 4 to 10 years after diagnosis (initial therapy not specified). Five patients (17.8%) developed metastatic carcinoma that proved fatal 1 to 4 years after diagnosis. One of these patients had axillary nodal metastases and four had negative axillary nodes. Overall primary tumor size in the fatal cases ranged from 1 to 8 cm (mean 3 cm).

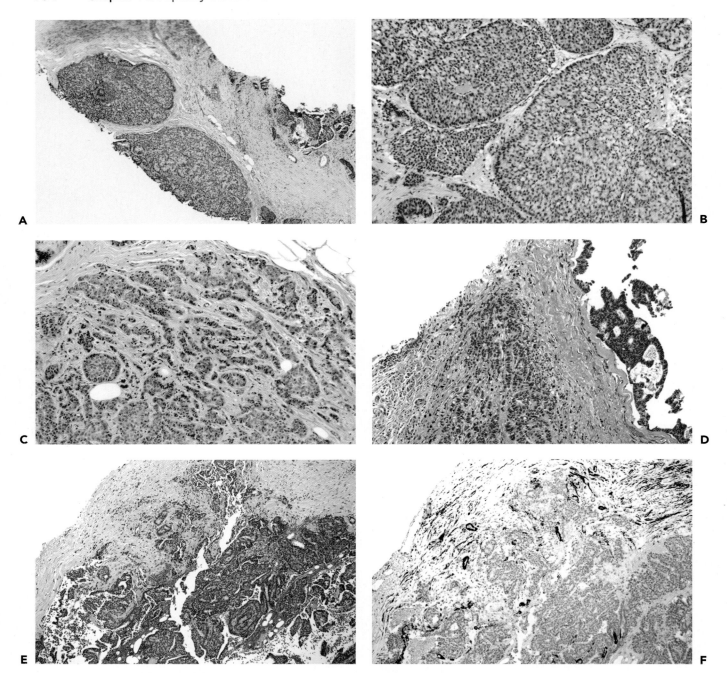

Figure 11.16 Solid papillary carcinoma with invasion. A, B: A needle core biopsy specimen showing solid papillary carcinoma with signet ring cells that were positive with the mucicarmine stain. Some glandular areas in the lower left of **(B)** have uneven borders, but invasion is not evident. **C:** The subsequent excisional biopsy specimen contained this area of invasive carcinoma. Note the distinctly different growth patterns of the in situ and invasive components. **D:** This needle core biopsy sample shows intracystic papillary carcinoma with cribriform architecture **(right)** and invasive carcinoma **(left)**. **E, F:** This needle core biopsy sample from a breast tumor in a 68-year-old woman shows a papillary carcinoma with invasion. Absence of myoepithelium is demonstrated by the actin immunostain in the in situ component **(below)** and in the invasive glands **(above)** (immunoperoxidase).

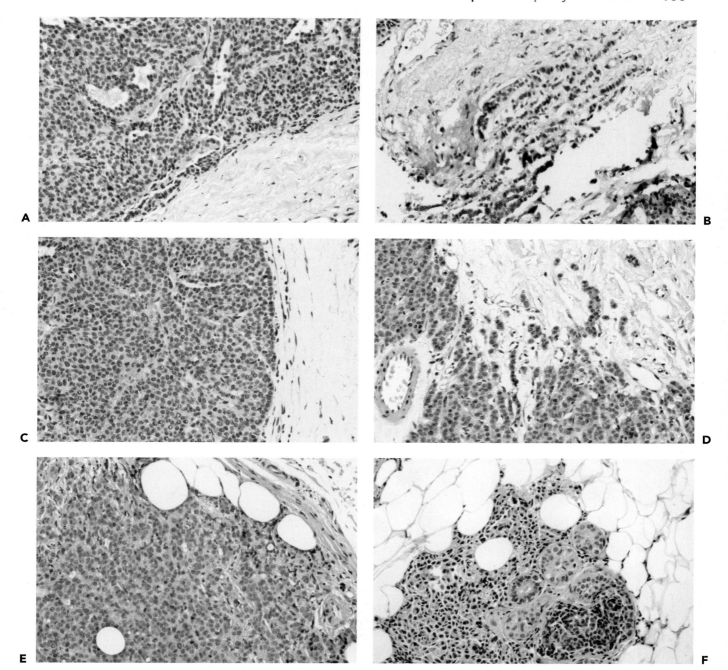

Figure 11.17 Solid papillary carcinoma with invasion. A: This needle core biopsy specimen shows solid papillary carcinoma. **B:** Another part of the specimen contained this fragment of tissue, in which were seen infiltrating carcinoma cells with a linear pattern suggestive of lobular carcinoma. **C:** Solid papillary carcinoma as it appeared in the excisional biopsy specimen. **D:** Infiltrating carcinoma at the edge of the excised lesion with the same appearance as in the needle core biopsy specimen in **(B). E:** An area of excised tumor in which there is invasion of fat with a solid growth pattern. **F:** Carcinoma in fat around a lobule in another biopsy specimen of solid papillary carcinoma. The absence of hemorrhage or fat necrosis and the delicate manner in which the carcinoma cells surround lipocytes support interpreting this as true invasive carcinoma.

REFERENCES

1. Fisher ER, Palekar AS, Redmond C, et al. Pathologic findings from the National Surgical Adjuvant Breast Project (Protocol No. 4). VI. Invasive papillary cancer. *Am J Clin Pathol.* 1980;73:313–320.

2. Carter D, Orr SL, Merino MJ. Intracystic papillary carcinoma of the breast after mastectomy, radiotherapy or excisional biopsy alone. *Cancer.* 1983;52:14–19.

3. Lefkowitz M, Lefkowitz W, Wargotz ES. Intraductal (intracystic) papillary carcinoma of the breast and its variants: a clinicopathological study of 77 cases. *Hum Pathol.* 1994;25:802–809.

4. Masood S, Barwick K. Estrogen receptor expression of the less common breast carcinomas. *Am J Clin Pathol.* 1990;93:437.

5. Meyer JS, Bauer WC, Rao BR. Subpopulations of breast carcinoma defined by S-phase fraction, morphology and estrogen receptor content. *Lab Invest.* 1978;39:225–235.

6. Estabrook A, Asch T, Gump F, et al. Mammographic features of intracystic papillary lesions. *Surg Gynecol Obstet.* 1990;170:113–116.

7. Schneider JA. Invasive papillary breast carcinoma: mammographic and sonographic appearance. *Radiology.* 1989;171:377–379.

8. Silva R, Ferrozi F, Paties C. Invasive papillary carcinoma in elderly women: sonographic and mammographic features. *Am J Roentgenol.* 1992;159:898–899.

9. McCulloch GL, Evans AJ, Yeoman L, et al. Radiological features of papillary carcinoma of the breast. *Clin Radiol.* 1997;52:856–868.

10. Soo MS, Williford ME, Walsh R, et al. Papillary carcinoma of the breast: imaging findings. *Am J Roentgenol.* 1995;164:321–326.

11. Liberman L, Bracero N, Vuolo M, et al. Percutaneous large core biopsy of papillary breast lesions. *Am J Roentgenol.* 1999;172:331–337.

12. Papotti M, Gugliotta P, Eusebi V, Bussolati G. Immunohistochemical analysis of benign and malignant papillary lesions of the breast. *Am J Surg Pathol.* 1983;7:451–461.

13. Papotti M, Gugliotta P, Ghiringhello B, Bussolati G. Association of breast carcinoma and multiple intraductal papillomas: an histological and immunohistochemical investigation. *Histopathology.* 1984;8:963–975.

14. Stefanou D, Bastistatou A, Nonni A, et al. P63 expression in benign and malignant breast lesions. *Histol Histopathol.* 2004;19:465–471.

15. Hill CB, Yeh I-T. Myoepithelial cell staining patterns of papillary breast lesions: from intraductal papillomas to invasive papillary carcinoma. *Am J Clin Pathol.* 2005;123;36–44.

16. Collins LC, Carlo VP, Hwang H, et al. Intracystic papillary carcinomas of the breast: A reevaluation using a panel of myoepithelial cell markers. *Am J Surg Pathol.* 2006;30:1002–1007.

17. Nicolas MM, Wu Y, Middleton LP, Gilcrease MZ. Loss of myoepithelium is variable in solid papillary carcinoma of the breast. *Histopathology.* 2007;51:647–665.

18. Rabban JT, Koerner FC, Lerwill MF. Solid papillary ductal carcinoma in situ versus usual ductal hyperplasia in the breast: a potentially difficult distinction resolved by cytokeratin 5/6. *Hum Pathol.* 2006;37:787–793.

19. Tan PH, Aw MY, Yip G, et al. Cytokeratins in papillary lesions of the breast. Is there a role in distinguishing intraductal papilloma from papillary ductal carcinoma in situ? *Am J Surg Pathol.* 2005;29:625–632.

20. Rosen PP, Oberman HA. Papillary carcinoma. In: Rosen PP, Oberman HA, eds. *Tumors of the Mammary Gland (Fasc. 7, 3rd series).* Washington, DC: Armed Forces Institute of Pathology; 1993:217.

21. Raju U, Vertes D. Breast papillomas with atypical ductal hyperplasia: a clinicopathologic study. *Hum Pathol.* 1996;27:1231–1238.

22. Page DL, Salhany KE, Jensen RA, Dupont WD. Subsequent breast carcinoma risk after biopsy with atypia in a breast papilloma. *Cancer.* 1996;78:258–266.

23. Cross AS, Azzopardi JG, Krausz T, et al. A morphologic and immunocytochemical study of a distinctive variant of ductal carcinoma in situ of the breast. *Histopathology.* 1985;9:21–37.

24. Youngson B, Cranor M, Rosen PP. Epithelial displacement in surgical breast specimens following needling procedures. *Am J Surg Pathol.* 1994;18:896–903.

25. Solorzano CC, Middleton LP, Hunt KK, et al. Treatment and outcome of patients with intra-cystic papillary carcinoma. *Am J Surg.* 2002;184:364–368.

26. Mulligan AM, O'Malley FP. Metastatic potential of encapsulated (intracystic) papillary carcinoma of the breast: a report of 2 cases with axillary lymph node micrometastases. *Int J Surg Pathol.* 2007;15:143–147.

27. Esposito NN, Dabbs DJ, Bhargava R. Are encapsulated papillary carcinomas of the breast in situ or invasive? *Am J Clin Pathol.* 2009;131:228–242.

28. Grabowski J, Salzstein SL, Sadler GR, Blair S. Intracystic papillary carcinoma. A review of 917 cases. *Cancer.* 2008;113:916–920.

29. Nassar H., Qureshi H., Adsay NV, Visscher D, Clinicopathologic analysis of solid papillary carcinoma of the breast and associated invasive carcinomas. *Am J Surg Pathol.* 2006;39:501–507.

Medullary Carcinoma 12

Medullary carcinoma is a "well-circumscribed carcinoma composed of poorly differentiated cells with scant stroma and prominent lymphoid infiltration" (1). It accounts for less than 5% of breast carcinomas (2–4). The mean age in several series ranged from 45 to 54 years (5–8). Bilateral carcinoma is uncommon in patients with medullary carcinoma in one breast, and synchronous or metachronous medullary carcinoma involving both breasts is rare event (3,6,9). The size distribution of medullary carcinomas is not appreciably different from that of nonmedullary infiltrating duct carcinomas (5,6).

Because they have circumscribed margins grossly and a firm consistency, medullary carcinomas can be mistaken clinically and radiologically for fibroadenomas (10). There are no ultrasound or mammographic criteria specific for medullary carcinoma or for distinguishing medullary from circumscribed nonmedullary carcinoma (10,11). However, a tumor with an irregular or "jagged" margin on ultrasonography is unlikely to be a true medullary carcinoma (12).

Ipsilateral axillary lymph nodes tend to be enlarged in medullary carcinoma patients, even when no nodal metastases are present, a phenomenon that may complicate clinical staging (13). The average number of lymph nodes recovered from the axillary dissection specimen of a patient with medullary carcinoma is greater than for other types of carcinoma (14). This difference probably results from the greater ease of finding enlarged, hyperplastic lymph nodes that exhibit reactive changes when examined microscopically. Medullary carcinoma arising in the axillary tail of the breast can be mistaken for metastatic carcinoma in a lymph node. Residual uninvolved lymph node tissues or in situ carcinoma nearby are useful for distinguishing features.

The typical intact medullary carcinoma is a moderately firm, discrete tumor. A distinct margin usually outlines the tumor when bisected and distinguishes it from the surrounding breast tissue but some small medullary carcinomas have poorly circumscribed borders resulting from an intense lymphoplasmacytic reaction extending beyond the immediate perimeter of the tumor (5). The tumor has a lobulated or nodular structure that might be apparent on the cut surface. Necrosis is not unusual. As the amount of necrosis increases, there is a greater likelihood that the tumor will have cystic foci.

Medullary carcinoma is defined by a constellation of microscopic histopathologic features: prominent lymphoplasmacytic reaction, microscopic circumscription, growth of tumor cells in sheets (syncytial pattern), poorly differentiated nuclear grade, and high mitotic rate. When most but not all of these components are present, the tumor may be termed an *invasive duct carcinoma with medullary features*. A carcinoma is not medullary if it has one or more of the following features: invasive growth at the periphery of the tumor, a diminished lymphoplasmacytic reaction, nuclear cytology that is not poorly differentiated, or conspicuous glandular or papillary growth.

The diagnosis of medullary carcinoma cannot be made conclusively by needle core biopsy because of the limited sample provided by such materials. It is appropriate to report that the findings raise the possibility of medullary carcinoma and that the final classification depends on complete evaluation of the excised tumor.

The *lymphoplasmacytic reaction* must involve the periphery and be present diffusely in the substance of the tumor. The internal lymphoplasmacytic infiltrate tends to be limited to fibrovascular stroma between syncytial zones of tumor cells. In a minority of tumors, the lymphoplasmacytic infiltrate mingles intimately with carcinoma cells (Fig. 12.1).

The microscopic features of medullary carcinoma with an exceptionally abundant lymphoplasmacytic reaction resemble those of lymphoepithelial carcinomas that arise at other sites. These and other characteristics have suggested that the Epstein–Barr virus (EBV) might play a role in pathogenesis of medullary carcinoma. However, a study of 10 tumors using immunohistochemistry, in situ hybridization, and the polymerase chain reaction failed to detect evidence of EBV (15). A lymphoepithelioma-like tumor studied by Naidoo and Chetty (16) was also negative for EBV (15). This lesion was accompanied by sclerosing lymphocytic lobulitis in the surrounding breast tissue. Kulka et al. (17) reported finding molecular evidence of human papilloma virus (HPV) in a mammary lymphoepithelioma-like carcinoma. The patient previously had carcinoma of the uterine cervix with the same HPV type.

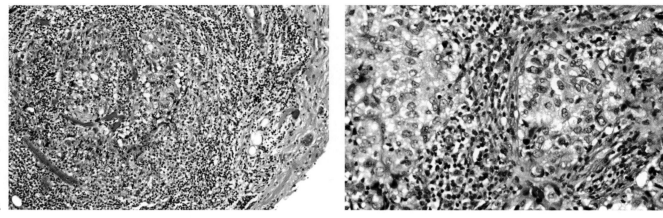

Figure 12.1 **Medullary carcinoma. A, B:** This needle core biopsy sample shows a diffuse lymphoplasmacytic infiltrate between syncytial masses of poorly differentiated carcinoma cells. Excisional biopsy revealed a typical medullary carcinoma.

The lymphoplasmacytic reaction usually encompasses surrounding ducts and lobules occupied by in situ carcinoma and more remote ducts and lobules not involved by carcinoma. The infiltrate may be composed almost entirely of either lymphocytes or plasma cells or a mixed population of these cell types. Intense lymphoplasmacytic infiltrates can occur in nonmedullary infiltrating duct carcinomas, but when plasma cells predominate, the tumor is more likely to be a medullary carcinoma. Rarely, the lymphocytic infiltrate gives rise to germinal centers within or around the tumor. The presence of germinal centers cannot be relied upon as the sole evidence that one is dealing with metastatic carcinoma in an intramammary or axillary lymph node.

Microscopic circumscription describes the edge of the carcinoma that should have a well-defined, pushing contour rather than infiltrate the breast parenchyma (Fig. 12.2). Glandular or fatty breast tissue should not be found within the substance of the invasive tumor but ducts, lobules, or islands of fat cells may be trapped in the surrounding lymphoplasmacytic reaction or between nodular components of the tumor.

A *syncytial growth pattern* is present as broad irregular sheets or islands in which the borders of individual cells are indistinct (18) (Figs. 12.2 and 12.3). A tumor that is otherwise characteristic may be accepted as a medullary carcinoma if it has minor components of trabecular, glandular, alveolar, or papillary growth. This judgment cannot be made with a needle core biopsy sample. It has been reported that overall and relapse-free survival are directly related to the extent of the syncytial component (18). Although there was not a significant difference in outcome between patients with 75% and 90% synctial growth, survival was diminished when less than 75% of a tumor was synctial, with the difference most marked at or less than the 50% level. These data substantiate the currently employed requirement for at least a 75% synctial component.

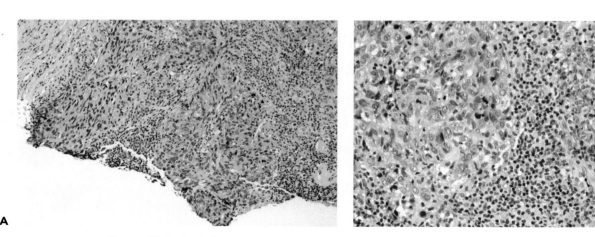

Figure 12.2 **Medullary carcinoma. A:** The well-defined tumor border is shown in this needle core biopsy sample from a medullary carcinoma. **B:** The round cell infiltrate is lymphoplasmacytic, and the tumor cells have poorly differentiated nuclei.

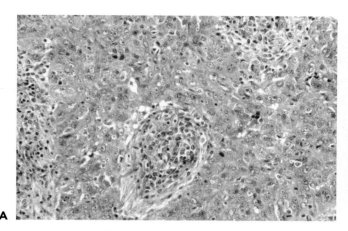 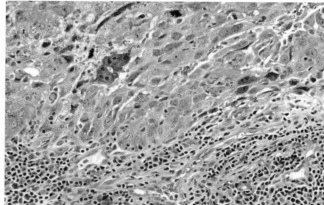

Figure 12.3 Medullary carcinoma. A: The carcinoma cells form bands surrounded by a reaction composed predominately of plasma cells. The borders of individual cells are indistinct, and they have poorly differentiated nuclei. **B:** A multinucleated giant cell is present.

Epidermoid differentiation is not unusual in medullary carcinomas and a small proportion of these tumors have fully developed foci of squamous metaplasia. Necrosis is more common in medullary carcinomas with squamous elements. Osseous, cartilaginous, and spindle cell metaplasia are much less common and bizarre epithelial giant cells can be found in an otherwise typical medullary carcinoma (Fig. 12.3). The tumor cells have a poorly differentiated nuclear grade and a high mitotic rate (Figs. 12.2 and 12.3). Pyknotic nuclei of degenerating cells are easily found, as are mitotic figures.

Intraductal carcinoma with lobular extension is found at the periphery of many medullary carcinomas. Foci of intraductal carcinoma occur more frequently with increasing tumor size and they are accompanied by the same prominent mononuclear cell infiltrate that one finds in the main tumor. The in situ carcinoma in ducts and lobules is composed of cells with the same poorly differentiated nuclei as the invasive portion of the medullary carcinoma. The intraductal carcinoma has comedo or solid growth patterns, and it can contain calcifications.

The majority of medullary carcinomas exhibit nuclear expression of p53. Membrane reactivity for epidermal growth factor receptor (EGFR) and HER2/*neu* are usually lacking. The characteristic immunophenotype of medullary carcinoma is p53(+)/HER2/*neu*(−), EGFR(−) (19,20). Vimentin expression was reported to be more frequent in medullary carcinomas and in duct carcinomas with medullary features than in ordinary invasive duct carcinomas (21). When compared with poorly differentiated invasive duct carcinomas of no special type, invasive duct carcinomas with medullary features reportedly display a basal-like immunophenotype significantly more often (62.9% vs. 18.9%) (22). Less than 10% of medullary carcinomas have nuclear immunoreactivity for estrogen and progesterone receptors (23). Although Larsimont et al. (24) reported that medullary carcinomas lacked expression of CK19, other investigators found no

significant difference in the expression of CK19 between medullary and poorly differentiated nonmedullary carcinomas (25,26).

Patients with medullary carcinoma have axillary lymph node metastases less often than patients with infiltrating duct carcinoma with medullary features or usual infiltrating duct carcinoma. When nodal metastases are present, they usually involve no more than three lymph nodes (3,5,6,27). Tumor size and nodal status are significant determinants of disease-free survival. The prognosis of patients with node-negative medullary carcinoma treated by mastectomy is particularly favorable if the tumor is not larger than 3 cm in diameter, with a disease-free survival of 90% or better (5,6,28). The survival results for stage II, $T_1N_1M_0$ medullary carcinoma have also been exceptionally good after 20 years of follow-up (28). Recurrences tend to occur early in the clinical course of patients with medullary carcinoma and recurrence is rare 5 years or more after diagnosis. Patients whose tumors are larger than 3 cm or who have four or more involved lymph nodes have high recurrence rates that are not appreciably different from the recurrence rates of patients with usual infiltrating duct carcinoma and equivalent stage.

There is presently little reported experience with breast-conserving surgery and radiotherapy of medullary carcinoma. In one study of 27 women with medullary carcinoma treated by breast conserving surgery and radiotherapy, the mammary recurrence rate was 4%, the 5 year overall survival was 90%, and relapse-free survival was 92% at 5 years (29). Haffty et al. (30) reported that 5 of 17 (29%) patients with medullary carcinoma treated by breast conserving therapy had local breast recurrences after a median follow-up of nearly 17 years, with the longest interval to recurrence being 18 years. In this study, the 10 years' actuarial breast recurrence-free survival was lower for medullary carcinoma (75%) than for usual infiltrating duct carcinoma (85%). No patient developed a systemic recurrence.

Sentinel lymph node mapping is an appropriate procedure for staging the axillary lymph nodes in patients with true medullary carcinoma. Indications for systemic adjuvant therapy include tumor size, nodal status, and the presence of lymphatic tumor emboli.

REFERENCES

Medullary Carcinoma

1. World Health Organization. Histological typing of breast tumors. *Tumori.* 1982;68:181–198.
2. Bloom HJG, Richardson WW, Fields JR. Host resistance and survival in carcinoma of breast: a study of 104 cases of medullary carcinoma in a series of 1511 cases of breast cancer followed for 20 years. *Br Med J (Clin Res).* 1970;3:181–188.
3. Rapin V, Contesso G, Mouriesse H, et al. Medullary carcinoma. A re-evaluation of 95 cases of breast cancer with inflammatory stroma. *Cancer.* 1988;61:2503–2510.
4. Rosen PP, Saigo PE, Braun Jr DW, et al. Predictors of recurrence in Stage 1 ($T_1N_0M_0$) breast carcinoma. *Ann Surg.* 1981;193:15–25.
5. Ridolfi R, Rosen P, Port A, et al. Medullary carcinoma of the breast. A clinicopathologic study with 10-year follow-up. *Cancer.* 1977;40:1365–1385.
6. Wargotz ES, Silverberg SG. Medullary carcinoma of the breast. A clinicopathologic study with appraisal of current diagnostic criteria. *Hum Pathol.* 1988;19:1340–1346.
7. Rosen PP, Lesser ML, Senie RT, Duthie K. Epidemiology of breast carcinoma. IV. Age and histologic tumor type. *J Surg Oncol.* 1982;19:44–47.
8. Rosen PP, Lesser ML, Kinne DW. Breast carcinoma at the extremes of age: a comparison of patients younger than 35 years and older than 75 years. *J Surg Oncol.* 1985;28:90–96.
9. Lesser ML, Rosen PP, Kinne DW. Multicentricity and bilaterality in invasive breast carcinoma. *Surgery.* 1982;1:234–240.
10. Meyer JE, Amin E, Lindfors KK, et al. Medullary carcinoma of the breast: mammographic and US appearance. *Radiology* 1989;170:79–82.
11. Kopans DB, Rubens J. Medullary carcinoma of the breast. *Radiology* 1989;171:876.
12. Cheung YC, Chen SC, Lee KF, et al. Sonographic and pathologic findings in typical and atypical medullary carcinomas of the breast. *J Clin Ultrasound.* 2000;28:325–331.
13. Neuman ML, Homer MJ. Association of medullary carcinoma with reactive axillary adenopathy. *Am J Roentgenol* 1996;167:185–186.
14. Rosen PP, Lesser ML, Kinne DW, Beattie Jr EJ. Discontinuous or "skip" metastases in breast carcinoma. *Ann Surg.* 1983;197:276–283.
15. Lespagnard L, Cochaux P, Larsimont D, et al. Absence of Epstein-Barr virus in medullary carcinoma of the breast as demonstrated by immunophenotyping *in situ* hybridization and polymerase chain reaction. *Am J Clin Pathol.* 1995;103:449–452.
16. Naidoo P, Chetty R. Lymphoepthelioma-like carcinoma of the breast with associated sclerosing lymphomcytic lobulitis. *Arch Pathol Lab Med.* 2001;125:669–672.
17. Kulka J, Kovalszky I, Svatics E, et al. Lymphoepithelioma-like carcinoma of the breast: not Epstein–Barr virus-, but human papilloma virus-positive. *Hum Pathol.* 2008;39:298–301.
18. Pedersen L, Schiodt T, Holck S, Zedeler K. The prognostic importance of syncytial growth pattern in medullary carcinoma of the breast. *APMIS.* 1990;98:921–926.
19. Rosen PP, Lesser ML, Arroyo CD, et al. Immunohistochemical detection of HER2/neu in patients with axillary lymph node negative breast carcinoma: a study of epidemiologic risk factors, histologic features and prognosis. *Cancer.* 1995;75:1320–1326.
20. Jacquemier J, Padovani L, Rabarol L, et al. Typical medullary breast carcinomas have a basal/myoepithelial phenotype. *J Pathol.* 2005;207:260–268.
21. Holck S, Pedersen L, Schiodt T, et al. Vimentin expression in 98 breast cancers with medullary features and its prognostic significance. *Virchows Arch (A).* 1993;422:475–479.
22. Rodriguez-Pinilla SM, Rodriguez-Gil Y, Moreno-Bueno G, et al. Sporadic invasive duct carcinomas with medullary features display a basal-like phenotype. An immunohistochemical and gene amplification study. *Am J Surg Pathol.* 2007;31:501–508.
23. Rosen PP, Menendez-Botet CJ, Nisselbaum JS, et al. Pathological review of breast lesions analyzed for estrogen receptor protein. *Cancer Res.* 1975;35:3187–3194.
24. Larsimont D, Lespagnard L, Degeyter M, Keimann R. Medullary carcinoma of the breast: a tumour lacking keratin 19. *Histopathology.* 1994;24:549–552.
25. Dalal P, Shousha S. Keratin 19 in paraffin sections of medullary carcinoma and other benign and malignant breast lesions. *Mod Pathol.* 1995;8:413–416.
26. Jensen ML, Kiaer H, Melsen F. Medullary carcinoma vs. poorly differentiated ductal carcinoma: an immunohistochemical study with keratin 19 and oestrogen receptor staining. *Histopathology.* 1996;29:241–245.
27. Reinfuss M, Stelmach A, Mitus J, et al. Typical medullary carcinoma of the breast: a clinical and pathological analysis of 52 cases. *J Surg Oncol.* 1995;60:89–94.
28. Rosen PP, Groshen S, Saigo PE, et al. A long-term follow-up study of survival in Stage I ($T_1N_0M_0$) and Stage II ($T_1N_1M_0$) breast carcinoma. *J Clin Oncol.* 1989;7:355–366.
29. Kurtz JM, Jacquemier J, Torhorst J, et al. Conservation therapy for breast cancers other than infiltrating ductal carcinoma. *Cancer.* 1989;63:1630–1635.
30. Haffty BG, Perrotta PL, Ward B, et al. Conservatively treated breast cancer: outcome by histologic subtype. *Breast J.* 1997;3:7–14.

Carcinoma with Metaplasia

13

The term *metaplastic carcinoma* has traditionally been reserved for carcinomas with microscopic structural features that diverge from glandular differentiation. In the breast, these phenotypic structural alterations are the expression of genotypic properties not manifested by normal mammary epithelium. Therefore metaplastic carcinoma represents patterns of gene expression rather than histogenesis. This conclusion is supported by the finding of the same p53 point mutation in several components of a metaplastic carcinoma that was studied by Wang et al. (1).

The frequency of metaplastic change in mammary carcinoma is probably underreported because inconspicuous foci are easily overlooked or ignored (Fig. 13.1). Squamous metaplasia was present in 3.7% of 1665 invasive carcinomas reviewed by Fisher et al. (2). Heterologous or sarcomatoid metaplasia was detected in 26 of 12,045 (0.2%) breast carcinomas in another study (3). Carcinomas with metaplasia usually have low levels of estrogen receptor and are classified as receptor negative (4–6).

The range of age at diagnosis and the clinical features of metaplastic mammary carcinoma are not appreciably different from those of invasive mammary carcinoma generally (3,6). The first symptom is typically a palpable tumor. The patient usually describes rapid growth and short duration before diagnosis (6). The radiologic appearance of metaplastic carcinoma is not specific except that bone formation in tumors with osseous metaplasia may be detectable by mammography (7). The tumors tend to have circumscribed contours radiologically and grossly. The results of magnetic resonance imaging (MRI) have been reported (8). The mean or median size (3–4 cm) reported in various series tends to be greater than that of ordinary infiltrating duct carcinomas.

Several lines of evidence support the view that metaplastic carcinoma arises from altered epithelial and/or myoepithelial cells. Cytogenetic and molecular studies have demonstrated clonality in the epithelial and pseudosarcomatous components of these tumors, a finding that indicates origin from a common stem cell (9,10). The concurrent presence of ordinary intraductal and invasive duct carcinoma in many of these tumors and transitions observed from carcinomatous foci to metaplastic components has led to the conclusion that these neoplasms are carcinomas derived from mammary glandular epithelial cells. Immunohistochemical studies that revealed coexpression of S-100, vimentin, and cytokeratin in components with epithelial and sarcomatoid phenotypes were interpreted as evidence for the epithelial origin of both elements by some investigators (11). Others pointed to these same observations as suggesting myoepithelial origin (3).

Recent studies that employed newly developed markers suggest that the sarcomatoid components of metaplastic carcinomas derive from myoepithelial cells. p63, a p53 homologue, found in the nuclei of myoepithelial and squamous cells, and only rarely in glandular epithelial cells (12,13), is expressed in almost all sarcomatoid metaplastic carcinoma of the breast (13–15). Koker and Kleer (15) detected p63 expression in 100% of spindle and squamous metaplastic carcinomas and in one of three tumors with chondroid differentiation. In the same study p63 was expressed in 1 of 174 (0.6%) nonmetaplastic carcinomas. There was no p63 reactivity in sarcomas or the stroma of phyllodes tumors. Other myoepithelial-associated markers such as CD10, myosin, and maspin, as well as smooth muscle actin (SMA), are also expressed in sarcomatoid components of many of these tumors but less consistently than p63 (16,17). Absence of p63 reactivity in the stroma of phyllodes tumors, almost all stromal sarcomas, fibromatasis, and myofibroblastic tumors is very useful for distinguishing these lesions from metaplastic carcinoma. At present, it appears likely that tumors included in the category of metaplastic carcinoma may be a heterogeneous group of neoplasms. Some may originate solely from the epithelium, others from the myoepithelium and a few may arise from both cell types. When distinct intraductal carcinoma or invasive ductal adenocarcinoma elements are not evident and the tumor is diffusely p63 positive, myoepithelial histogenesis is likely.

It has been customary to subdivide metaplastic carcinomas into two categories on the basis of histologic constituents: squamous and heterologous or pseudosarcomatous. These distinctions are somewhat arbitrary since some tumors exhibit both types of growth. A common pattern of metaplastic carcinoma is focal squamous metaplasia in an otherwise typical invasive duct carcinoma. A

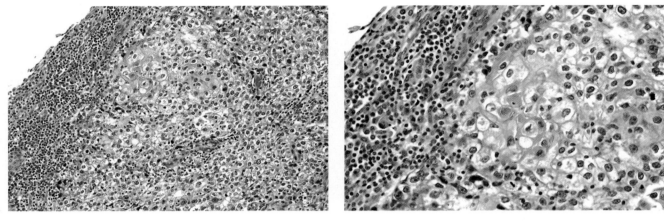

Figure 13.1 Invasive carcinoma with squamoid traits. This tumor is not classified as metaplastic carcinoma. **A, B:** A needle core biopsy specimen showing focal squamous differentiation in a poorly differentiated infiltrating duct carcinoma.

spectrum of differentiation may be found in squamous metaplasia. Mature keratinizing epithelium, sometimes with keratohyaline granules may be associated with poorly differentiated carcinoma or spindle cell, pseudosarcomatous areas (Fig. 13.2). Spindle cell carcinoma of the breast is a subset of carcinomas with squamous metaplasia in which most or virtually all of the neoplasm has assumed a pseudosarcomatous growth pattern that resembles fibrosar-

coma or fibromatosis (6,18) (Fig. 13.3). A moderate round cell infiltrate is almost always present in carcinomas with squamous and spindle cell metaplasia. This is such a common feature of these tumors that a diagnosis of metaplastic carcinoma should rarely be made when there is no inflammatory cell infiltrate. In some instances the nature of the lesion can be obscured by an inflammatory reaction that may suggest a nonneoplastic condition such as

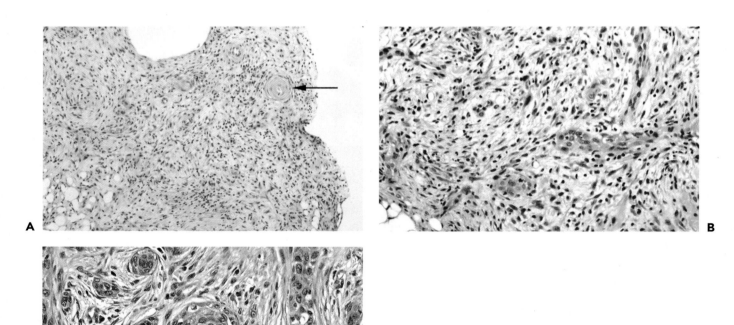

Figure 13.2 Metaplastic carcinoma, spindle cell and squamous type. A, B: This lesion might be misinterpreted as fibromatosis or as an inflammatory tumor. The needle core biopsy specimen shows a moderately cellular spindle cell lesion infiltrating fat with scattered lymphocytes. The spindle cells have bland cytologic features. A discrete squamous cell focus is present *(arrow)*. Indistinct cords and nests of polygonal carcinoma cells are shown. **C:** Squamous differentiation is better developed in this tumor.

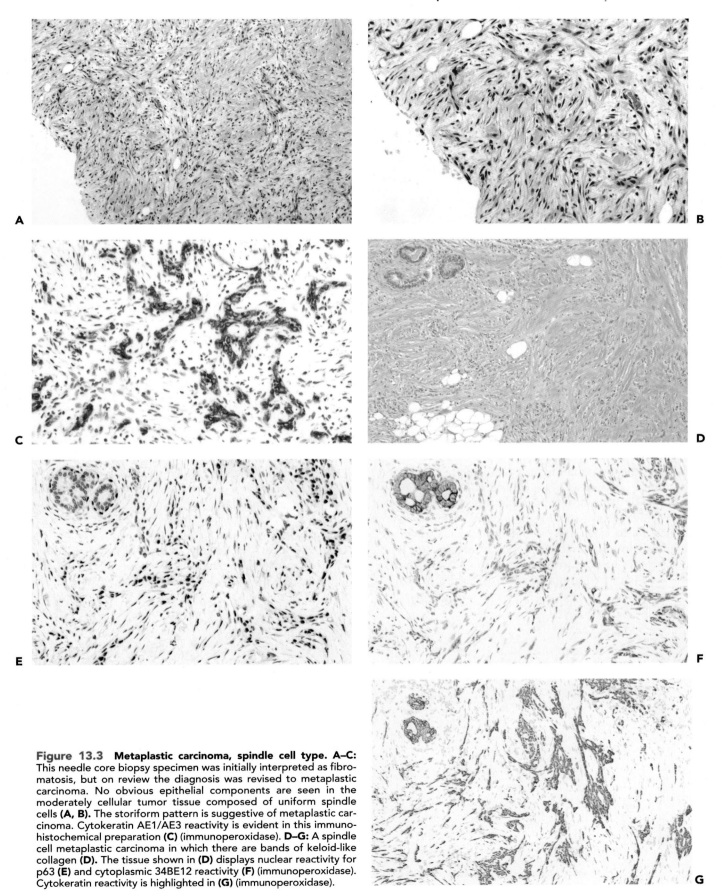

Figure 13.3 Metaplastic carcinoma, spindle cell type. A–C: This needle core biopsy specimen was initially interpreted as fibromatosis, but on review the diagnosis was revised to metaplastic carcinoma. No obvious epithelial components are seen in the moderately cellular tumor tissue composed of uniform spindle cells **(A, B)**. The storiform pattern is suggestive of metaplastic carcinoma. Cytokeratin AE1/AE3 reactivity is evident in this immunohistochemical preparation **(C)** (immunoperoxidase). **D–G:** A spindle cell metaplastic carcinoma in which there are bands of keloid-like collagen **(D)**. The tissue shown in **(D)** displays nuclear reactivity for p63 **(E)** and cytoplasmic 34BE12 reactivity **(F)** (immunoperoxidase). Cytokeratin reactivity is highlighted in **(G)** (immunoperoxidase).

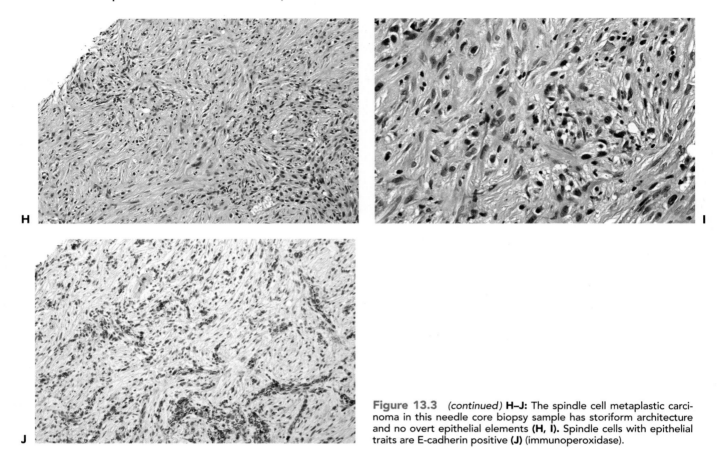

Figure 13.3 *(continued)* **H–J:** The spindle cell metaplastic carcinoma in this needle core biopsy sample has storiform architecture and no overt epithelial elements **(H, I).** Spindle cells with epithelial traits are E-cadherin positive **(J)** (immunoperoxidase).

inflammatory pseudotumor or fasciitis (Fig. 13.4). Another variant is characterized by dense, keloid-like areas of fibrosis in which the spindle cells and stroma often have a storiform pattern (Fig. 13.5). If immunostains performed on a limited needle core biopsy sample from such a spindle cell tumor are not diagnostic of metaplastic carcinoma, it is usually necessary to await an opportunity to study multiple portions of the excised tumor to arrive at a specific diagnosis.

Low-grade adenosquamous carcinoma is an unusual form of metaplastic duct carcinoma that is morphologically similar to adenosquamous carcinoma of the skin (19). These tumors are typically smaller than other varieties of metaplastic carcinoma (0.5–3.4 cm, average about 2.0 cm). They form hard nodules with grossly ill-defined borders. Microscopically, the invasive carcinoma exhibits variable amounts of epidermoid and glandular differentiation

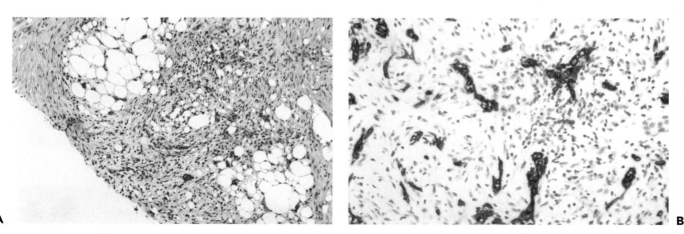

Figure 13.4 **Metaplastic carcinoma, spindle cell type.** A tumor with features that resemble an inflammatory lesion. **A:** The pattern of infiltration into fat and lymphocytic reaction shown in this needle core biopsy specimen were mistaken for fat necrosis. **B:** Cytokeratin 34BE12 expression is demonstrated in some of the spindle cells (immunoperoxidase).

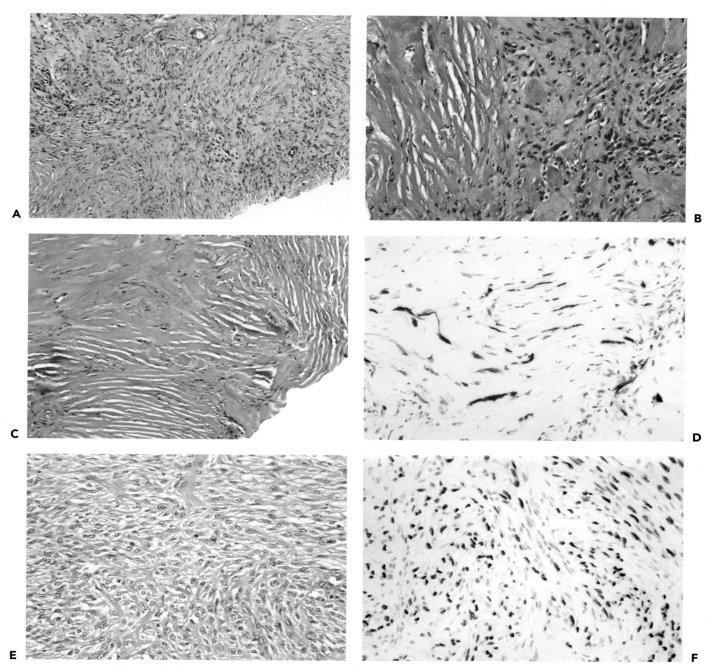

Figure 13.5 **Metaplastic carcinoma, spindle cell type. A:** This area in the needle core biopsy specimen has a storiform pattern. **B:** Another region with a component that resembles **(A)** on the right. A keloidal area composed of dense collagen and a pseudoangiomatous appearance is shown on the left. These findings resemble an area of scarring. **C:** A fully developed keloid-like area with prominent spaces between collagen bands. **D:** Some spindle cells among the collagen bands are immunoreactive for cytokeratin 34BE12 (immunoperoxidase). **E:** A densely cellular metaplastic spindle cell carcinoma. **F:** Nuclear reactivity for p63 is present in the carcinoma shown in **(D)** (immunoperoxidase).

in collagenous stroma. Foci of lymphocytic reaction are often present. A tendency to grow between and around ducts and lobules is most prominent at the periphery of the lesion, and it is not unusual to find a central area of sclerosing proliferation such as a radial scar or sclerosing adenosis. Conventional intraductal carcinoma is inconspicuous. Squamous metaplasia is found in varying patterns

including extensive epidermoid growth, syringoma-like differentiation (Fig. 13.6), and isolated inconspicuous squamous foci (Fig. 13.7). Large keratinizing cysts are uncommon but microcysts that may contain keratotic debris with calcification are sometimes present. Osteocartilaginous foci have been encountered in primary tumors and in recurrent lesions. Rarely, low-grade adenosquamous

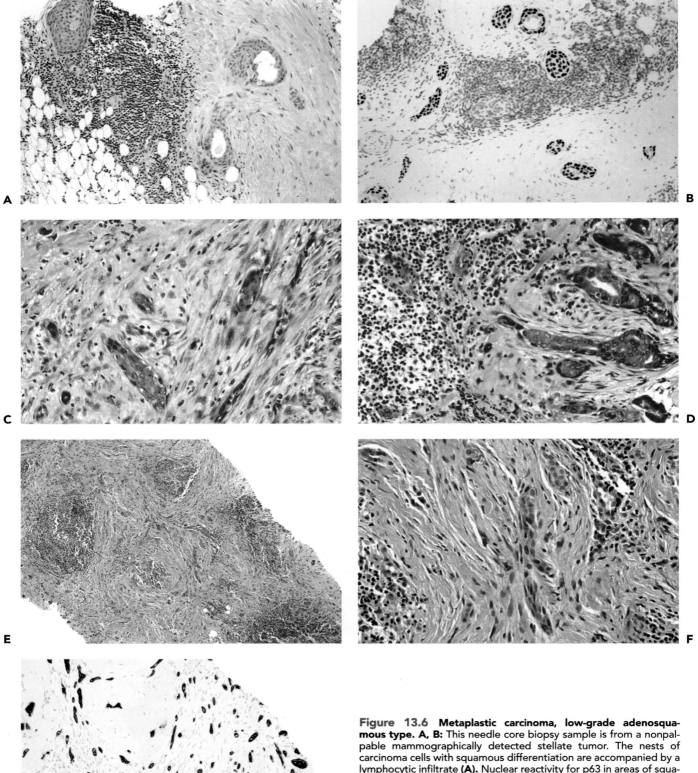

Figure 13.6 Metaplastic carcinoma, low-grade adenosquamous type. A, B: This needle core biopsy sample is from a nonpalpable mammographically detected stellate tumor. The nests of carcinoma cells with squamous differentiation are accompanied by a lymphocytic infiltrate **(A).** Nuclear reactivity for p63 in areas of squamous differentiation **(B)** (immunoperoxidase). **C, D:** The excisional biopsy of the tumor shown in **(A, B)** revealed cords and clusters of cells with squamoid **(C)** and glandular **(D)** differentiation. The lymphocytic aggregates shown in **(A, D)** are a characteristic feature of low-grade adenosquamous carcinoma. **E–G:** The needle core biopsy from another tumor showing prominent lymphocytic infiltrates **(E)** and attenuated strands of squamoid epithelial cells **(F)** that were reactive for the cytokeratin 34BE12 **(G)** (immunoperoxidase).

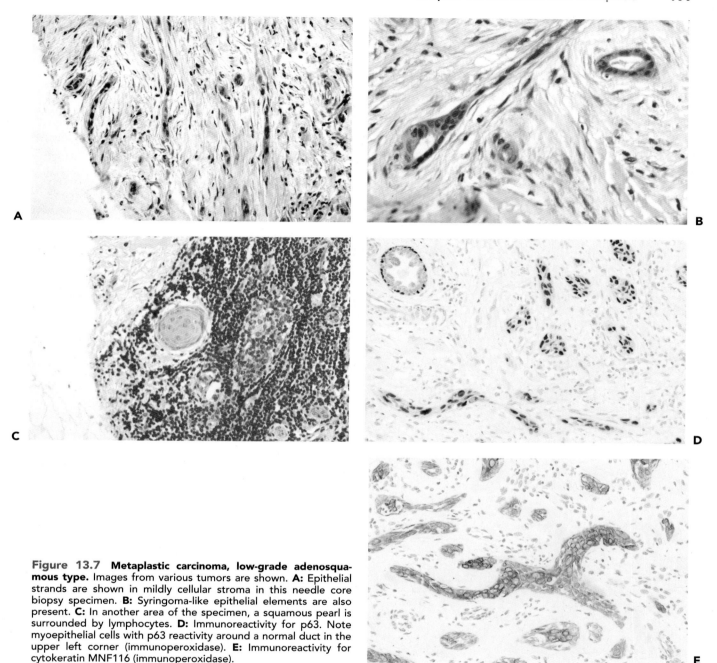

Figure 13.7 Metaplastic carcinoma, low-grade adenosquamous type. Images from various tumors are shown. **A:** Epithelial strands are shown in mildly cellular stroma in this needle core biopsy specimen. **B:** Syringoma-like epithelial elements are also present. **C:** In another area of the specimen, a squamous pearl is surrounded by lymphocytes. **D:** Immunoreactivity for p63. Note myoepithelial cells with p63 reactivity around a normal duct in the upper left corner (immunoperoxidase). **E:** Immunoreactivity for cytokeratin MNF116 (immunoperoxidase).

carcinoma shows transitions to conventional high-grade spindle cell and squamous metaplastic carcinoma. The epithelium of low-grade adenosquamous carcinoma is strongly reactive for p63 (Figs. 13.5–13.7), an observation that is consistent with squamous differentiation and myoepithelial histogenesis.

The distinction between spindle cell carcinoma and primary sarcoma of the breast may be difficult, and the neoplasm may be mistaken for a sarcoma, especially in a needle core biopsy specimen (20). Extensive sampling of the excised tumor is sometimes necessary to identify areas of squamous differentiation and to search for foci of

intraductal or invasive adenocarcinoma at the periphery. An unusual variant of spindle cell mammary carcinoma with squamous metaplasia has been described as pseudoangiosarcomatous or acantholytic carcinoma (21,22) (Fig. 13.8). The resemblance to angiosarcoma is a consequence of degeneration of the squamous epithelial component resulting in a pseudovascular pattern of anastomosing spaces. Cells lining these spaces are immunoreactive for cytokeratin and other epithelial markers and they do not stain for factor VIII or CD34, which characterize endothelial cells. Spindle cell and acanthoytic variants of metaplastic carcinoma are almost always immunoreactive for 34BE12(K903) and

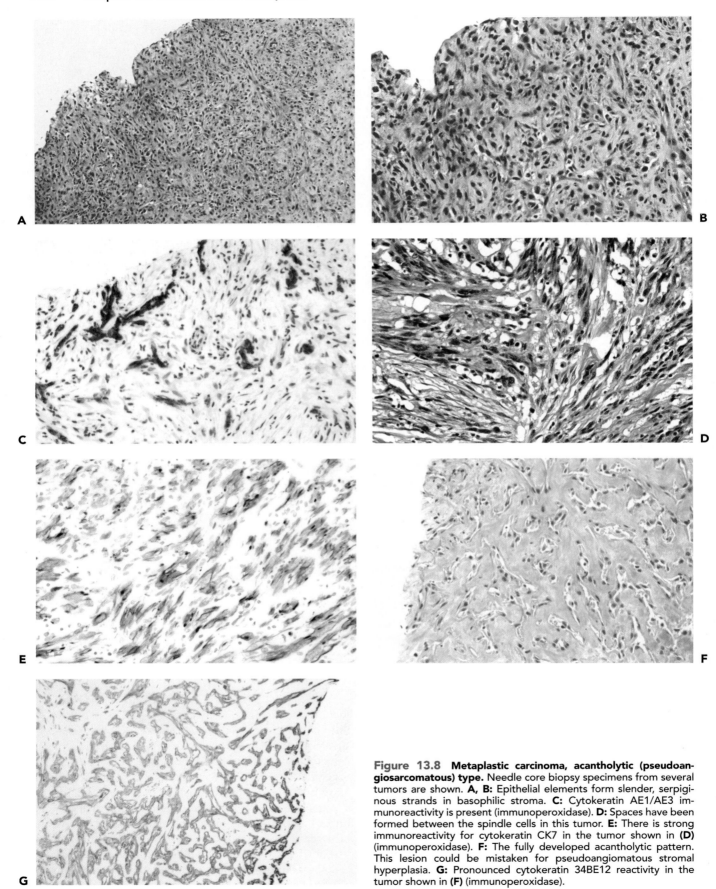

Figure 13.8 Metaplastic carcinoma, acantholytic (pseudoangiosarcomatous) type. Needle core biopsy specimens from several tumors are shown. **A, B:** Epithelial elements form slender, serpiginous strands in basophilic stroma. **C:** Cytokeratin AE1/AE3 immunoreactivity is present (immunoperoxidase). **D:** Spaces have been formed between the spindle cells in this tumor. **E:** There is strong immunoreactivity for cytokeratin CK7 in the tumor shown in **(D)** (immunoperoxidase). **F:** The fully developed acantholytic pattern. This lesion could be mistaken for pseudoangiomatous stromal hyperplasia. **G:** Pronounced cytokeratin 34BE12 reactivity in the tumor shown in **(F)** (immunoperoxidase).

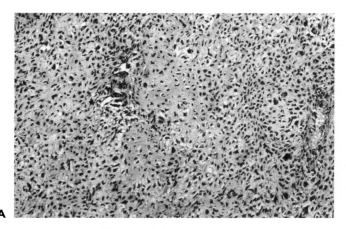
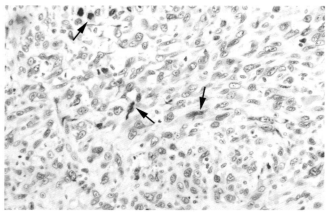

Figure 13.9 **Metaplastic carcinoma, osteocartilaginous metaplasia. A:** The tumor has poorly formed osteoid and chondroid matrix. **B:** Cytokeratin CAM5.2 expression is demonstrated in the spindle and round cells *(arrows)* (immunoperoxidase).

other high-molecular cytokeratins even when other keratin markers are negative. The presence of p63 reactivity in a malignant spindle cell tumor is indicative of metaplastic carcinoma except for the exceedingly rare occurrence of spindle cell myoepithelial sarcoma. Laminin 5 expression detected in metaplastic carcinomas and other triple-negative basal-like carcinomas may prove to be an additional useful marker (23).

Metaplastic carcinoma must be considered in the differential diagnosis of virtually any spindle lesion encountered in a needle core biopsy specimen. Immunohistochemistry should be employed in an effort to detect evidence of epithelial differentiation or p63 reactivity. If this effort is not successful, the report given for the needle core biopsy sample should indicate the need to study the excised tumor to establish a specific diagnosis. The distinction between a sarcoma and metaplastic carcinoma has important implications for therapy.

Heterologous metaplasia is most commonly encountered as bone and/or cartilage (Figs. 13.9, 13.10). Benign

heterologous metaplasia in the form of bone or cartilage may be found in radial sclerosing lesions, adenomyoepitheliomas, and rarely in apparently normal breast tissue (24). In metaplastic carcinoma these foci often coexist with areas composed of undifferentiated round or spindle cells. Zones of spindle cell metaplasia usually intervene between the adenocarcinomatous and heterologous elements (Fig. 13.10). Heterologous metaplastic carcinomas that have multinucleated giant cells resembling osteoclasts often exhibit osseous or cartilaginous metaplasia (3,5). This type of metaplastic carcinoma does not have the diffuse stromal hemorrhage and prominent adenocarcinoma found in carcinomas with osteoclast-like giant cells and should be distinguished from the latter type of carcinoma. Lee et al. (25) studied the p53 gene in a metaplastic carcinoma with osteoclast-like giant cells. They found strong p53 reactivity and the same point mutation in the p53 gene in the intraductal carcinoma and in the sarcomatoid component, but not in the osteoclast-like giant cells. These observations led the authors to conclude that the

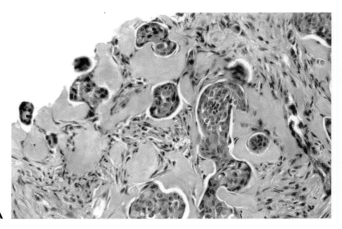
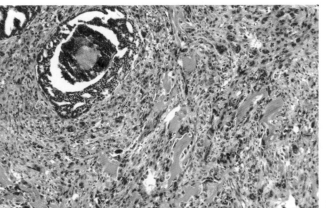

Figure 13.10 **Metaplastic carcinoma with osteosarcomatous differentiation. A:** The needle core biopsy specimen shows poorly differentiated carcinoma and osteoid. **B:** Intraductal carcinoma was found in the midst of the tumor in the excisional biopsy specimen.

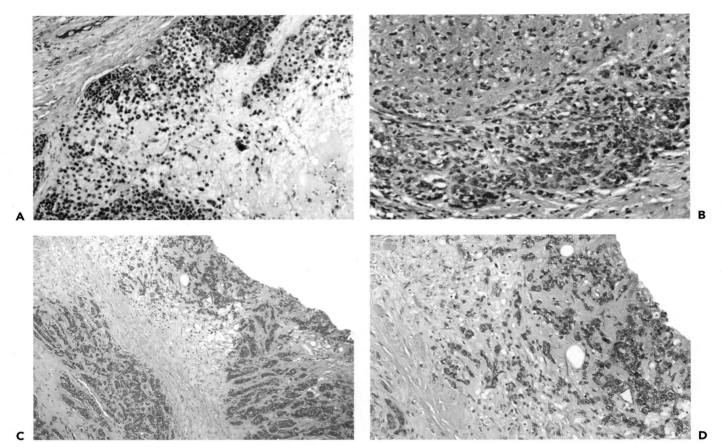

Figure 13.11 **Metaplastic carcinoma, matrix-producing type. A, B:** Undifferentiated carcinoma cells are seen blending with matrix material. The lacunar structure of cartilage is not present. **C, D:** The needle core biopsy sample from a poorly differentiated invasive duct carcinoma with focal matrix-forming differentiation. Taken out of context, the matrix-forming component could be mistaken for mucinous carcinoma **(D).**

carcinomatous and sarcomatoid elements arose from a common progenitor cell, and that the giant cells were reactive constituent.

Matrix-producing carcinoma is a variant of heterologous metaplastic carcinoma composed of "overt carcinoma with direct transition to a cartilaginous and/or osseous stromal matrix without an intervening spindle cell zone or osteoclastic cells" (26) (Fig. 13.11). The majority of matrix-producing carcinomas are circumscribed or nodular. The carcinomatous element is moderately to poorly differentiated adenocarcinoma (27). Mucin positivity is demonstrated in the carcinomatous areas, but the matrix-forming cells do not contain mucin. The cartilaginous matrix has the histochemical properties of a sulfated acid mucopolysaccharide, consistent with chondroitin sulfate. The carcinoma cells stain positively for keratin, epithelial membrane antigen, and S-100 in adenocarcinoma areas. A few tumors exhibit actin immunoreactivity, especially within metaplastic spindle cells, and actin myofilaments have been observed in the lesion by electron microscopy. Focal reactivity

for sox9 and p63 has been found in carcinomatous areas and the stroma contains types I and IV collagen (28).

Immunohistochemical studies have attempted to elucidate the relationship between epithelial and heterologous elements in metaplastic carcinomas, but the reported results have been inconsistent. It is very likely that there are intrinsic differences in the phenotypic expression of these markers that reflect the variable nature of genetic alterations in individual tumors. Rather than a single pattern of cytokeratin expression, these neoplasms appear to have a range of cytoskeletal phenotypes that express differing proportions and types of cytofilaments. A series of markers is usually required in order to detect cytokeratin expression (16). Most helpful in this regard are low- and high-molecular-weight cytokeratins including CAM 5.2, CK7, 34BE12, and the AE1/AE3 combination. In a given tumor, one marker will stain more strongly and more diffusely than the others but the pattern of expression tends to be unpredictable in a given tumor. Many spindle cell metaplastic carcinomas are also reactive for SMA. On the basis of data currently available, a spindle cell malignant tumor of the breast that is reactive for p63 and in which cytokeratin reactivity cannot be demonstrated with multiple markers, should be considered most likely to be metaplastic carcinoma. Epidermal growth factor receptor (EGFR) is expressed in squamous metaplastic carcinomas (29). Sheridan et al. (30) reported that metaplastic carcinomas of the breast and urinary bladder typically lack abnormally long telomeres, that are a characteristic feature of adult sarcomas.

Metastases derived from a metaplastic carcinoma can consist entirely of adenocarcinoma, entirely of metaplastic elements, or they may contain a mixture of these components. Tumors with squamous metaplasia often give rise to metastases with squamous differentiation in axillary lymph nodes and other sites. On the other hand, axillary lymph node metastases from some tumors with heterologous metaplasia are composed entirely of adenocarcinoma or the axillary metastases consist mainly of heterologous elements. Heterologous elements are expressed with greater frequency in local recurrences on the chest wall and in visceral sites than in nodal metastases (3,6). There does not appear to be a consistent relationship between the type and the amount of heterologous elements in the primary tumor and their representation in metastases. When metaplastic foci occur in metastatic deposits, they usually duplicate at least some of the components found in the primary tumor. It is also possible for metaplastic changes to develop within a metastasis or local recurrence, although corresponding metaplasia may not be detected in the primary tumor even after generous sampling (31).

Prognostic data thus far have been based largely on patients treated by mastectomy, usually with axillary dissection. Because of the rarity of metaplastic carcinomas and the relatively low frequency of axillary metastases, especially in patients with spindle cell metaplastic tumors, it is difficult to assemble a sufficient number of cases to stratify them by major prognostic factors, such as tumor size, nodal status, and pattern of metaplasia. Axillary lymph node metastases were reported in 6% to 14% of patients with squamous and spindle cell metaplastic carcinoma. The frequency of positive axillary lymph nodes associated with heterologous metaplastic carcinoma, including matrix-producing tumors, ranges from 6% (26) to 31% (20). Disease-free survival, generally reported for 5 or more years of follow-up, ranged from 33% to 65% for various types of metaplastic carcinoma in studies of at least 25 patients.

On the basis of reported data, it appears reasonable to conclude that the prognosis of metaplastic carcinoma is determined by the stage at diagnosis. It is not clear that the type of metaplasia has a significant effect on prognosis, although tumors with spindle metaplasia have a relatively low frequency of axillary nodal metastases when compared to those with matrix-producing or osteocartilaginous metaplasia.

REFERENCES

1. Wang X, Mori I, Tang W, et al. Metaplastic carcinoma of the breast: p53 analysis identified the same point mutation in the three histologic components. *Mod Pathol.* 2001;14:1183–1186.
2. Fisher ER, Gregorio RM, Palekar AS, Paulson JD. Mucoepidermoid and squamous cell carcinomas of breast with reference to squamous metaplasia and giant cell tumors. *Am J Surg Pathol.* 1984;7:15–27.
3. Kaufman MW, Marti JR, Gallager HS, Hoehn JL. Carcinoma of the breast with pseudosarcomatous metaplasia. *Cancer.* 1984;53:1908–1917.
4. Wargotz ES, Norris HJ. Metaplastic carcinoma of the breast. IV. Squamous cell carcinoma of ductal origin. *Cancer.* 1990;65:272–276.
5. Wargotz ES, Norris HJ. Metaplastic carcinomas of the breast. V. Metaplastic carcinoma with osteoclastic giant cells. *Hum Pathol.* 1990;21:1142–1150.
6. Oberman HA. Metaplastic carcinoma of the breast. A clinicopathologic study of 29 patients. *Am J Surg Pathol.* 1987;11:918–929.
7. Park JM, Han BK, Moon WK, et al. Metaplastic carcinoma of the breast: mammographic and sonographic findings. *J Clin Ultrasound.* 2000;28:179–186.
8. Velasco M, Santamaria G, Ganau S, et al. MRI of metaplastic carcinoma of the breast. *Am J Roentgenol.* 2005;184:1274–1278.
9. Wada H, Enomoto T, Tsujimoto M, et al. Carcinosarcoma of the breast: molecular-biological study for analysis of histogenesis. *Hum Pathol.* 1998;29:1324–1328.
10. Teixeira MR, Qvist H, Bohler PJ, et al. Cytogenetic analysis shows that carcinosarcomas of the breast are of monoclonal origin. *Genes Chromosomes Cancer.* 1998;22:145–151.
11. Palmer JO, Ghiselli RW, McDivitt RW. Immunohistochemistry in the differential diagnosis of breast diseases. *Pathol Annu.* 1990;25(pt 2):287–315.
12. Reis-Filho JS, Schmitt FC. Taking advantage of basic research: p63 is a reliable myoepithelial and stem cell marker. *Adv Anat Pathol.* 2002;9:280–289.
13. Barbareschi M, Pecciarini L, Gangi MG, et al. p63, a p53 homologue, is a selective nuclear marker of myoepithelial cells of the human breast. *Am J Surg Pathol.* 2001;25:1054–1060.
14. Reis-Filho JS, Schmitt FC. p63 expression in sarcomatoid/metaplastic carcinomas of the breast. *Histopathology.* 2003;42:92–99.
15. Koker MM, Kleer CG. p63 expression in breast cancer. A highly sensitive and specific marker of metaplastic carcinoma. *Am J Surg Pathol.* 2004;28:1506–1512.
16. Dunne B, Lee AHS, Pinder SE, et al. An immunohistochemical study of metaplastic spindle cell carcinoma, phyllodes tumor and fibromatosis of the breast. *Hum Pathol.* 2003;34:1009–1015.
17. Popnikolov NK, Ayala AG, Graves K, Gatalica Z. Benign myoepithelial tumors of the breast have immunophenotypic characteristics similar to metaplastic matrix-producing and spindle cell carcinomas. *Am J Clin Pathol.* 2003;120:161–167.
18. Gersell DJ, Katzenstein A-L. Spindle cell carcinoma of the breast. A clinicopathologic and ultrastructural study. *Hum Pathol.* 1981;12:550–561.
19. Rosen PP, Ernsberger D. Low-grade adenosquamous carcinoma. A variant of metaplastic mammary carcinoma. *Am J Surg Pathol.* 1987;11:351–358.
20. Pitts WC, Rojas VA, Gaffey MJ, et al. Carcinomas with metaplasia and sarcomas of the breast. *Am J Clin Pathol.* 1991;95:623–632.
21. Banerjee SS, Eyden BP, Wells S, et al. Pseudoangiosarcomatous carcinoma: a clinicopathological study of seven cases. *Histopathology.* 1992;21:13–23.
22. Eusebi V, Lamovec J, Cattani MC, et al. Acantholytic variant of squamous cell carcinoma of the breast. *Am J Surg Pathol.* 1986;10:855–861.
23. Carpenter PM, Wang-Rodriguez J, Chano TM, Wilczynskis P. Laminin 5 expression in metaplastic breast carcinomas. *Am J Surg Pathol.* 2008;32:345–353.
24. Gal-Gombos EC, Esserman LE, Poniecka AW, et al. Osseous metaplasia of the breast: diagnosis with stereotactic core biopsy. *Breast J.* 2002;8:50–52.
25. Lee JS, Kim YB, Min KW. Metaplastic mammary carcinoma with osteoclast-like giant cells: identical point mutation of p53 gene only identified in both the intraductal and sarcomatous components. *Virchows Arch.* 2004;444:194–197.
26. Wargotz ES, Norris HJ. Metaplastic carcinomas of the breast. I. Matrix-producing carcinoma. *Hum Pathol.* 1989;20:628–636.
27. Downs-Kelly E, Nayeemuddin KM, Albarracin C, et al. Matrix-producing carcinoma of the breast: an aggressive subtype of metaplastic carcinoma. *Am J Surg Pathol.* 2009;33:534–541.
28. Kusafuka K, Muramatsu K, Kasami M, et al. Cartilaginous features in matrix-producing carcinoma of the breast: four cases report with histochemical and immunohistochemical analysis of matrix molecules. *Mod Pathol.* 2008;21:1282–1292.
29. Bissuyt V, Fadere O, Martel M, et al. Remarkably high frequency of EGFR expression in breast carcinomas with squamous differentiation. *Mod Pathol.* 2005;18 (suppl):27A.
30. Sheridan T, Meeker A, Hicks J, et al. Metaplastic (sarcomatoid) carcinomas of the breast lack the abnormally long telomeres of the pleomorphic sarcomas that they mimic morphologically. *Mod Pathol.* 2005;18(suppl):50A.
31. Chell SE, Nayar R, DeFrias DV, Bedrossian CW. Metaplastic breast carcinoma metastatic to the lung mimicking a primary chondroid lesion: report of a case with cytohistologic correlation. *Ann Diagn Pathol.* 1998;12:173–180.

Squamous Carcinoma

14

The term *squamous carcinoma* should be used for lesions in which more than 90% of the neoplasm is composed entirely of keratinizing squamous carcinoma. Squamous carcinoma of the breast is a metaplastic carcinoma since the mammary glandular epithelium is not normally keratinizing. Benign metaplastic squamous epithelium is the precursor of pure squamous carcinoma. Squamous metaplasia occurs in the epithelium of cysts (1), fibroepithelial tumors, papillomas, duct hyperplasia, and at the site of prior surgery, traumatic injury, or inflammation (Fig. 14.1). Extensive benign squamous metaplasia of duct and lobular epithelium has been described in association with fat necrosis and other lesions (2). When squamous metaplasia occurs in an inflamed cyst, metaplastic epithelium may be embedded in the reactive process, resulting in a pattern that is difficult to distinguish from invasive squamous carcinoma. Epithelium displaced into surrounding tissue by a needle core biopsy performed on benign lesions such as papillomas or fibroadenomas sometimes undergoes squamous metaplasia. Minor instances of squamous metaplasia are often found in damaged ducts around a surgical biopsy site, and rarely, there is extensive squamous metaplasia in healing biopsy site. Tissue or cells obtained by a needle core biopsy from a biopsy site subjected to irradiation in which there is benign squamous metaplasia may display substantial atypia and suggest carcinoma (3).

There are no clinical features that are specifically associated with intraductal or invasive squamous carcinoma of the breast. The tumors have indistinct or partially distinct margins on mammography but no specific mammographic findings have been described (4,5). In one review, the average age at diagnosis was 57 years and half of the patients were 60 years or older (6). Calcifications in necrotic squamous tissue can sometimes be seen radiographically. Involvement of the skin by invasive squamous carcinoma makes it difficult to distinguish between cutaneous origin and secondary skin involvement by an underlying mammary lesion. When the bulk of the tumor is in the breast and the clinical history indicates a breast mass preceded skin ulceration, the lesion may be considered to be a mammary carcinoma. The presence of intraductal squamous carcinoma is very helpful for establishing that

the tumor is primary in the breast (Fig. 14.2). Since squamous epithelium is p63-positive, this stain is not useful for detecting myoepithelium in intraductal squamous carcinoma. Intraductal and invasive squamous carcinomas are estrogen receptor-negative and epidermal growth factor receptor-positive (7).

Invasive squamous carcinomas tend to be somewhat larger than other types of breast carcinoma. Reported sizes vary from 1 to 10 cm, with nearly half of the cases 5 cm or more in diameter (7). Central cystic degeneration is especially common in tumors larger than 2 cm, the cavity being filled with necrotic squamous debris.

Squamous carcinomas of the breast are differentiated sufficiently to form keratinized cells, and keratohyaline granules may be seen in the neoplastic epithelium (Fig. 14.3). Conversion of the squamous epithelium to spindle cell pseudosarcomatous growth can be found focally in some invasive squamous carcinomas of the breast. However, the distinction between myofibroblastic or fibroblastic stromal reaction and a neoplastic spindle cell component is not always easy to make. Evidence favoring pseudosarcomatous spindle cell carcinoma is mitotic activity, substantial cytologic atypia and demonstrable cytokeratin immunoreactivity in the spindle cells. Extensive sampling of the lesion following excisional biopsy is necessary to determine if the tumor is a metaplastic duct carcinoma with squamous differentiation or a pure squamous carcinoma. The latter diagnosis is made if there is extensive squamous differentiation of the epithelium with little or no spindle cell pseudosarcomatous element and no detectable adenocarcinoma. The strongest evidence in support of the diagnosis of primary mammary squamous carcinoma is the presence of in situ squamous carcinoma in ducts or in a cystic component of the tumor.

When invasive squamous carcinoma is found in the breast, it is necessary to consider the possibility that the tumor is metastatic from an extramammary primary. The most common sources of metastatic squamous carcinoma in the breast are the lung, esophagus, uterine cervix, and urinary bladder. The distinction between a primary tumor and metastatic squamous carcinoma may not be resolved with a needle core biopsy sample unless in situ squamous

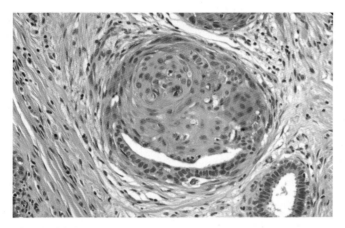

Figure 14.1   Squamous metaplasia in a hyperplastic duct. Benign metaplastic foci such as this may be the source of primary squamous carcinoma in the breast.

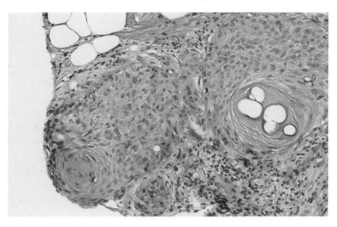

Figure 14.2   Intraductal squamous carcinoma. This needle core biopsy sample shows two contiguous ducts occupied by centrally keratinizing, well-differentiated squamous carcinoma.

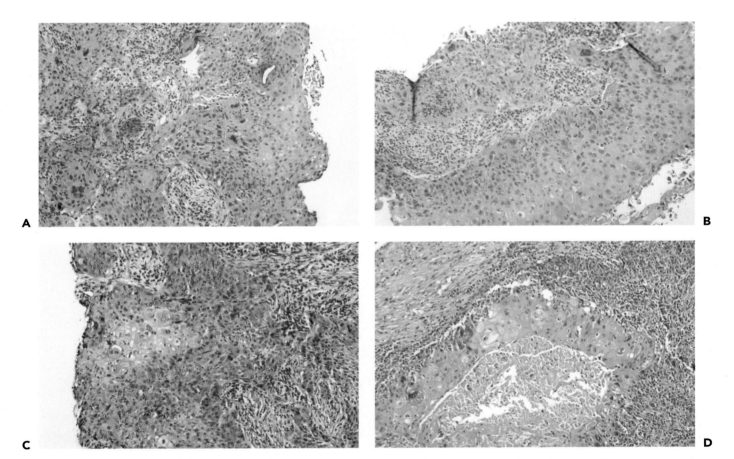

Figure 14.3   Invasive squamous carcinoma. A, B: A needle core biopsy specimen showing well to moderately differentiated invasive squamous carcinoma and invasive poorly differentiated carcinoma. **C:** A part of the same tumor with poorly differentiated squamous carcinoma. **D:** An area in the surgically excised tumor that duplicates the appearance of the needle core biopsy specimen. Note the cystic degeneration and the lymphoplasmacytic stromal infiltrate, frequent components of primary squamous carcinoma of the breast.

carcinoma is present. Consequently, the possibility of metastatic tumor must be considered if a needle core biopsy specimen from the breast contains squamous epithelium. Cystic degeneration occurs in primary squamous carcinoma of the breast, and it is not usual in metastatic squamous carcinoma that originates from various nonmammary sites. Isolated foci within a squamous carcinoma, whether primary or metastatic, may be so well differentiated that they are not distinguishable from benign epithelium in a limited core biopsy sample. Immunoreactivity for p63 is found in the nuclei of squamous carcinoma and in benign metaplastic squamous epithelium.

The prognosis of patients with primary squamous carcinoma of the breast is not well documented because the tumors are rare and authors have not always distinguished pure squamous carcinoma from metaplastic adenocarcinoma with squamous differentiation. In most patients, no axillary nodal metastases were found when an axillary dissection was performed (8). About one-third of patients with negative lymph nodes described in various reports died of metastatic carcinoma 4 to 30 months after diagnosis. Two patients with axillary lymph node metastases died 6 and 17 months after treatment, whereas two others were alive and well after 16 months and 6 years of follow-up. Local chest wall recurrence can occur.

REFERENCES

1. Kwak JY, Park HL, Kim JY, et al. Imaging findings in a case of epidermal inclusion cyst arising within the breast parenchyma. *J Clin Ultrasound.* 2004;32:141–143.
2. Hurt MA, Diaz-Arias AA, Rosenholtz MJ, et al. Posttraumatic lobular squamous metaplasia of breast. An unusual pseudocarcinomatous metaplasia resembling squamous (necrotizing) sialometaplasia of the salivary gland. *Mod Pathol.* 1988;1:385–390.
3. Saad RS, Silverman JF, Julian T, et al. Atypical squamous metaplasia of seromas in breast needle aspirates from irradiated lumpectomy sites: a potential pitfall for false-positive diagnoses of carcinoma. *Diagn Cytopathol.* 2002;26:104–108.
4. Tashjian J, Kuni CC, Bohn LE. Primary squamous cell carcinoma of the breast: mammographic findings. *J Canad Assoc Radiol.* 1989;40:228–229.
5. Samuels TH, Miller NA, Manchul LA, et al. Squamous cell carcinoma of the breast. *Can Assoc Radiol J.* 1996;47:177–182.
6. Rostock RA, Bauer TW, Eggleston JC. Primary squamous carcinoma of the breast: a review. *Breast.* 1984;10:27–31.
7. Bossuyt V, Fadare O, Martel M, et al. Remarkably high frequency of EGFR expression in breast carcinoma with squamous differentiation. *Mod Pathol.* 2005;18(suppl):27A.
8. Eggers JW, Chesney TMC. Squamous cell carcinoma of the breast: a clinicopathologic analysis of eight cases and review of the literature. *Hum Pathol.* 1984;15:526–531.

Mucinous Carcinoma

15

When the diagnosis is restricted to tumors consisting of pure or nearly pure mucinous carcinoma, not more than 2% of mammary carcinomas fall into this category (1–3). Focal mucinous differentiation occurs in up to 2% of additional carcinomas that are termed infiltrating duct carcinoma with mucinous differentiation or mixed mucinous carcinoma (3,4). Mucinous carcinoma occurs throughout the age range of breast carcinoma generally. Some studies found the mean age of women with mucinous carcinoma to be older than that of patients with nonmucinous carcinoma (2,3,5). Komenaka et al. (6) identified 65 patients (0.8%) with pure mucinous carcinoma among 7676 women with breast carcinoma treated in a single institution. The age range at diagnosis was 13 to 93 years (mean 67 years), and 85% of the patients were post menopausal. Mucinous carcinoma constitutes about 7% of carcinomas in women 75 years or older and only 1% among those younger than 35 years (7). Immunohistochemical studies have demonstrated nuclear estrogen receptor activity in about 90% of cases (8) and progesterone receptors in about 65% of tumors. Mucinous carcinomas may express WT1 weakly and rarely strongly (9).

Mucinous carcinoma can arise in ectopic breast tissue at sites that might be subject to needle biopsy such as the axilla or vulva (10). The differential diagnosis in these unusual locations will involve metastatic carcinoma from an extrinsic primary or mucinous carcinoma arising from sweat glands. It is necessary to document the presence of benign mammary glands to consider a diagnosis of mucinous carcinoma originating in ectopic breast tissue. The presence of in situ carcinoma in this tissue will firmly establish the diagnosis of primary mucinous carcinoma.

The initial symptom of mammary mucinous carcinoma is a breast mass in the majority of patients. A pure mucinous carcinoma typically has a mammographically and sonographically circumscribed border, whereas a mixed mucinous carcinoma tends to have an irregular, indistinct margin due to fibrosis and an infiltrative growth pattern (6,11). A spiculated contour is associated with a lesser mucinous component and a higher frequency of lymph node metastases. Mammographically detected calcifications occur in a minority of the tumors (6,12), involving

the invasive portion of approximately 20% of mucinous carcinomas (13,14). Calcifications are usually localized in associated intraductal carcinoma. The magnetic resonance imaging characteristics of mucinous carcinomas are reported not to be distinctive (15,16).

Mucinous carcinomas have been described ranging from less than 1 cm to more than 20 cm in diameter. In 1987, a nationwide study of Danish breast cancer patients found that only 16% of mucinous carcinomas were larger than 5 cm (1). A report from Japan found that 53.6% of mucinous carcinomas were 2.0 cm or less (T1) and 37.8% were 2.1 to 5.0 cm (T2) (4).

Histologically, pure mucinous carcinoma features the accumulation of extracellular mucin around invasive tumor cells (Fig. 15.1). The proportions of mucin and neoplastic epithelium vary from case to case but the distribution within a given tumor is fairly constant. Multiple sections can be necessary to detect carcinoma cells if a tumor is composed almost entirely of extracellular mucin. A carcinoma should not be classified as pure mucinous carcinoma if more than 10% of the invasive component is nonmucinous, or if the nonmucinous component is cytologically poorly differentiated.

With the exception of exceedingly rare examples that arise from signet ring cell lobular carcinoma, pure mucinous carcinomas are a type of ductal carcinoma. Intraductal carcinoma is associated with about 75% of the lesions, generally at the periphery. It can have any of the conventional patterns (cribriform, papillary, micropapillary, comedo) (Fig. 15.2). Occasionally, mucin is evident in the cytoplasm of intraductal carcinoma cells or in the duct lumen and one can find transitions from intraductal to invasive mucinous carcinoma. A difficult diagnostic problem arises in patients who have only this type of intraductal carcinoma when extravasated mucin is present in the adjacent stroma. Extravasation of mucin from intraductal carcinoma can be caused by a prior procedure or it may be spontaneous. Regardless of the mechanism by which it occurs, extravasated mucin devoid of carcinoma cells does not represent invasive mucinous carcinoma. It may be necessary to obtain multiple recuts and to do a cytokeratin stain to determine whether epithelial cells are present in

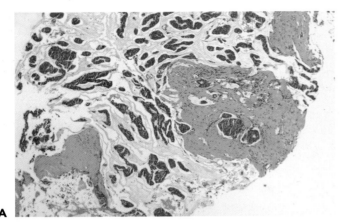
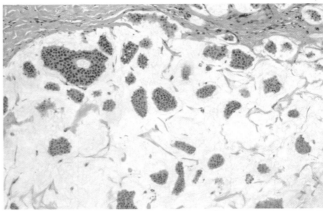

Figure 15.1 **Mucinous carcinoma. A, B:** Needle core biopsy specimens showing varying proportions of extracellular mucin and carcinoma cells. The epithelium forms small nests and trabeculae in **(A)** and nests in **(B)**.

the mucin. If carcinoma cells are found in the mucin, a diagnosis of invasive mucinous carcinoma is appropriate, unless there is compelling evidence to consider the alternative possibility of epithelial displacement caused by a prior procedure.

A minority of mucinous carcinomas do not have detectable intraductal carcinoma. These are typically large tumors but rarely a pure mucinous carcinoma smaller than 2 cm lacks intraductal carcinoma. Intraductal carcinoma may be absent from the limited samples of a needle core biopsy specimen.

Several patterns of epithelial distribution can be found in mucinous carcinomas (17). Lesions with epithelium arranged in clusters, trabeculae, or festoons have been associated with a younger age at diagnosis than tumors in which the carcinoma cells form larger clumps (Figs. 15.1 and 15.3). The latter lesions tend to have more abundant intracytoplasmic mucin, granular cytoplasm, and some of these tumors cells are argyrophilic. A micropapillary form of pure mucinous carcinoma has recently been described

(18). The presence of a micropapillary component in a mucinous carcinoma has been associated with an increased risk for nodal metastases and a less favorable prognosis (19). Areas with a cribriform structure are present in many mucinous carcinomas and a subset of the lesions have mixed growth patterns consisting of ribbons and clumps of cells. The margin of mucinous carcinoma is determined by the extent of the mucinous component, even if no epithelial cells are seen in the peripheral zone. The border is characterized as pushing in more than 70% of cases (14). It is difficult to recognize lymphatic tumor emboli in mucinous carcinomas because carcinoma cells suspended in mucin resemble intralymphatic carcinoma (Fig. 15.4). Immunostains for vascular endothelial markers such as CD31, CD34 factor VIII, and D2-40 may be helpful.

Argyrophilic granules are present in the cells of 25% to 50% of mucinous carcinoma (1–3,17). Mucinous carcinomas that contain these granules occur more frequently in women older than 60 years, and the tumor cells often grow in clumps, sheets, or trabeculae, suggestive of an endocrine

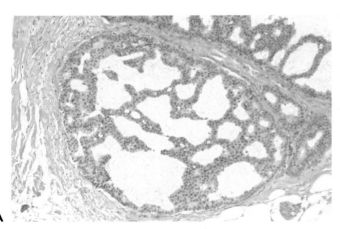
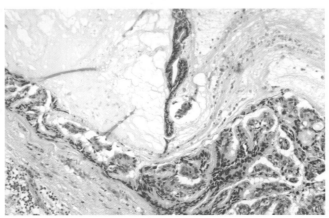

Figure 15.2 **Intraductal carcinoma. A:** Cribriform intraductal carcinoma that was present in the needle core biopsy specimen shown in Fig. 15.1B. Invasive mucinous carcinoma is present in the lower right corner. **B:** Papillary intraductal carcinoma with mucin formation in the duct lumen.

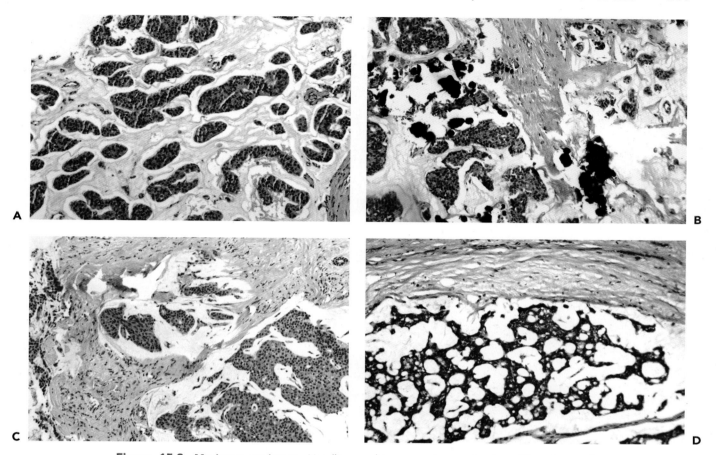

Figure 15.3 Mucinous carcinoma. Needle core biopsy specimens showing different growth patterns. **A:** Trabecular pattern. **B:** Irregular clusters of carcinoma cells and calcification in the mucin. **C:** Festoon growth pattern. **D:** Cribriform mucinous carcinoma.

growth pattern. The granules of some mucinous carcinomas contain immunohistochemically detectable serotonin, somatostatin, gastrin, and neuron-specific enolase (2,20). The presence or absence of argyrophilic granules is not

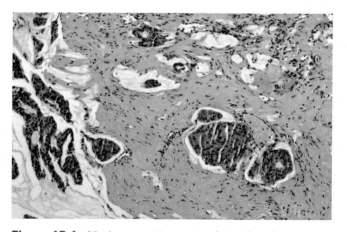

Figure 15.4 Mucinous carcinoma simulating lymphatic tumor emboli. A magnified view of a needle core biopsy specimen showing carcinoma cells surrounded by mucin in the stroma. This appearance simulates carcinoma in lymphatic spaces. Note the absence of endothelial cell nuclei around the mucin-filled spaces and infiltration into the collagenous stroma.

prognostically significant in pure mucinous tumors or in infiltrating duct carcinomas with focal mucinous differentiation (1,2,21).

Mucocele-like lesions must be considered in the differential diagnosis of mucinous carcinoma (22). The final classification of a mucocele-like tumor depends on the pattern of epithelial growth that may include atypical duct hyperplasia with or without atypia, or intraductal carcinoma (23,24). Mucocele-like lesions present as palpable tumors, or they are detected by mammography as well-circumscribed, lobulated tumors. Large and granular calcifications formed in many mucocele-like lesions lead to mammographic detection (25–27). The finding of this type of calcification in a needle core biopsy specimen is sufficient evidence to suggest the diagnosis of a mucocele-like tumor, especially if mucin is also present (Fig. 15.5).

A mucocele-like tumor is composed of mucin-containing cysts and ducts, some of which have ruptured and discharged mucin into the adjacent stroma. The epithelium lining the cysts and ducts in a typical benign mammary mucocele-like tumor is flat or cuboidal, but low columnar and minor papillary elements may be present (Figs. 15.6 and 15.7). A mucocele-like tumor that originated in a mucin-producing cystic papilloma has been described (22) and

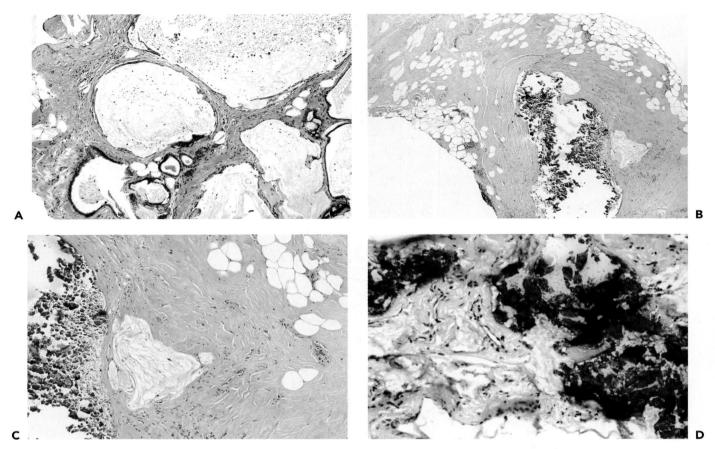

Figure 15.5 **Mucocele-like lesion. A:** A mucocele-like lesion with mucin and finely granular calcification in cysts. **B, C:** Granular calcification with adjacent mucin in a needle core biopsy specimen. **D:** A needle core biopsy sample from a benign mucocele-like lesion consisting of mucin and coarse calcifications.

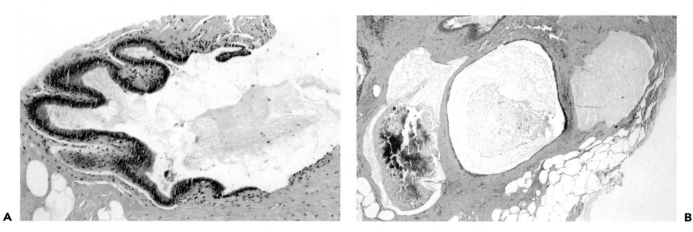

Figure 15.6 **Mucocele-like lesion. A:** This cystically dilated, partially disrupted duct was present in a needle core biopsy specimen performed for nonpalpable calcifications. The duct is lined by benign, low columnar epithelium. Note the epithelium curled back toward the duct lumen near the upper border at the site of disruption. This is a characteristic feature of mucocele-like lesions. **B:** Another specimen with an intact cyst flanked by extruded mucin. Coarse granular calcification is present in the mucin on the left.

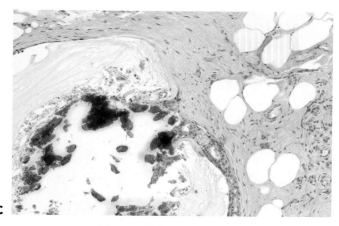

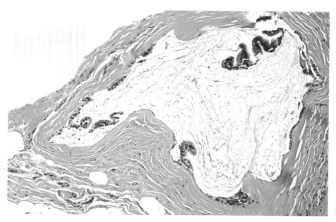

Figure 15.6 *(continued)* **C:** Slight epithelial hyperplasia in a cyst with calcification in extruded mucin. **D:** This mucin-filled duct in a needle core biopsy specimen from a patient with mucocele-like lesion has strips of detached benign epithelium in mucin. This finding should not be interpreted as invasive mucinous carcinoma.

rarely a mucocele-like tumor arises from benign lobules composed of mucin-secreting cells. Detached benign epithelial cells are rarely found in the secretion within the cysts or in secretion extruded into the stroma, and when present, they are usually in cohesive strips. Histiocytes and inflammatory cells may be present in the extruded mucin. Atypical duct hyperplasia is present in some mucocele-like lesions (23) (Fig. 15.8). Liebman et al. (27) reported intraductal carcinoma was found by excisional biopsy in 25% of patients with a benign mucocele-like lesion, and in 75% with an atypical mucocele-like lesion, respectively, diagnosed by needle core biopsy.

Hamele-Bena et al. (24) reviewed a series of mucinous tumors that included benign mucocele-like lesions and mucocele tumors associated with intraductal and invasive carcinoma (Figs. 15.9 and 15.10). The age range for the entire group was 24 to 79 years (mean 48 years), without significant differences in the age distributions of patients with benign and malignant lesions. Breast recurrences occurred

in one patient with a benign and one with a carcinomatous lesion. There were no instances of systemic metastases and no deaths due to carcinoma associated with a mucocele-like lesion.

Some benign and malignant mucinous tumors of the breast can be distinguished by needle core biopsy sampling (28,29). It is not difficult to identify mucinous carcinoma in a needle core biopsy specimen if the sample consists of neoplastic epithelial cells surrounded by mucin. However, the distinction between pure and mixed mucinous carcinoma cannot be assured histologically without a more thorough examination of the excised tumor. A mucocele-like lesion can usually be recognized in a needle core biopsy sample, especially if epithelium is absent and characteristic calcifications are present in the mucin. However, this limited material cannot be relied upon to exclude paucicellular mucinous carcinoma or coexisting in situ carcinoma. The risk of coexisting intraductal carcinoma is increased when the core biopsy specimen shows atypical duct hyperplasia or if the

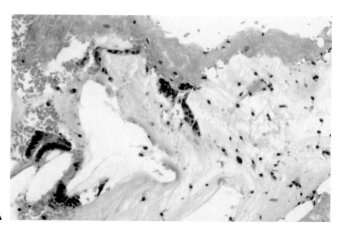

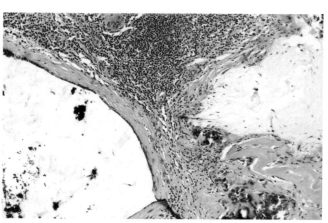

Figure 15.7 Mucocele-like lesion. A: This needle core biopsy specimen contains extruded mucin with histiocytes and small fragments of detached epithelium. **B:** A needle core biopsy specimen with mucin in the stroma accompanied by calcifications and by an inflammatory reaction. Note calcification in the cyst **(left).**

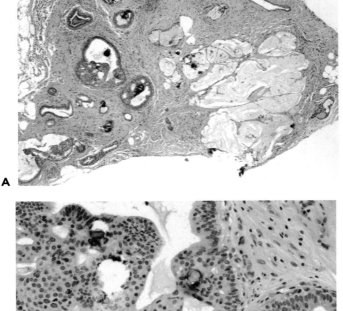

A

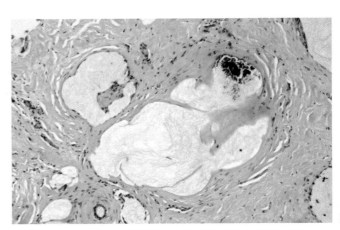

B

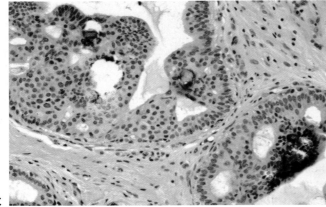

C

Figure 15.8 Mucocele-like lesion with atypical duct hyperplasia.
A: Ductal hyperplasia with calcifications and extruded mucin are evident at low magnification. **B:** Extruded mucin with calcification in the stroma. **C:** Atypical micropapillary and cribriform hyperplasia with calcifications. Note the regular low columnar epithelium focally present at the periphery of the duct in the lower right corner.

presenting signs include a mass lesion (25). Excisional biopsy is recommended for mucocele-like lesions diagnosed by needle core biopsy, especially if a mass is apparent radiologically, or by palpation, or if the sample exhibits atypical hyperplasia (25,30).

Women with pure mucinous carcinoma have had a better relapse-free survival 5 and 10 years after mastectomy than those with mixed mucinous carcinoma containing infiltrating duct carcinoma components and those who

have nonmucinous infiltrating duct carcinoma (2,5,31). Pure mucinous carcinomas tend to be smaller than tumors with a mixed pattern, and these patients have a lower frequency of axillary lymph node metastases (2,4,31,32). The frequency of negative axillary lymph nodes in patients with pure mucinous carcinoma is about 75% and about 50% in patients with mixed mucinous carcinomas (2–4,31). Recurrence is least likely with smaller tumors and in the absence of lymph node metastases (3,6,33).

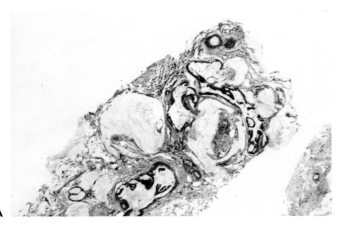

A

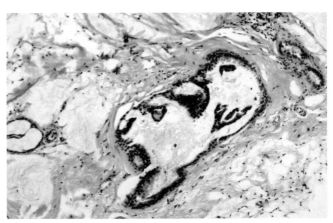

B

Figure 15.9 Mucocele-like lesions with intraductal carcinoma. A, B: A needle core biopsy specimen with micropapillary intraductal carcinoma in one duct and adjacent acellular extruded mucin.

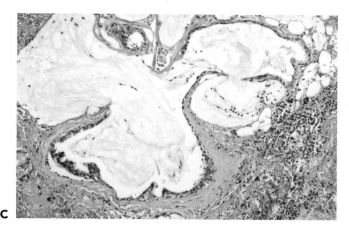

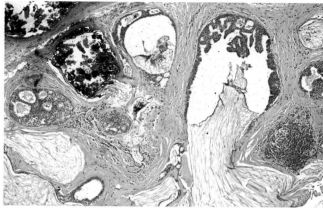

C

D

Figure 15.9 *(continued)* **C:** The excisional biopsy specimen revealed disruption of ducts with extrusion of mucin. **D:** Another needle core biopsy specimen with micropapillary **(left)** and cribriform **(right)** intraductal carcinoma in a mucocele-like lesion with large calcifications.

Komaki et al. (4) described a 90% 10-year survival for patients with pure mucinous carcinoma and 60% for those with mixed duct and mucinous carcinoma. In another report, the 15-year disease-free survival was 85% and 63% for pure mucinous and mixed mucinous-duct carcinoma patients, respectively (3). A series of 1008 women treated by breast conservation with radiotherapy at Yale University from 1970 to 1990 included 16 patients with mucinous carcinoma (34). After a median follow-up of 11.2 years, there were no breast recurrences, and a systemic recurrence developed in one patient 11 years after initial therapy. Combined data from two institutions included 10 patients with mucinous carcinoma who remained disease-free after excision and radiation therapy with a median follow-up of 79 months (35).

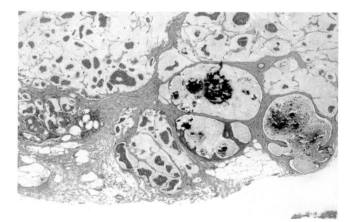

Figure 15.10 Mucinous carcinoma associated with a mucocele-like lesion. This needle core biopsy specimen demonstrates mucinous carcinoma surrounding a mucocele-lesion. The mucocele-like lesion consists of extruded mucin containing prominent basophilic calcification to the right of center and a cyst with mucin and finely granular calcification in the lower right corner. Calcification is absent and epithelium is present in the regions involved by carcinoma.

REFERENCES

1. Rasmussen BB, Rose C, Christensen I. Prognostic factors in primary mucinous breast carcinoma. *Am J Clin Pathol.* 1987;87:155–160.
2. Scopsi L, Andreola S, Pilotti S, et al. Mucinous carcinoma of the breast. A clinicopathologic, histochemical and immunocytochemical study with special reference to neuroendocrine differentiation. *Am J Surg Pathol.* 1994;18:702–711.
3. Toikkanen S, Kujari H. Pure and mixed mucinous carcinomas of the breast: a clinicopathologic analysis of 61 cases with long-term follow-up. *Hum Pathol.* 1989;20:758–764.
4. Komaki K, Sakamoto G, Sugano H, et al. Mucinous carcinoma of the breast in Japan. A prognostic analysis based on morphologic features. *Cancer.* 1988;61:989–996.
5. Rosen PP, Wang T-Y. Colloid carcinoma of the breast. Analysis of 64 patients with long-term follow-up. *Am J Clin Pathol.* 1980;73:30.
6. Komenaka IK, El-Tamer MB, Troxel A, et al. Pure mucinous carcinoma of the breast. *Am J Surg.* 2004;187:355–363.
7. Rosen PP, Lesser ML, Kinne DW. Breast carcinoma at the extremes of age: a comparison of patients younger than 35 years and older than 75 years. *J Surg Oncol.* 1985;28:90–96.
8. Shousha S, Coady AT, Stamp T, Alaghband-Zadeh J. Oestrogen receptors in mucinous carcinoma of the breast: an immunohistochemical study using paraffin wax sections. *J Clin Pathol.* 1989;42:902–905.
9. Domfeh, AB, Carley AL Striebel JM, et al. WT1 immunoreactivity in mucinous breast carcinoma: selective expression in pure and mixed subtypes. *Mod Pathol.* 2008;21:1217–1223.
10. Chung-Park M, Liu CZ, Giampoli EJ, et al. Mucinous adenocarcinoma of ectopic breast tissue of the vulva. *Arch Pathol Lab Med.* 2002;126:1216–1218.
11. Wilson TE, Helvie MA, Oberman HA, Joynt LK. Pure and mixed mucinous carcinoma of the breast: pathologic basis for differences in mammographic appearance. *Am J Roentgenol.* 1995;165:285–289.
12. Lam WWM, Chu WCW, Tse GM, Ma TK. Sonographic appearance of mucinous carcinoma of the breast. *Am J Roentgenol.* 2004;182:1069–1074.
13. Ruggieri AM, Scola FH, Schepps B, Esparza AR. Mucinous carcinoma of the breast: mammographic findings. *Breast Dis.* 1995;8:353–361.
14. Goodman DNF, Boutross-Tadross O, Jong RA. Mammographic features of pure mucinous carcinoma of the breast with pathological correlation. *Can Assoc Radiol J.* 1995;46:296–301.
15. Miller RW, Harris, SE. Mucinous carcinoma of the breast: potential false-negative MR imaging interpretation. *Am J Roentgenol.* 1996;167:539–540.
16. Orel SG, Schnall MD, LiVolsi VA, Troupin RH. Suspicious breast lesions: MR imaging with radiologic-pathologic correlation. *Radiology.* 1994;190:485–493.
17. Capella C, Eusebi V, Mann B, Azzopardi JG. Endocrine differentiation in mucoid carcinoma of the breast. *Histopathology.* 1980;4:613–630.
18. Ng WK. Fine-needle aspiration cytology findings of an uncommon micropapillary variant of pure mucinous carcinoma of the breast. Review of patients over an 8-year period. *Cancer Cytopathol.* 2002;96:280–288.
19. Shet T, Chinou R. Presence of a micropapillary pattern in mucinous carcinomas of the breast and its impact on the clinical behavior. *Breast J.* 2008;14:412–420.
20. Hull MT, Warfel KA. Mucinous breast carcinomas with abundant intracytoplasmic mucin and neuroendocrine features: light microscopic, immunohistochemical and ultrastructural study. *Ultrastruc Pathol.* 1987;11:29–38.
21. Coady AT, Shousha S, Dawson PM, et al. Mucinous carcinoma of the breast: further characterization of its three subtypes. *Histopathology.* 1989;15:617–626.

22. Rosen PP. Mucocele-like tumors of the breast. *Am J Surg Pathol.* 1986; 10:464–469.

23. Ro JY, Sneige N, Sahin AA, et al. Mucocele-like tumor of the breast associated with atypical duct hyperplasia or mucinous carcinoma. A clinicopathologic study of seven cases. *Arch Pathol Lab Med.* 1991;115:137–140.

24. Hamele-Bena D, Cranor ML, Rosen PP. Mammary mucocele-like lesions: benign and malignant. *Am J Surg Pathol.* 1996;20:1081–1085.

25. Carder, PJ, Murphy CE, Liston JC. Surgical excision is warranted following a core biopsy of mucocele-like lesion of the breast. *Histopathology.* 2004; 45:148–154.

26. Kim J-Y, HanB-K, Choe YH, Ko Y-H. Benign and malignant mucocele-like tumors of the breast: mammographic and sonographic appearances. *Am J Roentgenol.* 2005;185:1310–1316.

27. Liebman AJ, Staeger CN, Charney DA. Mucocelelike lesions of the breast: mammographic findings with pathologic correlation. *Am J Roentgenol.* 2006;186:1356–1360.

28. Renshaw AA. Can mucinous lesions of the breast be reliably diagnosed by core needle biopsy? *Am J Clin Pathol.* 2002;118:82–84.

29. Wang J, Simsir A, Mercado C, Cangiarella J. Can core biopsy reliably diagnose mucinous lesions of the breast? *Am J Clin Pathol.* 2007;127: 124–127.

30. Jacobs T, Connolly JL, Schnitt SJ. Nonmalignant lesion in breast core needle biopsies: to excise or not to excise? *Am J Surg Pathol.* 2007;127: 124–127.

31. Andre S, Cunha F, Bernardo M, et al. Mucinous carcinoma of the breast: a pathologic study of 82 cases. *J Surg Oncol.* 1995;58:162–167.

32. Rasmussen BB. Human mucinous carcinomas and their lymph node metastases. A histological review of 247 cases. *Pathol Res Pract.* 1985;180:377–382.

33. Rosen PP, Groshen S, Saigo PE, et al. A long-term follow-up study of survival in Stage I ($T_1N_0M_0$) and Stage II ($T_1N_1M_0$) breast carcinoma. *J Clin Oncol.* 1989;7:355–366.

34. Haffty BG, Perrotta PL, Ward B, et al. Conservatively treated breast cancer: outcome by histologic subtype. *Breast J.* 1997;3:7–14.

35. Kurtz, JM, Jacquemier J, Torhorst J, et al. Conservation therapy for breast cancer other than infiltrating duct carcinoma. *Cancer.* 1989;63: 1630–1635.

Apocrine Carcinoma

16

Some apocrine carcinomas probably arise from preexisting apocrine metaplasia (Fig. 16.1). In other cases apocrine traits appear to be an intrinsic property of the carcinoma. Apocrine metaplasia is particularly abundant and often atypical in the breasts of women with apocrine carcinoma (Fig. 16.2). Transitions from atypical hyperplastic apocrine lesions to carcinoma are evident in some but not all examples of apocrine carcinoma (1). A review of the pathology and clinical aspects of apocrine breast lesions was published by O'Malley and Bane (2). The clinical significance of the "loss of heterozygosity and allelic imbalance" in some examples of apocrine metaplasia remains to be determined (3). Absence of myoepithelium has been observed in benign apocrine epithelium and is by itself not an indication of in situ apocrine carcinoma when cytologic features of carcinoma are not present (4).

The diagnosis of apocrine carcinoma should be reserved for neoplasms in which all or nearly all of the epithelium has apocrine cytologic features. Not more than 1% of breast carcinomas qualify as true apocrine carcinomas (5). Apocrine carcinomas are usually classified as ductal. An apocrine variant of lobular carcinoma has been described, but these reports predate the availability of the E-cadherin immunostain (6–8). It has recently been observed that E-cadherin-positive apocrine intraductal carcinoma can involve the epithelium of ducts and lobules with a pagetoid distribution that mimics lobular carcinoma in situ.

There are no specific clinical or mammographic features associated with apocrine duct carcinomas (9). The reported age at diagnosis ranges from 19 to 86 years, with a distribution not significantly different from patients with nonapocrine duct carcinoma. In rare instances, the mammogram in a patient with extensive intraductal apocrine carcinoma displays diffuse "mixed form" linear and punctate calcifications "characterized by a strikingly wild, chaotic appearance with profuse deposition of calcium" (10). Patients who have invasive apocrine carcinoma usually present with a mass. The frequency of bilaterality in patients with apocrine carcinoma in one breast is not exceptional. Apocrine carcinoma of the male breast is very uncommon. One unusual apocrine male mammary carcinoma had a glandular structure and psammoma bodies (11). When studied by im-

munohistochemistry, 98% of 102 apocrine lesions, including benign conditions and carcinomas, were estrogen receptor (ER)-negative and progesterone receptor (PR)-negative (12). In the latter series, androgen receptors were present in 94% of benign lesions and 72% of carcinomas with apocrine differentiation. Apocrine carcinomas that are ER-negative by immunohistochemistry may express ER messenger ribonucleic acid (mRNA) (13).

The low frequency of ER expression applies to ER-α. Nearly 75% of apocrine carcinomas, intraductal or invasive, express ER-β as determined by immunohistochemistry and ER-β mRNA analysis (14).

The distinction between atypical apocrine hyperplasia and apocrine intraductal carcinoma is sometimes difficult (Fig. 16.3). Carter and Rosen (15) described sclerosing breast lesions with atypical apocrine epithelium characterized by nuclear atypia, varying degrees of cytoplasmic clearing, and rare mitoses. A critical feature that distinguishes atypical hyperplasia from apocrine intraductal carcinoma in a sclerosing lesion is the extent of epithelial expansion. In situ apocrine carcinoma is diagnosed when there is enough neoplastic epithelial proliferation to produce one of the characteristic growth patterns of intraductal carcinoma (Fig. 16.4). Rarely, cytologic features are so abnormal, and the mitotic rate is so elevated in a sclerosing apocrine lesion that a diagnosis of carcinoma can be made in the absence of a characteristic in situ structure.

The classification of atypical apocrine lesions on the basis of size as well as cytologic and structural criteria has been suggested. Tavassoli and Norris (16) considered apocrine ductal lesions that occupied an area of less than 2 mm to be atypical apocrine hyperplasia, regardless of cytologic and structural features. Larger histologically identical foci qualified as apocrine intraductal carcinoma. O'Malley et al. (17) used a combination of cytologic criteria and lesional diameter to define a "borderline" group of apocrine lesions. Foci with borderline cytologic features were considered to be apocrine intraductal carcinoma if larger than 8 mm. Borderline or atypical apocrine hyperplasias were proliferative foci smaller than 8 mm with nuclear atypia lacking the characteristic irregular nuclear membranes, coarse chromatin and large, often multiple nucleoli of apocrine carcinoma.

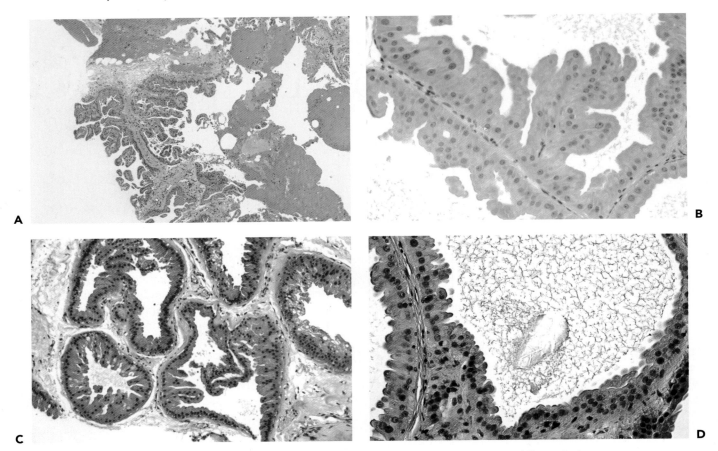

Figure 16.1   Apocrine metaplasia. Needle core biopsy specimens showing different lesions. **A, B:** Cystic papillary apocrine metaplasia is composed of cells with abundant eosinophilic cytoplasm, small round nuclei and punctate nucleoli. The nuclei are regularly and evenly distributed with respect to the basement membrane. **C:** These glands are lined by a single layer of columnar cells with evenly spaced, basally oriented nuclei. The eosinophilia seen in **(A)** and **(B)** and the basophilia in **(C)** reflect different staining properties encountered in benign and malignant apocrine lesions. **D:** Cystic apocrine metaplasia with oxalate calcification.

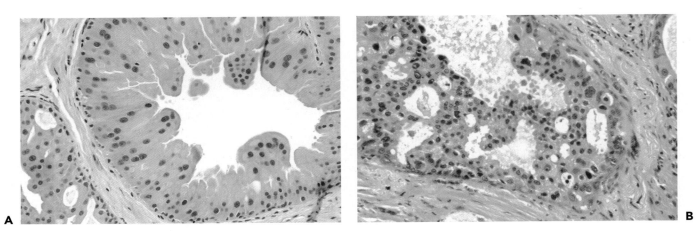

Figure 16.2   Apocrine metaplasia with atypia and apocrine intraductal carcinoma. A: Hyperplastic atypical apocrine epithelium arranged in micropapillary fronds is composed of cells with abundant eosinophilic cytoplasm and unevenly distributed nuclei with punctate nucleoli. **B:** Apocrine intraductal carcinoma in the same needle core biopsy specimen is characterized by cells arranged in a cribriform pattern with less abundant cytoplasm than in **(A)** and pleomorphic nuclei.

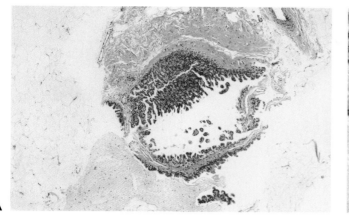

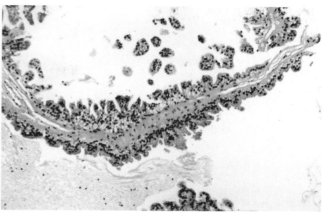

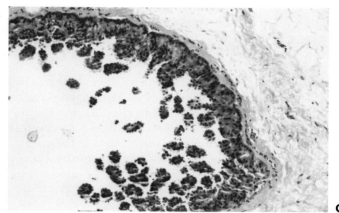

Figure 16.3 Cystic micropapillary apocrine metaplasia and cystic micropapillary apocrine intraductal carcinoma. A, B: This needle core biopsy specimen shows parts of the wall of a cystic apocrine lesion. A view of the epithelium in a perpendicular section is provided in **(B)**. Note the presence of subnuclear cytoplasmic clearing. **C:** Apocrine intraductal carcinoma with a micropapillary structure, shown here in a different needle core biopsy specimen, is characterized by a disorderly distribution of atypical hyperchromatic nuclei.

The 2-mm size criterion of Tavassoli and Norris was described by these authors as "arbitrary" (16), and the 4- to 8-mm rule of O'Malley et al. was stated by these authors to "require follow-up studies for . . . linkage to clinical outcomes." The precision of such measurements is highly unreliable. The diagnosis of apocrine lesions on the basis of size is not readily applicable to needle core biopsy specimens. The precision of the requisite measurements is highly unreliable and subject to many uncontrolled variables. A cluster of closely connected duct cross sections with little intervening stroma could occupy an area less than 2 mm, leading to a diagnosis of atypical apocrine hyperplasia on the basis of the 2-mm "rule," whereas the same group of duct sections separated by more stroma would encompass an area greater than 2 mm and qualify as intraductal carcinoma. Since these microscopic lesions

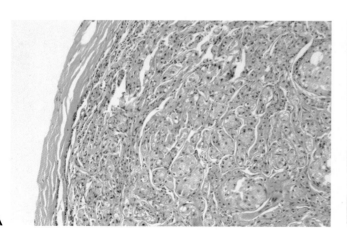

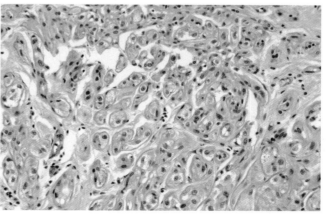

Figure 16.4 Apocrine intraductal carcinoma arising in apocrine adenosis. A, B: This part of a needle core biopsy specimen shows apocrine metaplasia in sclerosing adenosis.

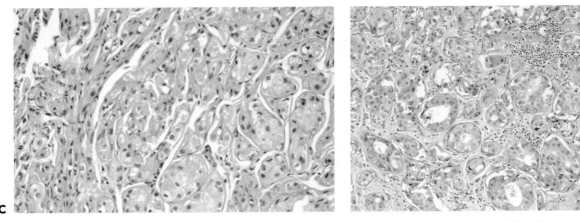

C   D

Figure 16.4 *(continued)* **C:** A transitional area with apocrine adenosis on the left and a more florid, atypical apocrine proliferation on the right. **D:** Enlarged adenosis glands occupied by apocrine intraductal carcinoma. There is nuclear pleomorphism and lymphocytes are present in the stroma.

are rarely appreciated grossly, there is no assurance that the tissue is oriented in a paraffin block so that the plane of section represents the maximum diameter. These issues are further compounded in a needle core biopsy specimen if the lesion is seen in more than one tissue core because the spatial relationship of the pieces is indeterminate. Consequently, these so-called criteria cannot be accepted as guidelines for the interpretation of apocrine lesions in surgical or needle core biopsy specimens.

Cytologic features of in situ and invasive apocrine carcinomas are manifested in the nuclei and in the cytoplasm. The nuclei are enlarged and pleomorphic when compared with the nuclei of benign apocrine cells. They usually contain prominent and eosinophilic or basophilic nucleoli (Figs. 16.2 and 16.5). Nuclear membranes tend to be hyperchromatic and irregular. Some apocrine carcinomas have pleomorphic, deeply basophilic nuclei in which little or no internal structure can be discerned, while in other instances, the chromatin is coarse (Fig. 16.6). Nucleoli are usually obscured when the chromatin is dense and hyperchromatic.

The cytoplasm commonly exhibits eosinophilia that may be homogeneous or granular. Cytoplasmic vacuolization or clearing are features associated with atypical apocrine proliferations as well as apocrine carcinoma (Fig. 16.7). Apocrine carcinomas, especially the clear cell variant, tend to attract a lymphocytic or lymphoplasmacytic reaction.

The architecture of apocrine intraductal carcinoma exhibits the same structural patterns as nonapocrine intraductal carcinomas, including comedo, micropapillary, solid, and cribriform configurations (18) (Figs. 16.2–16.7). Apocrine intraductal carcinomas can be graded on the basis of nuclear cytology and the presence or absence of necrosis (19). In general, nuclei in low-grade lesions most closely resemble the nuclei found in benign apocrine metaplasia, except that they tend to be larger and have more prominent but uniform nucleoli. Pleomorphic, hyperchromatic nuclei and nucleoli of varying size are typical of high-grade lesions. Calcifications and necrosis are sometimes present in the affected ducts. Periductal fibrosis with inflammation is a common reactive change around the ducts and "foamy"

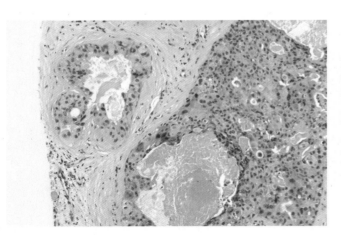

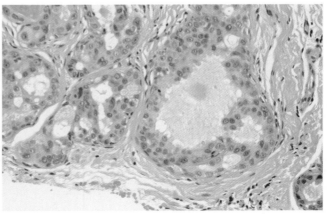

A   B

Figure 16.5 **Apocrine intraductal carcinoma.** Two different needle core biopsy specimens are shown. **A:** Solid intraductal carcinoma with necrosis. **B:** Cribriform intraductal carcinoma with extension into lobular glands on the left.

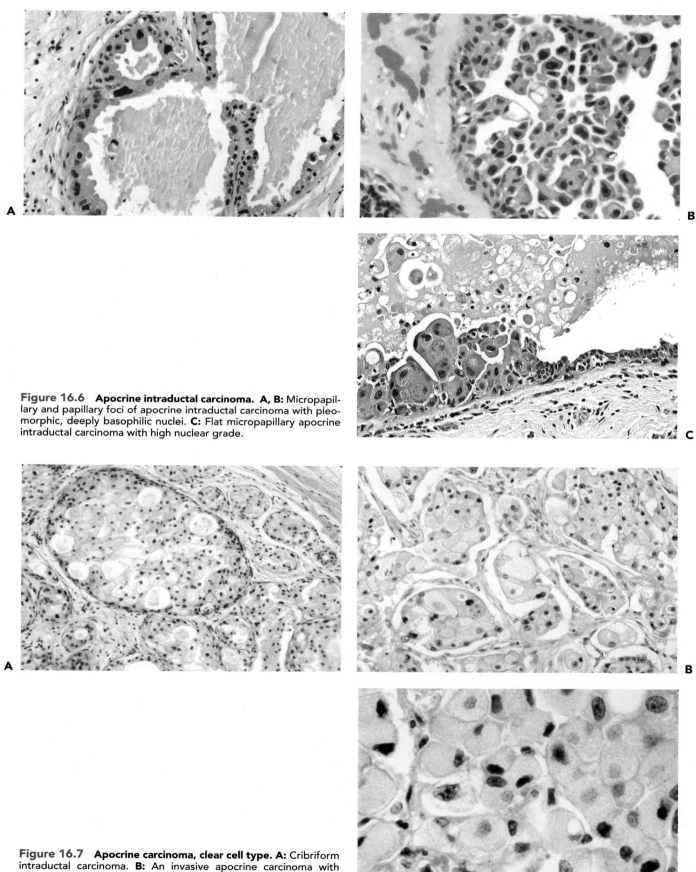

Figure 16.6   Apocrine intraductal carcinoma. A, B: Micropapillary and papillary foci of apocrine intraductal carcinoma with pleomorphic, deeply basophilic nuclei. **C:** Flat micropapillary apocrine intraductal carcinoma with high nuclear grade.

Figure 16.7   Apocrine carcinoma, clear cell type. A: Cribriform intraductal carcinoma. **B:** An invasive apocrine carcinoma with marked cytoplasmic clearing. **C:** Intracytoplasmic mucin is a magenta spot in one cell (mucicarmine stain).

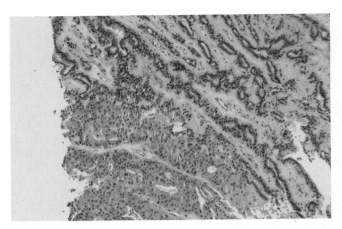

Figure 16.8 Apocrine metaplasia in a papilloma. Hyperplastic apocrine epithelium is present in the lower part of this needle core biopsy specimen from a papillary lesion.

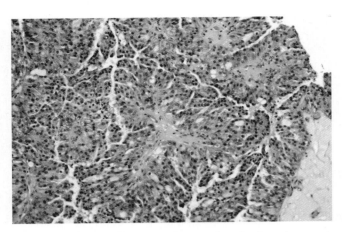

Figure 16.9 Papillary apocrine carcinoma. Apocrine carcinoma supported by fibrovascular stroma is present in this needle core biopsy specimen of a solid papillary carcinoma.

histiocytes with vacuolated cytoplasm in the reactive process can be mistaken for invasive carcinoma cells (20).

Atypical apocrine metaplasia may occupy part of a complex papillary lesion that has fully developed apocrine carcinoma in other areas (Fig. 16.8). The criteria for the diagnosis of apocrine carcinoma in a papillary lesion are the same as those outlined for the diagnosis of nonapocrine carcinoma in a papilloma. Pure cystic papillary apocrine carcinoma is infrequent (Fig. 16.9). Extension of carcinoma into the epithelium of lobules is more common in apocrine intraductal carcinoma than in other types of intraductal carcinoma, with the possible exception of nonapocrine comedocarcinoma (Fig. 16.10). Apocrine intraductal carcinoma that is predominantly distributed in a pagetoid manner in small ducts and lobules resembles lobular carcinoma in situ. The E-cadherin stain reveals diffuse membrane staining in this form of apocrine intraductal carcinoma, whereas when lobular carcinoma in situ has this distribution, E-cadherin reactivity is limited to residual ductal epithelial and myoepithelial cells. Fibrosis and chronic

inflammation are often present around ducts in foci of apocrine intraductal carcinoma (Fig. 16.11).

Infiltrating apocrine carcinomas may have any of the growth patterns of infiltrating duct carcinoma (Figs. 16.12 and 16.13), but they are often structurally poorly differentiated (Fig. 16.14). An uncommon variant of infiltrating apocrine carcinoma is composed of large polygonal cells with abundant foamy or granular cytoplasm (Fig. 16.15). Loss of cohesion is a characteristic feature of these carcinomas when a diffuse growth pattern is present. This type of apocrine carcinoma has been referred to as myoblastomatoid or histiocytoid (21). The distinction between dispersed invasive apocrine duct carincoma and invasive pleomorphic lobular carcinoma can be made with the E-cadherin stain, since the former is E-cadherin positive and the latter is negative. The expression of gross cystic disease fluid protein (GCDFP)-15 has been demonstrated in apocrine carcinomas by immunohistochemistry and by in situ hybridization (21). Invasive apocrine carcinoma in dense collagenous stroma may be difficult to identify, especially in a limited

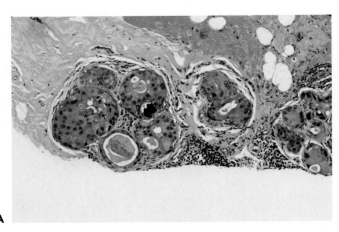

A

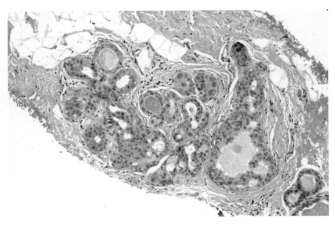

B

Figure 16.10 Apocrine intraductal carcinoma with lobular extension. Two different needle core biopsy specimens are shown. **A:** Apocrine intraductal carcinoma in lobular glands. Microcalcification is present in one lobular gland. **B:** A low magnification view of the lesion shown in Fig. 16.5B. Intraductal apocrine carcinoma involves some of the glands in the lobule.

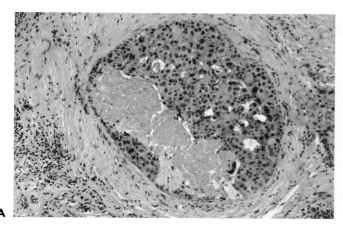

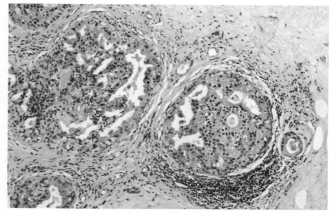

Figure 16.11   Apocrine intraductal carcinoma with stromal fibrosis and lymphocytic reaction.
A: Solid intraductal carcinoma with necrosis. **B:** Cribriform intraductal carcinoma.

needle core biopsy sample, and could be mistaken for a granular cell tumor or a histiocytic infiltrate.

Invasive apocrine carcinomas are prone to develop lymphatic tumor emboli (22). This may be manifested by clinical presentation as inflammatory carcinoma and in some cases predisposes to locally recurrent carcinoma with an inflammatory pattern (23). d'Amore et al. (22) found dermal invasion in 7 of 34 (21%) of their cases and in 4

(12%) there was associated lymphatic invasion within the breast.

Most apocrine carcinomas are negative for mucin or only a few cells contain mucicarmine-positive secretion (Fig. 16.7) (24). In exceptional tumors, there can be extensive intracytoplasmic mucin accumulation resulting in numerous, sometimes substantially enlarged cells of the signet ring type (Fig. 16.16). Benign and malignant

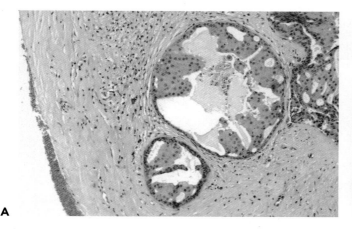

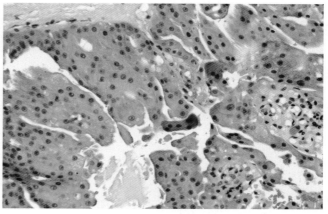

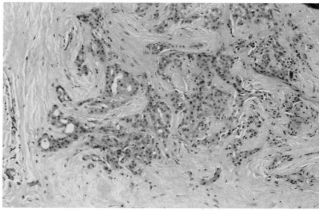

Figure 16.12   Apocrine carcinoma, intraductal and invasive.
A: This needle core biopsy specimen shows micropapillary intraductal carcinoma. Note the degenerated cells in the larger duct and the mild periductal reaction consisting of lymphocytes and histiocytes. **B:** Magnified view of the microscopic field contiguous with the right border of **(A)**. **C:** Moderately differentiated invasive apocrine carcinoma in the same needle core biopsy specimen.

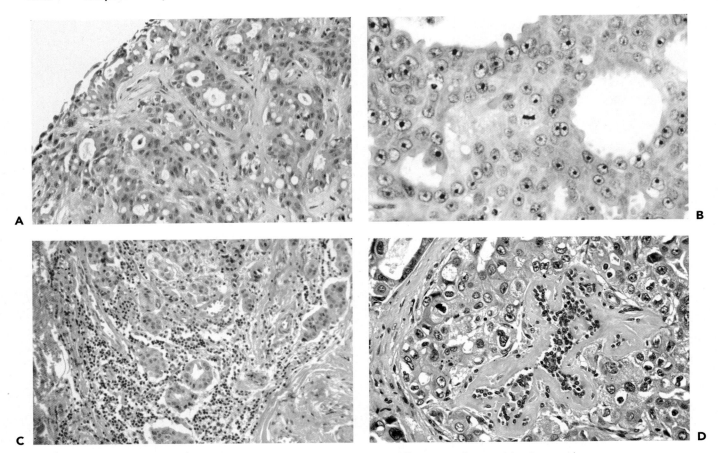

Figure 16.13 **Apocrine carcinoma, invasive.** Four different needle core biopsies are shown. **A:** Invasive apocrine duct carcinoma with a cribriform pattern and intermediate nuclear grade. **B:** Invasive apocrine duct carcinoma with a cribriform pattern and poorly differentiated nuclear grade. **C:** Invasive apocrine duct carcinoma forming small glands. A stromal lymphocytic reaction is evident. **D:** High-grade invasive apocrine duct carcinoma surrounds an atrophic lobule.

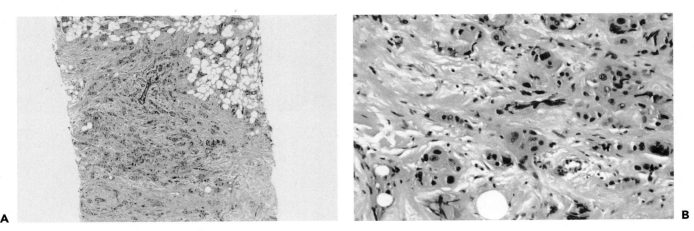

Figure 16.14 **Apocrine carcinoma, invasive. A, B:** The carcinoma in this needle core biopsy specimen is composed of cords and strands of cells without gland formation. The magnified view in **(B)** reveals the poorly differentiated nuclear grade.

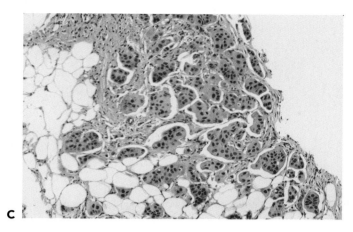

C

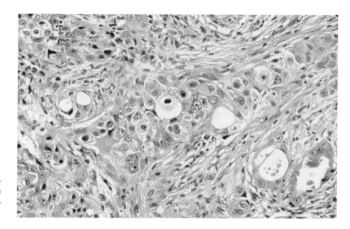

Figure 16.14 *(continued)* **C:** Another needle core biopsy specimen in which the carcinoma cells form papillary clusters.

Figure 16.15 Apocrine carcinoma with histiocytoid features. The tumor cells have abundant vacuolated and granular cytoplasm with pleomorphic, poorly differentiated nuclei. Traces of gland formation are evident.

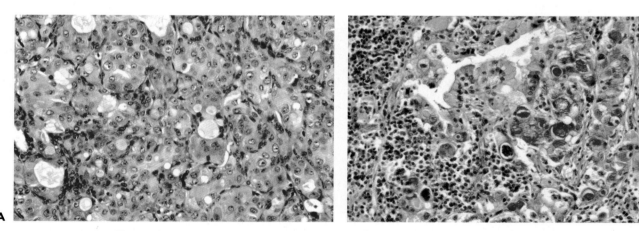

A   B

Figure 16.16 Apocrine carcinoma with mucin. A: Many of the cells in this apocrine carcinoma have discrete intracytoplasmic vacuoles that contain secretion. **B:** The secretion is stained red with the mucicarmine stain.

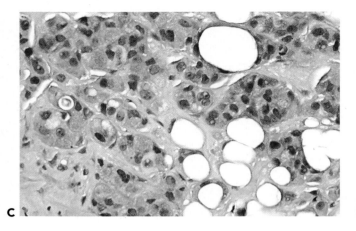

Figure 16.16 *(continued)* **C:** Invasive apocrine carcinoma with basophilic cytoplasmic mucin deposits.

apocrine cells are strongly immunoreactive for GCDFP-15. Staining for GCDFP-15 also occurs in nearly 25% of carcinomas that lack apocrine features (6,7).

Gatalica et al. (25) reported finding expression of epidermal growth factor receptor (EGFR) in 88% of apocrine carcinomas, a considerably higher frequency of expression than is found in breast carcinomas generally, except those of the basaloid type. Overexpression proved to be due to an increased number of chromosome 7 and therefore an increased number of EGFR copies rather than gene amplification.

Patients with intraductal apocrine carcinoma have generally had the same clinical course as women with nonapocrine intraductal carcinoma with equivalent-grade lesions (5). Comparison of patients with invasive apocrine and nonapocrine carcinomas has revealed no statistically significant differences in recurrence-free and overall survival between the two groups (18,22). The prognosis of apocrine carcinoma, whether intraductal or invasive, is determined mainly by conventional prognostic factors such as grade, tumor size, and nodal status (16,18,22). Apocrine differentiation should be mentioned as a descriptive feature, but presently it does not seem to be an important determinant of prognosis or of treatment (26).

Surgical biopsies of the conserved breast after radiotherapy are difficult to interpret in women with apocrine carcinoma because irradiation causes severe cytologic changes in nonneoplastic apocrine epithelium. In these cases, it is absolutely essential to have slides of the pretreatment carcinoma available for comparison with the posttreatment specimen, and this is also necessary when dealing with needle core biopsy samples of irradiated breast tissue.

REFERENCES

1. Yates AJ, Ahmed A. Apocrine carcinoma and apocrine metaplasia. *Histopathology.* 1988;13:228–231.
2. O'Malley FP, Bane AL. The spectrum of apocrine lesions of the breast. *Adv Anat Pathol.* 2004;11:1–9.
3. Selim AGA, Ryan A, El-Ayat G, Wells CA. Loss of heterozygosity and allelic imbalance in apocrine metaplasia of the breast: microdissection microsatellite analysis. *J Pathol.* 2002;196:287–291.
4. Csneri G. Lack of myopeithelium in apocrine glands of the breast does to necessarily imply malignancy. *Histopathology.* 2008:52:253–254.
5. Tanaka K, Imoto S, Wada N, et al. Invasive apocrine carcinoma of the breast: clincopathologic features in 57 patients. *Breast J.* 2008:14:164–168.
6. Mossler J, Barton TK, Brinkhous AD, et al. Apocrine differentiation in human mammary carcinoma. *Cancer.* 1980;46:2463–2471.
7. Eusebi V, Betts C, Haagensen DE, et al. Apocrine differentiation in lobular carcinoma of the breast: a morphologic, immunologic and ultrastructural study. *Hum Pathol.* 1984;15:134–140.
8. Walford N, Velden JT. Histiocytoid breast carcinoma: an apocrine variant of lobular carcinoma. *Histopathology.* 1989;14:515–522.
9. Gilles R, Lasnik A, Guinebretière J-M, et al. Apocrine carcinoma: clinical and mammographic features. *Radiology.* 1994;190:495–497.
10. Kopans DB, Nguyen PL, Koerner FC, et al. Mixed form, diffusely scattered calcifications in breast cancer with apocrine features. *Radiology.* 1990;177:807–811.
11. Bryant J. Male breast cancer: a case of apocrine carcinoma with psammoma bodies. *Hum Pathol.* 1981;12:751–753.
12. Tavassoli FA, Purcell CA, Bratthauer GL, Man Y-G. Androgen receptor expression along with loss of bcl-2, ER, and PR expression in benign and malignant apocrine lesions of the breast: implications for therapy. *Breast J.* 1996;2:261–269.
13. Bratthauer GL, Lininger RA, May YG, Tavassoli FA. Androgen and estrogen receptor mRNA status in apocrine carcinomas. *Diagn. Mol. Pathol.* 2002;11:113–118.
14. Homma N, Takubo K, Akiyama F, et al. Expression of estrogen receptor-β in apocrine carcinomas of the breast. *Histopathology.* 2007;50:425–433.
15. Carter D, Rosen PP. Atypical apocrine metaplasia in sclerosing lesions of the beast: a study of 51 patients. *Mod Pathol.* 1991;4:1–5.
16. Tavassoli FA, Norris HJ. Intraductal apocrine carcinoma: a clinicopathologic study of 37 cases. *Mod Pathol.* 1994;7:813–818.
17. O'Malley FP, Page DL, Nelson EH, Dupont WD. Ductal carcinoma in situ of the breast with apocrine cytology: definition of a borderline category. *Hum Pathol.* 1994;25:164–168.
18. Abati AD, Kimmel M, Rosen PP. Apocrine mammary carcinoma: a clinicopathologic study of 72 patients. *Am J Clin Pathol.* 1990;94:371–377.
19. Leal C, Henrique R, Monteiro P, Page DL. Apocrine ductal carcinoma in situ of the breast: histologic classification and expression of biologic markers. *Hum Pathol.* 2001;32:487–493.
20. Shousha S, Bull TB, Southall PJ, Mazoujian G. Apocrine carcinoma of the breast containing foam cells. An electron microscopic and immunohistochemical study. *Histopathology.* 1987;11:611–620.
21. Eusebi V, Foschini MP, Bussolati G, Rosen PP. Myoblastomatoid (histiocytoid) carcinoma of the breast. A type of apocrine carcinoma. *Am J Surg Pathol.* 1995;19:553–562.
22. d'Amore ESG, Terrier-Lacombe MJ, Travagli JP, et al. Invasive apocrine carcinoma of the breast: a long term follow-up study of 34 cases. *Breast Cancer Res Treat.* 1988;12:37–44.
23. Robbins GF, Shah J, Rosen PP, et al. Inflammatory carcinoma of the breast. *Surg Clin N Am.* 1974;54:801–810.
24. Bussolati G, Cattani MG, Gugliotta P, et al. Morphologic and functional aspects of apocrine metaplasia in dysplastic and neoplastic breast tissue. *Ann N.Y. Acad Sci.* 1986;464:262–274.
25. Gatalica Z, Lee L, Hatcher, L, et al. Pure apocrine carcinomas of the breast over express EGFR and have increased EGFR gene dosage due to polysomy of chromosome 7. *Mod Pathol.* 2007;20(suppl 2): 32A.
26. Bundred NJ, Walker RA, Everington D, et al. Is apocrine differentiation in breast carcinoma of prognostic significance? *Br J Cancer.* 1990;62:113–117.

Adenoid Cystic Carcinoma

17

The term *cylindroma*, previously used interchangeably with *adenoid cystic carcinoma*, refers to the histologic appearance that suggests entwined cylinders of stroma and epithelial cells. Less than 0.1% of mammary carcinomas have an adenoid cystic growth pattern. Adenoid cystic carcinoma occurs in adult women throughout the age distribution of mammary carcinoma, with patients between 25 and 80 years of age. The mean age varied from 50 to 63 years in several reports. Isolated instances have been encountered in men and in children (1,2). There is no predilection for adenoid cystic carcinoma to develop bilaterally but other types of carcinoma may occur in the contralateral breast (3,4) or in rare instances another carcinoma may be found elsewhere in the same breast (5).

Adenoid cystic carcinoma usually presents as a discrete firm mass. Calcifications can form in these tumors, leading to detection by mammography but in some instances the mammogram was reportedly negative (4). The typical mammographic image is that of a lobulated mass (6). In one case the tumor presented as an 8-mm hypoechoic nodule suggestive of an intramammary lymph node before periodic mammographic follow-up revealed increasing density and less discrete margins (7). Magnetic resonance imaging (MRI) of one tumor revealed an unusual pattern of enhancement (8). Pain or tenderness has been described in a minority of cases. The median duration of a symptomatic mass in one series was 24 months (4). Most adenoid cystic carcinomas have been described as hormone receptor-negative by biochemical and immunohistochemical analysis with occasional tumors positive for estrogen and/or progesterone receptors at relatively low levels (9–13). Adenoid cystic carcinomas are almost always diffusely reactive for c-K1T, p63, and CK5/6 (12,13).

Gross size of the lesions varies from 2 mm to 12 cm with the majority between 1 and 3 cm. Low-grade tumors tend to be smaller (mean 1.6 cm) than high-grade tumors (mean 3.5 cm). Many adenoid cystic carcinomas are circumscribed or nodular grossly, but most have an invasive growth pattern microscopically (Fig. 17.1). Microcystic areas formed by the coalescent spaces in dilated glands are found in some tumors.

Adenoid cystic carcinoma consists of a mixture of proliferating glands (adenoid component) and stromal or basement membrane elements ("pseudoglandular" or cylindromatous component). These elements are usually not distributed homogeneously in a given tumor (Fig. 17.2). Some regions may consist only of the adenoid elements, that are indistinguishable from cribriform carcinoma (14). Abundant stromal material in other parts of the tumor may produce a pattern that can be mistaken for scirrhous carcinoma. Because of this intratumoral heterogeneity, adenoid cystic carcinoma may be difficult to recognize in a needle core biopsy specimen if a characteristic sample has not been obtained (Figs. 17.2 and 17.3). Inspissated secretion and stromal fragments from benign lesions or other forms of carcinoma may be mistaken for cylindromatous material in needle core biopsy samples.

The microscopic growth patterns of mammary adenoid cystic carcinoma have been described as cribriform, solid, glandular (tubular), reticular (trabecular), and basaloid. Focal sebaceous and adenosquamous differentiation are variably present (4). Adenomyoepitheliomatous and syringomatous areas are further evidence of structural diversity. Perineural invasion is found in a minority of mammary tumors and lymphatic tumor emboli are extremely uncommon (Fig. 17.4). Shrinkage artifact, a relatively frequent occurrence in histologic sections of adenoid cystic carcinoma, may be mistaken for lymphatic tumor emboli.

Ro et al. (15) proposed stratifying adenoid cystic carcinomas into three grades on the basis of the proportion of solid growth within the lesion (I, or low grade—no solid elements; II, or intermediate grade—less than 30% solid; and III, or high grade—more than 30% solid). High-grade lesions are composed of poorly differentiated cells that have relatively large, hyperchromatic nuclei, mitoses, and sparse cytoplasm (Fig. 17.5). Intraductal carcinoma is sometimes a prominent feature of high-grade tumors with extensive intralobular and intraductal growth, whereas low-grade adenoid cystic carcinoma rarely has a distinct in situ component. Areas of cribriform and nearly confluent solid growth as well as typical adenoid cystic components may be present in a high-grade tumor. Prominent basaloid features are seen in some instances, a pattern that has been

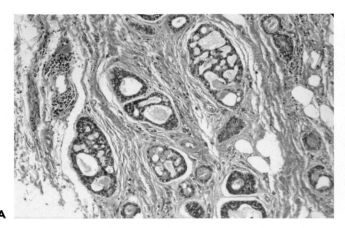
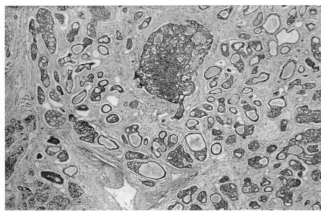

A

B

Figure 17.1 Adenoid cystic carcinoma. A: A needle core biopsy specimen showing nests of predominantly cribriform invasive carcinoma. **B:** The surgically excised tumor has a more heterogeneous growth pattern than the sample obtained in the needle biopsy procedure.

referred to as the solid variant of adenoid cystic carcinoma with basaloid features (16) (Fig. 17.6), or cylindroma of the breast of the skin adnexal type (17). Tumors with a solid component (grades II and III) tend to be larger than those without a solid element (grade I) and tumors with a solid element are more likely to have recurrences (15). The Ki67 labeling index is greater in high-grade than in low-grade tumors, but proliferative activity has not proven to be prognostically significant in adenoid cystic carcinoma of the breast (18). Mutations of the p53 gene occur more frequently in high-grade than in non-high-grade mammary adenoid cystic carcinomas (19).

Some conventional forms of mammary carcinoma may be incorrectly diagnosed as adenoid cystic carcinoma (14,20). When reexamined, about half of the cases recorded by the Connecticut Tumor Registry as adenoid cystic carcinoma were duct carcinomas with a prominent cribriform component (20). Because cribriform foci may be present in an adenoid cystic carcinoma, the limited sam-

ple in a needle core biopsy specimen may be misleading unless other components of adenoid cystic carcinoma are present (see Fig. 17.3).

Collagenous spherulosis must be considered in the differential diagnosis of adenoid cystic carcinoma (21). This stromal alteration usually found in benign papillary duct hyperplasia consists of nodular deposits of basement membrane components surrounded by myoepithelial cells between the glandular elements, a combination that mimics adenoid cystic carcinoma (Chapter 4). Immunohistochemical expression of c-Kit is found in adenoid cystic carcinoma but not in benign collagenous spherulosis (22). Rarely collagenous spherulosis is involved by in situ ductal or lobular carcinoma. Myoepithelium detected by immunostains such as p63 is present in adenoid cystic carcinoma, collagenous spherulosis, and in collagenous spherulosis involved by in situ carcinoma. p63 may be reduced in or absent from adenoid cystic carcinomas with a basaloid growth pattern (12).

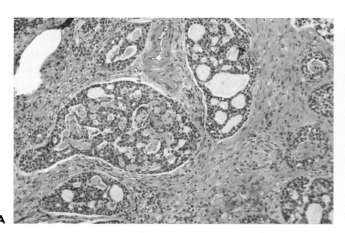
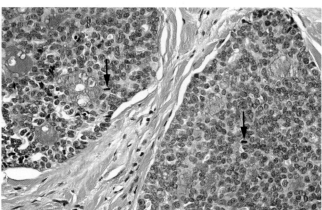

A

B

Figure 17.2 Adenoid cystic carcinoma with various growth patterns. A: In this needle core biopsy specimen some areas have prominent cylindromatous elements, whereas cribriform growth is accented in other foci. **B:** Solid basaloid areas with cribriform microlumens in another specimen. The arrows indicate mitotic figures.

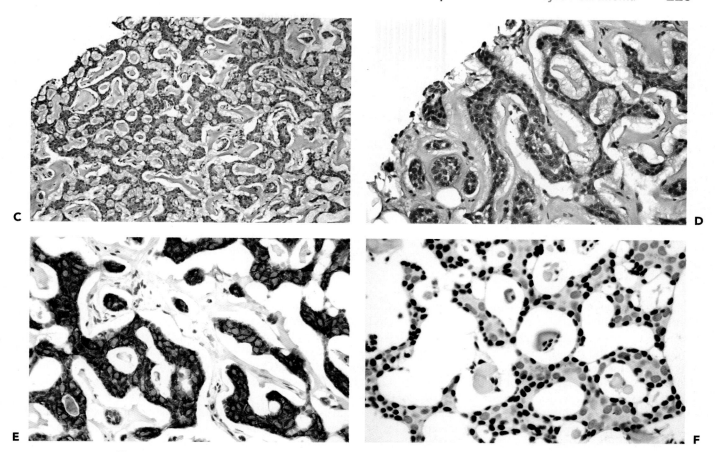

Figure 17.2 *(continued)* **C–F:** The tumor in this needle core biopsy specimen has an unusual trabecular structure **(C, D)** with reactivity for c-Kit **(E)** and p63 **(F)**.

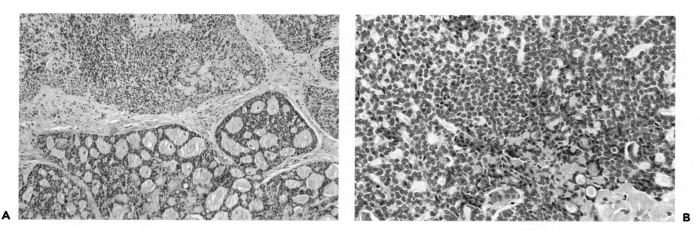

Figure 17.3 Adenoid cystic carcinoma. A: Two growth patterns are represented in this tumor. The lower area has glands filled with secretion reminiscent of cribriform carcinoma and inconspicuous eosinophilic cylindromatous material. The upper region is solid with some nodular cylindromatous material. **B:** Magnified view of the solid area with cylindromatous material in the lower right corner.

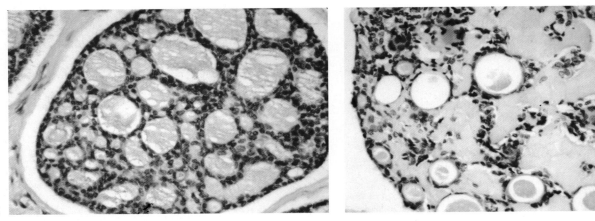

Figure 17.3 *(continued)* **C:** An area with cribriform growth. **D:** Cylindromatous and glandular growth are combined here.

Mucicarmine or alcian blue stains identify the secretion within adenoid cystic glands, whereas laminin and fibronectin, noncollagenous glycoproteins associated with basal lamina, and type IV collagen, can be demonstrated by immunohistochemistry in the cylindromatous elements (9). The spherules that occur in collagenous spherulosis have staining properties similar to those of the cylindromatous nodules in adenoid cystic carcinoma. The distinct myoepithelial layer surrounding the spherules in collagenous spherulosis can be highlighted with stains such as p63, CD10, myosin, and maspin.

Data on the prognosis of adenoid cystic carcinoma are based largely on patients usually treated by mastectomy (1–4,15,20,23). There have been a few isolated instances of systemic metastases after mastectomy (3,24–26). Most patients with metastases have had pulmonary involvement,

with recurrences in the lung being detected as late as 6 to 12 years after initial treatment in patients who had negative axillary lymph nodes (25,26). Axillary metastases were present at mastectomy in two other cases (15,27). The clinical follow-up of patients treated by lumpectomy and breast irradiation was equivalent to that of patients treated by mastectomy in one series (28). Axillary dissection is not indicated unless there is clinical evidence of nodal metastases but sentinel lymph node mapping would be prudent in most instances.

Radiotherapy may be used to supplement excisional surgery (13,29) especially when there is concern about the margin of excision, and for high-grade tumors. Systemic adjuvant chemotherapy is recommended for patients with axillary lymph node metastases and may be considered in patients with high-grade lesions or if the tumor is larger than 3 cm.

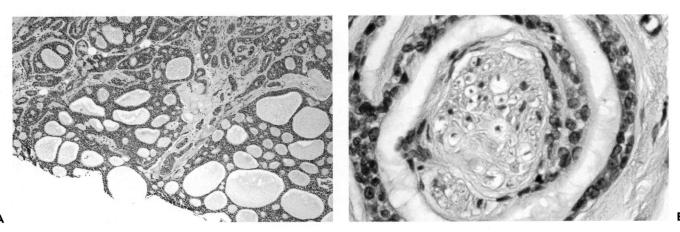

Figure 17.4 **Adenoid cystic carcinoma with perineural invasion. A:** This needle core biopsy specimen shows predominantly glandular adenoid cystic carcinoma. **B:** Perineural invasion in the specimen.

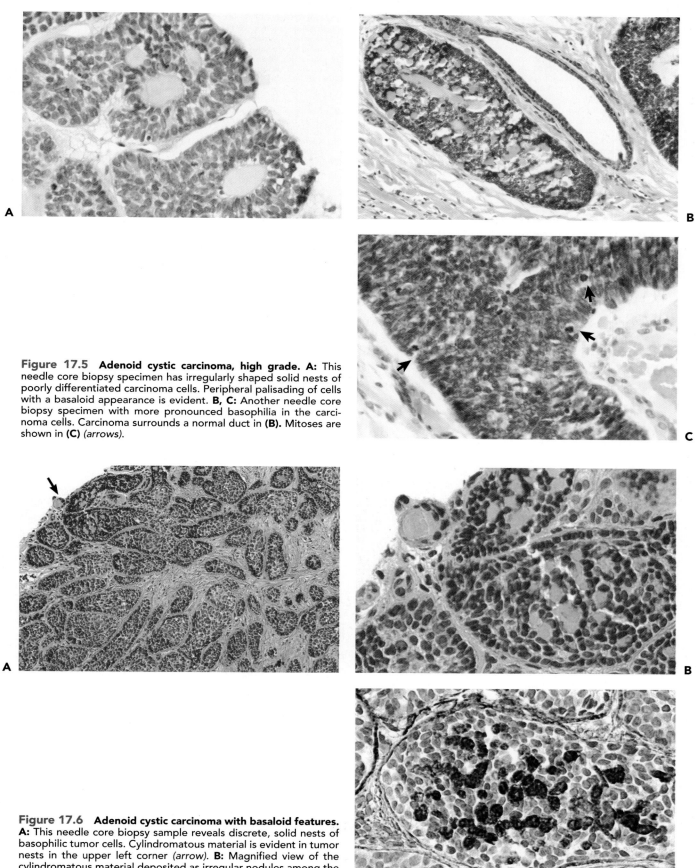

Figure 17.5 Adenoid cystic carcinoma, high grade. A: This needle core biopsy specimen has irregularly shaped solid nests of poorly differentiated carcinoma cells. Peripheral palisading of cells with a basaloid appearance is evident. **B, C:** Another needle core biopsy specimen with more pronounced basophilia in the carcinoma cells. Carcinoma surrounds a normal duct in **(B).** Mitoses are shown in **(C)** *(arrows)*.

Figure 17.6 Adenoid cystic carcinoma with basaloid features. A: This needle core biopsy sample reveals discrete, solid nests of basophilic tumor cells. Cylindromatous material is evident in tumor nests in the upper left corner *(arrow).* **B:** Magnified view of the cylindromatous material deposited as irregular nodules among the tumor cells. **C:** The cylindromatous material is immunoreactive for laminin (immunoperoxidase).

REFERENCES

1. Hjorth S, Magnusson PH, Blomquite P. Adenoid cystic carcinoma of the breast. *Acta Chir Scand.* 1977;143:155–158.
2. Qizilbash AH, Patterson MC, Oliveira KF. Adenoid cystic carcinoma of the breast. *Arch Pathol Lab Med.* 1977;101:302–306.
3. Peters GN, Wolff M. Adenoid cystic carcinoma of the breast; report of 11 new cases. *Cancer.* 1982;52:680–686.
4. Rosen PP. Adenoid cystic carcinoma of the breast. A morphologically heterogeneous neoplasm. *Pathol Annu.* 1989;(pt 2):237–254.
5. Koss LG, Brannan CD, Ashikari R. Histologic and ultrastructural features of adenoid cystic carcinoma of the breast. *Cancer.* 1970;26:1271–1279.
6. Bourke AG, Metcalf C, Wylie EJ. Mammographic features of adenoid cystic carcinoma. *Austral Radiol.* 1994;38:324–325.
7. Saqi, A, Mercado CL, Hamele-Bena D. Adenoid cystic carcinoma of the breast diagnosed by fine-needle aspiration. *Diagn Cytopathol.* 2004;30:271–274.
8. Tsuboi N, Ogawa Y, Inomata T, et al. Dynamic MR appearance of adenoid cystic carcinoma of the breast in a 67-year old female. *Radiat Med.* 1998;16:225–228.
9. Düe W, Herbst H, Loy V, Stein H. Characterization of adenoid cystic carcinoma of the breast by immunohistology. *J Clin Pathol.* 1989;42:470–476.
10. Lamovec J, Us-krasovec M, Zidar A, Kjun A. Adenoid cystic carcinomas of the breast: a histologic, cytologic and immunohistochemical study. *Sem Diagn Pathol.* 1989;6:153–164.
11. Pastolero G, Hanna W, Zbieranowski I, Kahn HJ. Proliferative activity and p53 expression in adenoid cystic carcinoma of the breast. *Mod Pathol.* 1996;9:215–219.
12. Mastropasqua MG, Maiorano E, Pruneri G, et al. Immuno-reactivity for c-KIT and p63 as an adjunct in the diagnosis of adenoid cystic carcinoma of the breast. *Mod Pathol.* 2005;18:1277–1282.
13. Azoulay S, Lae M, Freneaux P, et al. KIT is highly expressed in adenoid cystic carcinoma of the breast: a basal-like carcinoma associated with a favorable outcome. *Mod Pathol.* 2005;18:1623–1631.
14. Harris, M. Pseudoadenoid cystic carcinoma of the breast. *Arch Pathol Lab Med.* 1977;101:307–309.
15. Ro JY, Silva EG, Gallager HS. Adenoid cystic carcinoma of the breast. *Hum Pathol.* 1987;18:1276–1281.
16. Shin SJ, Rosen PP. Solid variant of mammary adenoid cystic carcinoma with basaloid features. *Am J Surg Pathol.* 2002;26:230–237.
17. Nonaka D, Rosai J, Spagnolo D, et al. Cylindroma of the breast of skin adnexal type: a study of 4 cases. *Am J Surg Pathol.* 2004;25:1070–1075.
18. Kloer CG, Oberman HA. Adenoid cystic carcinoma of the breast: value of histologic grading and proliferative activity. *Mod Pathol.* 1997;10:21A.
19. Yamamoto Y, Wistuba I, Kishimoto Y, et al. DNA analysis at p53 locus in adenoid cystic carcinoma: a comparison of molecular study and p53 immunostaining. *Pathol Intnl.* 1998;48:273–280.
20. Sumpio BE, Jennings TA, Merino MJ, Sullivan PD. Adenoid cystic carcinoma of the breast. Data from the Connecticut Tumor Registry and a review of the literature. *Ann Surg.* 1987;205:295–301.
21. Clement PB, Young RH, Azzopardi JG. Collagenous spherulosis of the breast. *Am J Surg Pathol.* 1987;11:411–417.
22. Rabban JT, Swain RS, Zaloudek CJ, et al. Immunophenotypic overlap between adenoid cystic carcinoma and collagenous spherulosis of the breast: potential diagnostic pitfalls using myoepithelial markers. *Mod Pathol.* 2006;19:1351–1357.
23. Zaloudek, C, Oertel, YC, Orenstein, JM. Adenoid cystic carcinoma of the breast. *Am J Clin Pathol.* 1984;81:297–307.
24. Nayer HR. Cylindroma of the breast with pulmonary metastases. *Dis Chest.* 1957;31:324–327.
25. Herzberg AJ, Bossen EH, Walter PJ. Adenoid cystic carcinoma of the breast metastatic to the kidney. A clinically symptomatic lesion requiring surgical management. *Cancer.* 1991;68:1015–1020.
26. Lim SK, Kovi J, Warner OG. Adenoid cystic carcinoma of breast with metastasis: a case report and review of the literature. *J Nat Med Assoc.* 1979; 71:329–330.
27. Wells CA, Nicoll, S, Ferguson, DJP. Adenoid cystic carcinoma of the breast: a case with axillary lymph node metastasis. *Histopathology.* 1986;10:415–424.
28. Arpino G, Clark GM, Mohsin S, et al. Adenoid cystic carcinoma of the breast. Molecular markers, treatment, and clinical outcome. *Cancer.* 2002; 34:2119–27.
29. Millar BA, Kerba M, Youngson, B, et al. The potential role of breast conservation surgery and adjuvant breast radiation for adenoid cystic carcinoma of the breast. *Breast Cancer Res Treat.* 2004;87:225–232.

Secretory Carcinoma

18

Secretory carcinoma was first described in children (1), but the majority of cases have been reported in adults (2). There have been reports of secretory carcinoma in children younger than 5 years (3), and in a 6-year-old boy (4). There is a dearth of cases of secretory carcinoma in girls 10 to 15 years of age, and with rare exceptions, affected males have been younger than 10 years (5–7). The term "secretory" is preferable to "juvenile," an appellation used in early descriptions of the tumor. The microscopic appearance of the lesion is the same regardless of patient age.

In most instances, the patient has a painless, circumscribed breast mass that may have been present for years before biopsy (2,3). Coexistence of juvenile papillomatosis and secretory carcinoma has been reported (8). Estrogen receptors (ERs) were negative in the majority of tumors, with only a few lesions positive for ERs and/or progesterone receptors (PRs) (2). HER2/*neu* expression is rarely present in secretory carcinoma (9). The characteristic ER(−), PR(−), and HER2/*neu*(−) "triple negative" immunophenotype of secretory carcinomas has led to the suggestion that these tumors are part of the "basal-like" carcinoma spectrum (10).

Secretory carcinoma is usually a circumscribed, firm mass that may be lobulated, but rarely, the tumor has infiltrative margins. The tumors tend to be 3 cm or less in diameter, with larger lesions up to 12 cm found mainly in adults. The lesions are typically unicentric and only rarely multicentric (11). Origin of secretory carcinoma in ectopic axillary breast tissue (12) and from axillary skin appendage glands (13) has been reported.

Imaging studies of secretory carcinoma were reviewed by Paeng et al. (14). On mammography, the tumor most often presents as rounded rather than distinctly spiculated. Calcifications may be present. The ultrasound appearance is that of a circumscribed hypoechoic tumor with no particular distinguishing features.

Secretory carcinoma has an intraductal component that exhibits the growth patterns associated with more conventional types of duct carcinoma. Most commonly, the intraductal carcinoma is papillary or cribriform, but solid foci and, rarely, comedo necrosis may be found (2). The invasive areas are relatively compact with papillary, microcystic, and cribriform structure. Microcalcifications are rarely seen in the neoplastic glands or in the stroma. The periphery of the carcinoma is usually circumscribed microscopically, but overtly infiltrative growth is sometimes present.

The tumor consists of cells with abundant, pale-to-clear, pink, or amphophilic cytoplasm and small, round, cytologically low-grade nuclei (Fig. 18.1). Signet ring cell forms may be present. Rarely, portions of the lesion have more granular or eosinophilic cytoplasm and the nuclear cytology of apocrine differentiation that has been mistaken for the cytologic appearance of acinic cell carcinoma (15) (Fig.18.2). The glands and microcystic spaces contain variable amounts of dense pink, amphophilic, or basophilic secretion that may be vacuolated or "bubbly." Rarely, the secretion resembles thyroid colloid or the secretion in a cystic hypersecretory lesion of the breast (Fig. 18.3). Strong staining of cells but not the secretion has been reported for α-lactalbumin as well as for S-100 protein and carcinoembryonic antigen (polyclonal) (4,5). No reactivity was observed for gross cystic disease fluid protein or for monoclonal carcinoembryonic antigen (4). The secretion reacts variably for mucin and with the periodic acid–Schiff (PAS) reaction (7).

Tognon et al. (16) and Euhus et al. (17) reported finding the ETV6-NTRK3 gene fusion in secretory carcinomas. ETV6-NTRK3 fusion has also been found in pediatric mesenchymal tumors, and it is capable of causing transformation in murine epithelial cells. This oncoprotein was found in 12 of 13 secretory carcinomas and in only 1 of 50 (2%) of ductal carcinomas studied by Tognon et al. (16). More recent studies have confirmed to specificity of the ETV6-NTRK3 gene fusion in secretory carcinoma of the breast (10,15).

STAT5a, mammary growth factor, is one of several molecules involved in the transcription of differentiation proteins. Activation of STAT5a in the breast occurs largely as a result of the binding of prolactin to its receptor (18). STAT5a expression is present in the majority of normal mammary gland cells and largely absent in atypical duct hyperplasia and carcinoma (19). Overexpression of STAT5a occurs in physiological secretory and lactating mammary epithelium as well as in secretory mammary carcinoma (20).

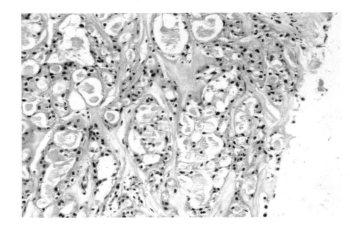

Figure 18.1   Secretory carcinoma. A needle core biopsy specimen from a circumscribed 2-cm tumor in a 68-year-old woman. The carcinoma has a characteristic microcystic architecture. In this example, the tumor cells have small, low-grade nuclei.

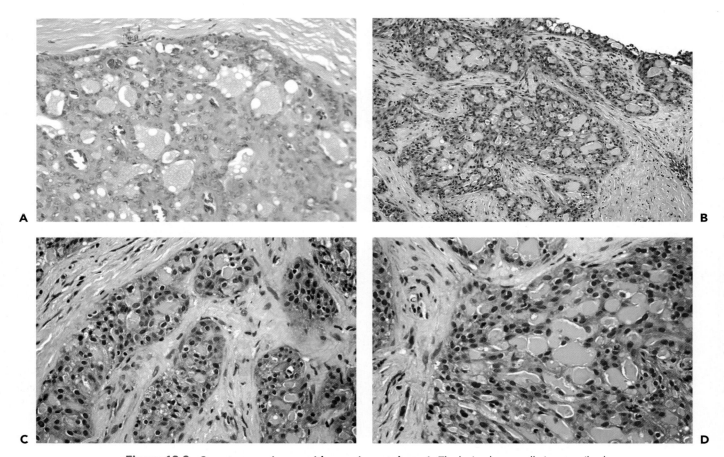

Figure 18.2   Secretory carcinoma with apocrine cytology. A: The lesion has a well-circumscribed border and a microcystic growth pattern. The nuclei in the tumor cells have prominent nucleoli typically associated with apocrine differentiation. **B–D:** Secretory carcinoma in needle core biopsy samples from a 41-year-old woman. Note apocrine cytology and irregular shapes of microcystic spaces filled with dense secretion.

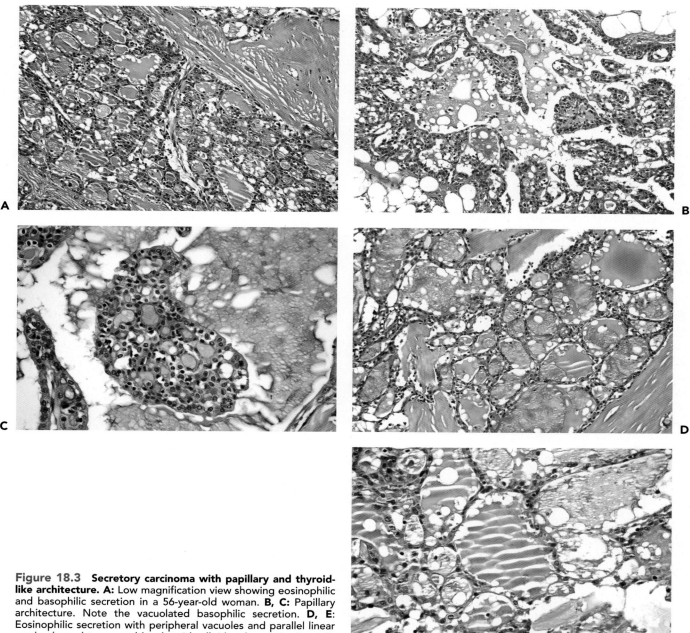

Figure 18.3 Secretory carcinoma with papillary and thyroid-like architecture. A: Low magnification view showing eosinophilic and basophilic secretion in a 56-year-old woman. **B, C:** Papillary architecture. Note the vacuolated basophilic secretion. **D, E:** Eosinophilic secretion with peripheral vacuoles and parallel linear cracks shown here resembles thyroid colloid and secretion in cystic hypersecretory lesions of the breast.

Surgical biopsy is usually necessary for the diagnosis of secretory carcinoma, although the lesion may be suspected in a needle core biopsy specimen (11). Local excision is the preferred initial treatment in children. Consideration should be given to preserving the breast bud in prepubertal patients but this cannot always be accomplished, and breast development may be impaired. In postmenarchal children, wide local excision may suffice for small lesions, but quadrantectomy can be necessary to obtain negative margins around larger tumors. Long-term follow-up data on the success of breast conservation therapy are lacking, and until recently, most children and adults were treated by mastectomy. Local

recurrence in residual breast tissue following a mastectomy has been reported (21).

Axillary metastases have been described and they rarely involve more than three lymph nodes. The risk of nodal involvement is at least as great among children with this tumor as it is for adults (2). Clinical examination is not a reliable guide to the status of axillary lymph nodes in children because nodal metastases were reportedly not palpable in most instances. Sentinel lymph node mapping may be an effective method for assessing the axilla in patients with secretory carcinoma.

In the majority of patients, secretory carcinoma has a low-grade clinical course with a very favorable prognosis.

The role of radiation therapy in adults after excisional biopsy remains to be determined. Radiation may inhibit normal breast development if administered to the pre-menarchal or menarchal breast. Because there have been few documented instances with follow-up of systemic adjuvant therapy, it is not possible to judge the effectiveness of this treatment in children or adults with secretory carcinoma.

REFERENCES

1. McDivitt RW, Stewart FW. Breast carcinoma in children. *JAMA.* 1966; 195:388–390.
2. Rosen PP, Cranor ML. Secretory carcinoma of the breast. *Arch Pathol Lab Med.* 1991;115:141–144.
3. Romdhane KB, Ayed B, Labbane N, et al. Carcinome secretant juvenile du sein. A propos d'une observation chez une fille de 4 ans. *Ann Pathol.* 1987;3:227–230.
4. Hartman AW, Magrish, P. Carcinoma of breast in children. Case report: six-year-old boy with adenocarcinoma. *Ann Surg.* 1955;141:792–797.
5. Lamovec J, Bracko M. Secretory carcinoma of the breast: light microscopical, immunohistochemical and flow cytometric study. *Mod Pathol.* 1994; 7:475–479.
6. deBree E, Askoxylakis J, Giannikaki E, et al. Secretory carcinoma of the male breast. *Ann Surg Oncol.* 2002;9:663–667.
7. Alenda C, Aranda I, Segui J, Laforga J. Secretory carcinoma of the male breast. *Diagn Cytopathol.* 2005;32:47–50.
8. Rosen PP, Holmes G, Lesser ML, et al. Juvenile papillomatosis and breast carcinoma. *Cancer.* 1985;55:1345–1352.
9. Diallo R, Schaefer K-L, Bankfalvi A, et al. Secretory carcinoma of the breast: a distinct variant of invasive ductal carcinoma assessed by comparative genomic hybridization and immunohistochemistry. *Hum Pathol.* 2003; 34:1299–1305.
10. Laé M, Fréneaux P, Sastre-Garau X, et al. Secretory breast carcinomas with ETV6-NTRK3 fusion gene belong to the basal-like carcinoma spectrum. *Mod Pathol.* 2009;22:291–298.
11. Beatty SM, Orel SG, Kim P, et al. Multicentric secretory carcinoma of the breast in a 35-year-old woman: mammographic appearance and the use of core biopsy in preoperative management. *Breast J.* 1998;4:200–203.
12. Shin SJ, Sheikh FS, Allenby PA, Rosen PP. Invasive secretory (juvenile) carcinoma arising in ectopic breast tissue of the axilla. *Arch Pathol Lab Med.* 2001;125:1372–1374.
13. Brandt SM, Swistel AJ, Rosen PP. Secretory carcinoma in the axilla. Probable origin from axillary skin appendage glands in a young girl. *Am J Surg Pathol.* 2009;33:950–953.
14. Paeng MH, Choi HY, Sung SH, et al. Secretory carcinoma of the breast. *J Clin Ultrasound.* 2003;31:425–429.
15. Reis-Filho JS, Natrajan R, Vatcheva R, et al. Is acinic cell carcinoma a variant of secretory carcinoma? A FISH study using ETV6 'split apart' probes. *Histopathology.* 2008;52:840–846.
16. Tognon C, Knezevich SR, Huntsman D, et al. Expression of the ETV6-NTRK3 gene fusion as a primary event in human secretory breast carcinoma. *Cancer Cell.* 2002;2:367–376.
17. Euhus DM, Timmons CF, Tomlinson GE. ETV6-NTRK-Trk-ing the primary event in human secretory carcinoma. *Cancer Cell.* 2002;2:347–348.
18. Nevalainen MT, Xie J, Bubendorf L, et al. Basal activation of transcription factor signal transducer and activator of transcription (STAT5) in non-pregnant mouse and human breast epithelium. *Mol Endocrinol.* 2002; 16:1108–1124.
19. Bratthauer GL, Strauss BL, Tavassoli FA. STAT5a expression in various lesions of the breast. *Virchows Arch.* 2006;448:165–171.
20. Strauss BL, Bratthauer GL, Tavassoli FA. STAT5a expression in the breast is maintained in secretory carcinoma, in contrast to other histologic types. *Hum Pathol.* 2006;37:586–592.
21. Mies C. Recurrent secretory carcinoma in residual mammary tissue after mastectomy. *Am J Surg Pathol.* 1993;17:715–721.

Cystic Hypersecretory Carcinoma

19

This variant of duct carcinoma was first described in 1984 (1). The majority of cases have been intraductal carcinomas. A benign proliferative lesion that resembles cystic hypersecretory carcinoma (CHC) has been termed *cystic hypersecretory hyperplasia* (CHH) (2). The age distribution of CHC ranges from 34 to 79 years, with a mean of 56 years (2). The presenting symptom is usually a palpable mass. Mammography in one case revealed a prominent ductal pattern and an irregular density in the breast (3). The mammogram in a patient with cystic hypersecretory intraductal carcinoma revealed "heterogeneous dense breast tissue with no indication of a mass or microcalcifications, and sonography revealed multiple small aggregated, anechoic cysts with good through transmission" (4). Two patients with invasive CHC were reported to have spiculated masses with calcifications on mammography (5).

Among 10 tumors studied biochemically, 8 had negative levels of estrogen and progesterone receptors. Two specimens were positive for both receptors. In situ and invasive components have been reported to be HER2/*neu*-positive (6).

The distinctive gross feature of CHC is the presence of numerous cysts measuring up to 1.5 cm. Secretion within cysts has been described as grossly sticky, mucinous, gelatinous, or as resembling thyroid colloid. It is usually not possible to distinguish grossly between cystic hypersecretory intraductal carcinoma and CHH. An invasive component associated with CHC produces a distinct, solid mass.

The microscopic hallmark of a cystic hypersecretory lesion is the presence of cysts that contain eosinophilic secretion that resembles thyroid colloid (Fig. 19.1). The homogeneous and virtually acellular secretion often retracts from the surrounding epithelium, resulting in a smooth or scalloped margin duplicating the contour of the epithelial proliferation. Folds, linear cracks, or small punched out holes occur in the secretion. There are no appreciable differences in the character of the secretion between CHC and CHH. Positive reactions for carcinoembryonic antigen, α-lactalbumin, periodic acid–Schiff (PAS), and mucin have been observed in the cyst contents which are consistently negative for thyroglobulin. Disruption of cysts results in discharge of cyst contents into the stroma, eliciting an intense inflammatory reaction consisting of lymphocytes and histiocytes.

The cysts in benign cystic hypersecretory lesions are lined by inconspicuous flat cells or a single layer of cuboidal to columnar cells (Fig. 19.2) (2). The cells in such lesions have uniform, cytologically bland nuclei, and scant cytoplasm. Atypical features in this setting are epithelial crowding sometimes resulting in micropapillary hyperplasia, hyperchromasia, and enlargement of nuclei that may contain nucleoli (Fig. 19.2). Lesions that lack fully developed intraductal carcinoma are diagnosed as *CHH with atypia*.

Lobules in and around the lesional areas in women with benign and carcinomatous cystic hypersecretory lesions often exhibit hypersecretory changes that include the accumulation of secretion in lobular gland lumens (Fig. 19.3). This lobular abnormality may occur as an isolated finding in the absence of a fully developed cystic hypersecretory lesion, an observation which suggests that the process may originate in such foci. The finding of cystic hypersecretory change in lobules in a needle core biopsy specimen should prompt consideration of excisional biopsy.

In CHC, the epithelium of some cysts and ducts grows as micropapillary intraductal carcinoma (Fig. 19.4). The spectrum of epithelial patterns in cystic hypersecretory intraductal carcinoma ranges from short, knobby epithelial tufts to complex branching fronds that may extend across the duct lumen. The so-called Roman arch, or bridging pattern, commonly seen in other forms of micropapillary intraductal carcinoma is uncommon in these lesions. Fibrovascular stroma is rarely found within the micropapillary fronds. Cytologically, the cells in the fronds of micropapillary intraductal carcinoma have crowded hyperchromatic nuclei with sparse cytoplasm. There is no secretion within the cytoplasm but frayed, apical cell borders, and cytoplasmic blebs are consistent with some degree of secretory activity. There are usually foci of CHH scattered in an area of CHC. A few examples of intraductal CHC have been encountered in which there is pronounced vacuolization of the cytoplasm of the carcinoma cells and secretion, a pattern reminiscent of pregnancy-like hyperplasia, and there are rare instances wherein CHH or CHC and pregnancy-like hyperplasia

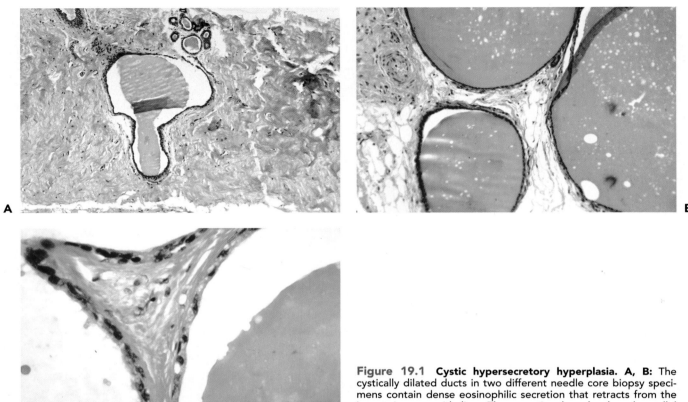

Figure 19.1 Cystic hypersecretory hyperplasia. A, B: The cystically dilated ducts in two different needle core biopsy specimens contain dense eosinophilic secretion that retracts from the inconspicuous epithelium The secretion has developed parallel cracks and small punctate holes. **C:** The cystic spaces are lined by flat cells distributed in a single layer.

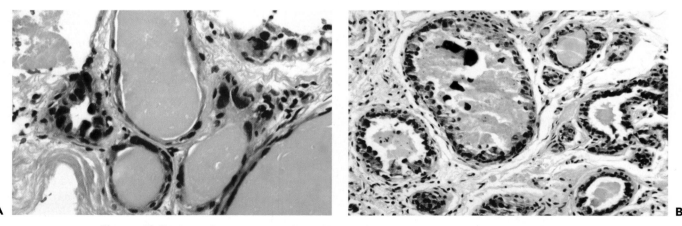

Figure 19.2 Cystic hypersecretory hyperplasia with atypia. A: The cells in this cystic hypersecretory lesion have hyperchromatic and pleomorphic nuclei. **B:** Cells with hyperchromatic, enlarged nuclei are present in this atypical cystic hypersecretory lesion. Calcification, shown in one cyst, is not often present in this condition.

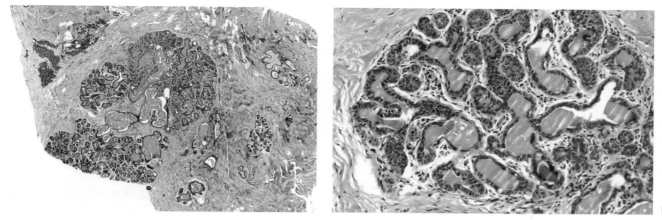

Figure 19.3 Cystic hypersecretory hyperplasia in lobules. A, B: Characteristic eosinophilic secretion is present in the terminal ducts and lobular glands of this needle core biopsy specimen.

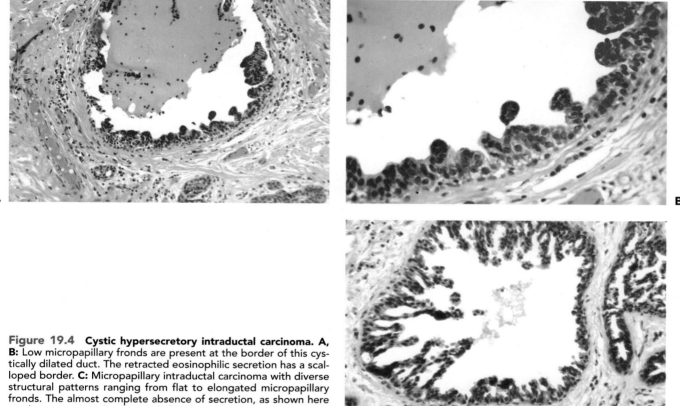

Figure 19.4 Cystic hypersecretory intraductal carcinoma. A, B: Low micropapillary fronds are present at the border of this cystically dilated duct. The retracted eosinophilic secretion has a scalloped border. **C:** Micropapillary intraductal carcinoma with diverse structural patterns ranging from flat to elongated micropapillary fronds. The almost complete absence of secretion, as shown here can be encountered in foci with florid cystic hypersecretory intraductal carcinoma.

coexist (7). Rarely, the proliferative and cytological abnormalities warrant a diagnosis of CHC arising in pregnancy-like hyperplasia (7).

Invasive CHC consists of intraductal CHC accompanied by an invasive component. Most invasive carcinomas encountered in this setting have been poorly differentiated duct carcinomas with a solid growth pattern. Nuclei in the invasive carcinoma cells usually have an "open" appearance similar to cells found in papillary thyroid carcinoma.

Excisional biopsy is required if CHH is present in a needle core biopsy because it is not possible to exclude focal carcinoma on basis of such a limited sample. Some lesions have been misclassified as "cystic disease," with the true nature of the process becoming apparent after there was a recurrence (1,3).

The finding of areas with the typical features of CHH, sometimes with atypia, associated with CHC suggests that these processes are related, but convincing evidence of progression through these stages has not yet been observed. Review of prior biopsies from women later found to have CHC has disclosed various lesions, including seemingly unrelated common proliferative changes as well as CHH and CHC. Follow-up of eight patients with CHH revealed subsequent breast carcinoma in two cases. One woman developed a fatal contralateral invasive duct carcinoma that lacked cystic hypersecretory features. The other patient had intraductal carcinoma separate from CHH in a biopsy, and residual CHH in the mastectomy specimen. Bogomoletz (8) described a 55-year-old woman who was well without recurrence 6 years after excisional biopsy of a 7-cm example of CHH.

The clinical course of intraductal CHC does not differ from that of other forms of intraductal carcinoma. Breast recurrence has been reported after lumpectomy alone. Too few patients have been treated by lumpectomy and radiotherapy to assess this form of treatment. There have been no recurrences in women treated by mastectomy after a mean follow-up of 8 years, extending in one case to 23 years. All had negative lymph nodes. Two of four women with invasive CHC had metastases in axillary lymph nodes, and a third patient presented with locally advanced or inflammatory carcinoma. Thus far, the one reported death due to CHC occurred in this latter patient. Adjuvant chemotherapy would be prudent when invasive carcinoma is present in view of the poorly differentiated character of these tumors.

REFERENCES

1. Rosen, PP, Scott, M. Cystic hypersecretory duct carcinoma of the breast. *Am J Surg Pathol.* 1984;8:31–41.
2. Guerry, P, Erlandson, RA, Rosen, PP. Cystic hypersecretory hyperplasia and cystic hypersecretory duct carcinoma of the breast. Pathology, therapy and follow-up of 39 patients. *Cancer.* 1988;61:1611–1620.
3. Colandrea JM, Shmookler BM, O'Dowd GJ, Cohen, MH. Cystic hypersecretory duct carcinoma of the breast. Report of a case with fine needle aspiration. *Arch Pathol Lab Med.* 1988;112:560–563.
4. Park C, Jung JI, Lee AW, et al. Sonographic findings in a patient with cystic hypersecretory duct carcinoma of the breast. *J Clin Ultrasound.* 2004;32:29–32.
5. Park JM, Seo MR. Cystic hypersecretory duct carcinoma of the breast: report of two cases. *Clin Radiol.* 2002;57:312–315.
6. Skalova A, Ryska A, Kajo K, et al. Cystic hypersecretory carcinoma: rare, poorly recognized variant of intraductal carcinoma of the breast. Report of five cases. *Histopathology.* 2005;46:43–49.
7. Shin SJ, Rosen PP. Carcinoma arising from pre-existing pregnancy-like and cystic hypersecretory hyperplasia lesions of the breast. *Am J. Surg Pathol.* 2004;28:789–793.
8. Bogomoletz, W-V. Hyperplasia hypersécrétoire kystique du sein. Un diagnostic rare en pathologie mammaire. *Ann Pathol.* 1994;14:131–132.

Other Special Types of Invasive Duct Carcinoma

20

MAMMARY CARCINOMA WITH OSTEOCLAST-LIKE GIANT CELLS

Since the first series was published in 1979, approximately 200 examples of this type of breast carcinoma have been reported (1). The clinical features are similar to those of breast carcinoma generally. Patients range in age from 28 to 88 years, with an average age at diagnosis of about 50 years (1–3). Mammographically and on ultrasonography the well-circumscribed margin of most tumors suggests a benign lesion such as a cyst or fibroadenoma (2). Bilateral primary mammary carcinomas with osteoclast-like giant cells are very rare (4). The gross appearance is quite striking due to the dark brown or red-brown color of the bisected tumor in most cases. Tumors with few giant cells may be tan or white. Reported diameters range from 0.5 to 10 cm, with most measuring 3 cm or less.

The mechanism by which osteoclast-like giant cells are formed in breast carcinoma is not known. In a case study Sano et al. (5) found that the carcinoma cells in one such tumor secreted excess vascular endothelial growth factor (VEGF). They hypothesized that VEGF "promotes tumor angiogenesis and migration of macrophages" that "fuse with each other," giving rise to osteoclast-like giant cells. Additional studies are needed to evaluate this interesting observation. Jimi et al. (6) demonstrated in vitro that multinucleation and functional osteoclastic differentiation of stromal cells could be induced by interleukin-1 (IL-1).

Most of these lesions are moderately or poorly differentiated invasive duct carcinomas (Fig. 20.1). A cribriform growth pattern is present relatively more often than among duct carcinomas generally. Osteoclast-like giant cells have been encountered in well-differentiated or tubular, infiltrating lobular (1,4), squamous, papillary (1), apocrine, mucinous (3), and metaplastic carcinomas (1–3) (Fig. 20.2). Rarely, the carcinoma has a glandular pattern reminiscent of infiltrating colonic carcinoma. The giant cells are located close to the edges of carcinomatous glands, and they may be found in the glandular lumens. Extravasated erythrocytes and hemosiderin are usually present in the intervening highly vascular stroma. Erythrophagocytosis by the giant cells is uncommon, and they contain scant hemosiderin that is detectable by light microscopy. Fibroblastic reaction, collagenization, and lymphocytic infiltration are variably present. When present, intraductal carcinoma has the appearance of one of the conventional variants, usually cribriform, solid, or papillary. Osteoclast-like giant cells are sometimes but not always present in the associated intraductal carcinoma and rarely osteoclast-like giant cells are found in intraductal carcinoma in the absence of an invasive lesion (7). Bone and cartilage are not found in mammary carcinomas with osteoclast-like giant cells.

The giant cells are stained by a variety of antibodies that react with macrophages and osteoclasts, exhibiting strong reactivity for acid phosphatase (4,8), α-1-antitrypsin (4), KP-1 (CD68) (4), and lysozyme (9,10) (Fig. 20.2). The tumors usually have low levels of estrogen receptor, but many had remarkably high progesterone receptors (2).

Axillary lymph node metastases have been reported in approximately a third of cases. Osteoclast-like giant cells are found in some but not all metastases in axillary lymph nodes or other sites, and within intralymphatic tumor emboli (1,2). Nearly two-thirds of patients have been reported to be alive and well with follow-up rarely reaching beyond 5 years (1,2,10). Data on breast conservation with radiation therapy and adjuvant systemic treatment for this neoplasm are anecdotal, but presently it would be appropriate to employ the same criteria as for the treatment of invasive mammary carcinoma generally.

CRIBRIFORM CARCINOMA

Invasive carcinomas with a cribriform pattern are termed *classical cribriform carcinomas*. Some of these tumors have cribriform and tubular components. The diagnosis of

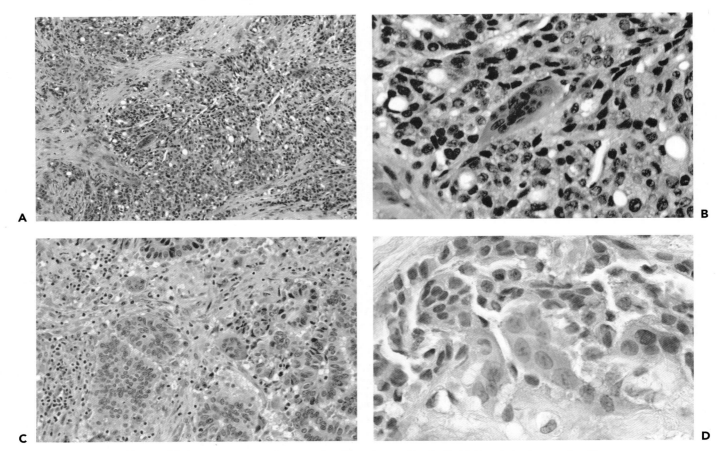

Figure 20.1 **Carcinoma with osteoclast-like giant cells. A, B:** Multinucleated osteoclast-like giant cells are scattered in an infiltrating, poorly differentiated duct carcinoma. The tumor shown in this needle core biopsy specimen is unusual because it lacks typical stromal elements, including red blood cells, hemosiderin, and lymphocytes. **C:** A moderately differentiated invasive duct carcinoma with osteoclast-like giant cells in stroma that contains red blood cells, lymphocytes, plasma cells, and hemosiderin. **D:** Two osteoclast-like giant cells are shown at the edge of invasive carcinoma. Nuclei in the giant cells differ from those in carcinoma cells.

mixed invasive cribriform carcinoma has been reserved for tumors in which less than 50% of the lesion has a cribriform pattern and the remainder of the tumor is composed of nontubular, less well-differentiated areas. Fewer than 6% of invasive mammary carcinomas have a cribriform component, with nearly equal proportions of pure and mixed lesions (11,12).

A mammographic study of eight cases revealed spiculated masses measuring 20 to 35 mm in four of the patients (13). Two of these lesions contained a few punctate calcifications. Four other tumors were not visualized radiographically. Venable et al. (14) reported that 16 classical and mixed cribriform carcinomas were estrogen receptor–positive and that 11 (69%) of the tumors were also progesterone receptor–positive. There was no appreciable difference in progesterone receptor positivity between classical and mixed cribriform tumors.

A small proportion of cribriform carcinomas occur as multifocal lesions (11,12). The invasive component of cribriform carcinoma duplicates the sieve-like growth pattern of conventional cribriform intraductal carcinoma (Fig. 20.3). The rounded and angular masses of uniform,

well-differentiated tumor cells are embedded in variable amounts of collagenous stroma (Fig. 20.4). Some tumors have areas of tubular growth that comprise up to 50% of the tumor. Page et al. (11) found tubular areas in 6 of 35 classical cribriform tumors (17%). Mucin-positive secretion is present in varying amounts within the cribriform lumina, and they may contain microcalcifications (15,16). The intraductal component has a cribriform pattern in most but not all classical cribriform carcinomas. When present, nodal metastases from classical tumors usually also have a cribriform structure, whereas metastases derived from mixed tumors are more likely to have a noncribriform pattern (11,14).

Cribriform carcinoma should be distinguished morphologically from adenoid cystic carcinoma. Cribriform growth produces a fenestrated structural pattern that lacks the cylindromatous components composed of basal lamina material characteristic of adenoid cystic carcinoma. However, cribriform areas are found in many adenoid cystic carcinomas in which glands are more prominent than cylindromatous elements (17). The glandular component of some carcinomas with osteoclast-like stromal giant cells

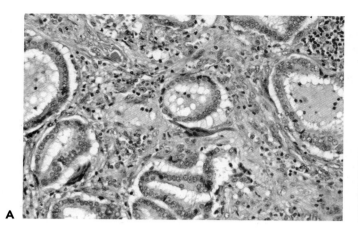

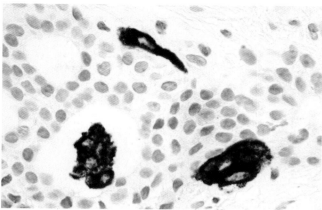

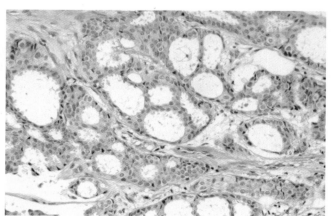

Figure 20.2 **Carcinomas with osteoclast-like giant cells. A:** Infiltrating duct carcinoma with a well-differentiated glandular pattern and characteristic stroma. The giant cells are attenuated and apposed to the outer surfaces of the glands. **B:** Osteoclast-like giant cells in and around the carcinoma glands are KP1-positive (immunoperoxidase). **C:** Low-grade invasive duct carcinoma with cribriform structure, osteoclast-like giant cells, and many red blood cells in the stroma.

shows a cribriform growth pattern. These tumors are classified as carcinomas with osteoclast-like giant cells.

The majority of patients have been treated by mastectomy and axillary dissection (11,14). Two studies concluded that patients with classical cribriform carcinoma were less likely to have axillary lymph node metastases than women with mixed cribriform (11) or ordinary invasive duct carcinoma (14). No deaths due to classical cribriform carcinoma occurred among 34 patients studied by Page et al. (11) with follow-up of 10 to 21 years. Among 16 women with mixed

cribriform carcinoma followed an average of 12.5 years, there were six deaths resulting from the breast carcinoma. Venable et al. (14) reported a disease-free survival of 100% among 45 patients with classical cribriform carcinoma followed for 1 to 5 years.

Pure invasive cribriform carcinoma has a favorable prognosis and a low frequency of axillary nodal metastases. If adequate excision can be performed, breast conservation therapy would appear feasible, although published prognostic data are presently largely based on treatment by

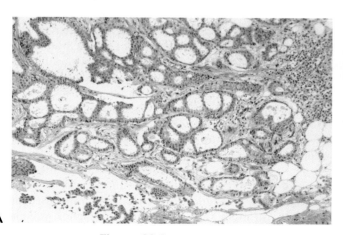

Figure 20.3 **Invasive cribriform carcinoma. A, B:** The invasive carcinoma in this needle core biopsy specimen has a cribriform structure composed of round or oval glandular spaces separated by thin, rigid bands of tumor cells with low-grade nuclei.

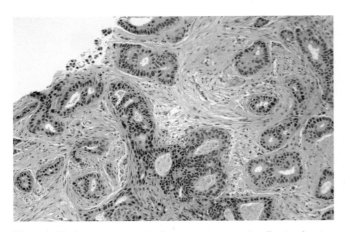

Figure 20.4 **Invasive cribriform carcinoma.** Small microlumina are separated by bands several cells thick in this example of cribriform carcinoma in a needle core biopsy specimen.

mastectomy. The possibility of encountering multifocal lesions should be borne in mind. In the absence of axillary nodal metastases, systemic adjuvant therapy is probably not warranted for tumors 1 cm or smaller unless there are specific unfavorable findings such as lymphatic tumor emboli. Axillary staging by sentinel lymph node mapping is appropriate.

SMALL CELL (OAT CELL) CARCINOMA

Carcinoma with neuroendocrine features that resembles small cell (oat cell) carcinoma of the lung is one of the most uncommon variants of breast carcinoma (18–21). The diagnosis of primary small cell mammary carcinoma can only be made with confidence if a nonmammary site is excluded clinically or if an in situ component can be demonstrated histologically in the breast. These criteria had not been met in all published descriptions of this rare neoplasm. Small cell carcinoma of the breast should be distinguished from more conventional forms of invasive carcinoma, usually ductal type, with immunohistochemical evidence of neuroendocrine differentiation (22,23). Expression of neuroendocrine markers by this latter group of tumors does not have a significant influence on their prognosis. Imaging studies in one patient with small cell mammary carcinoma revealed a solid, hypoechoic lobulated mass with both smooth and ill-defined contours (24).

Shin et al. (20) described the largest published series of small cell mammary carcinomas to date, consisting of nine patients of ages of 43 to 70 years. Two patients had prior cutaneous malignant melanoma and one had lobular carcinoma in situ in an earlier biopsy of the breast in which small cell carcinoma arose. Tumor size ranged from 1.3 to 5.0 cm (mean, 2.6 cm).

Intraductal carcinoma associated with small cell carcinoma may have various growth patterns including cribriform, solid, and micropapillary (Fig. 20.5). The tumor cells

are immunoreactive for cytokeratin (CAM5.2) and CD56 and may also be immunoreactive for synaptophysin, neuron-specific enolase (NSE), and stain with the Grimelius stain. Scattered neurosecretory granules were detected by electron microscopy in one tumor (18). Mammary small cell carcinoma is not reactive for TTF-1.

Small cell carcinoma can occur as part of a dimorphic intraductal carcinoma in which the small tumor cells in the center of the duct are surrounded at the periphery by large cells with abundant cytoplasm. Squamous metaplasia may occur in such lesions. Dimorphic structure is also represented in some small cell carcinomas by morule-like nests of eosinophilic cells that develop squamoid or glandular differentiation. These discrete foci are found scattered in the invasive small cell carcinoma component.

A minority of the primary mammary small cell carcinomas are associated with and appear to arise from in situ and invasive lobular carcinoma or invasive tubulolobular carcinoma. In these cases the small cell carcinoma will be E-cadherin-positive, variably reactive for neuroendocrine markers and negative for hormone receptors. Conversely, the lobular carcinoma component is not reactive for E-cadherin or neuroendocrine markers, and it is typically positive for hormone receptors.

There is no consistent pattern of immunoreactivity for neuroendocrine markers in mammary small cell carcinoma. The tumors are reactive for cytokeratin (AE1/AE3, CAM5.2, or CK7) and usually for NSE (25). Most are also positive with one or more indicators of neuroendocrine differentiation such as CD56, PGP9.5, synaptophysin, chromogranin (A or B), gastrin-releasing peptide (bombesin), serotonin, and Leu7 (25,26). In situ hybridization has been used to demonstrate chromogranin A and B messenger ribonucleic acid (mRNA) (27). Mammary small cell carcinomas are typically immunoreactive for E-cadherin (20), but those portions of the tumor with lobular features are E-cadherin-negative.

Some patients with mammary small cell carcinoma have large tumors, axillary lymph node metastases and an unfavorable prognosis. Treatment and follow-up for nine patients described in reports up to 1999 were summarized by Shin et al. (20). Six of the patients had axillary lymph node metastases. Four died of small cell carcinoma, two died of other causes, and three were alive without recurrence. In the series of nine new cases reported by Shin et al. (20) three women had axillary lymph node metastases. Mastectomy was performed in three cases, whereas six had lumpectomy with radiation or chemotherapy, or both. After follow-up of 3 to 35 months, two women had developed metastatic tumor and all were alive. These recent results suggest that the prognosis for relatively early-stage small cell carcinoma arising in the breast may be more favorable than was indicated by earlier reports based on patients with more advanced tumors at diagnosis. Mammary small cell carcinoma has been responsive to chemotherapy used for similar tumors at other sites such as VP-16 and cisplatin (24).

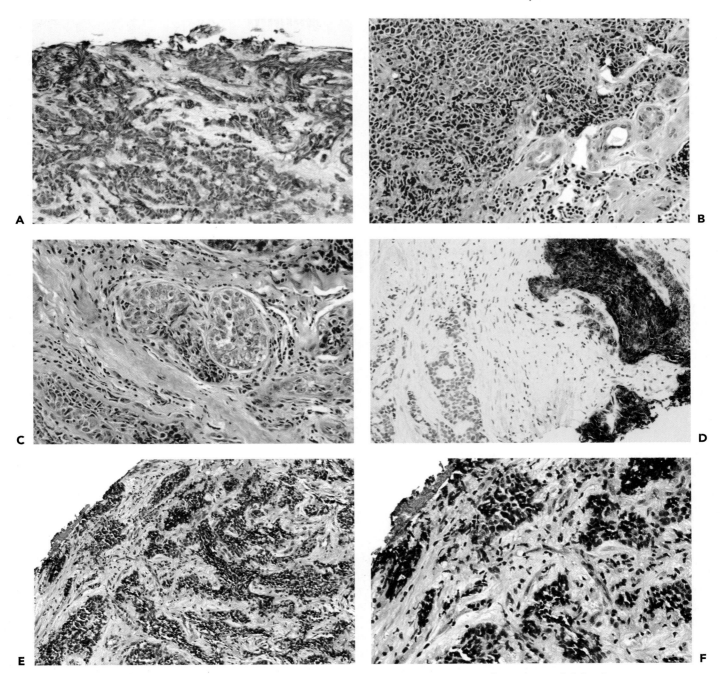

Figure 20.5   Small cell carcinoma.   A: Undifferentiated small carcinoma cells growing in ill-defined bands in a needle core biopsy specimen. Characteristic "crush artifact" is evident at the edge of the tumor tissue. **B, C:** The excisional biopsy specimen from the tumor shown in **A** with small cell carcinoma infiltrating mammary parenchyma and in situ carcinoma in a terminal duct–lobular unit **(C). D:** Small cell carcinoma is immunoreactive for CD56 **(right)**. The invasive duct carcinoma component **(left)** is CD56-negative (immunoperoxidase). **E, F:** Invasive small cell carcinoma with a trabecular growth pattern in a needle core biopsy sample.

Metastatic pulmonary oat cell carcinoma can involve the breast (28). In most cases, the existence of a pulmonary primary was previously documented, but the mammary metastasis may be the first manifestation of an occult pulmonary carcinoma. Pulmonary small cell carcinoma expresses TTF-1 that is absent from mammary small cell carcinoma.

LIPID-RICH CARCINOMA

This rare variant of infiltrating duct carcinoma is composed of cells containing abundant cytoplasmic lipid that is extracted when the tissue is processed for histologic sections, so that vacuolated cytoplasm is left (29–31) (Fig. 20.6). The tumor cells have small, dark nuclei (32). The presence of

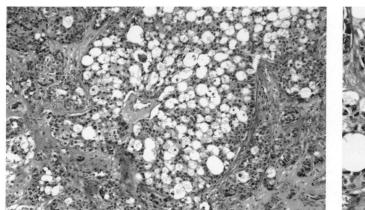
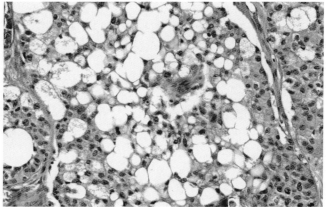

Figure 20.6   Lipid-rich carcinoma. A, B: Prominent cytoplasmic vacuoles are present due to extraction of cytoplasmic lipid during tissue processing (Courtesy of Frank Braza, MD).

lipid can be demonstrated in frozen sections of fresh tissue, by electron microscopy, or in tissue prepared by processes that preserve cytoplasmic lipids. The carcinoma is immunoreactive for epithelial membrane antigen, cytokeratin, and α-lactalbumin.

Ramos and Taylor (30) described 13 cases that had the growth pattern of lipid-rich carcinoma in routine histologic sections, but they were able to demonstrate lipid only in four tumors that were available as unfixed specimens. The other nine tumors were identified retrospectively among 900 carcinomas on the basis of histologic pattern alone. Eleven of the 12 patients treated by radical mastectomy had axillary lymph node metastases. Follow-up revealed that six patients died of metastatic carcinoma and two were alive with recurrent carcinoma. The rest were alive and recurrence free, with the majority followed less than 2 years.

GLYCOGEN-RICH CARCINOMA

Carcinomas that accumulate abundant cytoplasmic glycogen can arise in the breast. Extraction of the water-soluble glycogen during histologic processing causes the cytoplasm in these tumor cells to have a clear, vacuolated appearance in routine sections. In one series, 3% of 1555 tumors were classified as clear cell, glycogen-rich carcinomas (33). These investigators were able to find lesser amounts of intracytoplasmic glycogen in 58% of non–clear cell carcinomas. Others reported that glycogen-rich clear cell carcinoma accounted for less than 1% of mammary duct carcinomas (34).

The patients range in age from 34 to 78 years and present with a mass. Intraductal and invasive glycogen-rich lesions have been detected by mammography (35–37). Hormone receptor analysis revealed that approximately 50% of tumors were estrogen receptor-positive, but all lesions studied have been negative for progesterone receptor (35–38).

The lesions have basic structural features of conventional intraductal carcinoma alone or of intraductal and infiltrating duct carcinoma. The intraductal component has solid, comedo, cribriform, or papillary growth patterns (37). In invasive areas the tumor cells form cords, solid nests, or papillary structures. A linear pattern consisting of strands of cells resembling invasive lobular carcinoma may be seen.

Cytologically, the tumor cells have sharply defined borders and polygonal contours. The cytoplasm is clear and less often finely granular or foamy. The central or eccentrically placed nuclei are hyperchromatic, sometimes exhibiting clumped chromatin and nucleoli (Fig. 20.7). Mitotic figures are infrequent. The differential diagnosis includes clear cell apocrine and lipid-rich carcinomas of the breast and metastatic clear cell renal carcinoma. Apocrine cytologic features are identified focally in a majority of the tumors, and it has been suggested that glycogen-rich carcinoma may be a variant of apocrine carcinoma (37). The cytoplasm gives a positive, diastase-labile reaction with the periodic-acid–Schiff (PAS) stain. The cells stain only focally and faintly with alcian blue or mucicarmine (34,36), and the oil red O stain for lipid is negative (36).

Approximately 30% of the reported patients had metastatic tumor in their axillary lymph nodes. In one series, 50% of the patients treated by mastectomy died of

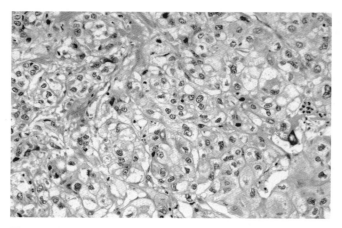

Figure 20.7   Glycogen-rich carcinoma. Typical clear cell cytology.

metastatic mammary carcinoma 1 to 175 months (median 15 months) after diagnosis, and one patient was alive with recurrent carcinoma 36 months after local excision and lymph node dissection (25). Hayes et al. (37) reported that three of eight patients with follow-up information died of metastatic carcinoma. These data suggest that the prognosis of patients with glycogen-rich carcinoma is not particularly favorable.

INVASIVE MICROPAPILLARY CARCINOMA

Invasive micropapillary carcinoma is a histologically distinctive form of duct carcinoma in which the tumor cells are arranged in morule-like clusters, referred to as an "exfoliative appearance" (39). This growth pattern may be found throughout the lesion (pure invasive micropapillary carcinoma) or as part of an otherwise conventional invasive duct carcinoma (mixed invasive micropapillary carcinoma). About 4% of invasive duct carcinomas studied by Kuroda et al. (40) were either pure or mixed forms by invasive micropapillary carcinoma. Luna-Moré et al. (41) found micropapillary differentiation in 27 of 986 (2.7%) consecutive breast carcinomas. In 15 of the tumors, the micropapillary component occupied more than 50% of the lesion. The distinction between pure and mixed invasive micropapillary carcinoma cannot be made with certainty in the limited sample obtained in a needle core biopsy. In practical terms, to be considered in the "pure" category at least 75% of the excised tumor should have the micropapillary growth pattern.

The reported age range at diagnosis was 25 to 89 years in several series with a median age of 52 to 62 years (39,40,42,43). Patients with lesions composed of more than 50% invasive micropapillary carcinoma tend to be older than patients with less extensive micropapillary involvement (41). The majority of patients present with a palpable mass, but an occasional lesion has been detected mammographically as a mammary soft tissue density or as a result of microcalcifications (42,44). Tumors with more than 50% of micropapillary growth tend to be larger (mean size 6 cm) than those with a lesser amount of this pattern (mean size 3.5 cm).

The carcinoma cells are cuboidal to columnar, containing finely granular or dense, eosinophilic cytoplasm with intermediate to high-grade nuclei. The tumor cells are arranged in small clusters that have a serrated peripheral border and sometimes surround a central lumen (Fig. 20.8). An uncommon variant features microcystic dilatation of lumina within cell clusters. A clear space surrounds each tumor cell cluster, defined by intervening stroma consisting of dense fibrocollagenous tissue or a more delicate network of reticular tissue. In some instances, a lymphoid infiltrate permeates the stroma. Guo et al. (45) reported a relative scarcity of cytotoxic T-lymphocytes in invasive micropapillary carcinoma when compared with medullary carcinoma. The sponge-like

pattern of spaces filled by tumor cell clusters occurs in metastatic lesions as well as in the primary tumors. The spaces within tumor cell clusters generally appear to be empty, but in some instances mucinous material has been demonstrated with special stains (41). Myxoid stroma has been noted in a minority of cases (42). Microcalcifications, sometimes with psammomatous features, are variably present. Foci of necrosis are found in large tumors.

By electron microscopy, microvilli have been found on the cell surfaces bordering the clear spaces, suggesting that these cells are oriented as though the spaces around the tumor cell clusters were glandular lumina (41). This has been referred to as an "inside-out growth pattern" (46). This impression is supported by the distribution of MUC-1 glycoprotein in these carcinomas. MUC-1 expression within ordinary gland forming carcinomas is localized to the apical cell surface where the glycoprotein is involved in lumen formation. In invasive micropapillary carcinoma MUC-1 was found to be localized to the external surfaces of papillary tumor clusters, adjacent to the surrounding stroma (47). This reversal of cell polarity has also been observed as a feature of lymphovascular tumor emboli (48).

It is difficult to identify true lymphatic tumor emboli in the vicinity of the primary tumor because of the intrinsic capacity of the neoplasm to grow in the sponge-like pattern. By using antibodies to define vascular endothelium (factor VIII, CD31), Pettinato et al. (43) demonstrated vascular invasion in 63% of tumors examined. When they are present, the intravascular tumor cells are arranged in the same papillary clusters that characterize the invasive part of the tumor (48).

Intraductal carcinoma, which is detected in most cases, is usually micropapillary, sometimes with cribriform elements. However, solid intraductal carcinoma can be found in these tumors. Cells in the intraductal and invasive parts of the tumor often have poorly differentiated, hyperchromatic nuclei rather than the bland nuclear cytology usually associated with low-grade micropapillary intraductal carcinoma. Calcifications and necrosis are sometimes found in intraductal foci.

The differential diagnosis of invasive micropapillary carcinoma includes primary mucinous carcinoma and metastatic serous ovarian carcinoma. Mucinous carcinoma features abundant extracellular mucin that is absent from invasive micropapillary carcinoma. Tumor cell clusters in mucinous carcinoma usually have a smooth rather than a serrated periphery. The presence of an intraductal component serves to exclude metastatic ovarian carcinoma. Serous ovarian carcinoma is immunoreactive for WT1, a marker that can also be present in invasive micropapillary breast carcinoma. Lee et al. (49) found that 21% of invasive micropapillary breast carcinomas expressed CA125, whereas this marker was identified in more than 90% of serous papillary ovarian carcinomas, usually in 80% to 100% of cells. WT1 nuclear expression was found in 26% of invasive micropapillary carcinomas, typically in less than 10% of cells, and there was cytoplasmic staining in

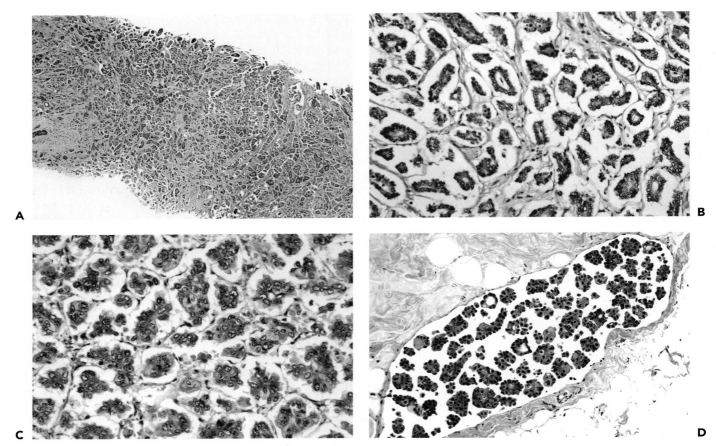

Figure 20.8 Invasive micropapillary carcinoma. A: This needle core biopsy specimen shows small nests of carcinoma cells outlined by a clear spaces. **B, C:** The "inside-out" pattern consists of morule-like solid clusters of tumor cells with a serrated outer border. The tumor cells show apocrine differentiation. Spaces between the carcinoma cells and the stroma are devoid of secretion. **D:** Invasive micropapillary carcinoma in a lymphatic channel.

59% of the tumors. Only one of 34 invasive micropapillary breast carcinomas displayed nuclear reactivity for WT1 and cytoplasmic reactivity for CA125. The presence of diffuse nuclear expression of WT1 and diffuse cytoplasmic staining for CA125 in a papillary breast tumor strongly favors metastatic serous papillary ovarian carcinoma.

In one study of invasive micropapillary carcinoma, immunoreactivity for prognostic markers was detected as follows: estrogen receptor—73% (+); progesterone receptor—45% (+); HER2/*neu*—36% (+); p53—12% (+) (50). Somewhat different results were obtained by Pettinato et al. (43): estrogen receptor—32% (+); progesterone receptor—20% (+); HER2/*neu*—95% (+); p53—70% (+). The latter investigators reported that E-cadherin was expressed between carcinoma cells but not on the outer surfaces of the cell clusters. Overexpression of N-cadherin, which has been associated with tumor invasiveness, has been found more frequently in invasive micropapillary carcinoma than in other types of carcinoma (51). Thirty-six invasive micropapillary carcinomas studied by Kim et al. (52) were not reactive for epidermal growth factor receptor (EGFR) or for c-Kit.

Data on prognosis are difficult to interpret because investigators have not clearly distinguished between pure and mixed invasive micropapillary carcinoma nor have they stratified cases by TNM stage for comparison with conventional duct carcinomas. The available evidence suggests that tumor size influences stage in this as in other types of breast carcinoma. Nonetheless, invasive micropapillary carcinoma appears to have a substantial likelihood of nodal metastasis, local recurrence, and of systemic recurrence (40,42,43,46,50,53).

Staging of the axilla can be achieved with sentinel lymph node mapping. Adjuvant chemotherapy is indicated when there are axillary lymph node metastases and in the absence of lymph node metastases for tumors larger than 1.0 cm. Invasive micropapillary carcinomas smaller than 1.0 cm are exceedingly unusual. The decision to give adjuvant systemic treatment in this latter situation will depend upon the circumstances in the individual case. Postmastectomy chest wall irradiation should be considered, especially for patients with tumors larger than 2 cm or if the tumor is multifocal.

REFERENCES

Mammary Carcinoma with Osteoclast-Like Giant Cells

1. Agnantis NT, Rosen PP. Mammary carcinoma with osteoclast-like giant cells. *Am J Clin Pathol.* 1979;72:383–389.
2. Holland R, Van Haelst VJGM. Mammary carcinoma with osteoclast-like giant cells. Additional observations on six cases. *Cancer.* 1984;53:1963–1973.
3. Nielsen BB, Kiaer HW. Carcinoma of the breast with stromal multinucleated giant cells. *Histopathology.* 1985;9:183–193.
4. Iacocca MV, Maia DM. Bilateral infiltrating lobular carcinoma of the breast with osteoclast-like giant cells. *Breast J.* 2001;7:60–65.
5. Sano M, Kikuchi K, Zhao C, et al. Osteoclastogenesis in human breast carcinoma. *Virchows Arch.* 2004;444:470–472.
6. Jimi E, Nakamura I, Duong LT, et al. Interleukin-1 induces multinucleation and bone-resorbing activity of osteoclasts in the absence of osteoblasts/stromal cells. *Exp Cell Res.* 1999;247:84–93.
7. Krishnan C, Longacre TA. Ductal carcinoma in situ of the breast with osteoclast-like giant cells. *Hum Pathol.* 2006;37:369–372.
8. Ichijima K, Kobashi Y, Ueda Y, Matsuo S. Breast cancer with reactive multinucleated giant cells: report of three cases. *Acta Pathol Jpn.* 1986; 36:449–457.
9. Phillipson J, Ostrzega N. Fine needle aspiration of invasive cribriform carcinoma with benign osteoclastlike giant cells of histiocytic origin. A case report. *Acta Cytol.* 1994;38:479–482.
10. Viacava P, Naccarato AG, Nardini V, Bevilacqua G. Breast carcinoma with osteoclast-like giant cells: immunohistochemical and ultrastructural study of a case and review of the literature. *Tumori.* 1995;81:135–141.

Cribriform Carcinoma

11. Page DL, Dixon JM, Anderson TJ, et al. Invasive cribriform carcinoma of the breast. *Histopathology.* 1983;7:525–536.
12. Marzullo F, Zito FA, Marzullo A, et al. Infiltrating cribriform carcinoma of the breast. A clinico-pathologic and immunohistochemical study of 5 cases. *Eur J Gynaecol Oncol.* 1996;17:228–231.
13. Stutz JA, Evans AJ, Pinder S et al. The radiological appearances of invasive cribriform carcinoma of the breast. *Clin Radiol.* 1994;49:693–695.
14. Venable JG, Schwartz AM, Silverberg SG. Infiltrating cribriform carcinoma of the breast: a distinctive clinicopathologic entity. *Hum Pathol.* 1990; 21:333–338.
15. Wells CA, Ferguson DJP. Ultrastructural and immunocytochemical study of a case of invasive cribriform breast carcinoma. *J Clin Pathol.* 1988; 41:17–20.
16. Shousha S, Schoenfeld A, Moss J, et al. Light and electron microscopic study of an invasive cribriform carcinoma with extensive microcalcification developing in a breast with silicone augmentation. *Ultrastruct Pathol.* 1994; 18:519–523.
17. Rosen PP. Adenoid cystic carcinoma of the breast: a morphologically heterogeneous neoplasm. *Pathol Annu.* 1989;24(pt 2):237–254.

Small Cell (Oat Cell) Carcinoma

18. Wade Jr PM, Mills SE, Read M, et al. Small cell neuroendocrine (oat cell) carcinoma of the breast. *Cancer.* 1983;52:121–125.
19. Francois A, Chatikhine VA, Chevallier B, et al. Neuroendocrine primary small cell carcinoma of the breast. Report of a case and review of the literature. *Am J Clin Oncol.* 1995;18:133–138.
20. Shin SJ, DeLellis RA, Ying L, Rosen PP. Small cell carcinoma of the breast: a clinicopathologic and immunohistochemical study of nine patients. *Am J Surg Pathol.* 2000;24:1231–1239.
21. Hoang MP, Maitra A, Gazdar AF, Albores-Saavedra J. Primary mammary small-cell carcinoma: a molecular analysis of 2 cases. *Hum Pathol.* 2001; 32:753–757.
22. Miremadi A, Pinder SE, Lee AHS, et al. Neuroendocrine differentiation and prognosis in breast adenocarcinoma. *Histopathology.* 2002;40:215–222.
23. Marketsov N, Gilks B, Coldman AJ, et al. Tissue microarray analysis of neuroendocrine differentiation and its prognostic significance in breast cancer. *Hum Pathol.* 2003;34:1001–1008.
24. Mariscal A, Balliu E, Diaz R, et al. Primary oat cell carcinoma of the breast: imaging features. *Am J Roentgenol.* 2004;183:1169–1171.
25. Adegbola T, Connolly CE, Mortimer G. Small cell neuroendocrine carcinoma of the breast: a report of three cases and review of the literature. *J Clin Pathol.* 2005;58:775–778.
26. Pappotti M, Gherardi G, Eusebi V, et al. Primary oat cell neuroendocrine carcinoma of the breast. Report of four cases. *Virchows Arch A Pathol Anat Histopathol.* 1992;420:103–108.

27. Shin SJ, DeLellis RA, Rosen PP. Small cell carcinoma of the breast: additional immunohistochemical studies. *Am J Surg Pathol.* 2001; 25:831–832.
28. Deeley TJ. Secondary deposits in the breast. *Br J Cancer.* 1965;19:738–743.

Lipid-Rich Carcinoma

29. Aboumrad MH, Horn RC, Fine G. Lipid-secreting mammary carcinoma: report of a case associated with Paget's disease of the nipple. *Cancer.* 1963;16:521–525.
30. Ramos CV, Taylor HB. Lipid-rich carcinoma of the breast. A clinicopathologic analysis of 13 examples. *Cancer.* 1974;33:812–819.
31. Van Bogaert L-J, Maldague P. Histologic variants of lipid-secreting carcinoma of the breast. *Virchows Arch (A).* 1977;375:345–353.
32. Mazzella FM, Sieber SC, Braza F. Ductal carcinoma of male breast with prominent lipid-rich component. *Pathology.* 1995;27:280–283.

Glycogen-Rich Carcinoma

33. Fisher ER, Tavares J, Bulatao IS, et al. Glycogen-rich, clear cell breast cancer: with comments concerning other clear cell variants. *Hum Pathol.* 1985;16:1085–1090.
34. Hull MT, Warfel KA. Glycogen-rich clear cell carcinomas of the breast. A clinicopathologic and ultrastructural study. *Am J Surg Pathol.* 1986;10:553–559.
35. Hull MT, Priest JB, Broadie TA, et al. Glycogen-rich clear cell carcinoma of the breast. A light and electron microscopic study. *Cancer.* 1981;48:2003–2009.
36. Sorensen FB, Paulsen SM. Glycogen-rich clear cell carcinoma of the breast: a solid variant with mucus. A light microscopic, immunohistochemical and ultrastructural study of a case. *Histopathology.* 1987;11:843–848.
37. Hayes MMM, Seidman JD, Ashton MA. Glycogen-rich clear cell carcinoma of the breast: a clinicopathologic study of 21 cases. *Am J Surg Pathol.* 1995;19:904–911.
38. Benisch B, Peison B, Newman R, et al. Solid glycogen-rich clear cell carcinoma of the breast (a light and ultrastructural study). *Am J Clin Pathol.* 1983;79:243–245.

Invasive Micropapillary Carcinoma

39. Fisher ER, Palekar AS, Redmond C, et al. Pathologic findings from the National Surgical Adjuvant Breast Project (Protocol No. 4). VI. Invasive papillary cancer. *Am J Clin Pathol.* 1980;73:313–322.
40. Kuroda H, Sakamoto G, Ohnisi K, Itoyama S. Clinical and pathologic features of invasive micropapillary carcinoma. *Breast Cancer.* 2004;11:169–174.
41. Luna-Moré S, Gonzalez B, Acedo C, et al. Invasive micropapillary carcinoma of the breast. A new special type of invasive mammary carcinoma. *Path Res Pract.* 1994;190:668–674.
42. Siriaunkgul S, Tavassoli FA. Invasive micropapillary carcinoma of the breast. *Mod Pathol.* 1993;6:660–662.
43. Pettinato G, Manivel CJ, Panico L, et al. Invasive micropapillary carcinoma of the breast. *Am J Clin Pathol.* 2004;121:857–866.
44. Middleton LP, Tressera F, Sobel ME, et al. Infiltrating micropapillary carcinoma of the breast. *Mod Pathol.* 1999;12:499–504.
45. Guo X, Fan Y, Lang R, et al. Tumor infiltrating lymphocytes differ in invasive micropapillary carcinoma and medullary carcinoma of the breast. *Mod Pathol.* 2008;21:1101–1107.
46. Petersen JL. Breast carcinoma with an unexpected inside out growth pattern, rotation of polarisation associated with angioinvasion. *Path Res Pract.* 1993;189:780.
47. Nassar H, Pansare V, Zhang H, et al. Pathogenesis of invasive micropapillary carcinoma: role of MUC1 glycoprotein. *Mod Pathol.* 2004;17:1045–1050.
48. Adams SA, Smith MEF, Cowley GP, Carr LA. Reversal of glandular polarity in the lymphovascular compartment of breast cancer. *J Clin Pathol.* 2004; 57:1114–1117.
49. Lee AHS, Paish EC, Marchio C, et al. The expression of Wilms' tumor-l and CA125 in invasive micropapillary carcinoma of the breast. *Histopathology.* 2007;51:824–828.
50. Luna-Moré S, de los Santos F, Breton JJ, Canadas MA. Estrogen and progesterone receptors, c-erb-2, p53, and BCL-2 in thirty-three invasive micropapillary breast carcinomas. *Pathol Res Pract.* 1996;192:27–32.
51. Nagi V, Guttman M. Jaffer S, et al. N-cadherin expression in breast cancer: correlation with aggressive histologic variant-invasive micropapillary carcinoma. *Breast Cancer Research and Treat.* 2005;94:225–235.
52. Kim M-J, Gong G, Joo HJ, et al. Immunohistochemical and clinicopathologic characteristics of invasive ductal carcinoma of breast with micropapillary carcinoma component. *Arch Pathol Lab Med.* 2005;129:1277–1282.
53. Acs G, Paragh G, Chuang S-T, et al. The presence of micropapillary features and retraction artifact in needle core biopsy material predicts lymph node metastases in breast carcinoma. *Am J Surg Pathol.* 2009;33:202–210.

Lobular Carcinoma In Situ and Atypical Lobular Hyperplasia

21

LOBULAR CARCINOMA IN SITU

Lobular carcinoma in situ (LCIS) is a microscopic lesion that by itself does not form a palpable tumor and is rarely detectable by mammography. It is typically discovered coincidentally in breast tissue removed for lesions that produce a mass or when processes that cause mammographic abnormalities lead to a biopsy. Calcifications are infrequently formed in LCIS (1), and when calcifications are present in LCIS they are usually associated with an underlying lesion such as sclerosing adenosis. Mammography has not been an effective method for detecting LCIS and cannot be depended upon to assess the multicentricity or bilaterality of the disease (2,3).

An exceptional situation exists in infrequent instances of florid LCIS that can cause marked expansion of ducts and lobules. This condition may be extensive, and it sometimes partially involves sclerosing adenosis. Necrosis and calcification frequently occur in florid LCIS with a pattern and distribution more commonly encountered in intraductal carcinoma or ductal carcinoma in situ (DCIS) (4). Florid LCIS may have classical or pleomorphic cytology. The resultant appearance on mammography is likely to suggest DCIS. The histologic diagnosis of these lesions is sometimes controversial. As discussed below in this chapter, the most compelling evidence supporting classification of these cases as LCIS is the cytologic appearance that is typical of LCIS, coexistent nonflorid LCIS in virtually all cases, association with invasive lobular carcinoma of the usual lobular type and lack of reactivity for E-cadherin.

In retrospective reviews, each involving several thousand breast specimens, the frequency of LCIS was 0.5% to 1.5% (5–7). Analysis of population-based data from 1978 to 1998 in the United States revealed an increase in the incidence rate of LCIS from 0.90 per 100,000 person years to 3.19 per 100,000 person years (8). Incidence rates increased continuously throughout the study period among postmenopausal women with the highest incidence rate among women 50 to 59 years of age in 1996 to 1998 (11.47/100,000 person years). The absence of consistent pathology review creates uncertainty about the reliability of the data, but if it is correct the increasing use of mammography leading to more frequent biopsies would probably be the most important factor responsible for this change. In particular, columnar cell duct hyperplasia, a condition predisposed to develop calcifications so often coexists with LCIS that this association is probably not coincidental (9,10). Columnar cell duct hyperplasia is a frequent benign abnormality responsible for mammographically detected calcifications in the absence of a palpable lesion.

Up to 25% of LCIS patients are postmenopausal when the lobular lesion is identified (11). LCIS occurs infrequently as an isolated lesion in women younger than 35 years or older than 75 years. In a consecutive series of more than 1,000 patients treated for breast carcinoma, the mean age of women with LCIS (53 years) was not significantly different from the mean age of patients who had infiltrating duct carcinoma (57 years) (12). LCIS is associated with a high frequency of multicentric ipsilateral carcinoma, including occult invasive foci in 4% to 6% of women who undergo mastectomy (13,14). The contralateral breast is found to harbor LCIS in 40% of cases when a random biopsy is performed on the opposite breast in the absence of a clinical abnormality (15).

The microscopic anatomic distribution of LCIS in lobules and terminal ducts, and alterations in the morphology of these structures, influence the histopathologic appearance of LCIS in any given case. In the typical lobular form, a population of neoplastic cells replaces the normal epithelium of acini and intralobular ductules (Figs. 21.1 and 21.2). The abnormal cells must be sufficiently numerous to cause expansion of these structures. There may be enlargement of the entire lobule in comparison with uninvolved lobules in the adjacent breast, but lobular enlargement is not an absolute diagnostic criterion. The trend to lobular atrophy in postmenopausal women makes expansion of

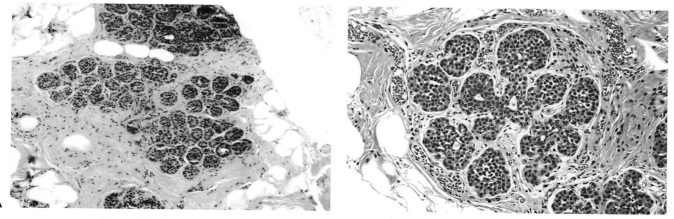

Figure 21.1 Lobular carcinoma in situ (LCIS). The normal lobular epithelium has been replaced by neoplastic cells that fill the acinar lumina in this needle core biopsy specimen. **A:** Two contiguous lobules are affected. The biopsy was performed for mammographically-detected calcifications which were present in lobular glands not involved by in situ carcinoma. **B:** Magnified view of classical LCIS in a lobule.

lobular glands on unreliable diagnostic feature in that patient group (Fig. 21.3). If the diagnosis of LCIS is to be meaningful because it identifies a lesion associated with a substantial risk of later carcinoma, then lobular enlargement cannot be regarded as the paramount diagnostic criterion in lesions that have reached an acceptable qualitative level of cytologic abnormality.

The issue of how much lobular involvement is necessary for the diagnosis of LCIS remains unanswered and is of questionable relevance in the diagnosis of needle core biopsy specimens that provide limited samples. Because the number of affected lobules in a biopsy specimen has not proven to be related to the risk for subsequent carcinoma among patients not treated by mastectomy (2,16), there is presently no reason for drawing a distinction between one and two or more involved lobules as a basis for the diagnosis of LCIS (2) (Fig. 21.4). In some instances, the only evidence of a neoplastic lobular proliferation is one lobule in which some, but not all, of the acini are involved.

At least 75% of one lobule should be involved to establish a diagnosis of LCIS (Fig. 21.5). Specimens with lesser lesions should be included in the category of atypical lobular hyperplasia (ALH).

Loss of cohesion is a characteristic of the neoplastic cells in LCIS, although this is not always readily apparent in acini filled and expanded by the process. When loss of cohesion is prominent and the neoplastic cells have a dissociated distribution, spaces may be created between them that can be mistaken for glandular lumina (Fig. 21.6). Degenerative changes may also disrupt the cellular composition of LCIS. In these situations the neoplastic cells are not arranged in the polarized fashion, which characterizes non-neoplastic cells persisting around true glandular lumina.

Loss of cohesion in lobular neoplastic lesions is largely attributable to genetic alterations in the E-cadherin gene that are manifested by greatly reduced, fragmented or absent membrane E-cadherin immunoreactivity in the neoplastic cells (17,18). Losses in chromosome 16q22.1, the site of the

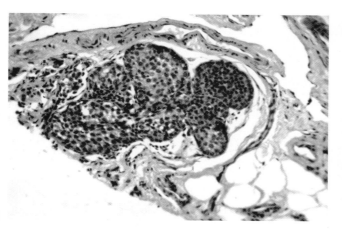

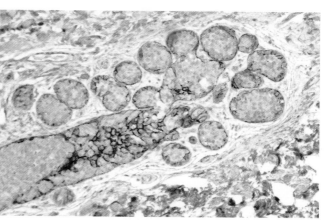

Figure 21.2 Lobular carcinoma in situ. A: A needle core biopsy specimen with a completely involved lobule. **B:** E-cadherin reactivity is present in residual duct epithelium and in lobular myoepithelial cells in this example of LCIS in a terminal duct–lobular unit. The neoplastic cells are not reactive (immunoperoxidase).

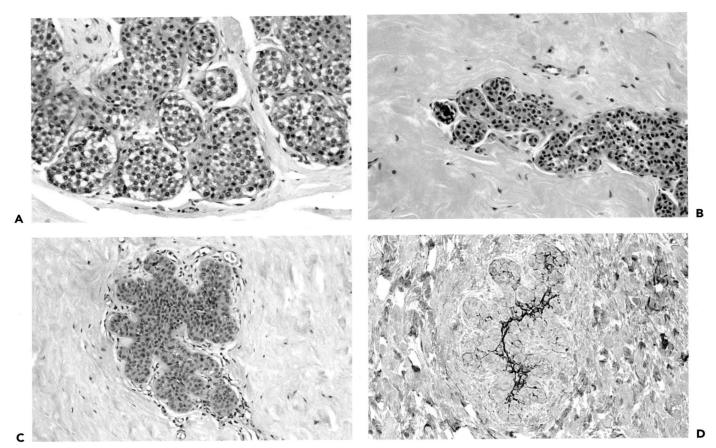

Figure 21.3   Lobular carcinoma in situ. A: LCIS as it appeared when the patient was pre-menopausal. The lobular glands are fully expanded. **B, C:** LCIS as it appeared in a biopsy specimen taken from the same breast after the menopause. The lobules are markedly shrunken. One lobular gland contains a calcification **(B). D:** The lobule shown in **(C)** stained for E-cadherin showing strong reactivity in residual nonneoplastic epithelium and weak, fragmented reactivity in the LCIS. Reactivity is present in residual duct epithelial cells in the center of the ductule. The LCIS cells are E-cadherin negative (immunoperoxidase).

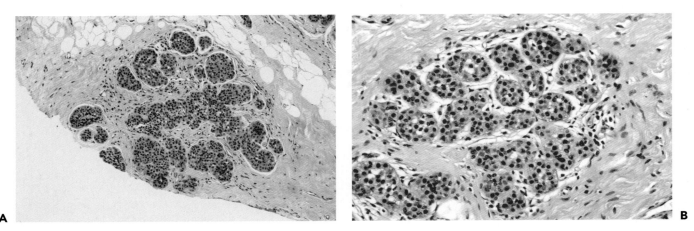

Figure 21.4   Lobular carcinoma in situ. A: The only pathologic lesion in this needle core biopsy specimen is this lobule with LCIS. **B:** This is one of several foci of LCIS found in the subsequent excisional biopsy specimen.

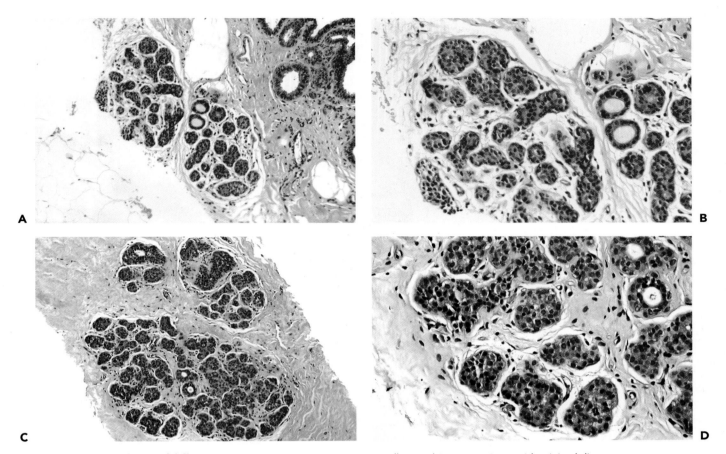

Figure 21.5   Lobular carcinoma in situ. A, B: A needle core biopsy specimen with minimal diagnostic evidence. Approximately 85% of the lobular glands are involved. **C, D:** Another example of minimal evidence for lobular carcinoma **in situ** in a needle core biopsy sample. Note the distinct lobular glands.

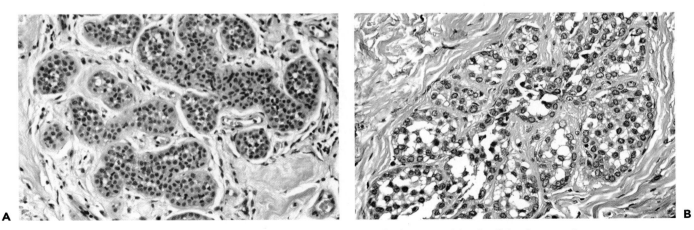

Figure 21.6   Lobular carcinoma in situ. A, B: Loss of cohesion and focal cellular degeneration have resulted in the formation of spaces in some lobular glands. These are not true acinar lumina. Extreme loss of cohesion in LCIS **(B).**

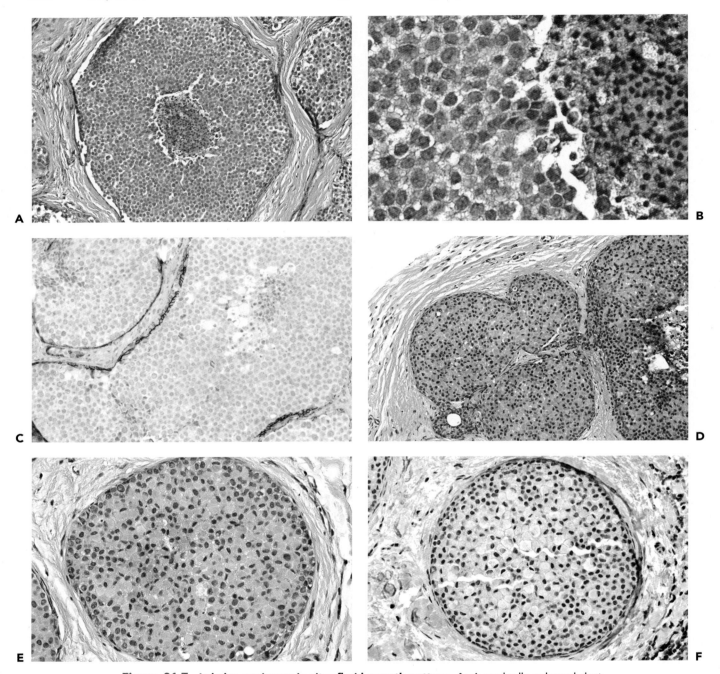

Figure 21.7 Lobular carcinoma in situ, florid growth pattern. A: A markedly enlarged duct is filled with a solid growth of florid, pleomorphic LCIS. Central comedo-type necrosis is evident. **B:** This magnified view of the carcinoma shows necrosis and loss of cohesion between tumor cells. **C:** The LCIS is E-cadherin negative (immunoperoxidase). Reactivity is demonstrated in persisting myoepithelium. **D–F:** Another example of florid LCIS composed of cells with cytoplasmic mucin. The LCIS is E-cadherin negative **(F)** (immunoperoxidase).

E-cadherin gene, are the most common cytogenetic abnormality found in LCIS (19). Despite the high frequency of somatic E-cadherin mutations in LCIS, germ line E-cadherin mutations are rarely detected in these patients (19,20).

Typically, the neoplastic cells in LCIS have scant cytoplasm and small, round, cytologically bland nuclei that lack nucleoli. This cytologic pattern has been referred to as type

A, or classical LCIS (Figs. 21.1, 21.2, and 21.4). When greater cytologic pleomorphism is encountered, the more varied cells have been classified as type B, or pleomorphic LCIS (Fig. 21.7). Pleomorphic LCIS cells have more abundant cytoplasm than cells of the classical type, as well as larger more pleomorphic nuclei that sometimes have prominent nucleoli. The cytologic features of pleomorphic LCIS cells

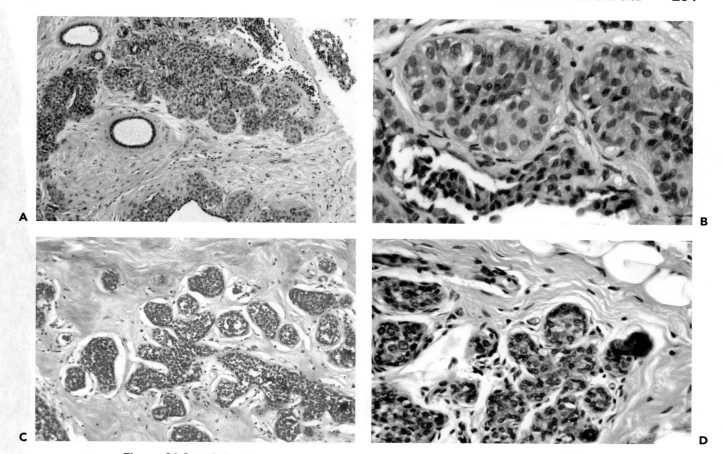

Figure 21.8 Lobular carcinoma in situ. A: The lesion in this needle core biopsy specimen involves lobular glands and a duct. **B:** Intracytoplasmic mucin is stained magenta with the mucicarmine stain. **C, D:** A focus of LCIS with minimal acinar expansion. Intracytoplasmic mucin is demonstrated with the mucicarmine stain **(D).**

in some instances resemble those of ductal carcinoma. When the lesion is composed entirely of pleomorphic LCIS cells, the distinction between pleomorphic LCIS and intralobular extension of DCIS may be difficult to establish. The E-cadherin immunostain is very useful in this situation because greatly reduced, fragmented or absent membrane reactivity is diagnostic of LCIS (21–24) (Fig. 21.7). Some examples of LCIS have classical and pleomorphic cell types, both of which are E-cadherin negative (17). Variable E-cadherin reactivity has been reported when different antibodies were used (24).

Intracytoplasmic vacuoles that contain mucinous secretion are usually present in some cells in LCIS, but the presence of mucin can be an inconspicuous feature that must be highlighted with a mucicarmine or alcian blue periodic acid–Schiff (PAS) stain (25,26) (Fig. 21.8). An extreme manifestation of this phenomenon is the formation of signet ring cells having a distended cytoplasmic vacuole that causes the nucleus to be eccentric or indented. Because intracytoplasmic mucin vacuoles are uncommon in the cells of ductal carcinoma and are virtually absent in hyperplastic lesions of duct or lobular epithelium, their presence is an important but not a necessary criterion for

the diagnosis of LCIS. Intracytoplasmic mucin is also present in LCIS with clear cell change.

Several uncommon cytologic features can be found in LCIS. Cytoplasmic pallor or cytoplasmic clearing occurs rarely in LCIS. These cells may have intracytoplasmic mucin that is not restricted to vacuoles. Apocrine metaplasia has been described in LCIS (27). Mucin in the cytoplasm of cells in apocrine LCIS is usually evident as cytoplasmic amphophilia or basophilia. Apocrine LCIS often has pleomorphic cytology, and it tends to grow in a pagetoid manner in small ducts where it is difficult to distinguish from apocrine DCIS. However, apocrine LCIS is E-cadherin negative, and it is often estrogen receptor (ER) positive, whereas apocrine DCIS is E-cadherin positive and almost always ER negative. LCIS in atrophic lobules and terminal ducts of postmenopausal women sometimes features cells with dark, eosinophilic-to-basophilic cytoplasm and deeply basophilic, eccentric nuclei (Fig. 21.9). This appearance is probably the result of cytoplasmic condensation associated with loss of cohesion and shrinkage of cells. These cells frequently have intracytoplasmic mucin. In another variant, the cells of LCIS have a *mosaic* appearance that results from the presence of distinct cell borders between cells and

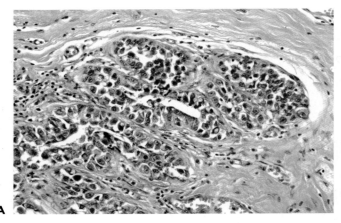
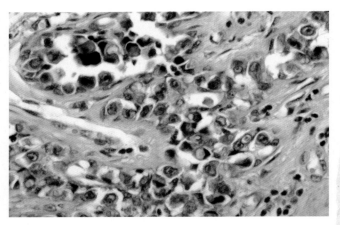

Figure 21.9 **Lobular carcinoma in situ postmenopausal. A, B:** The lesion is characterized by loss of cohesion and shrinkage of the tumor cells in lobular glands. Intracytoplasmic mucin is demonstrated with the mucicarmine stain **(B)**.

prominent, round, centrally placed nuclei surrounded by pale cytoplasm (Fig. 21.10). Intracytoplasmic mucin vacuoles can usually be found in this type of LCIS.

Lobular carcinoma in situ typically involves intralobular and extralobular or terminal ductules as well as acinar units within the lobule. In postmenopausal patients with atrophic lobules, duct involvement may be the only manifestation of LCIS (28). The irregular configuration of ductules affected by LCIS has been described as "saw-toothed" or as resembling a cloverleaf. Pagetoid LCIS cells growing beneath the nonneo-plastic ductal epithelium may be distributed continuously or discontinuously along the ductal system, undermining and ultimately displacing the normal ductal epithelium (Fig. 21.11). The myoepithelial layer is preserved to a variable extent, and it may require p63 and actin immunostains to confirm that it is present. There is also evidence that the cloverleaf pattern sometimes arises de novo in ducts rather than by pagetoid spread (Fig. 21.12). Pagetoid spread of LCIS may also be encountered in papillomas or radial scar lesions. In its most florid form of ductal involvement, LCIS may pro-liferate to form a solid mass of tumor cells that fill and e: pand the duct lumen (Fig. 21.13). Foci such as this ma develop central necrosis and calcifications that are detectabl in mammograms (Fig. 21.7). A negative, weak, or fragmented E-cadherin immunostain distinguishes this florid form of LCIS, from E-cadherin-positive comedo DCIS (21). Florid LCIS with necrosis may consist of classical, pleomorphic or both cell types. In some instances the abundant cytoplasm of pleomorphic LCIS cells has apocrine traits.

An unusual pattern of ductal involvement occurs when LCIS develops in ducts altered by collagenous spherulosis (29). This configuration mimics cribriform DCIS. However, myoepithelial cells outline spherule material that should be distinguished from the true microlumens of cribiform carcinoma. The carcinoma cells in such foci display loss of cohesion and intracytoplasmic vacuoles characteristic of lobular carcinoma. When LCIS involves collagenous spherulosis, myoepithelium can be highlighted with immunostains such as p63 and calponin. The LCIS will be E-cadherin negative.

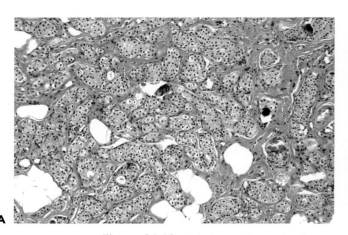
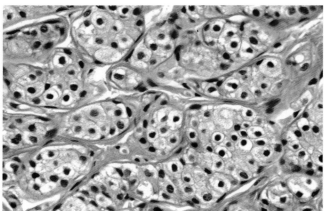

Figure 21.10 **Lobular carcinoma in situ, mosaic pattern. A, B:** The lesion involves sclerosing adenosis. Calcifications are shown in **(A)**. The cells have distinct cytoplasmic borders, abundant pale cytoplasm, and punctate centrally placed nuclei.

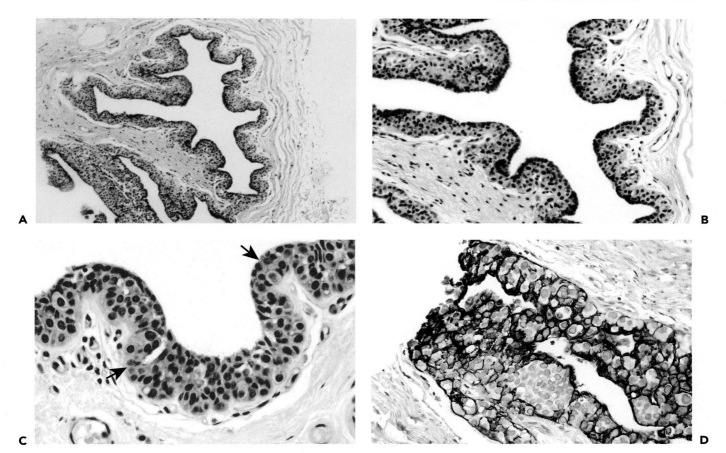

Figure 21.11 **Lobular carcinoma in situ, pagetoid ductal involvement. A, B:** These dilated ducts involved by pagetoid spread of LCIS were found in a needle core biopsy specimen. **C:** Intracytoplasmic mucin is demonstrated with the mucicarmine stain in carcinoma cells *(arrows)* but not in the overlying residual benign ductal epithelium. **D:** Pagetoid LCIS in this duct is highlighted by absence of E-cadherin reactivity. The hyperplastic ductal epithelium is E-cadherin positive (immunoperoxidase).

Two abnormalities in benign epithelium must be considered in the differential diagnosis of pagetoid LCIS: histiocytes in the epithelium and epitheloid myoepithelial cell hyperplasia. When examined at high magnification, intraepithelial histiocytes are found to have abundant foamy cytoplasm, sometimes with lipofuscin or hemosiderin pigment and small dark nuclei. Intracytoplasmic mucin is absent from histiocytes, and they are not immunoreactive for cytokeratin. The overlying nonneoplastic epithelium is attenuated and flattened over intraepithelial histiocytes as well as over pagetoid spread of LCIS. Intraepithelial histiocytes may be relatively sparse, or they may form a continuous layer one or more cells thick.

Epithelioid myoepithelial hyperplasia is more likely to be mistaken for pagetoid spread of LCIS than is the presence of intraepithelial histiocytes. Epithelioid myoepithelial cells have abundant clear vesicular cytoplasm. Except in papillomas, hyperplastic myoepithelial cells tend to be distributed in a single layer causing less attenuation of the overlying epithelium than pagetoid LCIS. Some myoid immunohistochemical properties are usually retained in epithelioid myoepithelial hyperplasia, but occasionally these

cells entirely lack myoid cytoplasmic reactivity. The p63 immunostain is most reliable in this circumstance because nuclear reactivity is retained in epithelioid myoepithelial cells, whereas LCIS cells are p63 negative.

Coexistence of LCIS and DCIS in a single duct is a very unusual phenomenon (Fig. 21.14). When this occurs, the LCIS often grows in a cloverleaf pattern around the perimeter of a duct lumen that contains structurally and cytologically different DCIS. When LCIS and DCIS coexist in a single duct–lobular unit, the LCIS is E-cadherin negative and the DCIS is E-cadherin positive (21).

The E-cadherin immunostain is usually strongly positive in ductal epithelium and lesions that derive from it. Normal and nonneoplastic lobular epithelium is also strongly E-cadherin positive. With rare exceptions, loss of E-cadherin reactivity denotes a lobular neoplastic process. The presence of residual nonneoplastic ductal or lobular epithelial cells or myoepithelial cells is responsible for traces of reactivity that can be found in some lobular neoplastic lesions. In a minority of instances, lobular neoplastic cells display fragmented and discontinuous E-cadherin reactivity that is substantially weaker than reactivity in ductal epithelium (22,30). The

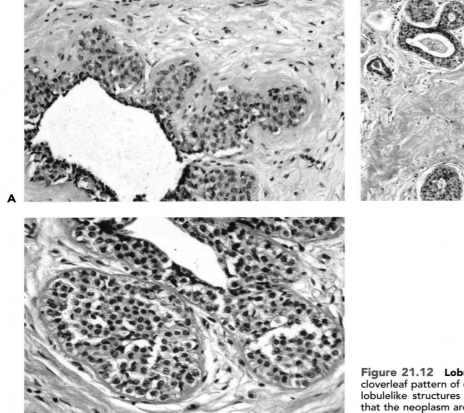

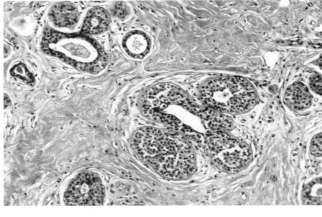

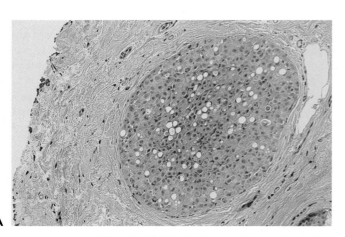

Figure 21.12 **Lobular carcinoma in situ, ductal origin. A:** The cloverleaf pattern of ductal involvement is shown. The presence of lobulelike structures around the perimeter of the duct suggests that the neoplasm arose de novo at this site. **B, C:** This small duct exhibits florid LCIS and pagetoid spread in adjacent ductules.

pattern of E-cadherin reactivity can be influenced by the particular antibody that is used (24).

Lobules structurally altered by various benign proliferative processes can harbor LCIS. As a consequence, LCIS has been encountered in fibroadenomas, sclerosing adenosis, papillary duct hyperplasia, collagenous spherulosis (29), and in radial sclerosing lesions (Fig. 21.15). The diagnosis of LCIS under these circumstances rests largely on the identification of the appropriate cytologic features and absence of E-cadherin reactivity. The demon-

stration of intracytoplasmic mucin droplets is helpful for distinguishing LCIS from florid adenosis because intracellular mucin is present in the former but not in the latter. LCIS in tubular adenosis has a striking histologic appearance (Fig. 21.16). In all of the foregoing situations, the most reliable method for confirming the presence of LCIS is the demonstration of weak, fragmented, or absent E-cadherin reactivity.

The lobular configuration is radically distorted in sclerosing lesions, and as a result it is difficult to exclude invasion

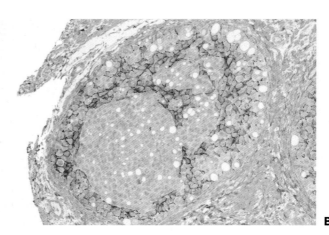

Figure 21.13 **Lobular carcinoma in situ in a duct. A:** A duct occupied by florid pleomorphic LCIS. **B:** E-cadherin reactivity highlights residual ductal epithelial cells. The LCIS cells are E-cadherin negative (immunoperoxidase).

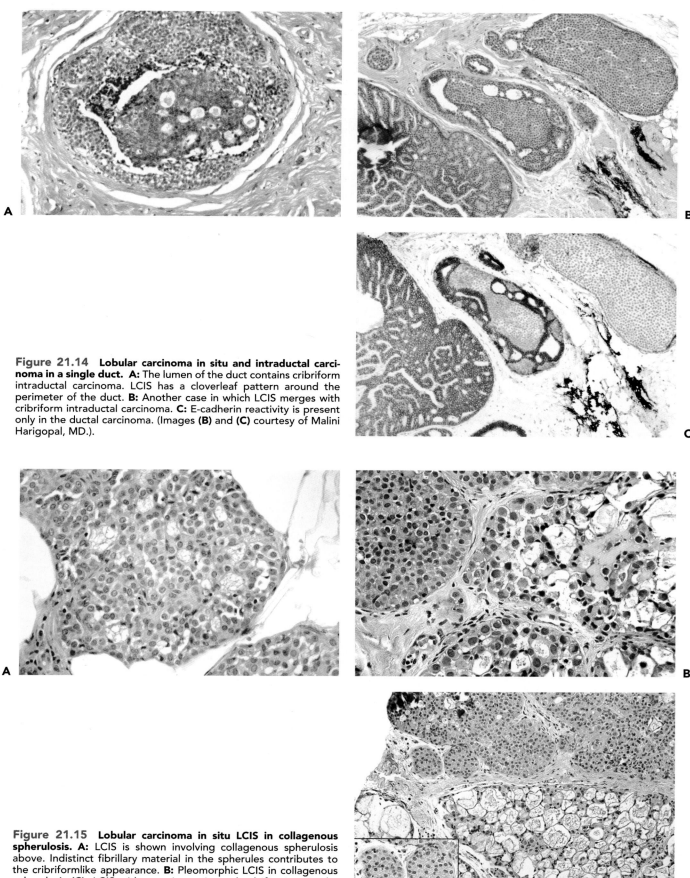

Figure 21.14 **Lobular carcinoma in situ and intraductal carcinoma in a single duct.** **A:** The lumen of the duct contains cribriform intraductal carcinoma. LCIS has a cloverleaf pattern around the perimeter of the duct. **B:** Another case in which LCIS merges with cribriform intraductal carcinoma. **C:** E-cadherin reactivity is present only in the ductal carcinoma. (Images **(B)** and **(C)** courtesy of Malini Harigopal, MD.).

Figure 21.15 **Lobular carcinoma in situ LCIS in collagenous spherulosis.** **A:** LCIS is shown involving collagenous spherulosis above. Indistinct fibrillary material in the spherules contributes to the cribriformlike appearance. **B:** Pleomorphic LCIS in collagenous spherulosis **(C).** LCIS with apocrine traits and calcifications in degenerative collagenous spherulosis. LCIS is shown in the inset.

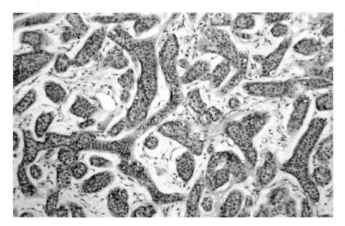

Figure 21.16 Lobular carcinoma in situ in tubular adenosis. LCIS inhabits a network of elongated adenosis tubules.

when LCIS occurs in such foci (31). Careful inspection usually reveals the underlying adenosis pattern in which glandular units are surrounded by a basement membrane, myoepithelial cells and stroma. Basement membrane can be highlighted with the reticulin stain and by the immunohistochemical demonstration of laminin or type IV collagen. Immunostains for p63, CD10, calponin, and actin highlight the myoepithelium. Attenuated, spindle-shaped myoepithelial cells that proliferate in sclerosing adenosis usually persist even when the lesion is colonized by LCIS (32). Invasion is rarely detectable as long as the neoplastic cells remain confined to the configuration of sclerosing adenosis. The diagnosis of invasion is more readily made by finding carcinoma cells without myoepithelial cells in the stroma outside the sclerotic process. The appearance of such invasive foci is no different from that of invasive lobular carcinoma in the absence of a sclerosing lesion. Microinvasive foci are more easily detected and can be highlighted with a cytokeratin immunostain such as CK7 or AE1/AE3.

Most lobules are surrounded by fibrous stroma, but infrequently lobules are distributed in mammary adipose tissue.

Lobules in fat are subject to the same pathologic alterations that occur in parenchymal lobules, including the development of sclerosing adenosis and LCIS. These conditions may resemble invasive carcinoma (Fig. 21.17). Important distinguishing features of LCIS in fat are the presence of well-circumscribed glands containing LCIS and myoepithelial cells. The lobular glandular pattern is lost when classical infiltrating lobular carcinoma involves fat. However, the distinction between LCIS and invasive alveolar lobular carcinoma in fat is sometimes difficult.

With few exceptions, follow-up studies of LCIS have consisted of patients who were biopsied for palpable clinical abnormalities in which LCIS was an incidental finding. The risk associated with not treating LCIS by mastectomy has been estimated in several retrospective studies. The frequency of subsequent carcinoma other than LCIS varies from 12% to 36.4% (1–3,33–37). Studies with longer follow-up tend to report a higher frequency of subsequent carcinoma. When compared with control populations, the relative risk to LCIS patients for the development of carcinoma other than LCIS has been 4.0 to 12.0. In most studies, the risk of subsequent carcinoma was slightly higher in the ipsilateral than in the contralateral breast, although the difference has not been great.

Several studies prospectively assessed the follow-up of patients with LCIS following a surgical biopsy. After approximately 5 years in three studies, subsequent ipsilateral carcinoma other than LCIS developed in 7% to 17% of patients managed by follow-up only (16,38,39). Ottesen et al. (39) evaluated 100 women with a median prospective follow-up of 120 months. Subsequent carcinoma was detected in 18 (18%), consisting of invasive carcinoma in 13 and DCIS in 5. Sixteen carcinomas occurred in the ipsilateral and two in the contralateral breast. The risk of subsequent carcinoma was significantly greater when the initial LCIS had "large" nuclear size when compared with those with "small" nuclear size. The terms *pleomorphic* and *classical LCIS* were not used by these authors, but they are probably equivalent.

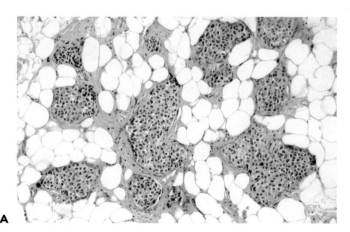

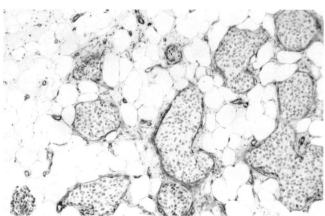

A

B

Figure 21.17 Lobular carcinoma in situ in adenosis. A: Glandular structures occupied by LCIS are shown in fat. This pattern suggests invasive carcinoma. **B:** Each glandular structure is outlined by an actin-positive border indicative of a myoepithelial cell layer. This confirms the in situ nature of the lesion (immunoperoxidase).

In this prospective study, the risk for developing subsequent carcinoma other than LCIS was not significantly related to the number of lobules with LCIS in the initial biopsy.

Zurrida et al. (40) reported the prospective follow-up of 157 patients in whom LCIS was detected in a biopsy performed for a mammographic or palpable lesion. The ipsilateral breast was conserved in 135 cases. After a mean follow-up of 5 years, eight patients (5%) had developed invasive carcinoma. The observed rate of carcinoma in the ipsilateral breast with LCIS (4 carcinomas per 639 person years at risk = 0.00625) was significantly greater ($p < 0.05$) than the expected rate (0.98 carcinomas per 639 person-years at risk = 0.00152), resulting in a relative risk of 4.1 (C.I., 1.1 to 10.5). The person years at risk for carcinoma in either breast was 865, with an expected rate of 0.0015, an observed rate of 0.00925 (8/865), and a relative risk of 5.93 (C.I., 2.6 to 11.7).

Reliable pathologic predictors of increased risk for the subsequent development of carcinoma after LCIS has been diagnosed by needle core or surgical biopsy have not been found. Three studies reported a greater risk in patients with LCIS that contained both classical and pleomorphic cells in comparison with patients who had LCIS with either cell type alone (2,16,33). Increased risk has also been associated with marked lobular distension (16). Lesions with marked duct distension, necrosis, and calcification are special concern because the authors have found an unexpectedly high frequency of microinvasion in such cases. Specimens with these features should be examined carefully with cytokeratin and E-cadherin immunostains accompanied by contemporaneous hematoxylin and eosin (H&E) recuts.

Goldstein et al. (30) conducted a retrospective study of 82 patients with LCIS who did not undergo mastectomy. The actuarial rates for subsequent carcinoma were 7.8% after 10 years of follow-up and 15.4% after 20 years. Six of the subsequent 21 carcinomas (29%) developed 20 or more years after diagnosis. No E-cadherin reactivity was present in 73 LCIS lesions (89%), and 9 had focal weak and discontinuous reactivity. When compared with patients with E-cadherin negative LCIS, the presence of focal E-cadherin reactivity was associated with a higher risk for developing subsequent carcinoma, earlier onset of carcinoma and more frequent ductal carcinoma. This observation based on a small number of cases with focal E-cadherin reactivity remains to be confirmed by other investigators.

The management of a patient with LCIS in a mammographically directed needle core biopsy specimen is a relatively recent concern. Liberman et al. (41) found LCIS as the only neoplastic lesion in 16 (1.2%) of 1,315 consecutive needle core biopsy specimens. Other significant proliferative lesions in the core biopsy specimens with LCIS included "radial scar" in three and atypical ductal hyperplasia in two cases. Subsequent excision revealed DCIS in the region of the LCIS in two cases and infiltrating carcinoma in a third. Florid LCIS involving markedly expanded ducts was present in two core biopsy specimens after which surgery revealed DCIS in one case and invasive carcinoma in the other. Atypical duct hyperplasia accompanied LCIS in another core biopsy specimen that was followed by DCIS at surgery. The authors concluded that surgical biopsy should be performed when a core biopsy specimen contains LCIS accompanied by a "high-risk" proliferative lesion, when florid LCIS resembling DCIS is present or if there is discordance between histologic and imaging findings.

A larger series of patients with LCIS and ALH diagnosed in needle core biopsies performed for mammographic indications was reported by Lechner et al. (42). This multi-institutional study of 32,424 biopsies revealed 89 (0.3%) examples of LCIS. Surgical biopsies were performed on 58 (65%) of the LCIS lesions yielding invasive lobular carcinoma in 8 (14%), invasive duct carcinoma in 2 (3%), tubular carcinoma in 8 (14%), and DCIS in 2 (3%). Thus, 20 of the 89 (22%) patients with LCIS in a core biopsy specimen had intraductal or invasive carcinoma in a subsequent surgical biopsy. Foster et al. (43) described 12 patients with LCIS in a core biopsy specimen who had a surgical excision performed. Four patients (25%) were found to have invasive carcinoma or DCIS. Crisi et al. (44) found invasive carcinoma in two of nine (22%) surgical specimens after a needle core biopsy specimen showed LCIS.

A summary of the foregoing reports and other studies including a total of 140 patients with LCIS diagnosed in a needle core biopsy specimen who underwent surgical biopsy was compiled by Arpino et al. (45). Carcinoma, either intraductal or invasive, was found in 40 (26%). These data support a recommendation to perform a surgical biopsy in most patients after LCIS is detected in a needle core biopsy specimen (46). The final decision for the management of individual patients may be influenced by clinical and radiologic factors. Londero et al. (47) and Brem et al. (48) reported that the likelihood of finding intraductal or invasive carcinoma in a surgical biopsy was greater if the mammogram was classified as BI-RADS 4 or 5 than if it was BI-RADS 3.

Reports of follow-up studies of LCIS diagnosed by needle core biopsy have not identified the LCIS as classical or pleomorphic type, and in some instances they have not clearly distinguished between LCIS and ALH. At this time, a report by Chivukula et al. (49) is the only one to describe a substantial series of patients with pleomorphic LCIS diagnosed by needle core biopsy. In this series of 12 cases, 11 (92%) were ER positive, 6 (50%) were progesterone receptor (PR) positive, 3 (25%) were HER2/*neu* positive and all were E-cadherin negative. Subsequent surgical excisions revealed residual pleomorphic LCIS in 10 (83%) and invasive lobular carcinoma in 3 (25%). One invasive carcinoma was classified as classical, one as pleomorphic, and one as classical/pleomorphic.

ATYPICAL LOBULAR HYPERPLASIA

There are no specific clinical features associated with the diagnosis of ALH. The clinical indications for biopsy are the same as those that lead to the detection of LCIS: a palpable lesion or a mammographic abnormality. ALH is

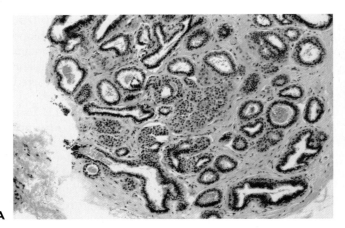
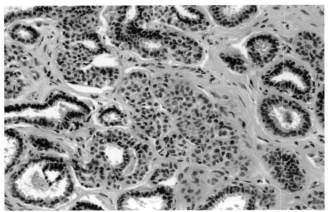

Figure 21.18   Atypical lobular hyperplasia. A, B: A needle core biopsy specimen obtained for calcifications revealed tubular carcinoma. One of the additional tissue samples had this focus of atypical lobular hyperplasia in adenosis.

usually an incidental finding not specifically associated with the abnormality that prompted the biopsy (Fig. 21.18).

The glandular proliferation in ALH has some features of LCIS, but they are not sufficiently developed to qualify for the latter diagnosis. There are no universally accepted criteria for the precise distinction between ALH and LCIS. Qualitative and quantitative factors must be considered. The cells that form ALH are E-cadherin negative.

Quantitative criteria for the diagnosis of LCIS influence the distribution of cases classified as ALH. The diagnosis of ALH is made if less than 75% of the only affected lobule shows the features of LCIS (Figs. 21.19 and 21.20). ALH is characterized by the presence, within one or more lobules, of abnormal cells similar to those found in LCIS. In the least conspicuous configuration, these cells replace a portion of the normal lobular glandular epithelium, effacing some lumina. Acinar units are not enlarged at this proliferative level (Fig. 21.21). As the process evolves, the accumulation of a greater number of cells causes progressive acinar expansion, but the borders of individual acinar units and intralobular ductules remain indistinct

in ALH (Fig. 21.22). Clear delineation of intralobular acinar units filled by the abnormal cell population is an important feature that characterizes LCIS and reflects the accumulation of enough neoplastic cells to cause the individual glands to have a distinct configuration.

Similar criteria apply to the diagnosis of lobular proliferations in terminal duct structures. These alterations tend to occur around rather than in the duct lumen, creating a cloverleaf pattern similar to LCIS (Figs. 21.22 and 21.23). The peripheral lobulelike bulges are sometimes inhabited by a mixture of normal and neoplastic cells. ALH of terminal ducts may also occur in a solid form that develops when the neoplastic growth is distributed in a continuous layer around the duct lumen. ALH is E-cadherin negative, a property it shares with LCIS (50).

Estimates of the risk for subsequent carcinoma in women with ALH are clouded by the absence of a clear definition for this lesion. Some investigators who did not distinguish between ALH and LCIS have reported relative risk estimates for both lesions under the heading of lobular neoplasia (33,34). The relative risk for

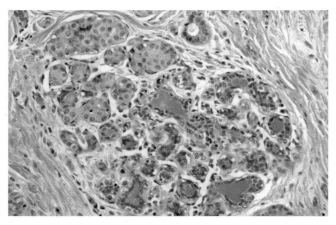
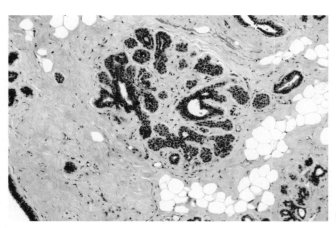

Figure 21.19   Atypical lobular hyperplasia. A, B: Examples of partially involved lobules that qualify as atypical lobular hyperplasia found in needle core biopsy specimens.

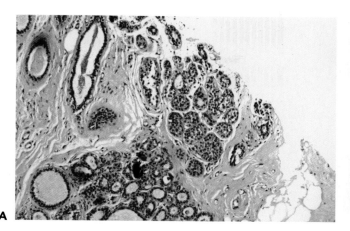
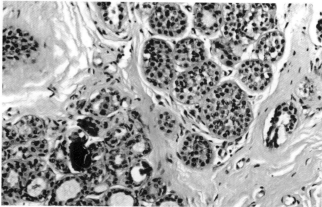

Figure 21.20 Atypical lobular hyperplasia. A, B: One partially involved lobule is present at the edge of this needle core biopsy specimen. The procedure was performed for calcifications that were present in sclerosing adenosis next to the atypical lobular hyperplasia in a premenopausal patient.

developing carcinoma after the finding of ALH is three to four times the expected frequency when compared to age-matched controls (35,36). The risk is higher in women with a family history of breast carcinoma, when there is ductal involvement by the ALH (51), and when there is coexistent atypical duct hyperplasia (36).

There is no consensus as to the optimal management of patients with ALH diagnosed by a needle core biopsy procedure. Lechner et al. (42) reported the results of a multi-institutional study that included 154 (0.5%) instances of ALH in 32,424 needle core biopsy specimens. Surgical biopsies performed in 84 cases of ALH (55%) revealed invasive lobular carcinoma in 3 (4%) and DCIS in 4 (5%) for a total yield of 9 (11%) carcinomas.

A review of 6,081 consecutive breast needle core biopsy procedures performed at 2 institutions uncovered 20 (0.3%) cases of ALH (43). Surgical biopsies performed in 14 cases revealed DCIS in 2. The six patients

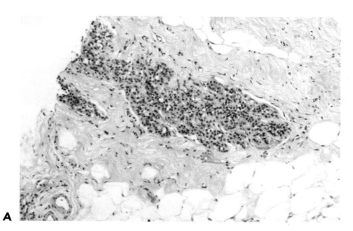
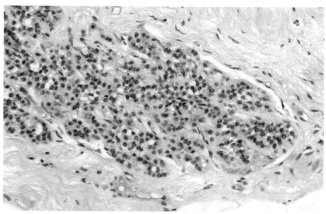
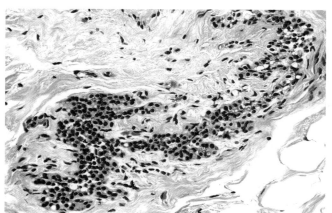

Figure 21.21 Atypical lobular hyperplasia. A, B: Atypical lobular hyperplasia in this needle core biopsy specimen involves an atrophic terminal duct–lobular unit from a postmenopausal woman. **C:** Another example of atypical lobular hyperplasia in an atrophic terminal duct–lobular unit.

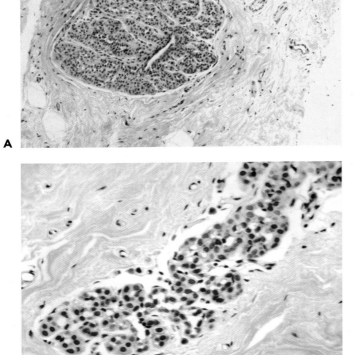

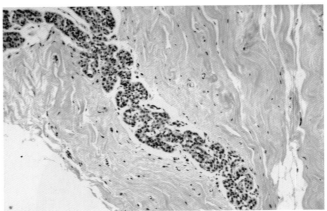

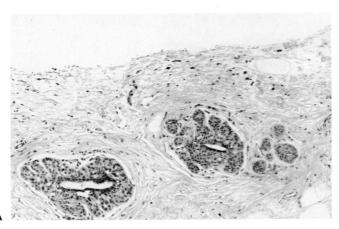

Figure 21.22 Atypical lobular hyperplasia, ductal involvement. A: A duct with the cloverleaf pattern cut transversely. **B, C:** Atypical lobular hyperplasia in a duct from a post menopausal patient cut in a longitudinal plane. Note the indistinct borders of the involved glands.

who did not have a surgical biopsy had not developed clinical evidence of carcinoma after a mean follow-up of 36 months.

Arpino et al. (45) reviewed 16 studies of patients with ALH diagnosed by needle core biopsy, included the foregoing reports. A total of 184 women had subsequent surgical excisions that revealed either intraductal or invasive carcinoma in 30 (16%). The frequency of carcinoma detected in these excisions was somewhat lower than for LCIS, but not inconsequential.

Surgical biopsy is not indicated in all cases on the basis of a diagnosis of ALH that is not accompanied by atypical duct hyperplasia. However, the final management decision should take into consideration the mammographic indications for the needle core biopsy procedure, clinical information, and physical exam findings.

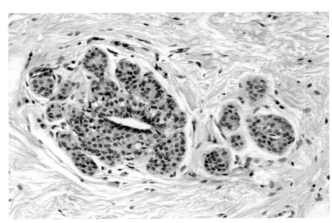

Figure 21.23 Atypical lobular hyperplasia. A, B: The lobular–terminal duct unit on the lower left in **(A)** shows atypical hyperplasia with a cloverleaf pattern. The unit on the right has a more distinct lobular pattern which approaches lobular carcinoma in situ.

IS LCIS A MARKER LESION OR A PRECUSOR TO INVASIVE CARCINOMA?

LCIS is a morphologically and clinically heterogeneous disease. The concept that LCIS is simply a "marker" lesion has been widely promulgated. The impression created by this idea is that LCIS is a proliferative abnormality associated with an increased risk for the development of breast carcinoma but, in contrast to DCIS, LCIS does not progress to invasive carcinoma. This misperception is unfortunate. Data set forth in this chapter support the conclusion that LCIS is a direct precursor to invasive lobular carcinoma, and possibly in a minority of instances to invasive duct carcinoma (e.g., ductolobular and tubulolobular), but that this progression is not observed in the lifetime of every patient with LCIS.

The data most closely linking LCIS to invasive lobular carcinoma come from molecular studies of the two lesions when they coexist. For example, Vos et al. (17) demonstrated that LCIS and invasive lobular carcinomas had losses of the same alleles in 16q22.1 and the same E-cadherin mutations. Similar results were obtained by Sarrió et al. (52) who found that coincidental LCIS and invasive lobular carcinomas shared the same E-cadherin mutations and the same distribution of loss of heterozygosity. Additional supporting studies were published by Nayar et al. (53) and Hwang (54).

It appears that progression of LCIS to the invasive phenotype is less frequent and that on average it takes longer than is the case for DCIS. LCIS and DCIS coexist in a substantial number of patients. It is not surprising that such patients might develop invasive ductal carcinoma sooner and therefore more frequently than invasive lobular carcinoma. This phenomenon most likely reflects differences in the rates of progression of the two diseases so that the earlier appearance of invasive ductal carcinoma results in treatment before the LCIS has had an opportunity to evolve into invasive lobular carcinoma.

LCIS is a heterogeneous disease cytologically and structurally. The relationships of these differences to prognosis or to the risk of progression have not been well characterized. Perhaps the greatest challenge to regarding LCIS as a "marker" lesion has come from the recent recognition of the florid and pleomorphic variants of LCIS characterized by marked gland expansion with a tendency to necrosis and calcification. Contrary to the widely held perception that LCIS is not detected by mammography except as an incidental lesion, the florid form of LCIS is likely to present with calcifications and a pattern that resembles DCIS. The paradigm of LCIS as an incidental "marker" lesion does not fit well with this clinical presentation and the histopathologic findings. On the basis of limited published and, admittedly anecdotal personal, observations, including a number of instances of microinvasive lobular carcinoma that arose in florid and/or pleomorphic LCIS, the authors are of the opinion that pleomorphic and florid forms of LCIS might in some cases be treated as if they were DCIS, at least with respect to local surgical control in the conserved breast. The effectiveness of radiotherapy for treating any of these forms of LCIS has not been determined.

REFERENCES

1. Hutter RVP, Snyder RE, Lucas J, et al. Clinical and pathologic correlation with mammographic findings in lobular carcinoma in situ. *Cancer.* 1969;23:826–839.
2. Mackaren G, Yacoub LK, Lee AKC, et al. Effects of screening on detection of lobular carcinoma in situ of the breast: nonspecificity of mammography and physical examination. *Breast Dis.* 1994;7:339–345.
3. Morris DM, Walker AP, Cocker DC. Lack of efficacy of xeromammography in preoperatively detecting lobular carcinoma in situ of the breast. *Breast Cancer Res Treat.* 1982;1:365–368.
4. Fadare O, Dadmanesh F, Alvarado-Cabrero I, et al. Lobular intraepithelial neoplasia (lobular carcinoma in situ) with comedo-type necrosis. A clinicopathologic study of 18 cases. *Am J Surg Pathol.* 2006;30:1445–1453.
5. Andersen J. Lobular carcinoma in situ: a long-term follow-up in 52 cases. *Acta Pathol Microbiol Scand Sect A.* 1974;82:519–533.
6. Rosen PP, Lieberman PH, Braun DW Jr, et al. F. Lobular carcinoma in situ of the breast. Detailed analysis of 99 patients with average follow-up of 24 years. *Am J Surg Pathol.* 1978;2:225–251.
7. Page DL, Kidd TE Jr, Dupont WD, et al. Lobular neoplasia of the breast: higher risk for subsequent invasive cancer predicted by more extensive disease. *Hum Pathol.* 1991;22:1232–1239.
8. Li CI, Anderson BO, Daling JR, Moe RE. Changing incidence of lobular carcinoma in situ of the breast. *Breast Cancer ResTreat.* 2002;75:259–268.
9. Rosen PP. Columnar cell hyperplasia is associated with lobular carcinoma in situ and tubular carcinoma. *Am J Surg Pathol.* 1999;23:1561.
10. Carley AM, Chivukula M, Carter GJ, et al. Frequency and clinical significance of simultaneous association of lobular neoplasia and columnar cell alterations in breast tissue specimens. *Am J Clin Pathol.* 2008;130:254–258.
11. Rosen PP, Senie R, Ashikari R, Schottenfeld D. Age, menstrual status, and exogenous hormone usage in patients with lobular carcinoma in situ (LCIS). *Surgery.* 1979;85:219–224.
12. Rosen PP, Lesser ML, Senie RT, Duthie, KJ. Epidemiology of breast carcinoma IV: age and histologic tumor type. *J Surg Oncol.* 1982;19:44–47.
13. Shah JP, Rosen PP, Robbins GF. Pitfalls of local excision in the treatment of carcinoma of the breast. *Surg Gynecol Obstet.* 1973;136:721–725.
14. Carter D, Smith AL. Carcinoma in situ of the breast. *Cancer.* 1977;40:1189–1193.
15. Urban JA. Biopsy of the "normal" breast in treating breast cancer. *Surg Clin North Amer.* 1969;49:291–301.
16. Fisher ER, Costantino J, Fisher B, et al. Five-year observations concerning lobular carcinoma in situ. [For the National Surgical Adjuvant Breast and Bowel Project Collaborating Investigators. Pathologic findings from the National Surgical Adjuvant Breast Project (NSABP) Protocol B-17.] *Cancer.* 1996;78:1403–1416.
17. Vos CB, Cleton-Jones AM, Berx G, et al. E-cadherin in-activation in lobular carcinoma in situ of the breast: an early event in tumor genesis. *Br J Cancer.* 1997;76:1131–1133.
18. Moll R, Mitze M, Frixen UH, et al. Differential loss of E-cadherin expression in infiltrating ductal and lobular carcinomas. *Am J Pathol.* 1993;143:1737–1742.
19. Etzell JE, DeVries S, Chew K, et al. Loss of chromosome 16q in lobular carcinoma in situ. *Hum Pathol.* 2001;32:292–296.
20. Rahman N, Stone JG, Coleman G, et al. Lobular carcinoma in situ of the breast is not caused by constitutional mutations in the E-cadherin gene. *Br J Cancer.* 2000;82:568–570.
21. Acs G, Lawton TJ, Rebbeck TR, et al. Differential expression of E-cadherin in lobular and ductal neoplasms of the breast and its biological and diagnostic implications. *Am J Clin Pathol.* 2001;115:85–89.
22. Goldstein NS, Bassi D, Watts JC, et al. E-cadherin reactivity of 95 noninvasive ductal and lobular lesions of the breast. Implications for the interpretation of problematic lesions. *Am J Clin Pathol.* 2001;115:534–542.
23. Jacobs TW, Pliss N, Kouria G, Schnitt SJ. Carcinomas in situ of the breast with indeterminate features. Role of E- cadherin staining in categorization. *Am J Surg Pathol.* 2001;25:229–236.
24. Choi YJ, Pinto MM, Hao L, Riba AK. Interobserver variability and aberrant E-cadherin immunostaining of lobular neoplasia and infiltrating lobular carcinoma. *Mod Pathol.* 2008;21:1224–1237.
25. Andersen JA, Vendelhoe ML. Cytoplasmic mucous globules in lobular carcinoma in situ. Diagnosis and prognosis. *Am J Surg Pathol.* 1981;5:251–255.
26. Gad A, Azzopardi JG. Lobular carcinoma of the breast: a special variant of mucin secreting carcinoma. *J Clin Pathol.* 1975;28:711–716.
27. Chen Y, Fitzgibbons P, Jacobs T, et al. Pleomorphic apocrine lobular carcinoma in situ (PALCIS): phenotypic and genetic study of a distinct variant of lobular carcinoma in situ (LCIS). *Mod Pathol.* 2005;18(suppl.):29A.
28. Haagensen CD, Lane N, Lattes R. Neoplastic proliferation of the epithelium of the mammary lobules: adenosis, lobular neoplasia and small cell carcinoma. *Surg Clin North Amer.* 1972;52:497–524.
29. Sgroi D, Koerner FC. Involvement of collagenous spherulosis by lobular carcinoma in situ. Potential confusion with cribriform ductal carcinoma in situ. *Am J Surg Pathol.* 1995;19:1366–1370.

30. Goldstein NS, Kestin LL, Vicini FA. Clinicopathologic implications of E-cadherin reactivity in patients with lobular carcinoma in situ of the breast. *Cancer.* 2001;92:738–747.

31. Fechner RE. Lobular carcinoma in situ in sclerosing adenosis. A potential source of confusion with invasive carcinoma. *Am J Surg Pathol.* 1981;5:233–239.

32. Oberman HA, Markey BA. Noninvasive carcinoma of the breast presenting in adenosis. *Mod Pathol.* 1991;4:31–35.

33. Haagensen CD, Lane N, Lattes R, Bodian C. Lobular neoplasia (so-called lobular carcinoma in situ) of the breast. *Cancer.* 1978;42:737–769.

34. Bodian CA, Perzin KH, Lattes R, et al. Prognostic significance of benign proliferative breast disease. *Cancer.* 1993;71:3896–3907.

35. Page DL, Dupont WD, Rogers LW, Rados MS. Atypical hyperplastic lesions of the female breast. A long-term follow-up study. *Cancer.* 1985;55:2698–2708.

36. Page DL, Schuyler PA, Dupont WD, et al. Atypical lobular hyperplasia as a unilateral predictor of breast cancer risk: a retrospective cohort study. *Lancet.* 2003;361:125–129.

37. Bodian CA, Perzin KH, Lattes R. Lobular neoplasia. Long term risk of breast cancer and relation to other factors. *Cancer.* 1996;78:1024–1034.

38. Ciatto S, Cataliotti C, Cardona G, Bianchi S. Risk of infiltrating breast cancer subsequent to lobular carcinoma in situ. *Tumori.* 1992;78:244–246.

39. Ottesen GL, Graversen HP, Blichert-Toft M, et al. Lobular carcinoma in situ of the female breast. Short-term results of a prospective nationwide study. *Am J Surg Pathol.* 1993;17:14–21.

40. Zurrida S, Bartoli C, Galimberti V, et al. Interpretation of the risk associated with the unexpected finding of lobular carcinoma in situ. *Ann Surg Oncol.* 1996;3:57–61.

41. Liberman L, Sama M, Susnik B, et al. Lobular carcinoma in situ at percutaneous breast biopsy: surgical biopsy findings. *Am J Roentgenol.* 1999;173:291–299.

42. Lechner MD, Park SL, Jackman RJ, et al. Lobular carcinoma in situ and atypical lobular hyperplasia at percutaneous biopsy with surgical correlation: multi-institutional study. *Radiology.* 1999;213:106.

43. Foster MC, Helvie MA, Gregory NE, et al. Lobular carcinoma in situ or atypical lobular hyperplasia at core-needle biopsy: is excisional biopsy necessary? *Radiology.* 2004;231:813–819.

44. Crisi GM, Mandavilli S, Cronin E, Ricci A Jr. Invasive mammary carcinoma after immediate and short-term follow-up for lobular neoplasia on core biopsy. *Am J Surg Pathol.* 2003;27:325–333.

45. Arpino G, Allred DC, Mohsin SK, et al. Lobular neoplasia on core-needle biopsy-clinical significance. Cancer 2004;101:242–250.

46. Cohen MA. Cancer upgrades at excisional biopsy after diagnosis of atypical lobular hyperplasia or lobular carcinoma in situ at core-needle core biopsy: Some reasons why. *Radiology.* 2004;231:671–621.

47. Londero V, Zuiani C, Linda A, et al. Lobular neoplasia: core needle breast biopsy underestimation of malignancy in relation to radiologic and pathologic features. *The Breast.* 2008;17:623–630.

48. Brem RF, Lechner MC, Jackman RJ, et al. Lobular neoplasia at percutaneous breast biopsy: variables associated with carcinoma at surgical excision. *Am J Roentgenol.* 2008;190:637–641.

49. Chivukula M, Haynik DM, Brufsky A, et al. Pleomorphic lobular carcinoma in situ (PLCIS) on breast core needle biopsies. Clinical significance and immunoprofile. *Am J Surg Patho.* 2008;32:1721–1726.

50. Mastracci TL, Tjan S, Ban AL, et al. E-cadherin alterations in atypical lobular hyperplasia and lobular carcinoma in situ of the breast. *Mod Pathol,* 2005;18:741–751.

51. Page DL, Dupont WD, Rogers LW. Ductal involvement by cells of atypical lobular hyperplasia in the breast: a long-term follow-up study of cancer risk. *Hum Pathol.* 2003;34:201–207.

52. Sarrió D, Moreno-Bueno G, Hardisson E, et al. Epigenetic and genetic alterations of APC and CDH1 genes in lobular breast cancer: relationships with abnormal E-cadherin and catenin expression and microsatellite instability. *Int J Cancer.* 2003;106:208–215.

53. Nayar R, Zhuang Z, Merino MJ, Silverberg SG. Loss of heterozygosity on chromosome 11q13 in lobular lesions of the breast using microdissection and polymerase chain reaction. *Hum Pathol.* 1996;28:277–282.

54. Hwang ES, Nyante SJ, Chen YY, et al. Clonality of lobular carcinoma in situ and synchronous invasive lobular carcinoma. *Cancer.* 2004;100:2562–2572.

Invasive Lobular Carcinoma

22

When the diagnosis is restricted to tumors with the so-called classic histologic appearance, less than 5% of carcinomas qualify for a diagnosis of invasive lobular carcinoma (1–3). If the classification is broadened to include variant forms, the frequency of invasive lobular carcinoma has reportedly been as high as 10% to 14% of invasive carcinomas (4–6). Invasive lobular carcinoma occurs throughout virtually the entire age range of breast carcinoma in adult women (28–86 years). Most studies have placed the median age at diagnosis between 45 and 56 years (2,3,5–7). Invasive lobular carcinoma is relatively more common among women older than 75 years (11%) than in women 35 years or younger. A population-based study of women with invasive breast carcinoma diagnosed from 1987 through 1999 revealed that the incidence rate of lobular carcinoma increased during this period (8). The increased incidence rate of invasive lobular carcinoma was greatest in women 50 years of age or older. On the other hand, the incidence rate for invasive ductal carcinoma was relatively constant. In the absence of a systematic pathology review, these data have marginal reliability.

The presenting symptom in almost all patients is a mass, often with ill-defined margins. In some cases, the only evidence of the neoplasm is vague thickening or fine diffuse nodularity of the breast. Invasive lobular carcinoma is not prone to form calcifications, but they may be present coincidentally in benign proliferative lesions such as sclerosing adenosis (9). A lower frequency of calcifications detected by mammography has been reported in invasive lobular carcinomas than in duct carcinomas (10–12). One exception is invasive lobular carcinoma arising in florid or pleomorphic lobular carcinoma in situ with comedonecrosis and calcifications in ducts (see Chapter 21).

In a screening situation, invasive lobular carcinoma was found more often clinically during intervals between examinations than by mammography (13).

The mammographic estimate of tumor size tends to be less than the grossly measured size (14). Rodenko et al. (15) found that magnetic resonance imaging (MRI) was more effective than mammography in a significant proportion of cases for determining the extent of a primary invasive lobular carcinoma, but the presence of metastatic carcinoma in axillary lymph nodes was not detected in four cases examined. Yeh et al. (16) reported that tumor morphology seen on MRI combined with quantitative measurement of gadolinium uptake was effective for detecting invasive lobular carcinoma in most cases. However, in the absence of an enhancing mass, this type of carcinoma might not be detectable by MRI. Ultrasonography has been useful for detecting multifocal and multicentric invasive lobular carcinoma (17), and it may be more accurate than mammography for predicting tumor size (18). Selinko et al. (19) reported that the sensitivity of sonography for detecting invasive lobular carcinoma (98%) was substantially higher than the sensitivity of mammography (65%).

The most common mammographic manifestation of invasive lobular carcinoma is an asymmetric, ill-defined or irregular, spiculated mass (9,10,12,20). In one study, 46% of mammograms from patients who ultimately proved to have invasive lobular carcinoma were initially reported to be negative (11). The absence of well-defined margins and, in some cases, a tendency to form multiple small nodules throughout the breast are features that may hinder the radiologic detection of invasive lobular carcinoma and lead to a false-negative mammogram interpretation. Patients with a spiculated invasive lobular carcinoma are less likely to have residual carcinoma when re-excision is performed than are those with ill-defined or asymmetric lesions (20). A minority of invasive lobular carcinomas are mammographically round or oval tumors (21).

Patients with invasive lobular carcinoma are reported to have a relatively high frequency of bilateral carcinoma when compared with women who have other types of carcinoma (22–24). The reported relative risk for contralateral carcinoma in women with invasive lobular carcinoma when compared with those with ductal carcinoma ranged from 1.6 to 2 (25,26). Prior and concurrent contralateral carcinomas have been described in 6% to 28% of cases (5,7,27). The reported incidence of subsequent contralateral carcinoma ranges from 1.0 (27,28) to 2.38 (29) per 100 women per year. There is some evidence that the frequency of bilaterality is higher in patients with classical invasive lobular carcinoma than in patients with variant

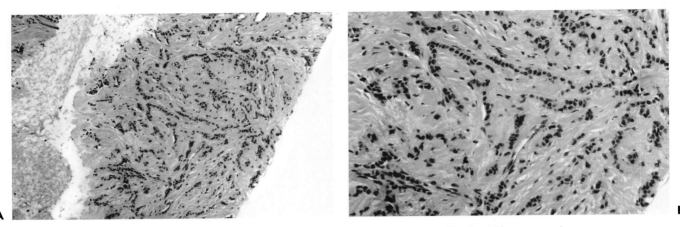

Figure 22.1 Invasive lobular carcinoma, classic type. A, B: The small cells with scant cytoplasm and dark, homogeneous nuclei are arranged in a linear pattern in this needle core biopsy specimen.

subtypes (29). A lobular component has been found in the majority of synchronous or metachronous contralateral carcinomas, and at least 50% of these have been invasive (7,27,28). In one series, random concurrent contralateral biopsies in 108 patients revealed intraductal carcinoma in 6% and invasive carcinoma in 10% of patients (30). Biopsies performed for clinical indications in an additional 22 cases yielded intraductal carcinoma in 5% and invasive carcinoma in 32%. The probability of detecting contralateral invasive carcinoma was significantly greater in women who had multicentric invasive lobular carcinoma in the ipsilateral breast or who had ipsilateral lymph node metastases.

Several growth patterns may be encountered in lesions classified as classical or pure invasive lobular carcinoma. The common denominator is the virtual absence of solid, alveolar, papillary, and gland-forming aggregates of cells. In the two-dimensional plane of a histologic section, the slender strands of cells are arranged in a linear fashion, one or two cells across (Fig. 22.1). If the tumor cells are arranged around ducts and lobules in a concentric fashion, the distribution is described as having a targetoid appearance (Fig. 22.2). In a minority of cases, the linear

strand-forming pattern is not conspicuous, and the tumor cells tend to grow mainly in dispersed, disorderly foci (Fig. 22.3). The small tumor cells in such foci may be mistaken for lymphocytes or plasma cells in areas of fibrosis or in fat when sections are examined at low magnification especially in a frozen section or in a needle core biopsy specimen (Figs. 22.4 and 22.5). Invasive lobular carcinoma is only rarely accompanied by a notable lymphocytic reaction (Fig. 22.6). The term "lymphoepithelioma-like carcinoma" has been applied to an invasive lobular carcinoma with prominent lymphocytic reaction (31). One tumor proved to be negative for Epstein–Barr virus.

Tumors with the cytologic features of invasive lobular carcinoma and substantial elements of nonlinear growth have been referred to as "variant" forms of invasive lobular carcinoma (2,5,6). Areas of classical invasive lobular carcinoma with a linear pattern are found in most variant forms, but they will not necessarily be present in a needle core biopsy specimen. These carcinomas are composed of cells with the cytologic features typically found in classical invasive lobular carcinoma (6). Solid, tubular, trabecular, and alveolar variants have been described, extending the

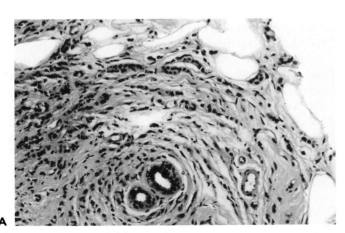
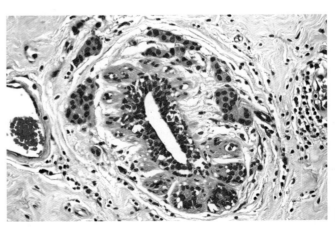

Figure 22.2 Invasive lobular carcinoma, classic type with targetoid growth. A, B: The linear infiltrates of carcinoma cells are distributed circumferentially around ducts.

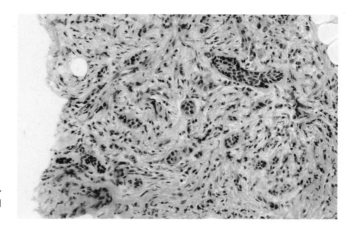

Figure 22.3   Invasive lobular carcinoma, classic type. The linear growth pattern is obscured by stromal reaction around a terminal duct and lobular glands in this needle core biopsy specimen.

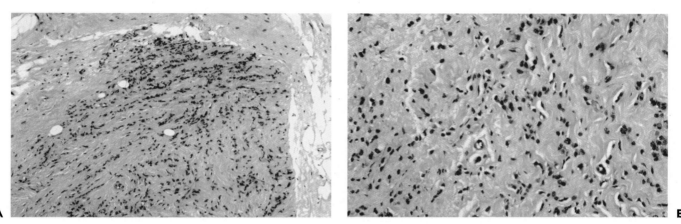

Figure 22.4   Invasive lobular carcinoma obscured by fibrosis.   A, B: The small invasive carcinoma cells in this needle core biopsy specimen are obscured by dense fibrosis and a subtle form of pseudoangiomatous stromal hyperplasia. The specimen was obtained from an area of increased density found by mammography at the site of prior breast conservation therapy for infiltrating duct carcinoma.

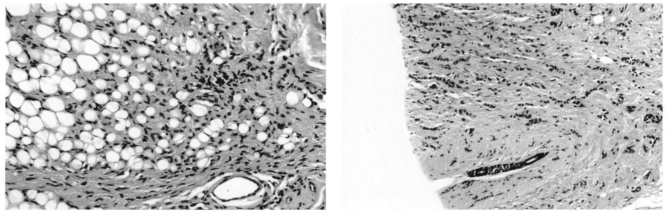

Figure 22.5   Invasive lobular carcinoma obscured by fat. A: Carcinoma cells infiltrating fat in this needle core biopsy specimen create an appearance that superficially resembles fat necrosis. **B:** Another portion of the specimen contained classic invasive lobular carcinoma.

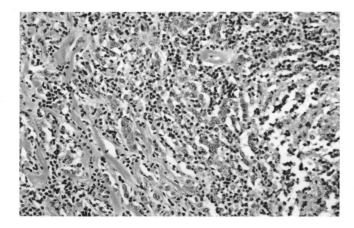

Figure 22.6 **Invasive lobular carcinoma with lymphocytic reaction.** The carcinoma cells have a linear growth pattern that is difficult to appreciate in the midst of the lymphocytic reaction.

diagnosis of invasive lobular carcinoma to a larger group of tumors. The solid type consists of compact nests of tumor cells (Fig. 22.7). Trabecular lobular carcinoma refers to tumors with prominent bands more than two cells broad (Fig. 22.8). Usually, the trabecular pattern is found in association with other variants, and the tumors are classified as mixed. The alveolar pattern is defined by rounded aggregates or clumps of cells, a configuration that overlaps somewhat with the solid pattern (Fig. 22.9). Lobular carcinoma in situ coexists with about 85% of variant tumors. The observation that many examples of classical invasive lobular carcinoma have minor components of alveolar, tubular, trabecular, or solid growth is further evidence for classifying neoplasms that express these features prominently as variants of invasive lobular carcinoma. This conclusion is also supported by the fact that variant forms are E-cadherin negative.

Occasionally, the sample obtained in a needle core biopsy procedure contains minimal, inconspicuous evidence of invasive lobular carcinoma that can easily be overlooked or mistaken for an inflammatory cell infiltrate (Figs. 22.10 and 22.11). When lobular carcinoma in situ is identified in a needle core biopsy specimen, all tissue

should be carefully inspected for occult invasion. A cytokeratin immunostain can be helpful for detecting inconspicuous invasive lobular carcinoma cells (Fig. 22.12).

All of the cytologic appearances found in lobular carcinoma in situ may also be present in invasive lobular carcinoma. Classical invasive lobular carcinoma consists of small, uniform cells with round nuclei and inconspicuous nucleoli. A variable proportion of cells have intracytoplasmic lumina (Fig. 22.13). Mucin is demonstrable in these vacuoles with the mucicarmine and Alcian blue stains (32,33). When the secretion is prominent, the cells have a signet ring configuration. The majority of so-called signet ring cell carcinomas are forms of invasive lobular carcinoma (5,32–34).

Some invasive lobular carcinomas consist entirely or in part of cells with relatively abundant cytoplasm and enlarged hyperchromatic nuclei (Fig. 22.14). These cells have been referred to as histiocytoid (35) and pleomorphic lobular carcinoma (36–38). The cytoplasm of the cells in pleomorphic lobular carcinoma may have apocrine traits (36,39) (Fig. 22.15). A low frequency of reactivity for estrogen and progesterone receptors is found in pleomorphic invasive lobular carcinoma (40), and apocrine carcinomas

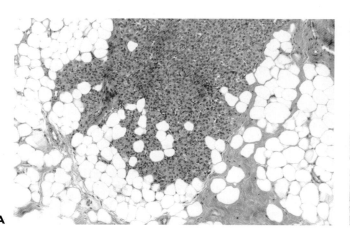

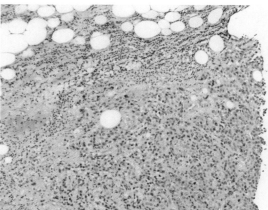

A   **B**

Figure 22.7 **Invasive lobular carcinoma, solid variant. A:** The tumor cells form a solid mass with uneven borders infiltrating fat (hematoxylin–phloxine–saffranin). **B:** A needle core biopsy specimen in which the border of solid invasive lobular carcinoma is defined by a lymphocytic reaction.

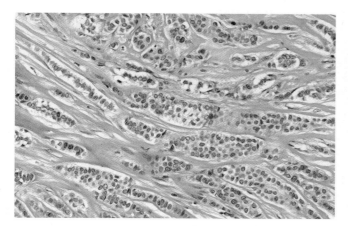

Figure 22.8 Invasive lobular carcinoma, trabecular variant. This tumor has a trabecular growth pattern formed by bands of cells arrayed two to four across.

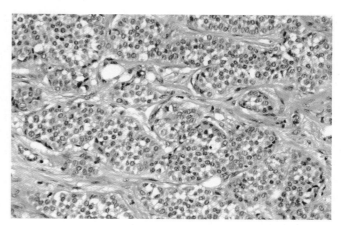

Figure 22.9 Invasive lobular carcinoma, alveolar type. The tumor cells form rounded masses that duplicate the appearance of lobular carcinoma in situ.

are also typically not reactive for these receptors. Androgen receptors have been detected in pleomorphic lobular carcinoma (41), and they are typically present in apocrine carcinomas.

Perineural invasion is uncommon in invasive lobular carcinoma but may occur when the lesion is very extensive. Lymphatic tumor emboli are also rarely found in this type of carcinoma, and in some situations shrinkage artifacts may simulate carcinoma in lymphatic spaces. When lym-

phatic tumor emboli are present, the tumor cells tend to form cohesive aggregates rather than being individually dispersed.

E-cadherin is an epithelium-associated molecule involved in cell-to-cell adhesion that acts as a tumor invasion–suppressor gene. When compared with invasive duct carcinoma, E-cadherin expression is markedly reduced or absent in the great majority of invasive lobular carcinomas when studied by immunohistochemistry

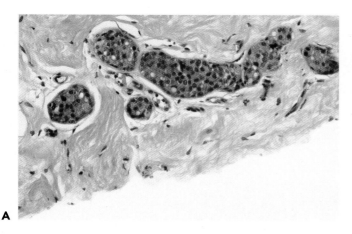

A

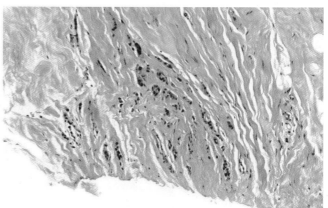

B

Figure 22.10 Invasive lobular carcinoma, minimal lesions. A–C: Lobular carcinoma in situ in one part of the needle core biopsy specimen **(A).** The only evidence of invasive carcinoma was this inconspicuous focus that measured less than 1 mm **(B, C).**

C

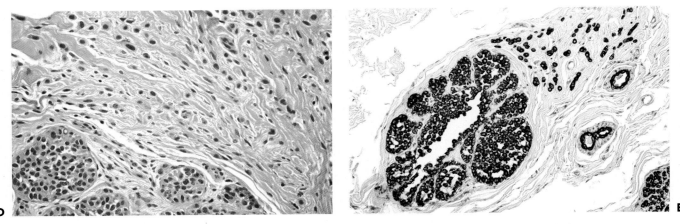

Figure 22.10 *(continued)* **D:** A 1 mm focus of classical invasive lobular carcinoma next to lobular carcinoma in situ. **E:** Microinvasive lobular carcinoma is highlighted by the CK7 cytokeratin stain (immunoperoxidase).

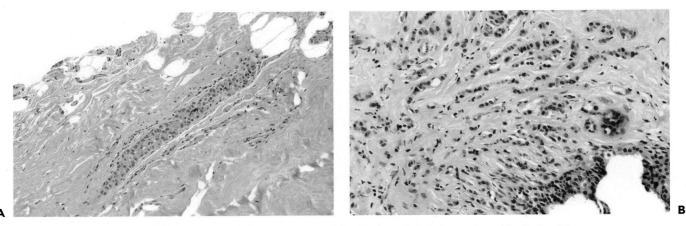

Figure 22.11 **Invasive lobular carcinoma, minimal lesion.** **A:** Lobular carcinoma in situ involving a terminal duct was present in this needle core biopsy specimen. **B:** This 1 mm focus of invasive lobular carcinoma was initially diagnosed incorrectly as a periductal lymphocytic reaction. No other evidence of carcinoma was found in the specimen that consisted of several tissue cores.

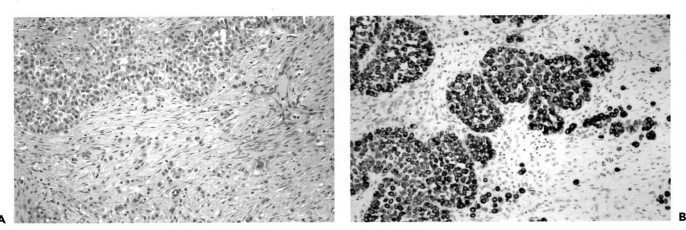

Figure 22.12 **In situ and invasive lobular carcinoma in a benign phyllodes tumor.** **A:** In situ carcinoma is shown in enlarged lobular glands. The stroma contains small round cells suggestive of invasive lobular carcinoma. **B:** Scattered invasive carcinoma cells are highlighted with a CK7 cytokeratin immunostain (immunoperoxidase).

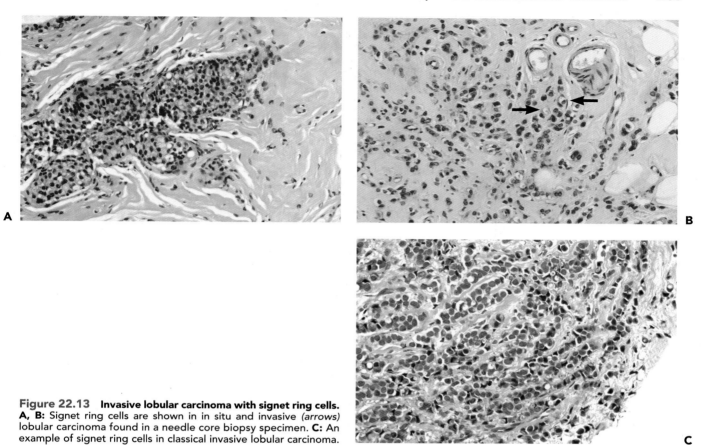

Figure 22.13   Invasive lobular carcinoma with signet ring cells.
A, B: Signet ring cells are shown in in situ and invasive *(arrows)* lobular carcinoma found in a needle core biopsy specimen. **C:** An example of signet ring cells in classical invasive lobular carcinoma.

(42–44) (Fig. 22.16). Loss of immunoreactivity for α, β, and λ catenins also occurs in invasive lobular carcinoma (43). Mutations have been reported in the E-cadherin gene in classical (45–47) and in pleomorphic (48) invasive lobular carcinoma. Loss of E-cadherin immunoreactivity is consistently observed in lobular carcinoma in situ of the classical and pleomorphic type in the presence of or in the absence of invasive lobular carcinoma (47–49). In one

study of paired in situ and invasive lobular carcinoma samples from 24 patients, loss of the entire 16q arm was detected in all specimens and it was concluded that "the striking similarity in genomic changes between the in situ and invasive components of these lesions clearly demonstrated the common clonality of the two lesions" (50). Because the E-cadherin staining pattern is so highly associated with histologic tumor type, lesions that depart from

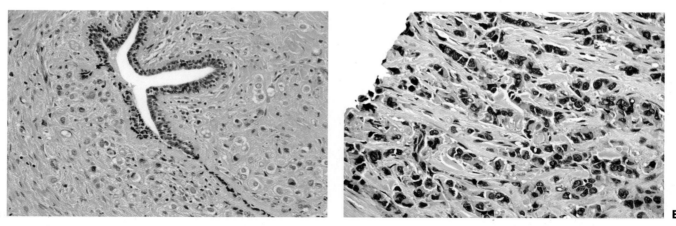

Figure 22.14   Invasive lobular carcinoma, pleomorphic type.   A: Invasive pleomorphic lobular carcinoma with histiocytoid features is shown surrounding a duct. The carcinoma cells have relatively abundant cytoplasm. Signet ring cell forms are present. **B:** Pleomorphic invasive lobular carcinoma with linear growth.

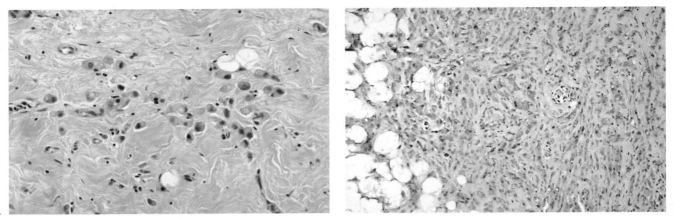

Figure 22.15 **Invasive lobular carcinoma, pleomorphic type with apocrine differentiation. A:** The carcinoma cells have relatively abundant eosinophilic cytoplasm and pleomorphic hyperchromatic nuclei. This example features cells with a prominent histiocytoid appearance and intracytoplasmic vacuoles. **B:** Intracytoplasmic mucin appears magenta and gross cystic disease fluid protein is brown in this combined staining reaction (mucicarmine reaction and immunoperoxidase).

expected E-cadherin reactivity are described as having aberrant E-cadherin staining (51). Da Silva et al. (52) reported that the cadherin–catenin complex may not be functional in lobular carcinomas with aberrant E-cadherin expression. They concluded that when the H&E histologic appearance is characteristic for lobular carcinoma, "positive staining for E-cadherin should not preclude a diagnosis of lobular in favor of ductal carcinoma."

The majority of invasive lobular carcinomas exhibit nuclear immunoreactivity for estrogen receptor, usually accompanied by progesterone receptor (Fig. 22.17). Histiocytoid or pleomorphic invasive lobular carcinoma is positive for gross cystic disease fluid protein-15 (GCDFP-15) (53). The HER2/*neu* gene product is only rarely detected immunohistochemically in classical in situ or invasive lobular carcinoma (26). Invasive lobular carcinoma is typically negative for p53 protein, p63, and vimentin (54). About 20% of invasive lobular carcinomas are positive for CK 5/6 (55). These carcinomas tend to be negative for estrogen receptors and may represent a basal-like subset.

Metastatic deposits of invasive lobular carcinoma tend to duplicate the cytologic features of the primary tumor (Fig. 22.18). Axillary lymph node metastases derived from invasive lobular carcinoma of the classical type may be distributed largely in sinusoids, sparing lymphoid areas. If lymph node involvement is sparse, the distinction between tumor cells and histiocytes may be difficult to appreciate in H&E sections.

Isolated metastatic lobular carcinoma cells in the bone marrow may resemble hematopoietic elements (56). When compared with ductal carcinoma, there is a statistically significant greater frequency of metastatic lobular carcinoma in the peritoneum and retroperitoneum, leptomeninges, gastrointestinal tract, and gynecologic organs, and a lower frequency of pulmonary or pleural metastases (57). In the uterus, the carcinoma cells blend with normal endometrial stromal cells and may be overlooked in endometrial curettings (58). Metastatic lobular carcinoma has been described in endometrial polyps associated with tamoxifen therapy (59). Metastases involving the stomach

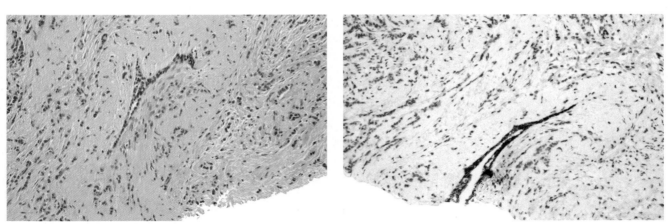

Figure 22.16 **Invasive carcinoma: E-cadherin stain. A:** Classical invasive lobular carcinoma infiltrates around a slit-shaped duct. **B:** The epithelium of the duct is E-cadherin positive. There is no E-cadherin reactivity in the invasive lobular carcinoma. (immunoperoxidase).

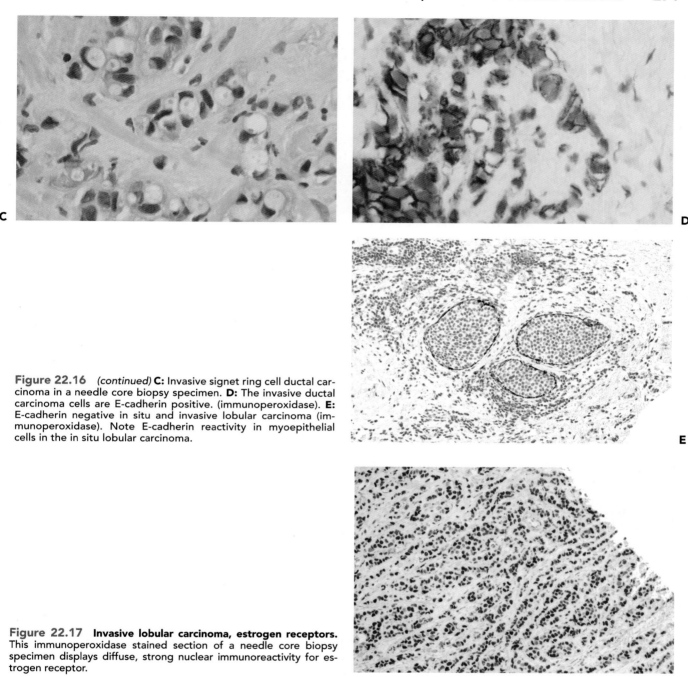

Figure 22.16 *(continued)* **C:** Invasive signet ring cell ductal carcinoma in a needle core biopsy specimen. **D:** The invasive ductal carcinoma cells are E-cadherin positive. (immunoperoxidase). **E:** E-cadherin negative in situ and invasive lobular carcinoma (immunoperoxidase). Note E-cadherin reactivity in myoepithelial cells in the in situ lobular carcinoma.

Figure 22.17 Invasive lobular carcinoma, estrogen receptors. This immunoperoxidase stained section of a needle core biopsy specimen displays diffuse, strong nuclear immunoreactivity for estrogen receptor.

Figure 22.18 Metastatic lobular carcinoma. Lobular carcinoma with a linear growth pattern is shown in skeletal muscle.

can produce clinical and pathologic findings indistinguishable from those of a primary gastric carcinoma (60). Estrogen receptors have been detected in gastric adenocarcinomas by immunohistochemical procedures but diffuse, strong staining would favor metastatic lobular carcinoma (61,62). No significant differences have been found in the distribution of metastases between patients with the classical and variant patterns of invasive lobular carcinoma (5).

Studies of prognosis in patients with invasive lobular carcinoma have not shown a consistent difference from patients with invasive duct carcinoma treated by mastectomy when stage at diagnosis is taken into consideration (2,5,29,63,64). Patients with classical invasive lobular carcinoma have a slightly better prognosis than those with variant forms as a group, but the differences have not been statistically significant. No reproducible differences in prognosis have been demonstrated among patients with different variant lesions, and it is evident that very large numbers of cases would be needed to document significant differences if they exist. Consequently, no distinction should be made between classical and variant forms of classical invasive carcinoma with regard to therapy. The most important determinants of prognosis and treatment are primary tumor size and nodal status. Data from several studies suggest that pleomorphic invasive lobular carcinoma may have a less favorable prognosis than classical variants (36–38).

Many reports of successful treatment by breast conservation with radiotherapy have appeared (20,65–72). These studies indicate that survival for patients with invasive lobular carcinoma treated by breast conservation is similar to the result obtained for duct carcinoma. Patients with multifocal invasive lobular carcinoma had a greater frequency of breast recurrence than those with unifocal tumors (70). Limited information is available about the treatment of invasive pleomorphic lobular carcinoma by conservation therapy. If this is done, it has been suggested that pleomorphic lobular carcinoma in situ be viewed as similar to intraductal carcinoma with respect to assessing margins.

Invasive lobular carcinoma responds poorly to neoadjuvant therapy when compared with the response rate for ductal carcinoma (73).

REFERENCES

1. Henson D, Tarone R. A study of lobular carcinoma of the breast based on the Third National Cancer Survey in the United States of America. *Tumori*. 1979;65:133–142.
2. Dixon JM, Anderson TJ, Page DL, et al. Infiltrating lobular carcinoma of the breast. *Histopathology*. 1982;6:149–161.
3. Ashikari R, Huvos AG, Urban JA, Robbins GF. Infiltrating lobular carcinoma of the breast. *Cancer*. 1973;31:110–116.
4. Martinez V, Azzopardi JG. Invasive lobular carcinoma of the breast: incidence and variants. *Histopathology*. 1979;3:467–488.
5. DiCostanzo D, Rosen PP, Gareen I, et al. Prognosis in infiltrating lobular carcinoma: an analysis of "classical" and variant tumors. *Am J Surg Pathol*. 1990;14:12–23.
6. Fechner RE. Histologic variants of infiltrating lobular carcinoma of the breast. *Hum Pathol*. 1975;6:373–378.
7. Fechner RE. Infiltrating lobular carcinoma without lobular carcinoma *in situ*. *Cancer*. 1972;29:1539–1545.
8. Li CL, Anderson BO, Daling JR, Moe RE. Trends in incidence rates of invasive lobular and ductal breast carcinoma. *JAMA*. 2003;289:1421–1424.
9. Mendelson EB, Harris KM, Doshi N, Tobon H. Infiltrating lobular carcinoma: mammographic patterns with pathologic correlation. *Am J Radiol*. 1989;153:265–271.
10. Helvie MA, Paramagul C, Oberman HA, Adler DD. Invasive lobular carcinoma: imaging features and clinical detection. *Invest Radiol*. 1993;28:202–207.
11. Krecke KN, Gisvold JJ. Invasive lobular carcinoma of the breast: mammographic findings and extent of disease at diagnosis in 184 patients. *Am J Roentgenol*. 1993;161:957–960.
12. Le Gal M, Ollivier L, Asselain B, et al. Mammographic features of 455 invasive lobular carcinomas. *Radiology*. 1992;185:705–708.
13. Porter PL, El-Bastawissi AY, Mendelson MT, et al. Breast tumor characteristics as predictors of mammographic detection: comparison of interval-and screen-detected cancers. *J Natl Cancer Inst*. 1999;91:2020–2028.
14. Yeatman TJ, Cantor AB, Smith TJ, et al. Tumor biology of infiltrating lobular carcinoma. Implications for management. *Ann Surg*. 1995;222:549–561.
15. Rodenko GN, Harms SE, Pruneda JM, et al. MR imaging in the management before surgery of lobular carcinoma of the breast: correlation with pathology. *Am J Roentgenol*. 1996;167:1415–1419.
16. Yeh ED, Slanetz PJ, Edmister WB, et al. Invasive lobular carcinoma: spectrum of enhancement and morphology on magnetic resonance imaging. *Breast J*. 2003;9:13–18.
17. Berg, WA, Gilbreath PL. Multicentric and multi-focal cancer: whole breast US in preoperative evaluation. *Radiology*. 2000;214:59–66.
18. Skaane P, Skjorken G. Ultrasonographic evaluation of invasive lobular carcinoma. *Acta Radiol*. 1999;40:369–375.
19. Selinko VL, Middleton LP, Dempsey PJ. Role of sonography in diagnosing and staging invasive lobular carcinoma. *J Clin Ultrasound*. 2004;32:323–332.
20. White JR, Gustafson GS, Wimbish K, et al. Conservative surgery and radiation therapy for infiltrating lobular carcinoma of the breast. The role of preoperative mammograms in guiding treatment. *Cancer*. 1994;74:640–647.
21. Evans WP, Burhenne LJW, Laurie L, et al. Invasive lobular carcinoma of the breast: mammographic characteristics and computer-aided detection. *Radiology* 2002;225:182–189.
22. Broët P, de la Rochefordière A, Scholl SM, et al. Contralateral breast cancer: annual incidence and risk parameters. *J Clin Oncol*. 1995;13:1578–1583.
23. Bernstein JL, Thompson WD, Risch N, Holford TR. Risk factors predicting the incidence of second primary breast cancer among women diagnosed with a first primary breast cancer. *Am J Epidemiol*. 1992;136:925–936.
24. Lesser ML, Rosen PP, Kinne DW. Multicentricity and bilaterality in invasive breast carcinoma. *Surgery*. 1982;1:234–240.
25. Horn PL, Thompson WD. Risk of contralateral breast cancer: Associations with factors related to initial breast cancer. *Am J Epidemiol*. 1988;128:309–323.
26. Kollias J, Ellis IO, Elston CW, Blamey RW. Clinical and histologic predictors of contralateral breast cancer. *Eur J Surg Oncol*. 1999;25:584–589.
27. Dixon JM, Anderson TJ, Page DL, et al. Infiltrating lobular carcinoma of the breast: an evaluation of the incidence and consequence of bilateral disease. *Br J Surg*. 1983;70:513–516.
28. Hislop TG, Ng V, McBride ML, et al. Incidence and risk factors for second breast primaries in women with lobular breast carcinoma. *Breast Dis*. 1990;3:95–105.
29. du Toit RS, Locker AP, Ellis IO, et al. Invasive lobular carcinomas of the breast—the prognosis of histopathological subtypes. *Br J Cancer*. 1989;60:605–609.
30. Simkovich AH, Sclafani LM, Masri M, Kinne DW. Role of contralateral breast biopsy in infiltrating lobular cancer. *Surgery* 1993;114:555–557.
31. Cristina S, Boldorini R, Brustia F, Monga G. Lymphoepithelioma-like carcinoma of the breast. An unusual pattern of infiltrating lobular carcinoma. *Virchows Arch*. 2000;437:198–202.
32. Breslow A, Brancaccio ME. Intracellular mucin production by lobular breast carcinoma cells. *Arch Pathol Lab Med*. 1976;100:620–621.
33. Gad A, Azzopardi JG. Lobular carcinoma of the breast: a special variant of mucin secreting carcinoma. *J Clin Pathol*. 1975;28:711–716.
34. Steinbrecher JS, Silverberg SG. Signet ring cell carcinoma of the breast. The mucinous variant of infiltrating lobular carcinoma. *Cancer*. 1976;37:828–840.
35. Allenby PL, Chowdhury LN. Histiocytic appearance of metastatic lobular breast carcinoma. *Arch Pathol Lab Med*. 1986;110:759–760.
36. Eusebi V, Magalhaes F, Azzopardi JG. Pleomorphic lobular carcinoma of the breast: an aggressive tumor showing apocrine differentiation. *Hum Pathol*. 1992;23:655–662.
37. Weidner N, Semple JP. Pleomorphic variant of invasive lobular carcinoma of the breast. *Hum Pathol*. 1992;23:1167–1171.
38. Bentz JS, Yassa N, Clayton F. Pleomorphic lobular carcinoma of the breast: clinicopathologic features of 12 cases. *Mod Pathol*. 1998;11:814–822.
39. Walford N, Ten Velden J. Histiocytoid breast carcinoma: an apocrine variant of lobular carcinoma. *Histopathology*. 1989;14:515–522.
40. Shimzu S, Kitamura H, Ito T, et al. Histiocytoid breast carcinoma. Histological, immunohistochemical, ultrastructural, cytological and clincopathological studies. *Pathol Int*. 1998;48:849–856.
41. Augros M, Buenerd A, Decouassoux-Shisheboran M, Berger G. Infiltrating lobular carcinoma of the breast with histiocytoid features. *Ann Pathol*. 2004;24:259–263.

42. Moll R, Mitze M, Frixen UH, Birchmeier W. Differential loss of E-cadherin expression in infiltrating ductal and lobular breast carcinomas. *Am J Pathol.* 1993;143:1731–1742.

43. DeLeeuw WJ, Berx G, Vos CB, et al. Simultaneous loss of E-cadherin and catenins in invasive lobular breast cancer and lobular carcinoma in situ. *J Pathol.* 1997;183:404–411.

44. Lehr HA, Folpe A, Yaziji H, et al. Cytokeratin 8 immunostaining pattern and E-cadherin expression distinguish lobular from ductal breast carcinoma. *Am J Clin Pathol.* 2000;114:190–196.

45. Kanai Y, Oda T, Tsuda H, et al. Point mutation of the E-cadherin gene in invasive lobular carcinoma of the breast. *Jpn J Cancer Res.* 1994;85:1035–1039.

46. Berx G, Cleton-Jansen AM, Strumane K, et al. E-cadherin is inactivated in a majority of invasive human lobular breast cancers by truncation mutations throughout its extracellular domain. *Oncogene.* 1996;13:1919–1925.

47. Huiping C, Sigurgeirdottir JR, Jonasson JG, et al. Chromosome alterations and E-cadherin gene mutations in human lobular breast cancer. *Br J Cancer.* 1999;81:1103–1110.

48. Palacios J, Sarrio D, Garcia-Macias MC, et al. Frequent E-cadherin gene inactivation by loss of heterozygosity in pleomorphic lobular carcinoma of the breast. *Mod Pathol.* 2003;16:674–678.

49. Wahed A, Connelly J, Reese T. E-cadherin expression in pleomorphic lobular carcinoma: an aid to differentiation from ductal carcinoma. *Ann Diagn Pathol.* 2002;6:349–351.

50. Hwang ES, Nyante SJ, Chen YY, et al. Clonality of lobular carcinoma in situ and synchronous invasive lobular carcinoma. *Cancer.* 2004;100:2562–2572.

51. Harigopal M, Shin SJ, Murray M, et al. Aberrant E-cadherin staining patterns in invasive mammary carcinoma. *World J Surg Oncol.* 2005;3:73–83.

52. Da Silva L, Parry S, Reid L, et al. Aberrant expression of E-cadherin in lobular carcinomas of the breast. *Am J Surg Pathol.* 2008;32:773–783.

53. Porter PL, Garcia R, Moe R, et al. C-erbB-2 oncogene protein in *in situ* and invasive lobular breast neoplasia. *Cancer.* 1991;68:331–334.

54. Domagala W, Markiewski M, Kubiak R, et al. Immunohistochemical profile of invasive lobular carcinoma of the breast: predominantly vimentin and p53 protein negative cathepsin D and oestrogen receptor positive. *Virchows Arch (A).* 1993;423:497–502.

55. Fadare O, Wang SA, Hileeto D. The expression of cytoberatin 5/6 in invasive lobular carcinoma of the breast: evidence of a basal-like subset? *Hum Pathol.* 2008;39:331–336.

56. Bitter MA, Fiorito D, Corkell ME, et al. Bone marrow involvement by lobular carcinoma of the breast cannot be identified reliably by routine histological examination alone. *Hum Pathol.* 1994;25:781–788.

57. Harris M, Howell A, Chrissohou M, et al. A comparison of the metastatic pattern of infiltrating lobular carcinoma and infiltrating duct carcinoma of the breast. *Br J Cancer.* 1984;50:23–30.

58. Kumar NB, Hart WR. Metastases to the uterine corpus from extragenital cancers. A clinicopathologic study of 63 cases. *Cancer.* 1982;50:2163–2169.

59. Houghton JP, Ioffe OB, Silverberg SG, et al. Metastatic breast lobular carcinoma involving tamoxifen-associated endometrial polyps: report of two cases and review of tamoxifen-associated polypoid uterine lesions. *Mod Pathol.* 2003;16:395–398.

60. Cormier WJ, Gaffey TA, Welch JM, et al. Linitis plastica caused by metastatic carcinoma of the breast. *Mayo Clin Proc.* 1980;55:747–753.

61. Harrison JD, Morris DL, Ellis IO, et al. The effect of tamoxifen and estrogen receptor status on survival in gastric carcinoma. *Cancer* 1989;64:1007–1010.

62. Yokozaki H, Takemura N, Takanashi A, et al. Estrogen receptors in gastric adenocarcinoma: a retrospective immunohistochemical analysis. *Virchows Arch (A).* 1988;413:297–302.

63. Frost AR, Terahata S, Siegel RS, et al. An analysis of prognostic features in infiltrating lobular carcinoma of the breast. *Mod Pathol.* 1995;8:830–836.

64. Jayasinghe VW, Bilous AM, Boyages J. Is survival from infiltrating lobular carcinoma different from that of infiltrating ductal carcinoma? *Breast J.* 2007;13:479–485.

65. Cha I, Weidner N. Correlation of prognostic factors and survival with classical and the pleomorphic variants of invasive lobular carcinoma. *Breast J.* 1996;2:385–393.

66. Kurtz JM, Jacquemier J, Torhorst J, et al. Conservation therapy for breast cancers other than infiltrating ductal carcinoma. *Cancer.* 1989;63:1630–1635.

67. Poen JC, Tran L, Juillard G, et al. Conservation therapy for invasive lobular carcinoma of the breast. *Cancer.* 1992;69:2789–2795.

68. Sastre-Garau X, Jouve M, Asselain B, et al. Infiltrating lobular carcinoma of the breast. Clinicopathologic analysis of 975 cases with reference to data on conservative therapy and metastatic patterns. *Cancer.* 1996;77:113–120.

69. Warneke J, Berger R, Johnson C, et al. Lumpectomy and radiation treatment for invasive lobular carcinoma of the breast. *Am J Surg.* 1996;172:496–500.

70. Schnitt SJ, Connolly JL, Recht A, et al. Influence of lobular histology on local tumor control in breast cancer patients treated with conservative surgery and radiotherapy. *Cancer* 1989;64:448–454.

71. Morrow M. Keeney K, Scholtens D, et al. Selecting patients for breast conserving therapy. The importance of lobular histology. *Cancer.* 2006;106:2563–2568.

72. Santiago RJ Harris EER, Quin L, et al. Similar long-term results of breast conservation treatment for Stage I and II invasive lobular carcinoma compared with invasive duct carcinoma of the breast. The University of Pennsylvania experience. *Cancer.* 2006;103:2447–2454.

73. Sullivan PS, Apple SK. Should histological type be taken into account when considering neoadjuvant chemotherapy in breast carcinoma? *Breast J.* 2009;15:146–154.

Mesenchymal Neoplasms

23

BENIGN MESENCHYMAL TUMORS

Fibromatosis is an infiltrating, histologically low-grade spindle cell neoplasm composed of fibroblastic cells and variable amounts of collagen.

Patients with mammary fibromatosis range in age from 13 to 80 years at diagnosis, averaging 37 to 49 years in three reported series (1–3). They usually present with a palpable, firm, painless mass that may suggest carcinoma on clinical examination. Bilateral fibromatosis is very uncommon. Mammography reveals a stellate tumor that may be indistinguishable from carcinoma (1,3–6). Calcifications are rarely formed in mammary fibromatosis, but they may be present in a coexisting benign proliferative lesion such as sclerosing adenosis that has been engulfed by the tumor. Rarely, the tumor may be nonpalpable and initially detected by mammography or ultrasonography (7). Antecedent injury or surgery has been reported at the site of fibromatosis in some patients, and an association with breast augmentation implants has been reported in several cases (2,8,9). Tumor size averages between 2.5 and 3.0 cm (2,3).

Rare examples of mammary fibromatosis have been associated with familial adenomatous polyposis (FAP), a condition in which somatic fibromatosis (desmoid tumor) frequently occurs (10). FAP is the result of germline mutations in the adenomatous polyposis coli or APC gene located on chromosome 5q. The APC gene product, the APC tumor suppressor protein, regulates β-catenin, a component of the cadherin cell-to-cell adhesion system and of the Wnt pathway (11). Altered regulation of β-catenin results in nuclear accumulation of β-catenin protein. In a study of 32 examples of sporadic mammary fibromatosis and 1 FAP-associated tumor, Abraham et al. (12) found β-catenin accumulation in tumor cell nuclei in 82% of the tumors but not in the nuclei of normal stromal cells or epithelial cells. In addition to this immunohistochemical evidence of nuclear translocation of β-catenin, most of the lesions had genetic alterations in the APC/β–catenin pathway, consisting of β-catenin gene mutation (15 cases) and mutation or 5q allelic loss (11 cases). However, β-catenin expression has not proven to be specific for fibromatosis (13).

A single lesion may have varied histologic growth patterns, a feature that complicates the diagnosis of fibromatosis in a needle core biopsy specimen. The microscopic components of the tumor are spindle cells and collagen. Areas in which the collagenous element is accentuated have a keloidal appearance (Fig. 23.1). More commonly, the lesion is composed of a moderately cellular spindle cell proliferation in which there is modest collagen deposition. Mitotic figures are very infrequent or undetectable. In most tumors, the cells have small, pale, oval, or spindly nuclei with little pleomorphism (Fig. 23.2). The tumor cells are usually distributed in broad sheets, sometimes in a storiform configuration or in the form of interlacing bundles. Actin and/or CD34-positive myofibroblasts are usually inconspicuous. In addition to varied amounts of collagenization, the stroma sometimes has localized myxoid areas. Focal lymphocytic infiltrates are found in nearly half of the tumors, especially at the periphery (Fig. 23.3). Regardless of how well demarcated the lesions seem to be grossly, all have at least some stellate, invasive extensions into the surrounding fat and glandular parenchyma. It is usually possible to find ducts and lobules engulfed by these extensions at the periphery of the tumor (Fig. 23.4). The differential diagnosis of mammary fibromatosis includes scarring from trauma or prior surgery, metaplastic spindle cell carcinoma, and other spindle cell mesenchymal neoplasms, including phyllodes tumor.

Recommended treatment is wide local excision. The frequency of local recurrence ranges from 21% to 27% (1–3). Histologic features such as cellularity, mitotic activity, and cellular pleomorphism are not helpful for predicting recurrence. Although the risk of recurrence is higher in patients with documented positive margins, recurrences have been observed in cases with apparently negative margins (3).

Fibrous tumor (focal fibrous disease) is a discrete breast tumor composed of collagenized mammary stroma (14). Fibrous tumor is a disease of premenopausal women. Mammography reveals an area of density with borders varying from irregular to smooth. Calcifications are not a feature of fibrous tumor. This benign stromal proliferation is treated by local excision.

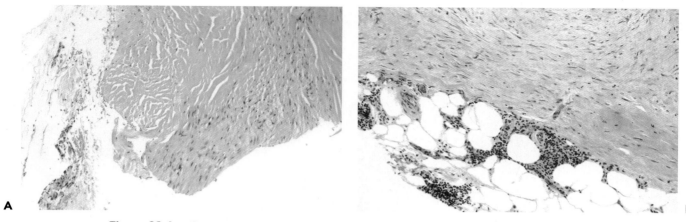

A

B

Figure 23.1 **Fibromatosis, keloidal. A:** This needle core biopsy specimen shows an area of dense collagenous tissue adjacent to a more cellular component of the lesion. The slit-shaped spaces in the keloidal tissue resemble pseudoangiomatous stromal hyperplasia. **B:** Fibromatosis with a peripheral lymphoid aggregate.

Harvey et al. (15) studied 14 patients with "fibrous nodules" that appear to correspond histologically to fibrous tumors. Of these, 10 patients (71%) were premenopausal and 3 of the 4 postmenopausal women were receiving hormone replacement therapy. The lesions measured 0.6 to 3.5 cm with a mean size of 1.8 cm. Twelve women had nonpalpable mammographically detected tumors. One woman had synchronous bilateral nonpalpable lesions. In mammograms, 11 of 13 nonpalpable tumors were round or oval, 6 of the 11 had circumscribed margins, and 5 had indistinct borders. Two tumors had irregular shapes and spiculated margins.

Histologic examination reveals normal-appearing, collagenous stroma that contains markedly decreased or absent ductal and lobular elements (14,16). The findings in a needle core biopsy specimen are not specific and are usually reported as "fibrosis" (Fig. 23.5). Capillaries, other vascular structures, and nerves are very sparse. Perivascular and perilobular inflammatory infiltrates are absent. Cysts,

apocrine metaplasia, sclerosing adenosis, pseudoangiomatous stromal hyperplasia (PASH), and duct hyperplasia are not features of fibrous tumor.

PASH can be mistaken for angiosarcoma. The term *pseudoangiomatous* was proposed to emphasize the fact that the histologic pattern mimics but does not constitute a vasoformative proliferation. PASH is a tumor formed by myofibroblasts with variable expression of myoid and fibroblastic features. Glandular hyperplasia is sometimes also present. Some examples of tumor-forming PASH have been misclassified as mammary hamartomas (17). It has been suggested that the pseudoangiomatous spaces in PASH are part of a prelymphatic pathway (18).

With rare exceptions, reported examples of tumor-forming PASH have been in women. PASH is a frequent incidental component of gynecomastia, having been found in 44 of 93 consecutive male breast biopsies (47.4%); 43 of the 44 male specimens with PASH were from patients with gynecomastia (19). The age at diagnosis in females

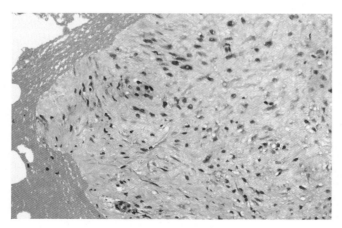

Figure 23.2 **Fibromatosis.** A needle core biopsy specimen showing average cellularity and slight stromal edema. The tumor cells have uniform round-to-oval nuclei.

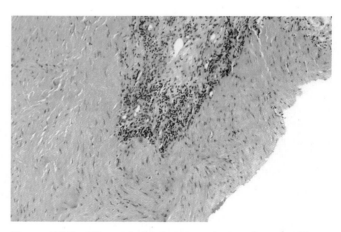

Figure 23.3 **Fibromatosis.** A perivascular lymphocytic infiltrate is apparent in this needle core biopsy specimen.

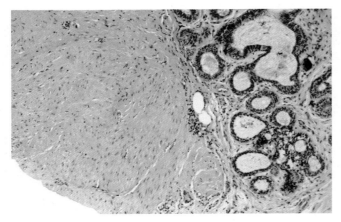

Figure 23.4 **Fibromatosis.** The tumor invades up to a lobule in this part of a needle core biopsy specimen.

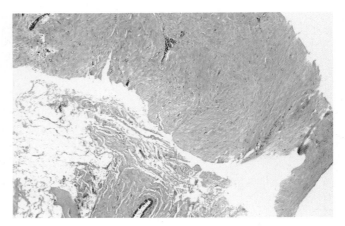

Figure 23.5 **Fibrous tumor.** The upper sample in this needle core biopsy specimen shows a broad expanse of collagenous tissue from the tumor. In the lower sample, a duct is surrounded by normal fibrofatty tissue.

ranges from the teens to the mid-50s with a median age in the mid-to-late 40s (20–22). Almost all patients have been premenopausal. Most women have a palpable, painless, unilateral mass that is firm or rubbery. Any part of the breast can be affected, including the nipple–areola complex (23). Palpable tumors average 5 cm in diameter. Skin necrosis has been observed in patients who have massive breast enlargement due to PASH during pregnancy.

PASH has been detected by mammography in patients who were asymptomatic (24–26). The lesion presents as a mass without calcification. The borders are usually smooth, but a minority of the tumors are spiculated or have ill-defined margins sometimes obscured by surrounding tissue. Ultrasound reveals a well-defined, usually hypoechoic mass (26,27). Clinically asymptomatic PASH detected by mammography may occur in postmenopausal patients (25), whereas palpable lesions are almost always found in premenopausal women or in postmenopausal women who have been treated with hormone replacement therapy.

The tumors are composed of intermixed stromal and epithelial elements in which lobular and duct structures are separated by an increased amount of stroma. Nonspecific proliferative epithelial changes include mild hyperplasia of duct and lobular epithelium, often with some accentuation of myoepithelial cells, and apocrine metaplasia with or without cyst formation. Gynecomastia-like hyperplasia may be present (25).

The most striking histologic finding is a complex pattern of anastomosing slit-shaped spaces in the intralobular as well as interlobular stroma (Fig. 23.6). Myofibroblasts that are present singly and intermittently at the margins of the spaces resemble endothelial cells. The nuclei of most of the myofibroblasts are attenuated, lack atypia, and do not show mitotic activity. Rarely, some of these cells are enlarged and have noticeably hyperchromatic nuclei. Also present in the stroma are round or oval blood-containing true blood vessels lined by endothelial cells (Figs. 23.6 and 23.7).

The myofibroblasts may accumulate in distinct bundles or fascicles in PASH (25) (Figs. 23.8 and 23.9). The most pronounced examples of the cellular or fascicular form of PASH have a growth pattern reminiscent of a myofibroblastoma. This is especially the case when the myofibroblasts have abundant cytoplasm and PASH occurs as a localized tumor rather than as a diffuse process. Myofibroblastoma and PASH are related conditions, representing the extremes of a spectrum of lesions, sharing a common histogenesis in the myofibroblasts. An atypical form of PASH has pleomorphic nuclei and infrequent mitotic figures (Fig. 23.10).

Basement membrane material is not present around the slit-like spaces in PASH. Myofibroblasts defining the pseudoangiomatous spaces exhibit strong immunoreactivity for vimentin and CD34. They are variably reactive for actin, CD31, desmin, and calponin and show no immunoreactivity for vascular markers. The nuclei of myofibroblasts in PASH are sometimes immunoreactive for progesterone receptor (20,28). Estrogen receptor is absent or only weakly present when the tissues are examined by immunohistochemistry (20,28).

PASH that forms a clinically palpable tumorous mass appears to be an exaggerated manifestation of physiologic changes commonly encountered microscopically. Ibrahim et al. (21) found microscopic foci of PASH in 23% of 200 consecutive breast specimens obtained for benign or malignant conditions. Eighty-nine percent of the patients were younger than 50 years. The majority of these specimens also exhibited epithelial hyperplasia, sometimes including secretory changes in lobules.

Most patients have remained well after excisional biopsy, but ipsilateral recurrences have occurred in some cases. Bilateral involvement, an infrequent occurrence, may be simultaneous or metachronous. Antiestrogen therapy may be beneficial in some cases (29,30).

Myofibroblastoma is a benign tumorous proliferation of myofibroblasts. These spindle-shaped or fusiform mesenchymal cells have cytoplasmic actin-like microfilaments

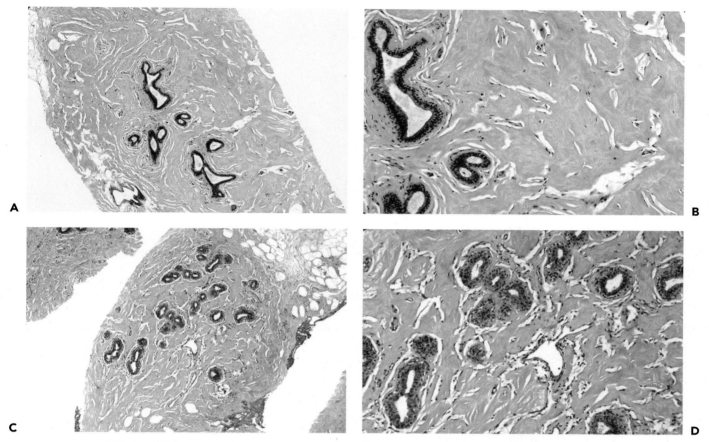

Figure 23.6 Pseudoangiomatous stromal hyperplasia. Needle core biopsy specimens from two patients. **A, B:** In this instance, myofibroblasts are inconspicuous, and the slit-shaped spaces are largely unconnected. Collagen fibrils extend across some of the spaces. **C, D:** This very pronounced pseudoangiomatous proliferation with connected spaces involves a lobule and the surrounding stroma.

measuring 5 to 7 nm in diameter with focal dense bodies and pinocytotic vesicles. Desmosomes are absent or poorly formed between myofibroblasts. Myofibroblasts exhibit variable expression of actin, calponin, desmin, and CD34 in various proliferative and neoplastic conditions. According to Chauhan et al. (31), in the normal breast and in the presence of most proliferative lesions myofibroblasts are CD34 positive and α-actin negative, whereas in invasive carcinoma they are CD34 negative and α-actin positive.

The patient with a myofibroblastoma typically presents with a solitary unilateral mass in the breast. The median age is about 65 years. Many patients reported to have

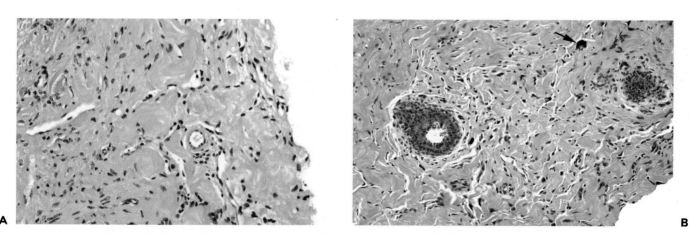

Figure 23.7 Pseudoangiomatous stromal hyperplasia. A: Small blood vessels are distributed among the pseudoangiomatous spaces in this needle core biopsy specimen. **B:** Another needle core biopsy specimen with enlarged and multinucleated *(arrow)* cells in PASH.

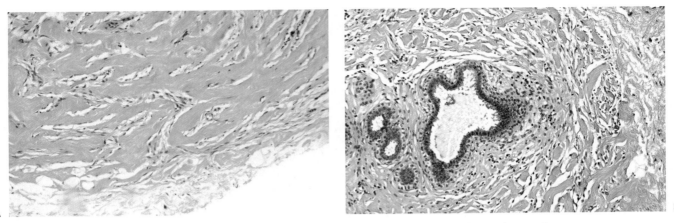

Figure 23.8 **Pseudoangiomatous stromal hyperplasia. A:** The lesion shown in this needle core biopsy specimen has a circumscribed border. The presence of myofibroblastic nuclei in some of the spaces is an early phase in the development of the fascicular pattern. **B:** Periductal growth with the early phase of the fascicular pattern.

myofibroblastoma have been men, but the lesion also occurs in women (32). Radiographically, the tumors are homogeneous, lobulated, well circumscribed, and lack microcalcifications (33–35). The average diameter of the tumor is about 2 cm with most smaller than 4 cm. Size extremes include one lesion that measured 0.9 cm (32) and one 10 cm tumor (36). Detection of nonpalpable myofibroblastomas by mammography has been reported (35). Excisional biopsy is adequate treatment in most cases, and local recurrence is infrequent.

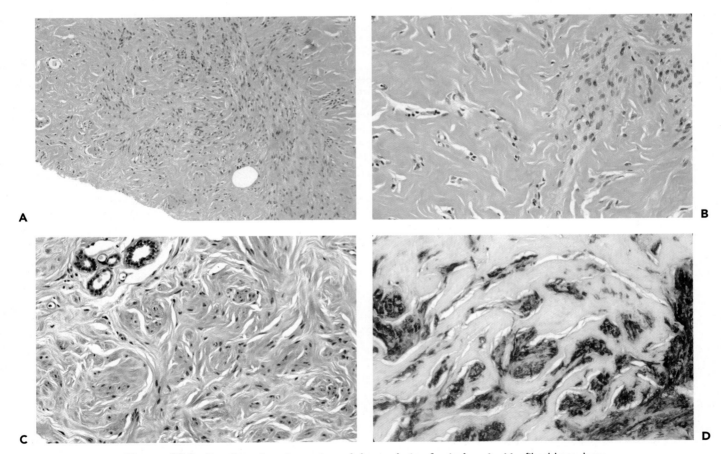

Figure 23.9 **Pseudoangiomatous stromal hyperplasia, fascicular. A:** Myofibroblasts have formed distinct bundles that are distributed in the pseudoangiomatous pattern in this needle core biopsy specimen. **B:** Another portion of the specimen showing pseudoangiomatous and fascicular elements. **C:** Fascicular pattern with myoid differentiation. **D:** The myofibroblasts are immunoreactive for actin (immunoperoxidase).

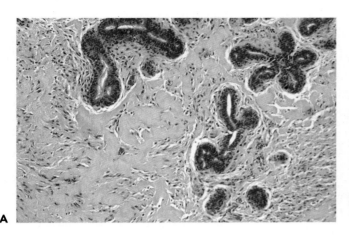

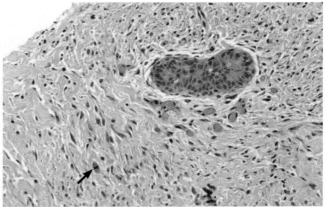

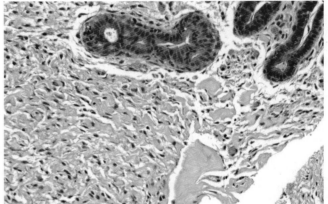

Figure 23.10 **Atypical pseudoangiomatous stromal hyperplasia, fascicular. A–C:** This needle core biopsy specimen was obtained from a 12-cm tumor in a 29-year-old woman. The stroma has occasional mitotic figures *(arrow)* and is focally very cellular. The pseudoangiomatous pattern is maintained in cellular foci. Ductal hyperplasia is also evident.

The classic type of myofibroblastoma is composed of bundles of slender, bipolar, uniform, spindle-shaped cells, typically arranged in clusters that are separated by broad bands of hyalinized collagen (37) (Fig. 23.11). Multinucleated giant cells are uncommon and mitotic figures are sparse or undetectable. Fat cells, ducts, and lobules are present in a minority of lesions. Usually, these components appear to have been incorporated from the surrounding tissue, especially if the tumor displays invasive growth. Rarely, fat cells are dispersed separately or in small groups throughout the tumor or there is abundant fat suggestive of a lipomatous element. The term *lipomatous myofibroblastoma* has been suggested for the latter group of lesions (38). The distinction between lipomatous myofibroblastoma and spindle cell lipoma is not clear, however. Gene rearrangements have been reported to affect 13q and 16q in spindle cell lipomas (39), and they have also been detected in myofibroblastomas (40). Spindle cell lipomas and myofibroblastomas both express CD10 (41).

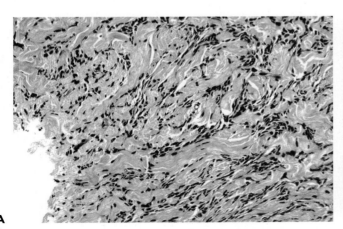

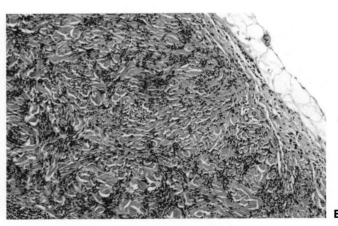

Figure 23.11 **Myofibroblastoma. A:** This needle core biopsy specimen shows the characteristic fascicles of myofibroblasts and intervening bands of collagen. **B:** The excised tumor had a circumscribed border.

Some lesions have foci of leiomyomatous differentiation and very rarely cartilage is formed (42,43). A perivascular lymphoplasmacytic infiltrate is sometimes identified. The border of the tumor is usually circumscribed microscopically, but in a minority of cases the tumor has an invasive margin. The majority of myofibroblastomas are immunoreactive for CD10, actin, and CD34. Many are also desmin positive. The tumors are not immunoreactive for cytokeratin or factor VIII and only rarely weakly reactive for S-100 protein.

Variant forms of myofibroblastoma have received little attention. In a *collagenized* myofibroblastoma, the spindle cells are distributed in diffusely collagenized stroma (Fig. 23.12). Irregular slit-shaped spaces formed between tumor cells and the stroma are reminiscent of PASH. The *epithelioid* variant features polygonal or epithelioid cells arranged in alveolar groups (Fig. 23.13), often mixed with classical myofibroblastoma elements (44). The term *epithelioid variant* is arbitrarily employed for tumors in which more than 50% of the lesion is composed of epithelioid cells. In sclerotic stroma, epithelioid myofibroblasts with a linear distribution resemble invasive lobular carcinoma. These cells are variably reactive for desmin, actin, and often for CD34 (44), but not for cytokeratin. Reactivity for estrogen, progesterone, and androgen receptors has been reported in epithelioid myofibroblastomas (44).

A *cellular variant* of myofibroblastoma features a dense proliferation of spindle-shaped neoplastic myofibroblasts. Collagenous bands may be absent in some parts of the lesion. These tumors tend to have infiltrative borders microscopically. The tumor cells are immunoreactive for actin and desmin. Rarely, cellular, and collagenous growth patterns are combined in a single tumor.

The *infiltrative variant of myofibroblastoma* is characterized by entirely invasive growth. These tumors consist not only of the lesional tissue but also fat, mammary stroma, ducts, and lobules (Fig. 23.14). This pattern differs from that of the classical and other foregoing variants of myofibroblastoma, which incorporate fat, glandular tissue, or both into what is essentially a discrete tumor composed of, in large measure, the lesional tissue. The infiltrative variant of myofibroblastoma consists of bundles of relatively evenly dispersed spindle, ovoid, and epithelioid cells embedded in collagenous stroma. Some of these lesions exhibit a peculiar tendency for the neoplastic myofibroblasts to be oriented around blood vessels.

Myxoid myofibroblastoma also displays infiltrative growth (Fig. 23.15). The sparse spindle cells in the myxoid stroma of these lesions are reactive for CD34 and actin, attributes consistent with myofibroblastic histogenesis.

Myofibroblastoma must be considered in the differential diagnosis of spindle cell mammary tumors. Sarcoma and metaplastic carcinoma are typically more cellular than myofibroblastomas and have frequent mitoses. Fasciitis and fibromatosis that also contain myofibroblasts tend to be stellate invasive lesions. Plump myoid cells and the inflammatory reaction of fasciitis are not seen in

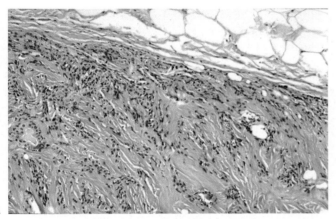

A

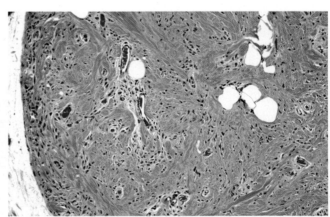

B

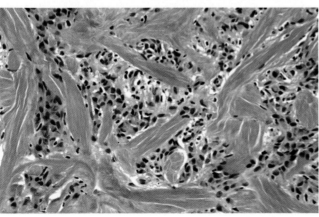

C

Figure 23.12 **Myofibroblastoma, collagenized. A:** Bundles of myofibroblasts are distributed between prominent bands of collagen. The tumor has a circumscribed border. **B, C:** Another tumor with dense collagen bands and epithelioid myofibroblasts.

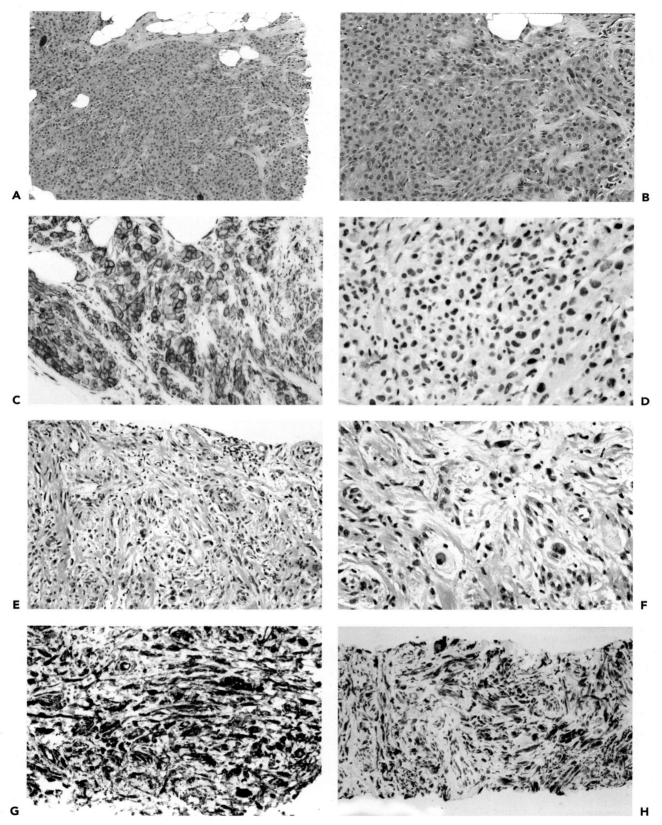

Figure 23.13   Myofibroblastoma, epithelioid. A, B: Epithelioid myofibroblasts form alveolar clusters and small bundles in this very cellular needle core biopsy specimen. This appearance could be mistaken for invasive carcinoma. **C:** The cells are strongly immunoreactive for smooth muscle actin (immunoperoxidase). **D:** Epithelioid myofibroblasts with nuclear reactivity for estrogen receptors (immunoperoxidase). **E–H:** This needle core biopsy sample is from a spindle and epithelioid cell myofibroblastoma with myxoid stroma. The tumor was strongly reactive for CD34 **(G)** and desmin **(H)**.

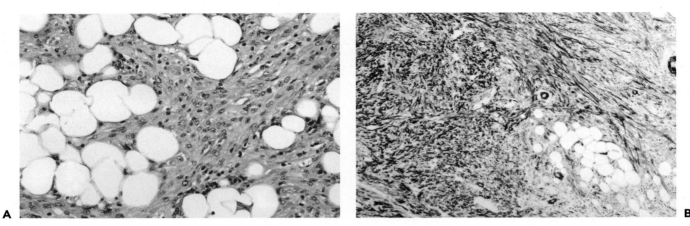

Figure 23.14 **Myofibroblastoma, infiltrating. A:** Tumor cells in fat might be mistaken for infiltrating carcinoma in this needle core biopsy specimen. **B:** The tumor cells are strongly immunoreactive for smooth muscle actin (immunoperoxidase).

myofibroblastoma. Fibromatosis exhibits abundant collagen and spindle cells arranged in broad bands rather than short fascicular clusters. Spindle cell lipomas also have a male predominance and sometimes may be well circumscribed. They have more abundant adipose tissue than myofibroblastomas. The distinction between a spindle cell

lipoma and infiltrative myofibroblastoma may not be possible in a limited needle core biopsy sample.

Virtually all patients are managed adequately by excisional biopsy. Complete excision is recommended when a myofibroblastoma is identified in a needle core biopsy sample. Wider excision should be performed in most cases

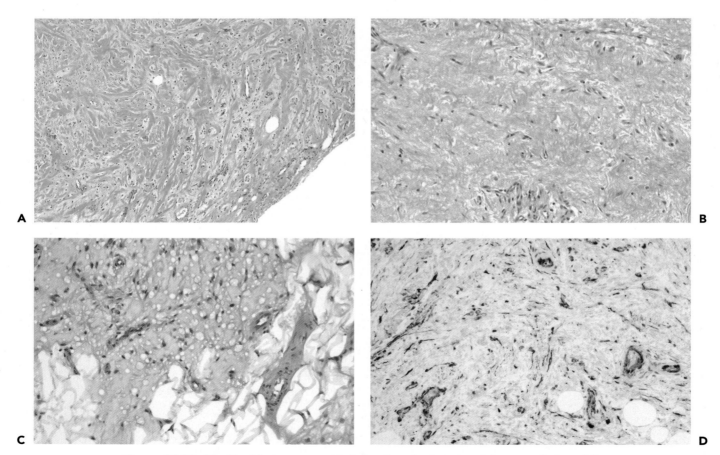

Figure 23.15 **Myofibroblastoma, myxoid. A:** A collagenized portion of the tumor. **B:** Basophilic myxoid material is evident in the tumor. **C:** Fully developed myxoid myofibroblastoma invading fat. **D:** The invasive myxoid portion of the tumor is immunoreactive for CD34 (immunoperoxidase).

if a myofibroblastoma is present at the margin of a lumpectomy specimen.

Granular cell tumors are derived from the Schwann cells of peripheral nerves. They occur throughout the body, with about 5% of them originating in the breast (45). The patient usually presents with a solitary firm or hard, painless mass, most often located in the upper and medial breast quadrants. On mammography, granular cell tumor of the breast (GCTB) is difficult to distinguish from carcinoma (46,47), and coexistence of the two lesions has been described (48). GCTB typically forms a stellate mass lacking calcifications, but circumscribed lesions have been reported (46,47,49,50).

Ultrasound usually reveals a solid mass with posterior shadowing suggestive of carcinoma (49,50). Benign GCTB is treated by wide excision. Local recurrence may occur after incomplete excision. Less than one percent of all granular cell tumors including mammary lesions are malignant.

Granular cell tumors of the breast have the same histologic appearance as these tumors at other sites. The tumor is composed of compact nests or sheets of cells that contain eosinophilic cytoplasmic granules (Fig. 23.16). In some lesions there is a tendency to cytoplasmic vacuolization and clearing. The cytoplasmic granules are positive for periodic acid–Schiff (PAS) and diastase resistant. The cells vary in

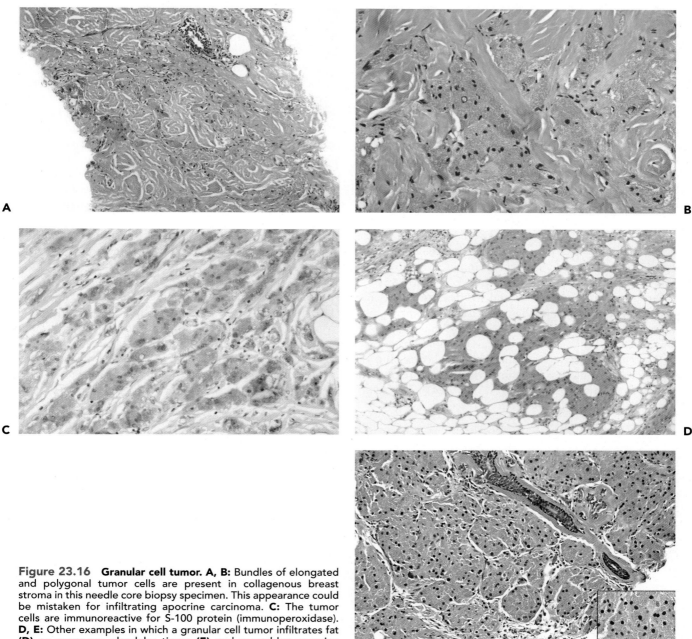

Figure 23.16 Granular cell tumor. A, B: Bundles of elongated and polygonal tumor cells are present in collagenous breast stroma in this needle core biopsy specimen. This appearance could be mistaken for infiltrating apocrine carcinoma. **C:** The tumor cells are immunoreactive for S-100 protein (immunoperoxidase). **D, E:** Other examples in which a granular cell tumor infiltrates fat **(D)** or mammary glandular tissue **(E)** and resembles apocrine carcinoma.

shape from polygonal to spindle. Variable amounts of collagenous stroma are present. Nuclei are round to slightly oval with an open chromatin pattern. Nucleoli tend to be prominent. A modest amount of nuclear pleomorphism, occasional multinucleated cells, and rare mitoses may be found, but these features should not be interpreted as evidence of a malignant neoplasm. Small nerve bundles are sometimes seen in the tumor or in close association with the peripheral invasive border. Ducts and lobules are typically surrounded by the invasive tumor cells and incorporated into the lesion.

The differential diagnosis of GCTB includes apocrine carcinoma and histiocytic or granulomatous lesions. The presence of intraductal carcinoma, often of the comedo type, as well as marked cytologic pleomorphism, usually serve to identify apocrine carcinoma, but these features may be absent from a needle core biopsy specimen. The lesions can be distinguished with confidence by histochemical studies. GCTB is not reactive for epithelial markers and does not contain mucin. Strong, diffuse immunoreactivity for S-100 protein and carcinoembryonic antigen (CEA) that characterizes granular cell tumors does not by itself distinguish these lesions from mammary carcinoma (47,51–53). A high proportion of granular cell tumors are reactive for vimentin, and they are estrogen and progesterone receptor negative. GCTB is immunohistochemically negative for histiocyte-associated antigens such as α_1-antitrypsin and muramidase (47,51). Apocrine carcinomas are immunoreactive for cytokeratin, androgen receptors, and usually for epithelial membrane antigen (EMA).

Tumors of nerve and nerve sheath origin of the breast have usually been diagnosed as "neurilemomas" (54–56) or as schwannomas. The age range at diagnosis is 15 to 78 years, with most patients in their 30s and 40s. The lesion presents as a painless, well-defined mass. One schwannoma was an asymptomatic 7-mm lesion detected by mammography (56). Microscopic examination reveals the typical histologic features of a benign nerve sheath tumor, consisting of spindle cells in bundles, sometimes with nuclei arranged in a palisading pattern (Antoni type A) (Fig. 23.17). Less cellu-

lar areas with thick-walled blood vessels, the Antoni B pattern, may be present as well. Vascular thrombi, hyalinized blood vessels, cells with atypical nuclei, and xanthomatous areas are found in sclerotic schwannomas. The diagnosis of a benign peripheral nerve sheath tumor is supported by a positive immunohistochemical stain for S-100 protein, negative immunostains for CEA and actin, and the absence of mitotic activity. Complete excision provides adequate therapy.

The tumor referred to as *hamartoma* of the breast occurs most often in premenopausal women, but it has been described in teenagers and in women in their 60s. The tumors have been as large as 17 cm, often resulting in substantial asymmetry. Mammography reveals a well-circumscribed, dense, round, or oval mass surrounded by a narrow lucent zone (57–59). Hamartomas of the breast were diagnosed in 16 of 10,000 mammography examinations reviewed by Hessler et al. (59). The ultrasonographic appearance of a mammary hamartoma is reported to be variable and not specific (60), probably because the term *mammary hamartoma* has been mistakenly applied to a variety of other entities such as tumor-forming PASH (17).

There are two common histologic variants of true mammary hamartoma. Radiologic exam of an *adenolipoma* demonstrates a sharply defined round or oval tumor that appears to be encapsulated and surrounded by a radiolucent ring. The mammographic appearance varies with the composition of the tumor. Predominantly fatty tumors may have the lucent structure of lipomas, whereas those with abundant glandular tissue are dense (61,62). Ultrasonography reveals a mixed pattern of echogenic and sonolucent regions (63). Microscopically, the tissue consists of mature fat and mammary parenchyma mixed in varying proportions, delimited by a pseudocapsule of compressed breast tissue (Fig. 23.18). Lobules and ducts present in the lesion appear structurally normal with little or no proliferative change, the most significant abnormality being the unusual tissue distribution. *Chondrolipomas* are composed of mature adipose tissue and hyaline cartilage (64,65). Mammography reveals a well-circumscribed mass without

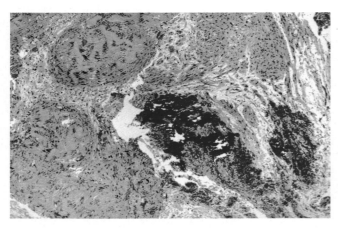

Figure 23.17 **Schwannoma.** The lesion has the Antoni type A pattern. Hemorrhage is at the site of a prior needle core biopsy procedure.

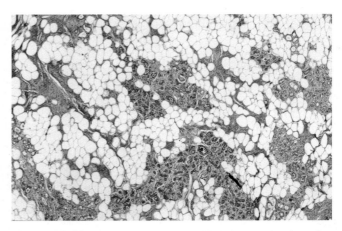

Figure 23.18 **Adenolipoma.** Normal lobules are distributed in lipomatous adipose tissue.

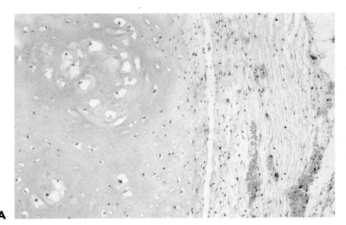

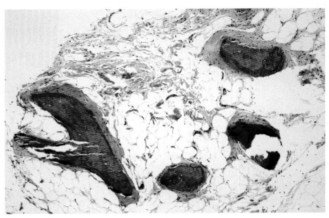

A   B

Figure 23.19   Chondrolipoma and osteolipoma. A: Mature hyaline cartilage in a chondrolipoma.
B: Mature bone is shown in this needle core biopsy sample from an osteolipoma.

calcification resembling a fibroadenoma (65). Histologically, the tumor is composed of islands of hyaline cartilage distributed in mature fat and fibrofatty glandular mammary parenchyma (Fig. 23.19).

Leiomyomas of the breast arise most often from smooth muscle in the nipple and areola (66). Parenchymal leiomyomas probably arise as a result of smooth muscle metaplasia of myoepithelial and myofibroblastic cells or from blood vessels. Radiologic examination reveals a circumscribed tumor without calcification (67,68). Complete excision is recommended. Local recurrence is very uncommon.

Microscopically, the growth pattern features interlacing fascicles of spindle cells with eosinophilic cytoplasm (Fig. 23.20). Cytologic atypia, mitoses, and necrosis that characterize leiomyosarcoma are absent. The tumor cells are immunoreactive for desmin and actin but not for S-100 protein.

The so-called *leiomyomatous ("myoid") hamartoma* is a tumorous form of sclerosing adenosis with leiomyomatous myoid metaplasia of the myoepithelial cell component (69). Mammography reveals a well-demarcated tumor of variable density (70–72). The histologic composition of a myoid hamartoma depends on the relative proportions of glandular, cystic, myomatous, and fibrous

elements. In most lesions, interlacing bundles of smooth muscle constitute a focal leiomyoma, but in a minority of tumors, the myoid component mingles more diffusely with adipose and fibrous tissue (Fig. 23.21). Epithelioid differentiation of myoepithelial cells can result in a pattern resembling infiltrating lobular carcinoma, especially in the limited sample of a needle core biopsy specimen (73). Adequate sampling reveals foci of sclerosing adenosis in virtually all examples of myoid hamartoma, and at these sites, the origin of the myoid element usually can be traced to myoepithelial cells. Associated "fibrocystic changes" include cystic apocrine metaplasia and duct hyperplasia (70,71).

Lipomas of the breast are usually solitary tumors, but multiple lipomas may be encountered. The tumors are circumscribed, well-defined masses of mature adipose tissue. On mammography, a lipoma often presents as a radiolucent homogeneous mass with a distinct border or capsule (74). However, lipomas may be difficult to detect in the mammogram of a fatty breast. In some instances, a clinically palpable lesion proves to be mature fat without the characteristic circumscription of a lipoma. It is not always possible to appreciate a pseudocapsule of compressed tissue around the lesion in needle core biopsy samples. The

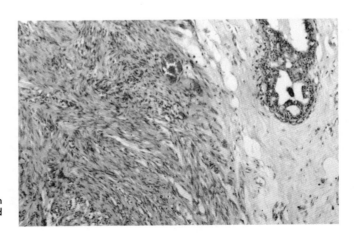

Figure 23.20   Leiomyoma. There is a suggestion of palisading in the arrangement of the smooth muscle cells in this circumscribed tumor. There is micropapillary hyperplasia in an adjacent duct.

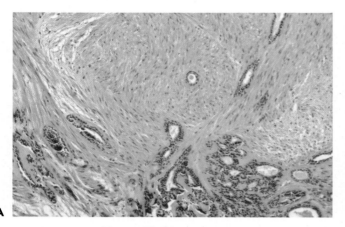

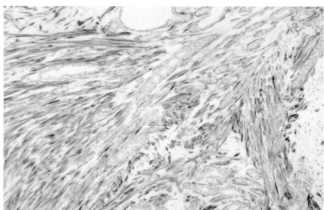

A

B

Figure 23.21 **Leiomyomatous ("myoid") hamartoma. A:** Myomatous proliferation of myoepithelial cells is present in this nodular focus of adenosis. **B:** Immunoreactivity for smooth muscle actin in the myomatous area (immunoperoxidase).

diagnosis of lipoma is established on the basis of a clinically palpable mass, the mammographic and sonographic appearance of a mass, and the presence of mature fat in the needle core biopsy specimen.

Hibernomas are composed of brown fat found in the axillary tail of the breast or in the axilla (Fig. 23.22). A *fibrolipoma* consists of mature adipose tissue in which collagenous stroma contains slightly prominent fibroblasts. Occasional ducts and lobular glands can be found in the substance of the tumor.

Spindle cell lipomas rarely occur in the breast (75–77). Biopsy reveals lipomatous tissue mixed with spindly myofibroblasts and variably collagenous stroma. CD10 and CD34 immunoreactivity can be demonstrated in the spindle cell myofibroblastic component (41,44), features thought to link spindle cell lipoma histogenetically to myofibroblastoma. Rearrangements in 13q and 16a have been reported in spindle cell lipomas and in myofibroblastomas (40).

The *perilobular hemangioma* is a microscopic benign vascular lesion detected coincidentally in sections of breast

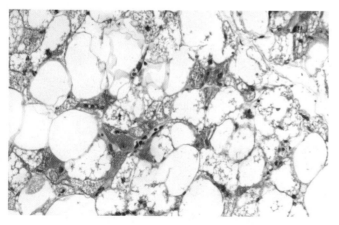

Figure 23.22 **Hibernoma.** Brown fat in a tumor from the axillary tail of the breast.

tissue taken to evaluate various unrelated benign and malignant lesions (78). A few have reportedly measured between 2 and 4 mm, but none were grossly or mammographically apparent (79,80). They have been found in 1.3% of mastectomies for carcinoma, 4.5% of biopsies for benign breast lesions, and in 11% of women whose breast tissue was sampled in forensic autopsies (78,79). Multiple perilobular hemangiomas may be found in one breast, and a number of patients have had these lesions in both breasts. There is no evidence that angiosarcomas arise from perilobular hemangiomas, although the existence of cytologically atypical variants leaves this issue open to speculation.

Microscopically, perilobular hemangiomas are not limited to a perilobular distribution. Many are partially or completely within the lobular stroma, whereas others are located in extralobular stroma sometimes in proximity to ducts or in no particular relationship to a duct or lobule. The lesion is typically a localized collection of distinct capillary-size vascular channels arranged in a meshwork fashion (Fig. 23.23). Anastomosing channels may be seen. The thin, delicate vessels consist of endothelial cells encased in inconspicuous stroma. Some perilobular hemangiomas have endothelial cells that appear cytologically atypical because they have prominent, hyperchromatic nuclei (78).

Hemangiomas are benign vascular tumors large enough to be clinically palpable or detected by mammography (78). A substantial number of hemangiomas are currently detected by mammography in the absence of a clinically palpable tumor. Hemangiomas range in size from 0.4 to 2.0 cm with a mean diameter of 0.9 cm. The majority of patients have been women 19 to 82 years of age (mean 60 years). The mammographic appearance is usually that of well-defined lobulated mass that may have fine or coarse calcifications (81,82). Almost all palpable vascular tumors of the male breast have been hemangiomas.

Rarely, it is possible to find extramedullary hematopoeisis (EMH) in the vascular channels of a breast hemangioma, especially those with cavernous or capillary components.

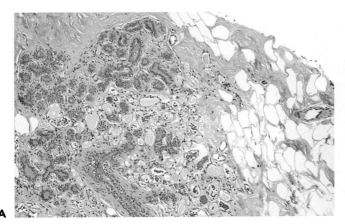

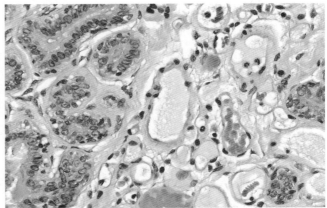

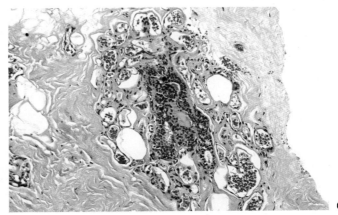

Figure 23.23 Perilobular hemangioma. A, B: This vascular lesion in intralobular stroma was an incidental finding in a needle core biopsy specimen. The procedure was done because of a nearby focus of calcifications. **C:** This microscopic hemangioma is centered around a duct in a needle core biopsy specimen.

This is an important diagnostic clue because EMH has not been reported in an angiosarcoma of the breast.

The Ki67 immunostain is a useful adjunct in the diagnosis of the mammary hemangiomas (83). The nuclear Ki67 labeling index in mammary hemangiomas is very low, rarely exceeding 5%. Focally higher rates of labeling may be found in hemangiomas at sites of organizing thrombi or where a biopsy was previously performed on the lesion. Therefore, it is important to have a hematoxylin and eosin (H&E)-stained section available to visualize structural details when the Ki67 stain is being interpreted. The Ki67 labeling index of mammary angiosarcomas is greater than in hemangiomas, typically exceeding 20% even in low-grade tumors. Because the distribution of labeling is not uniform in an angiosarcoma, it is possible by chance to obtain a needle core biopsy sample with less than 5% labeling from a low-grade angiosarcoma. A robust Ki67 labeling index in a needle core biopsy specimen from a mammary vascular lesion would strongly favor angiosarcoma. Very sparse labeling in such a limited sample can assist in making a diagnosis of hemangioma when correlated with the H&E appearance of the lesion.

Cavernous hemangiomas are the most common form of mammary hemangioma. On mammography and sonography a cavernous hemangioma presents as a round or ovoid nodule with an at least partially circumscribed margin (84). Microscopic examination reveals dilated vessels congested with red blood cells (Fig. 23.24). Small vessels of capillary dimension may be seen in portions of a cavernous hemangioma. The individual channels appear to be independent, there being few if any anastomosing vessels. Endothelial nuclei are inconspicuous and flat. Calcification may occur in the stroma. Thrombosis within cavernous channels sometimes elicits a lymphocytic reaction and endothelial proliferation may be seen within the organizing clot. These alterations can result in papillary endothelial hyperplasia that should not be mistaken for angiosarcoma. There is considerable variability in the degree of circumscription seen microscopically. In many cavernous hemangiomas, vascular channels drift into the fatty parenchyma, becoming smaller at the periphery (Fig. 23.25). This pattern duplicates the histologic appearance of peripheral parts of well-differentiated angiosarcoma.

Capillary hemangiomas tend to be cellular, with an average size of 1 cm. Many of these lesions have been detected by mammography. Fibrous septae frequently divide capillary hemangiomas into segments resulting in a lobulated structure (Fig. 23.26). Some of the tumors have prominent anastomosing vascular channels or spindle cells. Papillary endothelial hyperplasia may be present at sites of organizing thromboi. The small vascular channels are lined by endothelial cells that may have hyperchromatic nuclei (Fig. 23.27). Muscular blood vessels may be found within and

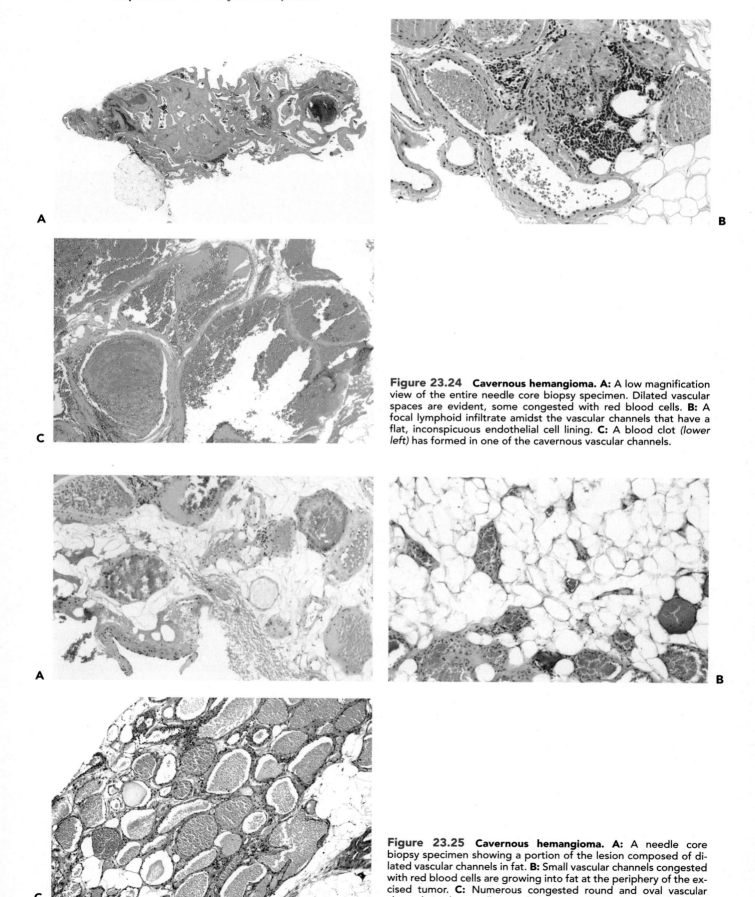

Figure 23.24 Cavernous hemangioma. A: A low magnification view of the entire needle core biopsy specimen. Dilated vascular spaces are evident, some congested with red blood cells. **B:** A focal lymphoid infiltrate amidst the vascular channels that have a flat, inconspicuous endothelial cell lining. **C:** A blood clot *(lower left)* has formed in one of the cavernous vascular channels.

Figure 23.25 Cavernous hemangioma. A: A needle core biopsy specimen showing a portion of the lesion composed of dilated vascular channels in fat. **B:** Small vascular channels congested with red blood cells are growing into fat at the periphery of the excised tumor. **C:** Numerous congested round and oval vascular channels in the needle core biopsy sample from another patient.

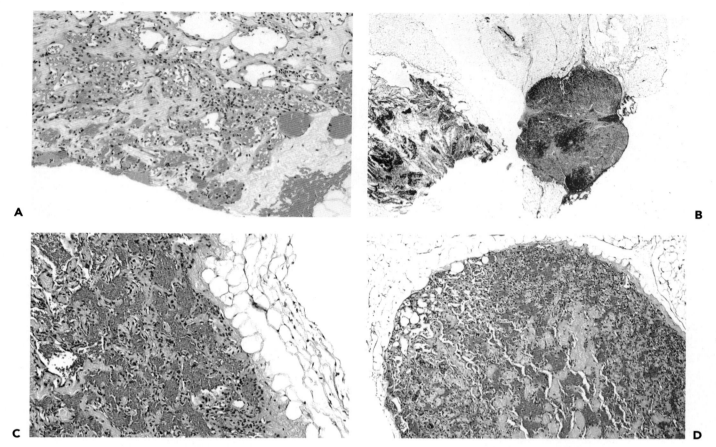

Figure 23.26 Capillary hemangioma. A: Capillary vessels in the needle core biopsy specimen. **B:** The excised tumor has a lobular configuration. **C, D:** Congested anastomosing capillary vessels in the needle core biopsy sample **(C)** from the excised 5 mm tumor shown in **(D).**

at the periphery of the tumor, apparently constituting the vessel that gave origin to the lesion ("feeding vessel").

Complex hemangiomas consisting of dilated vascular channels of varying size as well as compact, dense aggregates of capillary structures may also be detected by mammography. These lesions have an average size of 0.7 cm. Some complex hemangiomas have conspicuous anastomosing vascular channels (Fig. 23.28).

Hemorrhage and infarction can occur in hemangiomas, especially lesions detected radiologically and subjected to needle biopsy or needle localization. This should not be confused with the pattern of hemorrhagic necrosis that results in the formation of "blood lakes," characteristically found in angiosarcomas. Calcification may occur in organized thrombi, sometimes associated with endothelial hyperplasia, or in fibrous septae between vascular spaces.

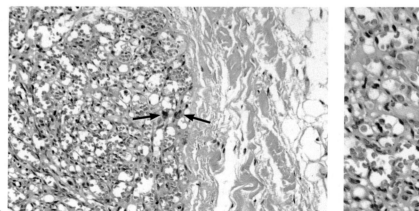
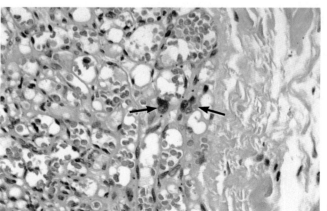

Figure 23.27 Capillary hemangioma. A, B: This needle core biopsy specimen shows the circumscribed border of the tumor. Some endothelial cells have prominent hyperchromatic nuclei *(arrows).*

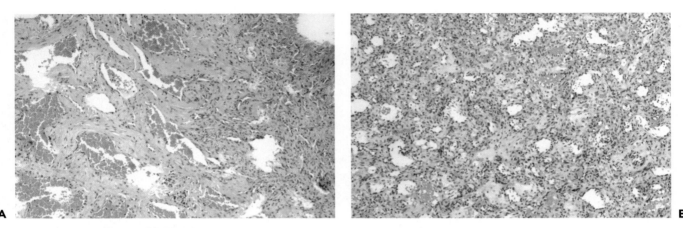

A

B

Figure 23.28 Complex hemangiomas. A: Vessels on the left have a cavernous appearance, whereas on the right there is a more cellular capillary network. **B:** Another hemangioma in which cellular fibrous stroma is distributed between capillary vessels.

Marked septal fibrosis is sometimes found in hemangiomas. Sites of hemorrhage or organizing blood clot usually display enhanced Ki67 reactivity that should not be misinterpreted as evidence of angiosarcoma.

Because of their relatively large size, atypical cytologic features with mitoses in some instances, and concern that they might be precursors of angiosarcoma, some vascular lesions have been characterized as *"atypical"* hemangiomas (78,85) (Fig. 23.29). Additional follow-up has demonstrated that so-called *atypical* angiomas are not borderline or low-grade variants of angiosarcoma and provides no evidence that they predispose to the development of angiosarcoma (85).

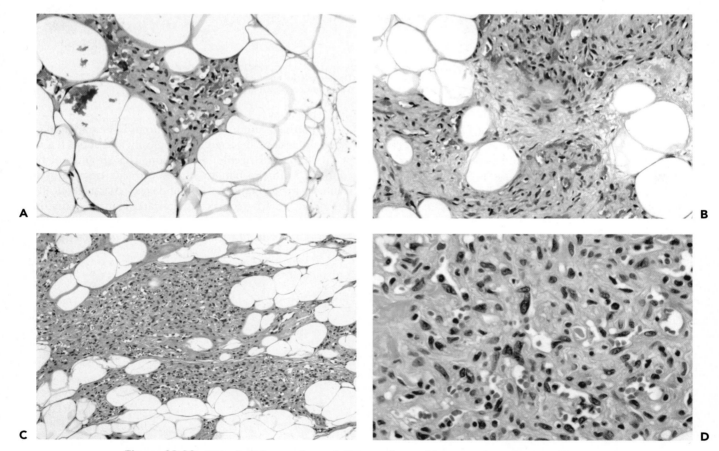

A

B

C

D

Figure 23.29 "Atypical" hemangioma. A: This needle core biopsy specimen shows capillary vessels in fat. **B:** A more compact portion of the same specimen. **C, D:** The excised tumor has an invasive growth pattern. Endothelial cell nuclei in the anastomosing capillary channels are pleomorphic and hyperchromatic. No mitotic figures were identified.

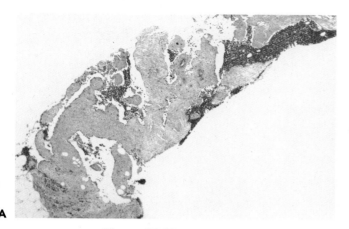

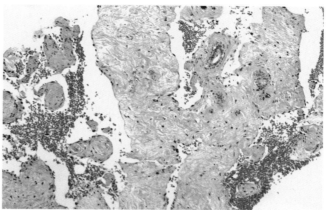

A

B

Figure 23.30 Angiomatosis. A, B: This needle core biopsy specimen reveals anastomosing dilated vascular spaces in fibrous breast stroma that contains small ducts.

Complete excision is necessary for accurate diagnosis. The material obtained in a needle core biopsy specimen is not always sufficient for this purpose. Peripheral portions of a cavernous hemangioma may be indistinguishable from a low-grade angiosarcoma in a small sample. Until recently, it has been possible to rely on the observation that hemangiomas rarely exceed 2.0 cm in diameter, whereas few angiosarcomas are smaller than 3.0 cm. This conclusion has been based primarily on data obtained from clinically palpable tumors. Currently, the availability of needle core biopsy samples from small nonpalpable vascular tumors has created a situation in which lesions smaller than 3 cm with the histologic characteristics of angiosarcoma can be encountered.

Complete excision of a hemangioma is necessary for accurate diagnosis. The material obtained with a needle core biopsy is usually not sufficient for this purpose. Peripheral portions of a cavernous hemangioma may be indistinguishable from low-grade angiosarcoma in a small sample. As a consequence, it is prudent to perform an excisional biopsy after a needle core biopsy reveals a vascular lesion. In cases where postbiopsy imaging indicates that the procedure removed most or all of a histologically benign lesion and a clip has been left at the biopsy site, follow-up by mammography can be an alternative to excisional biopsy.

Angiomatosis is a diffuse benign vascular lesion that produces a mass (86). The tumors have measured 9 to 11 cm and are grossly cystic. Microscopically they are composed of anastomosing, large vascular channels extending diffusely in the breast parenchyma. They surround ducts and lobules but do not invade into the lobular stroma. The vessels are lined by flat inconspicuous endothelium with sparse supporting mural tissue that is virtually devoid of smooth muscle (Fig. 23.30). The lesions consist predominantly of hemangiomatous erythrocyte-containing channels or lymphangiomatous empty channels accompanied by lymphoid aggregates, or a mixture of the two. Angiomatosis may occur in breast tissue involved by other conditions, such as fibroadenoma.

The microscopic distinction between low-grade angiosarcoma and angiomatosis may be difficult, especially in a small biopsy sample, because anastomosing channels that are "empty" or contain erythrocytes occur in both lesions. In angiosarcomas, the vascular channels grow into lobules that are consequently destroyed, whereas lobules are spared in angiomatosis as the vascular proliferation surrounds but does not invade them.

Mitoses are not found in angiomatosis, and it has a very low Ki67 labeling index.

Venous hemangiomas usually present as palpable tumors in patients averaging 40 years of age, but the lesion may be small enough to be detected only by mammography (87). The tumors have measured from 1.0 to 5.3 cm in greatest diameter (average 3.2 cm). All have open venous channels with smooth muscle walls of varying structural completeness (Fig. 23.31). Red blood cells are present in the lumens of some vascular spaces. Others are empty or contain lymph and lymphocytes. Thick-walled arterial channels and capillaries are usually not conspicuous. Lobules and

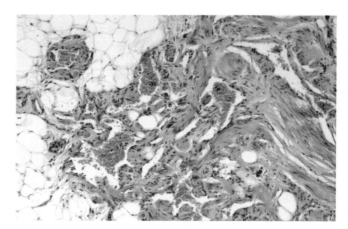

Figure 23.31 Venous hemangioma. The lesion shown in this needle core biopsy specimen is composed of vascular structures of various sizes with mural smooth muscle.

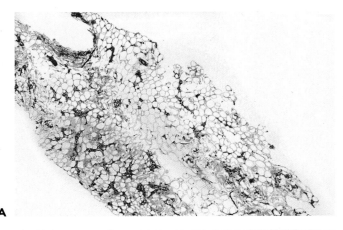

A

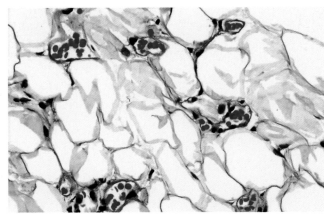

B

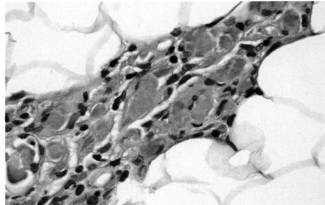

C

Figure 23.32   Nonparenchymal angiolipoma. A, B: Capillaries are dispersed in fat in this needle core biopsy specimen. Areas with a very similar histologic appearance can be found at the periphery of an angiosarcoma. **C:** Microthrombi in an angiolipoma.

ducts can be found distributed in the mammary stroma between the vascular channels and focal, perivascular lymphocytic infiltrates are usually present in the stroma.

Nonparenchymal mammary hemangiomas occur in the mammary subcutaneous tissue (88). Some are found in the inframammary region, whereas others are distributed in various quadrants. The presenting symptom is a mass in most cases, but nonpalpable lesions have been detected by mammography. Sonography is useful for determining whether a vascular lesion is located in subcutaneous tissue or in the breast parenchyma (89). Tumor size ranges from 0.8 to 3.2 cm, averaging 1.8 cm. Breast parenchyma may be included in the biopsy specimen. The lesion is classified as nonparenchymal if the neoplastic vessels are not in glandular tissue. In most cases, the specimen consists entirely of subcutaneous fat. Several types of nonparenchymal hemangiomas have been identified: angiolipoma, cavernous hemangioma, papillary endothelial hyperplasia, and capillary hemangiomas (Figs. 23.32 and 23.33). The histologic appearances of various types of hemangiomas in the mammary subcutaneous tissue does not differ from comparable lesions in other subcutaneous locations or in the breast parenchyma. Some hemangiomas found in mammary subcutaneous tissue feature interconnected vascular channels. Areas in which the septae between these channels are disrupted have a pseudopapillary pattern.

Encapsulation that characterizes many hemangiomas cannot always be reliably assessed in a core biopsy sample. Complete removal of the tumor may be necessary to exclude the possibility that the benign-appearing vascular lesion in a biopsy is a subcutaneous extension from an underlying low-grade angiosarcoma.

SARCOMAS

The diagnosis of mammary sarcomas should be reported in the same histogenetic terms used for soft part sarcomas occurring elsewhere in the body. The relative frequency of different types of breast sarcomas is difficult to determine from the literature because these lesions have sometimes been referred to by the general term *stromal sarcoma* (90). However, some differences in frequency exist. Angiosarcoma, the most common form of mammary sarcoma, is proportionately less frequent among somatic sarcomas. Other distinct mammary sarcomas include liposarcoma, fibrosarcoma, leiomyosarcoma, sarcomas with bone and cartilage, and malignant fibrous histiocytoma. A review of the reported incidence of local recurrence in relation to primary treatment suggests that total mastectomy should be recommended for most sarcomas of the breast. When a total mastectomy or a more extensive operation was the

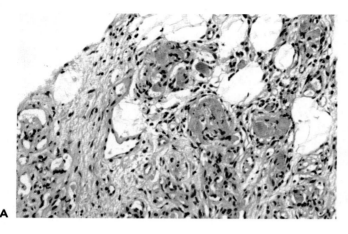

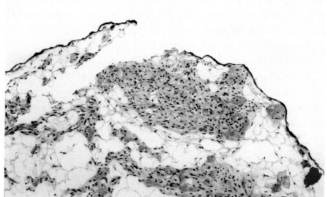

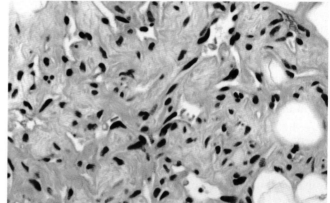

Figure 23.33 Nonparenchymal angiolipoma with atypia. A: This needle core biopsy specimen displays a compact area of capillary proliferation. Some cells have hyperchromatic nuclei. Microthrombi that characterize an angiolipoma are present. **B:** The excised tumor extended to an inked margin. **C:** This part of the excised tumor resembles the needle core biopsy specimen. Prominent hyperchromatic nuclei are shown.

initial treatment, 8% had local failures, whereas recurrence in the breast was reported in 53% of patients treated by excisional surgery. Axillary lymph node metastases are exceedingly uncommon at the time of primary therapy, and therefore routine axillary dissection is not indicated (90–92).

In a group of 83 women with primary breast sarcomas studied by Zelek et al. (93) with a median follow-up of 7.8 years, the 10 year overall survival and disease-free survival rates were 62% and 50%, respectively. Tumor size (less than 5 cm, 5–10 cm, larger than 10 cm) and tumor grade were significantly related to 10-year disease-free survival. Angiosarcoma was the only histologic type of tumor associated with a significantly poor prognosis. Another series of 25 women with primary breast sarcomas and a mean follow-up of 10.5 years was reported by Adem et al. (94). Local recurrence occurred in 11 patients after a mean follow-up of 15 months and 10 patients (40%) had systemic metastases. The five-year disease-free survival was 90% for tumors 5 cm or less and 50% for tumors larger than 5 cm. In this series disease-free survival was not significantly related to tumor grade. Multimodal therapy including radiation and chemotherapy may reduce the frequency of local and systemic recurrence in somatic sarcomas, but the results are inconclusive for mammary sarcomas.

A diagnosis of mammary sarcoma can be established only after metaplastic carcinoma is excluded. Perhaps the most difficult distinction lies between fibrosarcoma and a metaplastic spindle cell carcinoma. Immunohistochemical studies for cytokeratin, especially K903 and CK7, can detect foci of epithelial expression in a carcinoma that has undergone virtually complete conversion into a spindle cell neoplasm. Almost all spindle cell metaplastic carcinomas express p63, a marker associated with myoepithelial cells.

Angiosarcoma arises in the breast more often than in any other organ. With rare exceptions, the initial clinical finding is a painless mass. Blue or purple discoloration of the skin accompanies large or superficial tumors, but in some cases there are no external features to suggest angiosarcoma. Mammographic examination reveals an ill-defined, lobulated tumor, with areas of high and low echogenicity on sonography (95,96). Rarely, nonpalpable angiosarcomas measuring less than 3 cm have been detected by mammography. Some angiosarcomas are not visualized by mammography (96,97) but may be evident on ultrasonography or magnetic resonance imaging (MRI) (97,98). MRI is also helpful for determining the extent of the lesion (98).

Age at diagnosis ranges from the teens to older than 80 years, with a mean age at diagnosis of about 35 to 40 years. A statistically significant correlation between age at diagnosis and tumor grade was reported in one study (99).

The median ages of patients with low-, intermediate-, and high-grade tumors were 43, 34, and 29 years, respectively. Because of the relative youth of patients with mammary angiosarcoma, it is not unexpected that a number of the patients were also pregnant (99,100).

A substantial number of angiosarcomas have been described in the breast after breast-conserving surgery and irradiation for carcinoma (101–104). The interval between radiation and the diagnosis of angiosarcoma ranged from 3 to 12 years, with the many occurring within 6 years after radiotherapy (102). Almost all of these women were more than 50 years of age when treated for mammary carcinoma (102,105). Cutaneous presentation of angiosarcoma of the breast is more frequent after therapeutic irradiation for mammary carcinoma than is parenchymal angiosarcoma in the conserved breast (106). Many patients who present with angiosarcoma in the skin also have parenchymal involvement (107–110). MRI appears to be a more sensitive method than mammography for detecting parenchymal involvement (111). The estimated risk of cutaneous or parenchymal angiosarcoma of the breast after breast conservation and radiation for carcinoma is about 0.4% (103). With at least 1 year of follow-up, nearly 75% of these patients develop local recurrences, followed shortly thereafter by systemic metastases (104). Rarely, angiosarcoma has been found in a breast affected by mammary carcinoma without a history of radiotherapy (112).

Primary angiosarcomas not associated with radiation average about 5 cm, and very few are smaller than 2 cm. There is not a significant difference in the average size of high- and low-grade lesions.

Studies in the past decade have shown mammary angiosarcoma to be a morphologically heterogeneous group of neoplasms in which grade is prognostically significant (100,113–115). Three histologic patterns of growth in the primary tumor have been described. Low-grade (type I) tumors are composed of open, anastomosing vascular channels that have proliferated diffusely in mammary glandular tissue and fat (Fig. 23.34). Infiltration into lobules is characterized by spread of the vascular channels within the intralobular stroma, a process that leads to separation and atrophy of the lobular glandular units (Fig. 23.35). Endothelial cells are distributed in a flat single-cell layer around the vascular spaces, with papillary formations absent or at most very infrequent. Some prominent, hyperchromatic endothelial nuclei may be found, but the endothelial cells often have inconspicuous nuclei. Mitotic figures are rarely seen in the neoplastic endothelial cells. The vascular lumina are usually open and interanastomosing. The mean Ki67 labeling index is less than 30%. Red blood cells are typically present in small numbers but occasional lesions are congested. If mitoses are found with ease in an angiosarcoma that is structurally low grade, the tumor is likely to have the clinical course of a high-grade angiosarcoma and thorough sampling may disclose a structurally high-grade component. Ki67 labeling will be greater than is typical for low-grade angiosarcoma.

Low-grade components are found in intermediate- and high-grade lesions. This is particularly true for intermediate-grade (type 2) angiosarcomas that are distinguished from low-grade tumors by having scattered focal areas of cellular proliferation consisting of small buds or papillary fronds of endothelial cells that project into the vascular lumens (Fig. 23.36). Less often, the focally cellular areas feature polygonal and spindle cells, or there are foci that combine spindle cell and papillary elements (Fig. 23.37). Mitoses may be found in papillary or spindle cell cellular areas. Some spindle cell foci resemble lesions encountered in Kaposi sarcoma. Ki67 labeling is most evident in the focally cellular areas, whereas the remainder of the tumor exhibits labeling similar to that found in low-grade angiosarcoma. The mean Ki67 labeling index is about 40% in cellular areas.

Part of a high-grade (type 3) angiosarcoma may consist of low- and intermediate-grade elements, but in many cases more than half of the tumor has high-grade malignant features. These consist of prominent endothelial tufting and solid papillary formations that contain cytologically malignant endothelial cells, or conspicuous solid and spindle cell

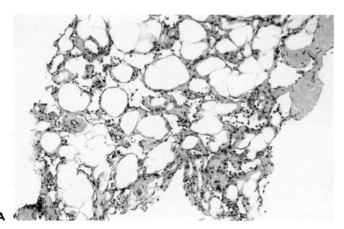
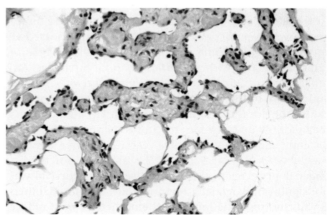

A   **B**

Figure 23.34 **Angiosarcoma, low grade. A, B:** Open, empty irregularly shaped vascular channels are distributed diffusely in this needle core biopsy specimen. The endothelial layer is flat with slightly prominent nuclei.

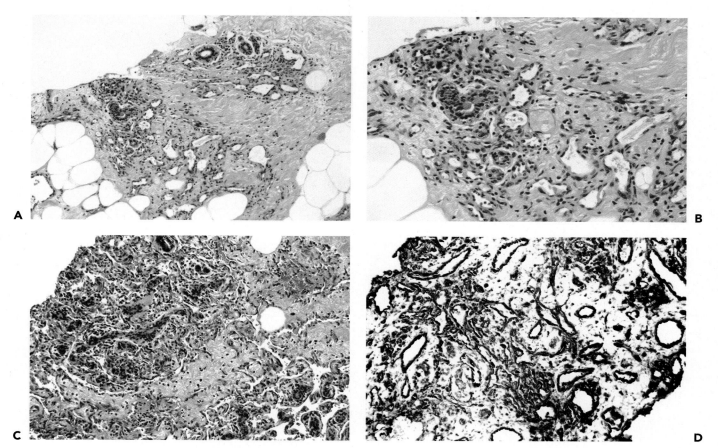

Figure 23.35   Angiosarcoma, low grade. A, B: Neoplastic vascular channels invade around and into lobules in this needle core biopsy specimen. **C, D:** Lobules partially destroyed by angiosarcoma in a needle core biopsy sample. In **(D)** the neoplastic vessels are reactive for CD31 and remnants of a lobule are highlighted by the blue hematoxylin counterstain (immunoperoxidase).

areas virtually devoid of vascular elements (Fig. 23.38). Mitoses are present. Necrosis is found only in high-grade angiosarcomas. Some high-grade angiosarcomas, especially those that arise after radiotherapy, are composed of cells with epithelioid cytology and vesicular nuclei with prominent nucleoli. The epithelioid appearance of these tumors may be mistaken for carcinoma (Fig. 23.39). Ki67 labeling is found in nearly 50% of the tumor cells (Fig. 23.40).

With few exceptions, angiosarcomas have infiltrative borders composed of well-formed or low-grade vascular channels. In some cases the peripheral vascular component is so orderly that the neoplastic vascular channels are structurally indistinguishable from existing capillaries in the normal parenchyma or resemble angiolipoma. The tendency for peripheral portions to have a low-grade structure is likely to be misleading when a superficial biopsy has been obtained from an intermediate- or high-grade tumor (116). If the initial sample does not indicate a high-grade lesion, thorough histologic evaluation of the entire tumor is required before the differentiation or grade of the tumor can be determined.

Two studies of mammary angiosarcomas reported more intense staining for factor VIII in well-differentiated than in poorly differentiated portions of the tumor (114,116). Angiosarcomas also exhibit reactivity for CD34 and CD31.

Tumor grade is an important prognostic factor (99,113). The majority of patients with orderly or low-grade lesions treated by mastectomy remain disease-free, whereas virtually all women with high-grade tumors have died of recurrent sarcoma within five years. Analysis of survival curves for patients stratified on the basis of tumor grade revealed the following estimated probabilities of disease-free survival 5 to 10 years after treatment: low grade: 76%; intermediate grade: 70%; and high grade: 15%. The median duration of disease-free survival was also correlated with tumor grade (low, >15 years; intermediate, >12 years; high, 15 months). The prognosis of angiosarcoma arising in the breast after radiotherapy is also determined by the degree of differentiation of the tumor, and when stratified for grade does not appear to differ substantially from that of parenchymal angiosarcoma. Total mastectomy is the recommended primary surgical therapy. Axillary dissection is not indicated, since metastases rarely involve these lymph nodes.

Leiomyosarcoma of the breast usually originates from blood vessels or the smooth muscle of the nipple–areolar

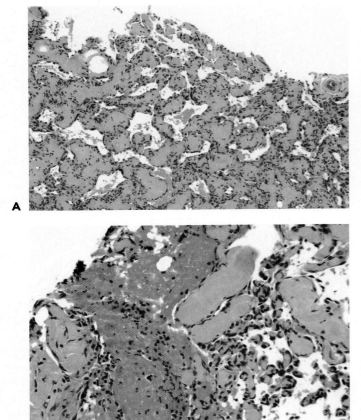

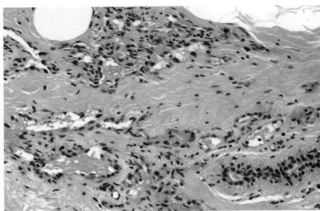

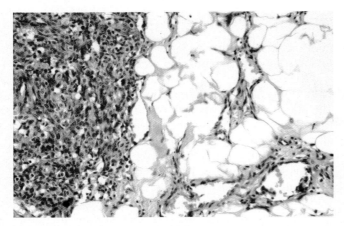

Figure 23.36 Angiosarcoma, intermediate grade. A, B: This needle core biopsy sample shows a low-grade area with fibrous stroma between anastomosing vascular channels. **C:** This region in the specimen shows focal papillary endothelial growth and thrombosis.

Figure 23.37 Angiosarcoma, intermediate grade. Low-grade growth is shown on the right and a nodular focus of spindle cell angiosarcoma on the left in this needle core biopsy specimen. These findings are compatible with an intermediate-grade tumor if the nodular element is found to be limited to isolated foci in the excised tumor.

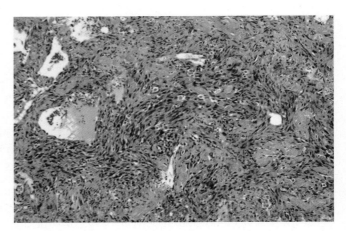

Figure 23.38 Angiosarcoma, high grade. A relatively solid spindle cell area is shown.

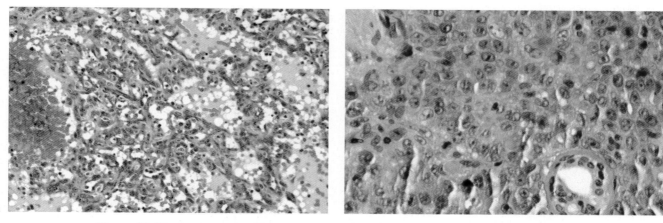

Figure 23.39 Angiosarcoma, high-grade epithelioid. A: This angiosarcoma arose in the breast 4 years after conservative surgery and radiotherapy. **B:** High-grade postradiation angiosarcoma with an epithelioid appearance. The tumor cells have characteristic vesicular nuclei and prominent nucleoli.

complex. A predisposition of smooth muscle in the nipple to give rise to neoplasms is evidenced by reports of leiomyomata and leiomyosarcomas at this site (117–120). The presenting symptom is a mass averaging about 4 cm. Mammography reveals a dense, noninvasive lesion. Approximately 25% of patients with mammary leiomyosarcoma with reported follow-up died of metastatic sarcoma (120,121). Microscopically, the neoplasm consists of in-terlacing bundles of fusiform cells characteristic of a smooth muscle tumor with typical blunt end nuclei (Fig. 23.41). Cells with an epithelioid phenotype are variably present. Malignant cytologic features are nuclear hyperchromasia, pleomorphism (sometimes with multinucleated giant cells), and readily identified mitoses. Focal areas of necrosis or hyalinized stromal fibrosis may be encountered. Immunohistochemical stains are positive for desmin and actin.

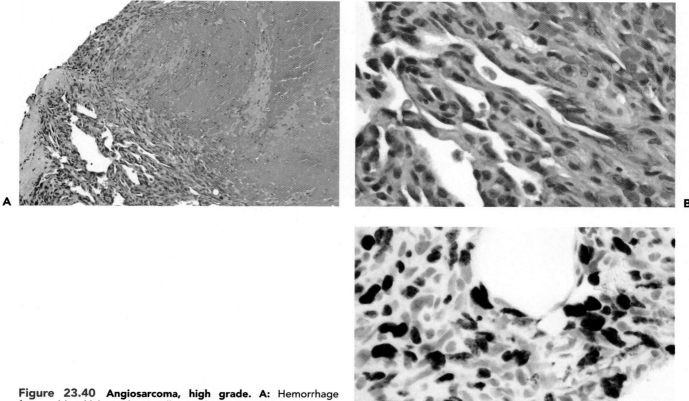

Figure 23.40 Angiosarcoma, high grade. A: Hemorrhage forms a blood lake in this needle core biopsy specimen. **B:** Hyperchromatic tumor cell nuclei. **C:** Many of the nuclei are reactive for Ki67 (immunoperoxidase).

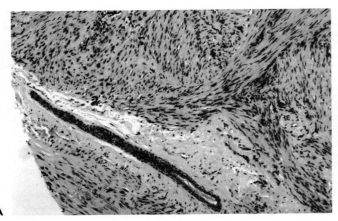

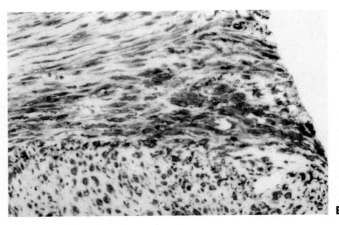

A

B

Figure 23.41 Leiomyosarcoma. A: A needle core biopsy specimen showing sarcoma infiltrating around a duct. **B:** The sarcoma is immunoreactive for smooth muscle actin (immunoperoxidase).

Liposarcoma of the breast occurs in patients 26 to 76 years of age at the time of diagnosis, with an average age of 49 years (122). The average size of mammary liposarcomas is 8 cm.

The histologic features of liposarcoma in the breast are identical to those of liposarcoma arising in the extremities or trunk. Among 25 mammary tumors classified in these terms, 12 (48%) were myxoid, 6 (24%) were well differentiated, 4 (76%) were pleomorphic, and 3 (12%) were poorly differentiated (122–124) (Fig. 23.42).

Osteogenic and chondrosarcomas of the mammary stroma are very uncommon. The precise frequency of these neoplasms is difficult to determine because some case reports do not clearly exclude metaplastic carcinoma or cystosarcoma. Mammography reveals a dense mass that may exhibit calcifications (125). One tumor was positive in a ^{99}Tc diphosphonate scan (126). Age at diagnosis averages 55 years (125–128).

The tumors have had an average size of 10 cm. Histologic examination reveals osteogenic and chondrosarcoma associated with a prominent component of high-grade spindle cell sarcoma that has a variable mitotic rate (Fig. 23.43).

Chondrosarcomas are less frequent than sarcomas with osseous differentiation. Multinucleated osteoclastic giant cells are usually present in areas of bone formation. Rarely, giant cells constitute a conspicuous element, and they may be associated with hemorrhagic cysts with a telangiectatic appearance. Special stains, including immunohistochemistry for cytokeratin, are helpful in ruling out an epithelial component. Areas with cartilaginous differentiation can be immunoreactive for EMA and staining for S-100 is sometimes found in spindle cell portions of the lesion (128).

Malignant fibrous histiocytoma including tumors recently characterized as undifferentiated pleomorphic sarcomas presents as a mass averaging 7 cm in diameter (129,130). Necrosis and calcification are infrequent. The microscopic hallmark of malignant fibrous histiocytoma is a storiform growth pattern in which the spindle cells are arranged in a pinwheel pattern (Fig. 23.44). Capillaries or small blood vessels may be found at the center of the storiform complex. Giant cells, usually with multiple nuclei, myxoid change, and a chronic inflammatory cell infiltrate are variably present. High-grade lesions are characterized by easily identified mitoses, marked cellular pleomorphism, and necrosis. Low-grade tumors have little mitotic activity, as well as minimal pleomorphism or necrosis.

Fibrosarcoma is a tumor in which the dominant growth pattern is formed by elongated spindle cells arranged in broad interdigitating sheets, bands, or fascicles (so-called *herringbone pattern*) (130). Some fibrosarcomas lacking the classic herringbone pattern consist of a loosely structured fibroblastic proliferation. Fibrosarcomas with the herringbone pattern tended to be low-grade histologically and to have a better prognosis than sarcomas with the malignant fibrous histiocytoma pattern.

Hemangiopericytoma of the breast is an uncommon neoplasm (131–133). Mammography in one case revealed a well-circumscribed dense mass that was hypoechogenic with posterior enhancement on sonography (133). Reported follow-up in 15 cases varied from less than a year to 276 months, averaging 5 years. Approximately equal numbers of

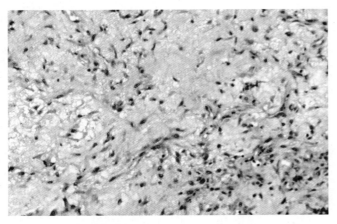

Figure 23.42 Liposarcoma. Myxoid liposarcoma with a characteristic network of capillaries.

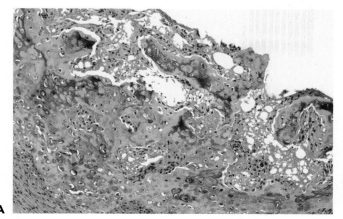

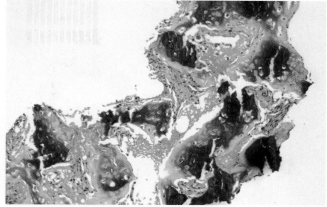

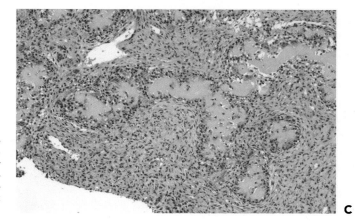

Figure 23.43 Osteochrondrosarcoma. A: This needle core biopsy specimen shows moderately differentiated cartilage with ossification. No epithelial differentiation was detected in the tumor with cytokeratin immunostains. **B:** This part of the needle core biopsy specimen revealed bone trabeculae. **C:** Another area in the specimen, with high-grade spindle cell sarcoma, osteoid, and giant cells.

patients were treated by mastectomy and local excision. None of the patients developed local recurrence or systemic metastases whether treated by local excision or mastectomy. As a consequence, mammary hemangiopericytomas that lack high-grade features such as necrosis or numerous mitoses should be considered low-grade neoplasms. Histologically, the tumor is composed of round, plump, oval, and spindle cells oriented around vascular channels of varying caliber (Fig. 23.45). The vessels often have a branching or "staghorn"

configuration. More compact zones have a spongiform appearance. The endothelium is supported by a delicate reticulin stroma without appreciable collagen or smooth muscle cells. Mitoses are infrequent, and the cells lack other cytologic features of high-grade sarcomas, such as anaplasia and pleomorphic cells. Endothelial cells of the capillaries stain for factor VIII, CD34, and CD31, but no reactivity has been found in the tumor cells. Reactivity for vimentin and variable staining for actin has been reported (131,132).

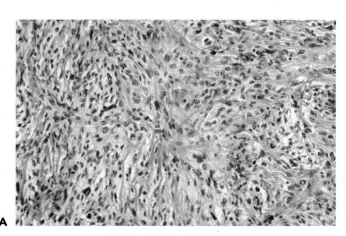

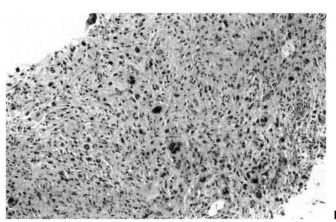

Figure 23.44 Malignant fibrous histiocytoma. A: The spindle cell tumor has a typical storiform structure. No epithelial differentiation was detected. **B:** This needle core biopsy specimen from another tumor shows giant cells.

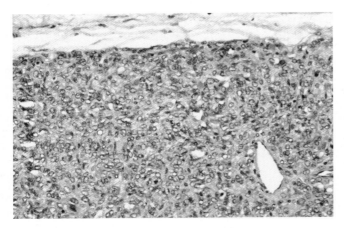

Figure 23.45 Hemangiopericytoma. The tumor has a circumscribed border. Numerous capillaries contain red blood cells. The dilated, empty vascular space in the lower right corner is a characteristic element.

Other sarcomas described in the breast include *malignant myofibroblastoma* (134), *angioblastic sarcoma, malignant peripheral nerve sheath tumors* (135), and *rhabdomyosarcoma* (136).

REFERENCES

Benign Mesenchymal Tumors

1. Gump FE, Sternschein MJ, Wolff M. Fibromatosis of the breast. *Surg Gynecol Obstet.* 1981;15:57–60.
2. Rosen PP, Ernsberger D. Mammary fibromatosis. A benign spindle cell tumor with significant risk for local recurrence. *Cancer.* 1989; 63:1363–1369.
3. Wargotz ES, Norris HJ, Austin RM, Enzinger FM. Fibromatosis of the breast. A clinical and pathological study of 28 cases. *Am J Surg Pathol.* 1987;11:38–45.
4. Cederlund CG, Gustavsson S, Linell F, et al. Fibromatosis of the breast mimicking carcinoma at mammography. *Br J Radiol.* 1984;57:98–101.
5. Kalisher L, Long JA, Peyster RG. Extra-abdominal desmoid of the axillary tail mimicking breast carcinoma. *Am J Roentgenol.* 1976;126:903–906.
6. Leal SM, Poppiti RJ, Surujon I, Matallana R. Fibromatosis of the breast mimicking infiltrating carcinoma on mammography. *Breast Dis.* 1989; 1:277–282.
7. El-Naggar A, Abdul-Karim FW, Marshalleck JJ, Sorensen K. Fine needle aspiration of fibromatosis of the breast. *Diagn Cytopathol.* 1987;3:320–322.
8. Balzer BL, Weiss SW. Implant-associated mesenchymal tumors (IAMT) of the breast: a fortuitous or causal association. *Mod Pathol.* 2005; 18(suppl):25A.
9. Aaron AD, O'Mara JW, Legendre KE, et al. Chest wall fibromatosis associated with silicone breast implants. *Surg Oncol.* 1996;5:93–99.
10. Haggitt RC, Booth JL. Bilateral fibromatosis of the breast in Gardner's syndrome. *Cancer.* 1970;25:161–166.
11. Barth AI, Nathke IS, Nelson WJ. Cadherins, catenins, and APC protein: interplay between cytoskeletal complexes and signaling pathways. *Curr Opin Cell Biol.* 1997;9:683–690.
12. Abraham SC, Reynolds C, Lee JH, et al. Fibromatosis of the breast and mutations involving the APC/β-catenin pathway. *Hum Pathol.* 2002; 33:39–46.
13. Carlson JW, Fletcher CDM. Immunohistochemistry for β-catenin in the differential diagnosis of spindle cell lesions: analysis of a series and review of the literature. *Histoathology.* 2007;51:509–514.
14. Rivera-Pomar JM, Vilanova JR, Burgos-Bretones JJ, Arocena G. Focal fibrous disease of breast. A common entity in young women. *Virchow Arch (A).* 1980;386:59–64.
15. Harvey SC, Denison CM, Lester SC, et al. Fibrous nodules found at large-core needle biopsy of the breast: imaging features. *Radiology.* 1999; 211:535–540.
16. Puente JL, Potel J. Fibrous tumor of the breast. *Arch Surg.* 1974; 109:391–394.
17. Tse GMK, Law BKB, Ma TKF, et al. Hamartoma of the breast: a clinico-pathological review. *J Clin Pathol.* 2002;55:951–954.
18. Asioli S, Eusebi V, Gaetano L, et al. The pre-lymphatic pathway, the roots of the lymphatic system in breast tissue: a 3D study. *Virchows Arch.* 2008;453:401–406.
19. Badve S, Sloane JP. Pseudoangiomatous hyperplasia of male breast. *Histopathology.* 1995;26:463–466.
20. Anderson C, Ricci A Jr, Pedersen CA, Cartun RW. Immunocytochemical analysis of estrogen and progesterone receptors in benign stromal lesions of the breast. Evidence for hormonal etiology in pseudoangiomatous hyperplasia of mammary stroma. *Am J Surg Pathol.* 1991;15:145–149.
21. Ibrahim RE, Sciotto CG, Weidner N. Pseudoangiomatous hyperplasia of mammary stroma. Some observations regarding its clinicopathologic spectrum. *Cancer.* 1989;63:1154–1160.
22. Vuitch MF, Rosen PP, Erlandson RA. Pseudoangiomatous hyperplasia of mammary stroma. *Hum Pathol.* 1986;17:185–191.
23. Iancu D, Nochomovitz LE. Pseudoangiomatous stromal hyperplasia: presentation as a mass in the female nipple. *Breast J.* 2001;7:263–265.
24. Polger MR, Denison CM, Lester S, Meyer JE. Pseudoangiomatous stromal hyperplasia: mammographic and sonographic appearances. *Am J Roentgenol.* 1996;166:349–352.
25. Ferreira M, Albarcacin T, Resetkova E. Pseudoangiomatous stromal hyperplasia tumor: a clinical, radiologic and pathologic study of 26 cases. *Mod Pathol.* 2008;21:201–207.
26. Cohen MA, Morris EA, Rosen PP, et al. Pseudoangiomatous stromal hyperplasia: mammographic, sonographic and clinical patterns. *Radiology.* 1996;198:117–120.
27. Mercado CL, Naidrich SA, Hamele-Bena D, et al. Pseudoangiomatous stromal hyperplasia of the breast: sonographic features with histopathologic correlation. *Breast J.* 2004;10:427–432.
28. Powell CM, Cranor ML, Rosen PP. Pseudoangiomatous stromal hyperplasia (PASH): A mammary stromal tumor with myofibroblastic differentiation. *Am J Surg Pathol.* 1995;19:270–277.
29. Pruthi S, Reynolds C, Johnson RE, Gisvold JJ. Tamoxifen in the management of pseudoangiomatous stromal hyperplasia. *Breast J.* 2001;6:434–439.
30. Seltzer MH, Kintiroglou M. Pseudoangiomatous hyperplasia and response to tamoxifen therapy. *Breast J.* 2003;9:344.
31. Chauhan H, Abraham A, Phillips JRA, et al. There is more than one kind of myofibroblast: analysis of CD34 expression in benign, in situ, and invasive breast lesions. *J Clin Pathol.* 2003;56:271–276.
32. Hamele-Bena D, Cranor ML, Sciotto C, et al. Uncommon presentation of mammary myofibroblastoma. *Hum Pathol.* 1996;9:786–790.
33. Ordi J, Riverola A, Solé M, et al. Fine needle aspiration of myofibroblastoma of the breast in a man: a report of two cases. *Acta Cytol.* 1992;36:194–198.
34. Rebner M, Raju U. Myofibroblastoma of the male breast. *Breast Dis.* 1993;6:157–160.
35. Greenberg JS, Kaplan SS, Grady C. Myofibroblastoma of the breast in women: imaging appearances. *Am J Roentgenol.* 1998;171:71–72.
36. Ali S, Teichberg S, Derisi DC, Urmacher C. Giant myofibroblastoma of the male breast. A case report. *Am J Surg Pathol.* 1994;18:1170–1176.
37. Wargotz ES, Weiss SW, Norris HJ. Myofibroblastoma of the breast. Sixteen cases of a distinctive benign mesenchymal tumor. *Am J Surg Pathol.* 1987;11:493–502.
38. Magro G, Michal M, Vasquez E, Bisceglia M. Lipomatous myofibroblastoma: a potential diagnostic pitfall in the spectrum of the spindle cell lesions of the breast. *Virchows Arch.* 2000;437:540–544.
39. Dal C, Sciot R, Polito P, et al. Lesions of 13q may occur independently of 16q in spindle cell/pleomorphic lipomas. *Histopathology.* 1997;31:222–225.
40. Pauwels P, Sciot R, Croiset F, et al. Myofibroblastoma of the breast: genetic link with spindle cell lipoma. *J Pathol.* 2000;191:282–285.
41. Magro G, Catalbiano R, Di Cataldo A, Puzzo L. CD10 is expressed in mammary myofibroblastoma and spindle cell lipoma of soft tissue: an additional evidence of their histogenetic linking. *Virchows Arch.* 2007;450:727–728.
42. Fukunaga M. Ushigome S. Myofibroblastoma of the breast with diverse differentiations. *Arch Pathol Lab Med.* 1997;121:599–603.
43. Thomas TNM, Myina A, Mak CKL, Chan JKC. Mammary myofibroblastoma with leiomyomatous differentiation. *Am J Clin Pathol.* 1997;107:52–55.
44. Magro G. Epitheloid cell myofibroblastoma of the breast: expanding the morphologic spectrum. *Am J Surg Pathol.* 2009;33:1085–1092.
45. Turnbull AD, Huvos AG, Ashikari R, Strong EW. Granular-cell myoblastoma of the breast. *N.Y. State J Med.* 1971;71:436–438.
46. Bassett LW, Cove HC. Myoblastoma of the breast. *Am J Roentgenol.* 1979;132:122–123.
47. Willen R, Willen H, Balldin G, Albrechtsson V. Granular cell tumor of the mammary gland simulating malignancy. *Virchows Arch (A).* 1984; 403:391–400.
48. Tai GD, Costa H, Lee D, et al. Case report: coincident granular cell tumour of the breast with invasive ductal carcinoma. *Br J Radiol.* 1995; 68:1034–1036.
49. Vos LD, Tham RTOTA, Vroegindweij D, et al. Granular cell tumor of the breast: mammographic and histologic correlation. *Eur J Radiol.* 1994; 19:56–59.
50. Green DH, Clark AH. Case report: granular cell myoblastoma of the breast: a rare benign tumour mimicking breast carcinoma. *Clin Radiol.* 1995;50:799.

51. Buley ID, Gatter KC, Kelly PMA, et al. Granular cell tumours revisited. An immunohistochemical and ultrastructural study. *Histopathology.* 1988;12:263–274.

52. Hahn HJ, Iglesias J, Flenker H, Kreuzer G. Granular cell tumor in differential diagnosis of tumors of the breast. *Path Res Pract.* 1992;188:1091–1094.

53. Ingram DL, Mossler JA, Snowhite J, et al. Granular cell tumors of the breast. Steroid receptor analysis and localization of carcinoembryonic antigen, myoglobin and S-100 protein. *Arch Pathol Lab Med.* 1984;108:897–901.

54. Majmudar B. Neurilemoma presenting as a lump in the breast. *South Med J.* 1976;69:463–464.

55. van der Walt JD, Reid HA, Shaw JHF. Neurilemoma appearing as a lump in the breast. *Arch Pathol Lab Med.* 1982;106:539–540.

56. Gultekin SH, Cody HS III, Hoda SA. Schwannoma of the breast. *South Med J.* 1996;89:238–239.

57. Linell F, Ostberg G, Soderstrom J, et al. Breast hamartomas. An important entity in mammary pathology. *Virchows Arch (A).* 1979;383:253–264.

58. Evers K, Yeh I-T, Troupin RH, et al. Mammary hamartomas. The importance of radiologic–pathologic correlation. *Breast Dis.* 1992;5:35–43.

59. Hessler C, Schnyder P, Ozzello L. Hamartoma of the breast: Diagnostic observation of 16 cases. *Radiology.* 1978;126:95–98.

60. Adler DD, Jeffries DO, Helvie MA. Sonographic features of breast hamartomas. *J Ultrasound Med.* 1990;9:85–90.

61. Crothers JG, Butler NF, Fortt RW, Gravelle IH. Fibroadenolipoma of the breast. *Br J Radiol.* 1985;58:191–202.

62. Jackson FI, Lalani Z, Swallow J. Adenolipoma of the breast. *Can Assoc Radiol J.* 1988;39:288–289.

63. Yasuda S, Kubota M, Noto T, et al. Two cases of adenolipoma of the breast. *Tokai J Exp Clin Med.* 1992;17:139–144.

64. Lugo M, Reyes JM, Putony PB. Benign chondrolipomatous tumor of the human female breast. *Arch Pathol Lab Med.* 1982;106:691–692.

65. Marsh WL Jr, Lucas JG, Olsen J. Chondrolipoma of the breast. *Arch Pathol Lab Med.* 1989;113:369–371.

66. Nascimento AG, Rosen PP, Karas M. Leiomyoma of the nipple. *Am J Surg Pathol.* 1979;3:151–154.

67. Diaz-Arias AA, Hurt MA, Loy TS, et al. Leiomyoma of the breast. *Hum Pathol.* 1989;20:396–399.

68. Velasco M, Ubeda B, Autonel F, Serra C. Leiomyoma of the male areola infiltrating the breast tissue. *Am J Roentgenol.* 1995;164:511–512.

69. Eusebi V, Cunsolo A, Fedeli F, et al. Benign smooth muscle cell metaplasia in breast. *Tumori.* 1980;66:643–653.

70. Huntrakoon M, Lin F. Muscular hamartoma of the breast. *Virchows Arch (A).* 1984;403:307–312.

71. Shepstone BJ, Wells CA, Berry AR, Ferguson JDP. Mammographic appearance and histopathological description of a muscular hamartoma of the breast. *Br J Radiol.* 1985;58:459–461.

72. Fiirgaard B, Kristensen S. Muscular hamartoma of the breast. A case report. *Acta Radiol.* 1992;33:115–116.

73. Garfein CF, Aulicino MR, Leytin A, et al. Epithelioid cells in myoid hamartoma of the breast. *Arch Pathol Lab Med.* 1996;120:676–680.

74. Pui MH, Movson IJ. Fatty tissue breast lesions. *J Clin Imaging.* 2003;27:150–155.

75. Chan KW, Chadially FN, Alagarantnam TT. Benign spindle cell tumor of breast—a variant of spindle cell lipoma or fibroma of breast? *Pathology.* 1984;16:331–336.

76. Lew WY. Spindle cell lipoma of the breast. A case report and literature review. *Diagn Cytopathol.* 1993;9:434–437.

77. Smith DN, Denison CM, Lester SC. Spindle cell lipoma of the breast. A case report. *Acta Radiol.* 1996;37:893–895.

78. Jozefczyk MA, Rosen PP. Vascular tumors of the breast II. Perilobular hemangiomas and hemangiomas. *Am J Surg Pathol.* 1985;9:491–503.

79. Lesueur GC, Brown RW, Bhathal PS. Incidence of perilobular hemangioma in the female breast. *Arch Pathol Lab Med.* 1983;107:308–310.

80. Rosen PP, Ridolfi RL. The perilobular hemangioma. A benign vascular lesion of the breast. *Am J Clin Pathol.* 1977;68:21–23.

81. Webb LA, Young JR. Case report: haemangioma of the breast—appearances on mammography and ultrasound. *Clin Radiol.* 1996;51:523–524.

82. Tabar L, Dean PB. *Teaching Atlas of Mammography.* 2nd ed. New York: George Thieme Verlag Stuttgart; 1985:45, 209.

83. Shin SJ, Lesser MJ, Rosen PP. Hemangiomas and angiosarcomas of the breast: diagnostic utility of cell cycle markers with emphasis on Ki-67. *Arch Pathol Lab Med.* 2007;131:538–544.

84. Mesurolle B, Wexler M, Halwani F, et al. Cavernous hemangioma of the breast: Mammographic and sonographic findings and follow-up in a patient receiving hormone-replacement therapy. *J Clin Ultrasound.* 2003;31:430–436.

85. Hoda SA, Cranor ML, Rosen, PP. Hemangiomas of the breast with atypical histological features. Further analysis of histological subtypes confirming their benign character. *Am J Surg Pathol.* 1992;16:553–560.

86. Rosen PP. Vascular tumors of the breast. III. Angiomatosis. *Am J Surg Pathol.* 1985;9:652–655.

87. Rosen PP, Jozefczyk MA, Boram LH. Vascular tumors of the breast IV. The venous hemangioma. *Am J Surg Pathol.* 1985;9:659–665.

88. Rosen PP. Vascular tumors of the breast V. Non-parenchymal hemangiomas of mammary subcutaneous tissue. *Am J Surg Pathol.* 1985;9:723–729.

89. Siewert B, Jacobs T, Baum JK. Sonographic evaluation of subcutaneous hemangioma of the breast. *Am J Roentgenol.* 2002;178:1025–1027.

Sarcomas

90. Berg JW, DeCrosse JJ, Fracchia AA, Farrow J. Stromal sarcomas of the breast: a unified approach to connective tissue sarcomas other than cystosarcoma phyllodes. *Cancer.* 1962;13:419–424.

91. Gutman H, Pollock RE, Ross MI, et al. Sarcoma of the breast: implications for extent of therapy. The MD Anderson experience. *Surgery.* 1994;116:505–509.

92. McGregor GI, Knowling MA, Este FA. Sarcoma and cystosarcoma phyllodes tumors of the breast: a retrospective review of 58 cases. *Am J Surg.* 1994;167:477–480.

93. Zelek L, Llombart-Cussac A, Terrier P, et al. Prognostic factors in primary breast sarcomas: A series of patients with long-term follow-up. *J Clin Oncol.* 2003;21:2583–2588.

94. Adem C, Reynolds C, Ingle JN, Nascimento AG. Primary breast sarcoma: clinicopathologic series from the Mayo Clinic and review of the literature. *Br J Cancer.* 2004;91:237–241.

95. Grant EG, Holt RW, Chung B, et al. Angiosarcoma of the breast sonographic, xeromammographic and pathologic appearance. *Am J Roentgenol.* 1983;141:691–692.

96. Liberman L, Dershaw DD, Kaufman RJ, Rosen PP. Angiosarcoma of the breast. *Radiology.* 1992;183:649–654.

97. Yang WT, Hennessy BTJ, Dryden MJ, et al. Mammary angiosarcomas: imaging findings in 24 patients. *Radiology.* 2007;242:725–734.

98. Glazebrook KN, Magut MJ, Reynolds C. Angiosarcoma of the breast. *Am J Roentgenol.* 2008;190:533–538.

99. Rosen PP, Kimmel M, Ernsberger D. Mammary angiosarcoma. The prognostic significance of tumor differentiation. *Cancer.* 1988;62:2145–2151.

100. Chen KTK, Kirkeguard DD, Bocian JJ. Angiosarcoma of the breast. *Cancer.* 1980;46:368–371.

101. Del Mastro L, Garrone O, Guenzi M, et al. Angiosarcoma of the residual breast after conservative surgery and radiotherapy for primary carcinoma. *Ann Oncol.* 1994;5:163–165.

102. Cafiero F, Gipponi M, Peressini A, et al. Radiation-associated angiosarcoma. Diagnostic and therapeutic implications—two case reports and a review of the literature. *Cancer.* 1996;77:2496–2502.

103. Pendlebury SC, Bilous M, Langlands AO. Sarcomas following radiation therapy for breast cancer: a report of three cases and a review of the literature. *Int J Rad Oncol Biol Phys.* 1994;31:405–410.

104. Monroe AT, Feigenberg SJ, Mandenhall NP. Angiosarcoma after breast-conserving therapy. *Cancer.* 2003;97:1832–1840.

105. Billings SD, McKenney JK, Folpe AL, et al. Cutaneous angiosarcoma following breast-conserving surgery and radiation: An analysis of 27 cases. *Am J Surg Pathol.* 2004;28:781–788.

106. Strobbe LJ, Peterse HL, van Tinteren H, et al. Angiosarcoma of the breast after conservation therapy for invasive cancer, the incidence and outcome. An unforeseen sequela. *Breast Cancer Res Treat.* 1998;47:101–109.

107. Wijnmaalen A, van Ooijen B, van Geel BN, et al. Angiosarcoma of the breast following lumpectomy, axillary lymph node dissection, and radiotherapy for primary breast cancer: three case reports and a review of the literature. *Int J Rad Oncol Biol Phys.* 1993;26:135–139.

108. Fineberg S, Rosen PP. Angiosarcoma and atypical cutaneous vascular lesions after radiation therapy for breast carcinoma. *Am J Clin Pathol.* 1994;102:757–763.

109. Timmer SJ, Osuch JR, Colony LH, et al. Angiosarcoma of the breast following lumpectomy and radiation therapy for breast carcinoma: case report and review of the literature. *Breast J.* 1997;3:40–47.

110. Bolin DJ, Lukas GM. Low-grade dermal angiosarcoma of the breast following radiotherapy. *Am Surg.* 1996;62:668–672.

111. Marchant LK, Orel SG, Perez-Joffe LA, et al. Bilateral angiosarcoma of the breast on MR imaging. *Am J Roentgenol.* 1997;169:1009–1010.

112. Benda RA, Al-Jurf AS, Benson AJB III. Angiosarcoma of the breast following segmental mastectomy complicated by lymphedema. *Am J Clin Pathol.* 1987;87:651–655.

113. Donnell RM, Rosen PP, Lieberman PH, et al. Angiosarcoma and other vascular tumors of the breast. Pathologic analysis as a guide to prognosis. *Am J Surg Pathol.* 1981;5:629–642.

114. Merino MJ, Berman M, Carter D. Angiosarcoma of the breast. *Am J Surg Pathol.* 1983;7:53–60.

115. Britt LD, Lambert P, Sharma R, Ladaga LE. Angiosarcoma of the breast. Initial misdiagnosis is still common. *Arch Surg.* 1995;130:221–223.

116. Guarda LA, Ordonez NG, Smith JL Jr, Hanssen G. Immunoperoxidase localization of Factor VIII in angiosarcomas. *Arch Pathol Lab Med.* 1982;106:515–516.

117. Cameron HM, Stamperl H, Warambo W. Leiomyosarcoma of the breast originating from myothelium (myoepithelium). *J Pathol.* 1974;114:89–92.

118. Pardo-Mindan J, Garcia-Julian G, Altuna ME. Leiomyosarcoma of the breast. *Am J Clin Pathol.* 1974;62:477–480.

119. Hernandez FJ. Leiomyosarcoma of the male breast originating in the nipple. *Am J Surg Pathol.* 1978;2:299–304.

120. Parham DM, Robertson AJ, Hussein KA, Davidson AIG. Leiomyosarcoma of the breast: cytological and histological features, with a review of the literature. *Cytopathology.* 1992;3:245–252.

121. Callery CD, Rosen PP, Kinne DW. Sarcoma of the breast. A study of 32 patients with reappraisal of classification and therapy. *Ann Surg.* 1985;201:527–532.

122. Austin RM, Dupree WB. Liposarcoma of the breast: a clinicopathologic study of 20 cases. *Hum Pathol.* 1986;17:906–913.

123. Odom JW, Mikhailova B, Pryce E, et al. Liposarcoma of the breast. Report of a case and review of the literature. *Breast Dis.* 1991;4:293–298.

124. Pollard SG, Marks PV, Temple LN, Thompson HH. Breast sarcoma. A clinicopathologic review of 25 cases. *Cancer.* 1990;66:941–944.

125. Remadi S, Doussis-Anagnostopoulu I, Mac Gee W. Primary osteosarcoma of the breast. *Pathol Res Pract.* 1995;191:471–474.

126. Savage AP, Sagor GR, Dovey P. Osteosarcoma of the breast: a case report with an unusual diagnostic feature. *Clin Oncol.* 1984;10:295–298.

127. Going JJ, Lumsden AB, Anderson JJ. A classical osteogenic sarcoma of the breast: histology, immunohistochemistry and ultrastructure. *Histopathology.* 1986;10:631–641.

128. Muller AGS, Van Zyl JA. Primary osteosarcoma of the breast. *J Surg Oncol.* 1993;52:135–136.

129. Jones MW, Norris HJ, Wargotz ES, Weiss SW. Fibrosarcoma-malignant fibrous histiocytoma of the breast. A clinicopathologic study of 32 cases. *Am J Surg Pathol.* 1992;16:667–674.

130. Rossen K, Stamp I, Sorensen IM. Primary malignant fibrous histiocytoma of the breast. A report of four cases and review of the literature. *APMIS.* 1991;99:696–702.

131. Arias-Stella J, Rosen PP. Hemangiopericytoma of the breast. *Mod Pathol.* 1988;1:98–103.

132. Mittal KR, Gerald W, True LD. Hemangiopericytoma of breast: report of a case with ultrastructural and immunohistochemical findings. *Hum Pathol.* 1986;17:1181–1183.

133. van Kints MJ, Tham RT, Klinkhamer PJ, van den Bosch HC. Hemangiopericytoma of the breast: mammographic and sonographic findings. *Am J Roentgenol.* 1994;163:61–63.

134. Taccagni G, Rovere E, Masullo M, et al. Myofibroblastoma of the breast. Review of the literature on myofibroblastic tumors and criteria for defining myofibroblastic differentiation. *Am J Surg Pathol.* 1997;21:489–496.

135. Catania S, Pacifico E, Zurrida S, Cusumano F. Malignant schwannoma of the breast. *Eur J Surg Oncol.* 1992;18:80–81.

136. Barnes L, Pietruszka M. Sarcomas of the breast. A clinicopathologic analysis of 10 cases. *Cancer.* 1977;40:1577–1585.

Lymphoid and Hematopoietic Tumors

24

NON-HODGKIN LYMPHOMA

The diagnosis of primary mammary lymphoma is limited to patients without evidence of systemic lymphoma or leukemia at the time that the breast lesion is detected (1). Clinically, the disease should involve only the breast or the breast and ipsilateral lymph nodes. Fewer than 1% of all non-Hodgkin lymphomas and about 2% of extra- nodal lymphomas involve the breast (2). The occurrence of synchronous and metachronous lymphoma and breast carcinoma has been described (3). Mammary involvement by lymphoma occurs in some but not all of these patients.

With rare exceptions, patients described in the literature have been women ranging in age from 13 to 90 years at diagnosis, averaging about 55 years. Bilateral disease is present in about 10% of patients at the time of diagnosis.

The presenting symptom in virtually all cases is a mass located most often in the upper outer quadrant. However nonpalpable non-Hodgkin lymphoma, especially when low grade may be detected by mammography in the absence of a mass (4). A history of recent onset and rapid growth is not unusual. The tumor is often solitary but patients with multiple lesions and diffuse infiltration have been described. Enlarged axillary lymph nodes have been present clinically in 30% to 50% of patients (5–7).

Mammographically, the tumor may be well defined and circumscribed or irregular and thus difficult to distinguish from other lesions (8–10). Research suggests that diffuse infiltration and multiple ill-defined lesions are radiologic clues to the diagnosis of lymphoma (11). There is no association between specific subtypes of lymphoma and radiologic findings on mammography (11,12). Mammary lymphomas may be hypoechoic when studied by ultrasonography (12). PET/CT scans are helpful for postchemotherapy follow-up because response to treatment is manifested by a decrease in hypermetabolism (13).

The tumors have measured 1 to 12 cm, averaging about 3.0 cm. Histologic examination often reveals that the lymphomatous infiltrate extends into the breast parenchyma beyond the grossly evident mass. The largest subgroup of primary mammary lymphomas has been described as diffuse histiocytic when classified by the Rappaport system (1,5,6,8) or as diffuse large cell (14) (Fig. 24.1). Poorly differentiated

lymphocytic lymphomas, the majority of which are diffuse, and mixed lymphomas, equally nodular and diffuse, are the second and third most common types, respectively (6) (Fig. 24.2). Well-differentiated lymphocytic, lymphoblastic, undifferentiated, Burkitt and mucosa-associated lymphoid tissue (MALT) lymphomas account for 10% to 15% of mammary lymphomas in most series (Fig. 24.3). Diffuse large cleaved, diffuse small cleaved, and diffuse or follicular mixed cell lymphomas are the three most common cell types according to the International Working Formulation (6). The majority of mammary lymphomas are of the B-cell type, with infrequent examples of T-cell and histiocytic lymphoma described (10,14–19). Anaplastic large cell lymphoma, a T-cell lymphoma, has been found to arise in the seroma associated with breast implant capsules (20,21).

Domchek et al. (4) described the classification of 32 primary breast lymphomas based on the International Working Formulation. Nine low-grade lymphomas include the following: MALT (5), follicular center cell (3), and chronic lymphocytic leukemia/small cell lymphocytic lymphoma (1). All 17 intermediate-grade lymphomas were of the diffuse large cell type. Five of six high-grade lymphomas were "Burkitt-like" and one was lymphoblastic. The Burkitt-like lymphomas did not have genetic analysis or studies for Epstein–Barr virus antigen expression.

Lymphoma in the breast typically consists of a dense population of tumor cells that diffusely infiltrates the mammary parenchyma. Ducts and lobules in the central portion of the lesion are usually obliterated and in some cases, the stroma develops a dense sclerotic reaction that tends to be associated with blood vessels (Fig. 24.4). Ducts and lobules are better preserved away from the center of the lesion, where there is a tendency for the lymphomatous infiltrate to concentrate in and around these structures (Fig. 24.5). A reactive lymphoid infiltrate composed of small lymphocytes is very commonly present at the periphery of the tumor, often localized around epithelial elements and blood vessels. Germinal centers may be formed in these reactive infiltrates (Fig. 24.6). Calcifications are not usually an intrinsic feature of mammary lymphoma but they may occur coincidentally in epithelial lesions or in fat necrosis.

Extension of lymphoma cells into the glandular epithelium of ducts and lobules may mimic in situ carcinoma or

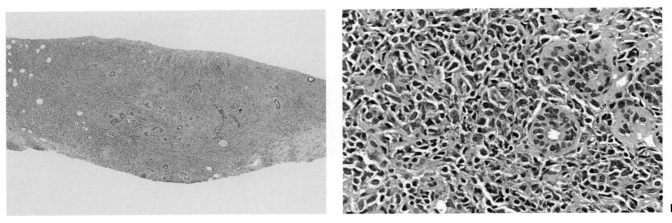

Figure 24.1   Malignant lymphoma. A, B: This 66-year-old patient presented with a periareolar breast mass. The needle core biopsy shown here revealed diffuse large cell B-cell lymphoma. Infiltration of lobular glands is evident in **(B)**.

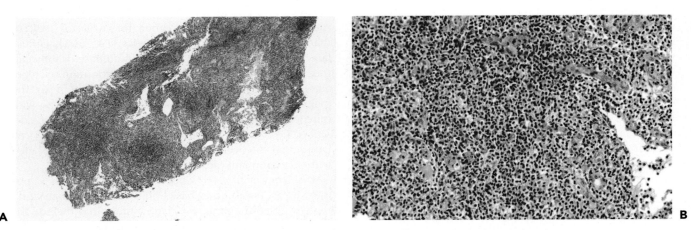

Figure 24.2   Malignant lymphoma. A, B: Diffuse poorly differentiated lymphocytic lymphoma in a needle core biopsy specimen of the breast.

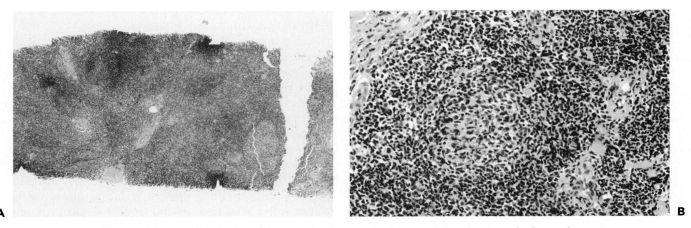

Figure 24.3   Malignant lymphoma. A, B: This lymphoplasmacytic lymphoma in the breast has nodular and diffuse areas. Focal perivascular fibrosis is evident **(A).**

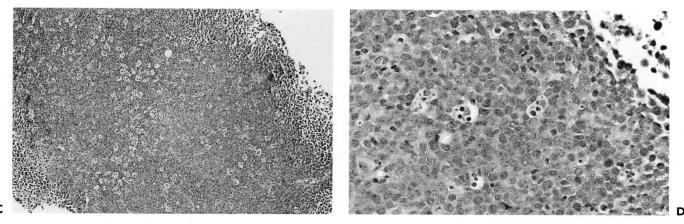

C

D

Figure 24.3 *(continued)* **C, D:** This needle core biopsy specimen from a large breast tumor in an 87-year-old woman shows Burkitt-like lymphoma with tingible body macrophages.

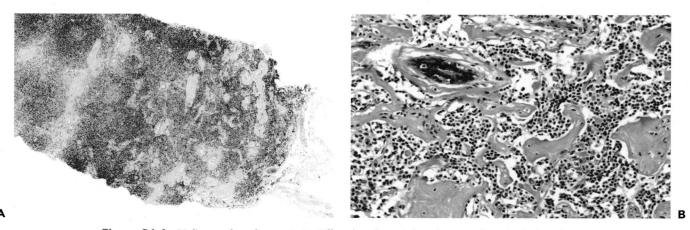

A

B

Figure 24.4 **Malignant lymphoma. A, B:** Diffuse lymphocytic lymphoma with perivascular sclerosis. A residual mammary duct is shown in **(B).**

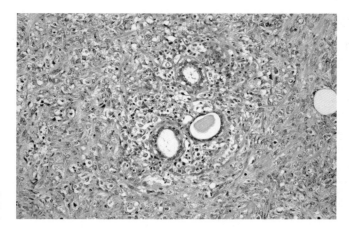

Figure 24.5 **Malignant lymphoma.** Diffuse large cell lymphoma has infiltrated and partially destroyed this lobular gland, creating an appearance that could be mistaken for infiltrating lobular carcinoma.

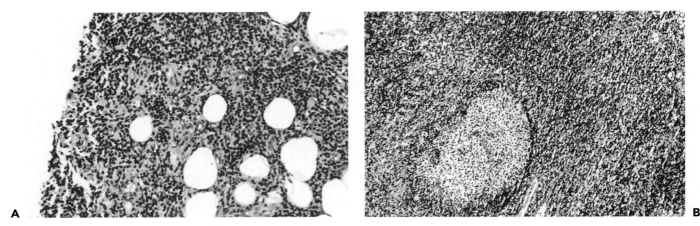

Figure 24.6 Malignant lymphoma. A, B: This needle core biopsy specimen contains small lymphocytes and germinal center formation in an atypical lymphoid infiltrate that is suggestive of lymphoma.

pagetoid spread of carcinoma. Signet ring cell lymphoma bears a striking resemblance to signet ring cell lobular carcinoma, and it may require immunostains for lymphoid and epithelial markers to distinguish between these entities. The appearance of lymphoma involving mammary stroma that is altered by pseudoangiomatous stromal hyperplasia may also be mistaken for invasive carcinoma

(14,15). This growth pattern arises when lymphoma cells insinuate themselves into the interstices of pseudoangiomatous stromal hyperplasia, a phenomenon not typical of inflammatory infiltrates (Fig. 24.7). Distinguishing large cell lymphoma from poorly differentiated carcinoma is sometimes difficult, especially when the tumor lacks an in situ carcinoma component (16). Large cell lymphoma may

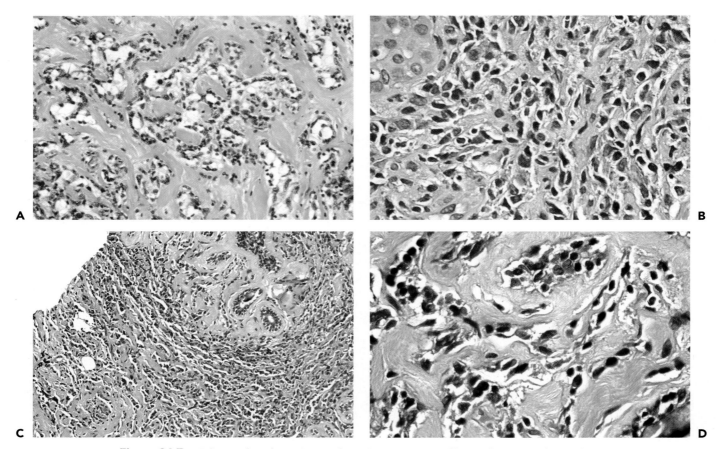

Figure 24.7 Malignant lymphoma in pseudoangiomatous stromal hyperplasia. A: Malignant lymphoma growing in mammary stroma altered by pseudoangiomatous hyperplasia can be mistaken for a vascular lesion or invasive lobular carcinoma. **B:** Diffuse large B-cell lymphoma growing in pseudoangiomatous stromal hyperplasia. A lobular gland is shown in the upper left corner. **C, D:** Diffuse large B-cell lymphoma shown here in pseudoangiomatous stroma resembles invasive lobular carcinoma.

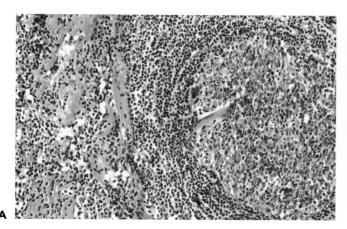

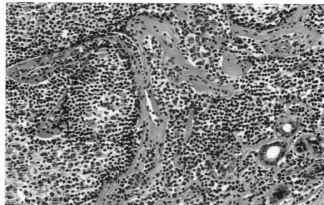

Figure 24.8   Pseudolymphoma. A, B: This atypical lymphoid lesion of the breast characterized by stromal fibrosis and prominent germinal centers proved to be a polyclonal infiltrate.

assume solid, diffuse, and sometimes alveolar growth patterns that resemble carcinoma. The limited samples of needle core biopsy specimens provide a setting where there is a risk of mistaking lymphoma for carcinoma. This is one of the many reasons why frozen section examination of needle core biopsy specimens is not recommended.

When immunostains are obtained to distinguish between carcinoma and lymphoma, it is important to employ a panel of cytokeratin markers (CK7, K903, AE1/AE3) because of the variable reactivity of mammary carcinoma for these reagents. A complete panel should also include E-cadherin, estrogen and progesterone receptors, and markers for B and T cells.

The term *pseudolymphoma* has been applied to tumor-forming lymphoid lesions assumed to be benign reactive conditions. Fewer than 20 cases have been reported in the breast (22,23). The number of patients initially diagnosed as having mammary pseudolymphoma who later developed malignant lymphoma is not known. Tumors described as pseudolymphomas have been characterized by an infiltrate composed largely of mature lymphocytes. Germinal centers are often present, especially at the periphery, and they are sometimes numerous (Fig. 24.8). The infiltrate tends to concentrate in the stroma, on occasion accompanied by fat necrosis and fibrosis. The epithelium of ducts and lobules is largely spared, although these structures can be surrounded by the infiltrative process. Analysis of the tissue for cell markers reveals a polyclonal cellular infiltrate. The sample obtained in a needle core biopsy is not a reliable basis for a diagnosis of mammary pseudolymphoma. Comparable foci of lymphocytic reaction are often encountered at the periphery of true lymphomas. Fragments of lymph node tissue may also be mistaken for a pseudolymphomatous lesion histologically.

Until fairly recently, there has been a tendency to treat patients with "primary" lymphoma clinically limited to the breast and axillary lymph nodes by mastectomy and to reserve excision for women with systemic disease. It has now been demonstrated that excellent local control in the breast and regional lymph nodes can be achieved with radiation and chemotherapy after partial mastectomy and, consequently, mastectomy is only recommended for specific clinical problems such as diffuse or bulky local disease or infected, ulcerated lesions (24–27).

Regardless of the type of local therapy, the majority of recurrences occur at distant sites or in the opposite breast. The role of various staging procedures including laparotomy in the selection of adjuvant systemic treatment remains uncertain. No prospective randomized trial has been performed to determine if any type of chemotherapy deemed effective for nonmammary lymphoma given in an adjuvant setting improves the prognosis of patients with mammary lymphoma.

To date, one of the largest reviews of treatment and prognosis was compiled by Jennings et al. (28), using reports published from 1972 to 2005. They identified 465 evaluable patients with primary breast lymphoma. Stage I patients defined as having disease limited to the breast and negative lymph nodes benefited from radiotherapy, with or without chemotherapy. Mastectomy did not improve survival, and patients who had a mastectomy were less likely to receive radiation or chemotherapy. In stage II patients, survival was more favorable among patients who received radiation and chemotherapy than when only one modality was used.

HODGKIN DISEASE

Hodgkin disease very rarely involves the breast. Mammary infiltration is usually the result of direct extension from axillary or mediastinal lymph nodes, part of regional disease with discontinuous axillary nodal involvement, or a manifestation of systemic disease (29). Most patients with primary mammary Hodgkin disease have been women and almost all of them ultimately developed systemic disease. The diagnosis of Hodgkin disease in the breast may be suspected in a needle core biopsy specimen. Reed–Sternberg cells are the diagnostic feature. The identification of Reed–Sternberg cells can be confirmed by immunohistochemical staining for Leu-M1 (CD15).

It is now a well-established observation that patients who receive extended field radiotherapy for Hodgkin disease are at increased risk to develop breast carcinoma (30–32). The risk is inversely related to age when Hodgkin disease was treated, being greatest in girls radiated prior to puberty or in adolescence. For patients treated before 21 years of age, the relative risk for developing breast carcinoma is about 15 to 25. Overall, there is a greater-than-expected frequency of bilateral carcinoma in these women. Histologically, the carcinomas tend to be ductal type, high grade, whether in situ or invasive, and they are often accompanied by a lymphocytic reaction (30). As would be expected for poorly differentiated tumors, the carcinomas are typically hormone receptor negative.

PLASMACYTIC TUMORS

Primary extramedullary plasmacytoma localized to the breast has been described in very few patients (Fig. 24.9). In one case, mammography revealed a circumscribed mass that was hypoechoic and solid on ultrasound (33). Solitary plasmacytomas of the breast have generally measured between 2 and 4 cm in diameter. In patients with multiple myeloma, the tumors have been composed of "abnormal" or "immature" plasma cells while solitary plasmacytomas

contain "a mixture of mature and immature plasma cells." Mitoses, nuclear pleomorphism, and multinucleated plasma cells may be seen in solitary plasmacytomas. Mammary glandular structures are largely effaced in the region where the plasma cell infiltrate is most concentrated. Mammary plasmacytoma should be distinguished from plasma cell mastitis, amyloid tumor, and plasma cell granuloma (34). If appropriate samples are available, immunohistochemical studies for immunoglobulins may be performed on the tissue to determine if the infiltrate has the monoclonal character of a neoplastic process or if it is a reactive polyclonal lesion (35).

LEUKEMIC INFILTRATION

Leukemic infiltration of the breast occurs not uncommonly at an advanced stage and only rarely as the initial manifestation of the disease or as the site of localized recurrence (36). Tumor involvement of the breast by *granulocytic leukemia* is referred to as granulocytic sarcoma (37). The term *chloroma* has been used to describe extramedullary, tumor-forming granulocytic leukemic infiltrates that develop a green color when the tissue is exposed to air as a result of the enzymatic action of myeloperoxidase (verdoperoxidase) contained in the neoplastic cells. Mammary infiltrates have also been

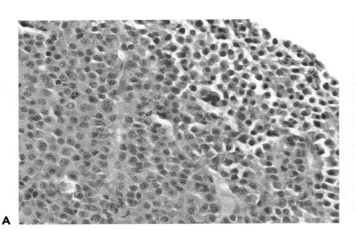

A

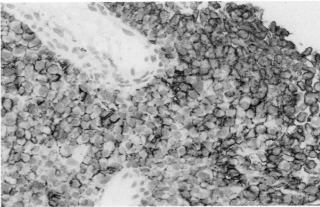

B

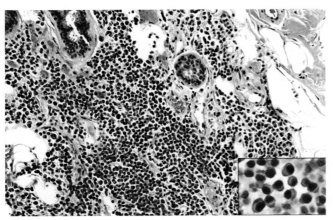

C

Figure 24.9   Plasmacytoma. A: This needle core biopsy specimen consists of mature and immature plasma cells. **B:** The tumor cells are immunoreactive for CD138 (immunoperoxidase). (Courtesy of K. Lewin, MD). **C:** This needle core biopsy sample from a breast tumor in a 41-year-old woman with known multiple myeloma shows a neoplastic infiltrate of small plasma cells. The tumor cells were immunoreactive for CD138 and kappa immunoglobulin but not for lambda immunoglobulin.

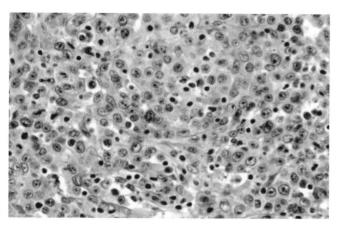

Figure 24.10 **Granulocytic leukemia.** The infiltrate consists of largely undifferentiated granulocytic cells.

described as a secondary manifestation in patients with established leukemia (38).

Microscopically, the growth pattern may simulate invasive lobular carcinoma or malignant lymphoma (4). The neoplastic cells forming broad sheets or cords invade into and around normal mammary parenchymal structures (Fig. 24.10). Intraepithelial extension of the leukemic infiltrate simulates in situ carcinoma. The diagnosis of granulocytic sarcoma may be suggested by cytoplasmic granules in maturing myeloid cells or by the presence of relatively numerous mature myeloid cells scattered throughout the lesion. The cells are reactive immunohistochemically for CD3, CD43, and CD117 (c-Kit). Myeloid granules in immature cells are reactive histochemically with the naphthol–ASD–chloroacetate esterase stain and immunohistochemically for lysozyme (muramidase) and myeloperoxidose. The differential diagnosis includes tumorous myeloid metaplasia in the breast, which is distinguished by the presence of abundant mature and maturing cells of all stem lines including megakaryocytes (39,40).

Mammary infiltration has been described in patients with lymphocytic leukemia (41,42) (Fig. 24.11). The

lesions tend to be bilateral. Coincidental bone marrow and hematogenous involvement are usually present.

EXTRANODAL SINUS HISTIOCYTOSIS WITH MASSIVE LYMPHADENOPATHY

The differential diagnosis of lymphohistiocytic infiltrative disease in the breast also includes *extranodal sinus histiocytosis with massive lymphadenopathy* (*Rosai–Dorfman disease*). Involvement of virtually every organ including the breast has been described (43). Mammography reveals a dense mass that may be nodular or ill defined (44,45). Axillary adenopathy is present in some but not all patients. Lymph node infiltration is characterized histologically by diffuse expansion of sinuses due to a histiocytic infiltrate. Subcutaneous lesions have been described in the breast, and there are rare examples of nodular unilateral or bilateral mammary parenchymal involvement (44,46). The lesion may have plasma cells, germinal centers and appear to be a reactive process when spindled histiocytic cells are associated with collagen deposition in a storiform pattern. The infiltrating histiocytic cells have single or multiple nuclei that contain one or more nucleoli, and there may be occasional mitotic figures. The histiocytes exhibit lymphophagocytosis or erythrophagocytosis. Aspiration cytology of the breast lesion is likely to suggest an inflammatory process or lymphoma (46). The infiltrating histiocytic cells are reactive for S-100 and histiocytic markers such as CD68 in almost all cases, but there is usually an inverse relationship in the intensity of staining for S-100 and CD68. The immunohistochemical phenotype will rule out most metastatic tumors, but lesions with strong S-100 staining and weak or absent histiocytic markers (CD68) may require more extensive study for HMB45, lysozyme, and other markers.

INTRAMAMMARY LYMPH NODES

The differential diagnosis of lymphoid tissue obtained in a needle core biopsy specimen includes intramammary lymph nodes that may be single or multiple (Fig. 24.12). Mammographic examination usually reveals a well-circumscribed mass that may have a lucent center and a peripheral "hilar" notch (47). Lymph nodes measuring 3 to 15 mm have been described (48). Enlargement of intramammary lymph nodes may be caused by lymphoid hyperplasia, sinus histiocytosis, involvement by or reaction to inflammatory conditions, HIV-associated lymph adenopathy, and neoplasms such as metastatic tumor or lymphoma (49–52) (Figs. 24.13–24.15). In one study of 1,655 retrospectively reviewed mammograms from patients with breast carcinoma, 16 (0.9%) had metastatic carcinoma in an intramammary lymph node detected radiologically (53). All lymph nodes with carcinoma were larger than

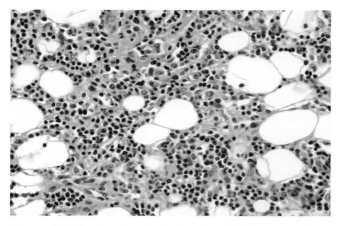

Figure 24.11 **Lymphocytic leukemia.** Well-differentiated lymphocytic leukemia.

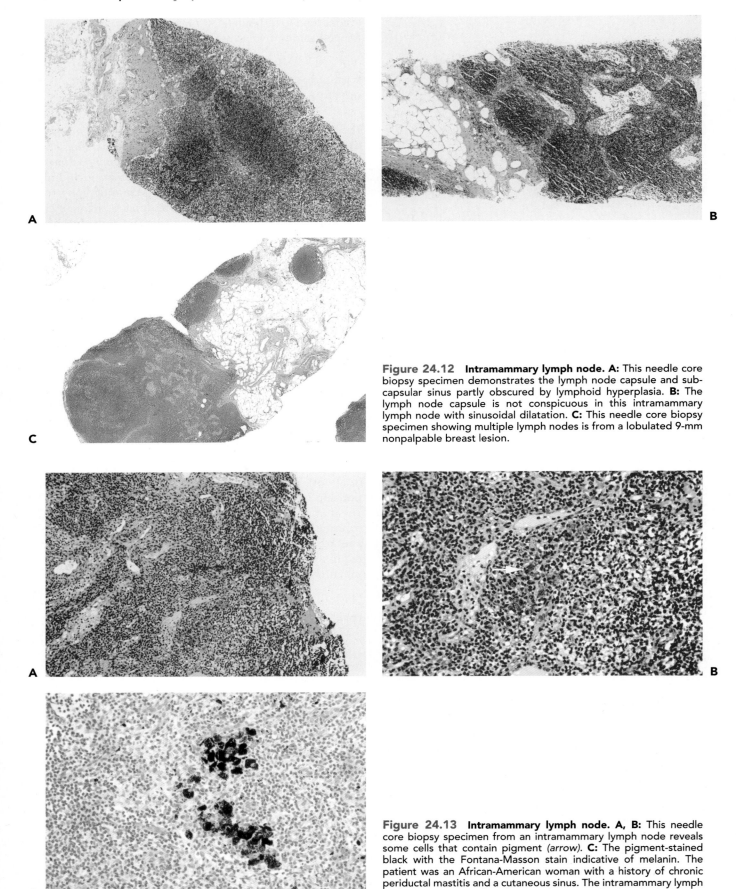

Figure 24.12 Intramammary lymph node. A: This needle core biopsy specimen demonstrates the lymph node capsule and sub-capsular sinus partly obscured by lymphoid hyperplasia. **B:** The lymph node capsule is not conspicuous in this intramammary lymph node with sinusoidal dilatation. **C:** This needle core biopsy specimen showing multiple lymph nodes is from a lobulated 9-mm nonpalpable breast lesion.

Figure 24.13 Intramammary lymph node. A, B: This needle core biopsy specimen from an intramammary lymph node reveals some cells that contain pigment *(arrow)*. **C:** The pigment-stained black with the Fontana-Masson stain indicative of melanin. The patient was an African-American woman with a history of chronic periductal mastitis and a cutaneous sinus. The intramammary lymph node was interpreted as showing dermatopathic lymphadenitis.

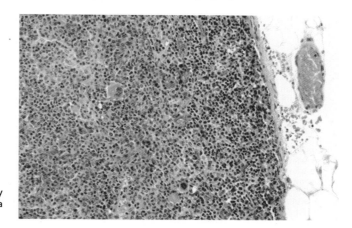

Figure 24.14 Intramammary lymph node. Extramedullary hematopoiesis is present in this intramammary lymph node from a patient with myelofibrosis. Megakaryocytes are evident.

1.0 cm and one had calcifications. Predictors of intramammary nodal metastases are tumor size greater than 1 cm, high-grade tumor, and positive axillary lymph nodes (54). Rampaul et al. (55) studied completion mastectomy specimens from 157 women who were not candidates for conservation therapy after wide local excision for invasive carcinoma because of findings such as extensive intraductal carcinoma or multifocal invasion. Intramammary lymph nodes were found in 44 of 70 (63%) women with negative axillary lymph nodes. Ten (14%) had a positive intramammary lymph node and were consequently converted from stage I to stage II.

Shen et al. (56) reported that the presence of metastatic carcinoma in an intramammary lymph node was usually associated with concurrent axillary nodal metastases. However, 2 (5%) of the 36 patients with positive intramammary lymph nodes had negative axillary lymph nodes. In this study, the presence of metastatic carcinoma in an intramammary lymph node was associated with a significantly less favorable prognosis when compared with patients with a negative intramammary lymph node. Nassar et al.

(54) found that the presence of positive intramammary lymph nodes was a predictor of poor prognosis in univariate analysis, but it was not an independent prognostic factor in multivariate analysis.

The distinction between medullary carcinoma and metastatic carcinoma in an intramammary lymph node is sometimes difficult and may not always be made with confidence in a needle core biopsy sample. This issue can arise in the breast proper and in the axillary region. The presence of a capsule and sinusoidal structure is the best evidence of a lymph node. Germinal centers suggest a lymph node but they are present rarely at sites of extranodal carcinoma. If the carcinoma lacks a syncytial growth pattern and is not cytologically high grade, it is not the medullary type.

Nevus cell aggregates that occur in the capsule or rarely in the parenchyma of axillary lymph nodes may be mistakenly interpreted as metastatic carcinoma (57,58). This possibility should be considered when examining a needle core biopsy sample from a mammary parenchymal lymph node.

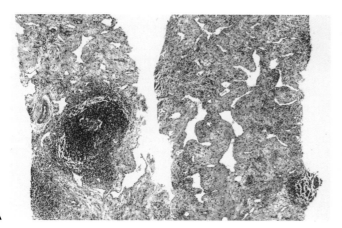 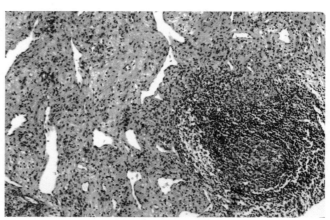

A

B

Figure 24.15 Intramammary lymph node. A, B: The patient had breast conservation treatment, including radiotherapy for invasive mammary carcinoma. A follow-up mammogram disclosed a non-palpable well-circumscribed nodule in the treated breast. The needle core biopsy specimen shown here reveals a lymph node with lymphoid depletion secondary to radiotherapy.

REFERENCES

1. Wiseman C, Liao KT. Primary lymphoma of the breast. *Cancer.* 1972; 29:1705–1712.
2. Giardini R, Piccolo C, Rilke F. Primary non-Hodgkin's lymphomas of the female breast. *Cancer.* 1992;69:725–735.
3. Sanford DB, Yeomans-Kinney A, McLaughlin PW, et al. Ninety-one cases of breast cancer and chronic lymphoproliferative neoplasm: a retrospective review of a population at high risk for multiple malignancies. *Breast J.* 1996;2:312–319.
4. Domchek SM, Hecht JL, Fleming MD, et al. Lymphomas of the breast. Primary and secondary involvement. *Cancer.* 2002;94:6–13.
5. Liu F-F, Clark RM. Primary lymphoma of the breast. *Clin Radiol.* 1986;37:567–570.
6. Brustein S, Filippa DA, Kimmel M, et al. Malignant lymphoma of the breast: a study of 53 patients. *Ann Surg.* 1987;205:144–150.
7. Lamovec J, Jancar J. Primary malignant lymphoma of the breast. Lymphoma of the mucosa-associated lymphoid tissue. *Cancer.* 1987;60:3033–3041.
8. Dixon JM, Lumsden AB, Krajewski A, et al. Primary lymphoma of the breast. *Br J Surg.* 1987;74:214–217.
9. Meyer JE, Kopans DB, Long JC. Mammographic appearance of malignant lymphoma of the breast. *Radiology.* 1980;135:623–626.
10. Wong WW, Schild SE, Halyard MY, Schomberg PJ. Primary non-Hodgkin lymphoma of the breast: The Mayo Clinic experience. *J Surg Oncol.* 2002;80:19–25.
11. Liberman L, Giess CS, Dershaw DD, et al. Non-Hodgkin lymphoma of the breast: imaging characteristics and correlation with histopathologic findings. *Radiology.* 1994;192:157–160.
12. DiPiro PJ, Lester S, Meyer JE, et al. Non-Hodgkin lymphoma of the breast: clinical and radiologic presentations. *Breast J.* 1996;2:380–384.
13. Yang WT, Lane DL, Le-Petross HT, et al. Breast lymphoma imaging findings in 32 tumors in 27 patients. *Radiology.* 2007;245:692–702.
14. Lin Y, Govindan R, Hess JL. Malignant hematopoietic breast tumors. *Am J Clin Pathol.* 1997;107:177–186.
15. Damiani S, Eusebi V, Peterse H. Malignant neoplasms infiltrating pseudoangiomatous stromal hyperplasia of the breast. *Histopathology.* 2002;41:208–215.
16. Pereira EM, Maeda SA, Reis-Filho JS. Sarcomatoid variant of anaplastic large cell lymphoma mimicking a primary breast cancer. A challenging diagnosis. *Arch Pathol Lab Med.* 2002;126:723–726.
17. Aozasa K, Ohsawa M, Saeki K, et al. Malignant lymphoma of the breast. Immunologic type and association with lymphocytic mastopathy. *Am J Clin Pathol.* 1992;97:699–704.
18. Kosaka M, Tsuchihashi N, Takishita M, et al. Primary adult T-cell lymphoma of the breast. *Acta Haematol.* 1992;87:202–205.
19. Bobrow LG, Richards MA, Happerfield LC, et al. Breast lymphomas: a clinicopathologic review. *Hum Pathol.* 1993;24:274–278.
20. Wong AK, Lopategui J, Clancy S, et al. Anaplastic large cell lymphoma associated with a breast implant capsule: a case report and review of the literature. *Am J Surg Pathol.* 2008;32:1265–1268.
21. Roden AC, Macon WR, Keeney GL, et al. Seroma-associated primary anaplastic large cell lymphoma adjacent to breast implants: an indolent T-cell lymphoproliferative disorder. *Mod Pathol.* 2008;21:455–463.
22. Lin JJ, Farha GJ, Taylor RJ. Pseudolymphoma of the breast I. In a study of 8,654 consecutive tylectomies and mastectomies. *Cancer.* 1980;45:973–978.
23. Jeffrey KM, Pantazis CG, Wei JP. Pseudolymphoma of the breast associated with Graves' thyrotoxicosis. *Breast Dis.* 1994;7:169–173.
24. Monfardin S, Banfi A, Bonadonna G, et al. Improved five year survival after combined radiotherapy-chemotherapy for stage I-II non-Hodgkin's lymphoma. *Int J Radiat Oncol Biol Phys.* 1980;6:125–134.
25. DeBlasio D, McCormick B, Straus D, et al. Definitive irradiation for localized non-Hodgkins lymphoma of breast. *Int J Radiat Oncol Biol Phys.* 1989;17:843–846.
26. Smith MR, Brustein S, Straus DJ. Localized non-Hodgkins lymphoma of the breast. *Cancer.* 1987;59:351–354.
27. Nissen NJ, Ersbol J, Hansen HS, et al. A randomized study of radiotherapy versus radiotherapy plus chemotherapy in stage I-II non-Hodgkin's lymphoma. *Cancer.* 1183;52:1–7.
28. Jennings WC, Baker RS, Murray SS, et al. Primary breast lymphoma. The role of mastectomy and the importance of lymph node status. *Am Surg.* 2007;245:784–789.
29. Shehata WM, Pauke TW, Schleuter JA. Hodgkin's disease of the breast. A case report and review of the literature. *Breast.* 1985;11:19–21.
30. Yahalom J, Petrek JA, Biddinger PW, et al. Breast cancer in patients irradiated for Hodgkin's disease: a clinical and pathologic analysis of 45 events in 37 patients. *J Clin Oncol.* 1992;10:1974–1981.
31. Dershaw DD, Yahalom J, Petrek JA. Breast carcinoma in women previously treated for Hodgkin's disease: mammographic evaluation. *Radiology.* 1992;184:421–423.
32. Horwich A, Swerdlow AJ. Second primary breast cancer after Hodgkin's disease. *Br J Cancer.* 2004;90:294–298.
33. Kim EE, Sawwaf ZW, Sneige N. Multiple myeloma of the breast: magnetic resonance and ultrasound imaging findings. *Breast Dis.* 1996;9:229–233.
34. Pettinato G, Manivel JC, Insabato L, et al. Plasma cell granuloma (inflammatory pseudo-tumor) of the breast. *Am J Clin Pathol.* 1988;90:627–632.
35. Alhan E, Calik A, Kucuktulu U, et al. Solitary extramedullary plasmacytoma of the breast with kappa monoclonal gammopathy. *Pathologica.* 1995;87:71–73.
36. Weinblatt ME, Kochen J. Breast nodules as the initial site of relapse in childhood leukemia. *Med Pediatr Oncol.* 1990;18:510–512.
37. Sears HF, Reid J. Granulocytic sarcoma. Local presentation of a systemic disease. *Cancer.* 1976;37:1808–1813.
38. Pascoe RH. Tumors composed of immature granulocytes occurring in breast in chronic granulocytic leukemia. *Cancer.* 1970;25:697–704.
39. Martinelli G, Santini D, Bazzocchi F, et al. Myeloid metaplasia of the breast. A lesion which clinically mimics carcinoma. *Virchows Arch (A).* 1983;401:203–207.
40. Zonderland HM, Michiels JJ, Tenkate FJW. Mammographic and sonographic demonstration of extramedullary hematopoiesis of the breast. *Clin Radiol.* 1991;44:64–65.
41. Gogoi PK, Stewart ID, Keane PF, et al. Chronic lymphocytic leukemia presenting with bilateral breast involvement. *Clin Lab Haemat.* 1989;11:57–60.
42. Seale DL, Riddervoid HO, Tears CD, Stone DD. Roentgenographic appearance of chronic lymphatic leukemia involving the female breast. *Am J Roentgenol.* 1972;115:808–810.
43. Foucar E, Rosai J. Dorfman R. Sinus histiocytosis with massive lymphadenopathy (Rosai–Dorfman disease): review of the entity. *Semin Diagn Pathol.* 1990;7:19–73.
44. Green I, Dorfman RF, Rosai J. Breast involvement by extranodal Rosai–Dorfman disease: report of seven cases. *Am J Surg Pathol.* 1997;21:664–668.
45. Hammond LA, Keh C, Rowlands DC. Rosai–Dorfman disease in the breast. *Histopathology.* 1996;29:582–584.
46. Soares FA, Llorach-Velludo AS, Andrade JM. Rosai–Dorfman's disease of the breast. *Am J Surg Pathol.* 199;23:359–360.
47. Kopans DB, Meyer JE, Murphy GF. Benign lymph nodes associated with dermatitis presenting as breast masses. *Radiology.* 1980;137:15–19.
48. McSweeney MB, Egan RL. Prognosis of breast cancer related to intramammary lymph nodes. *Recent Results Cancer Res.* 1984;90:166–172.
49. Arnaout AH, Shousha S, Metaxas N, Husain OAN. Intramammary tuberculous lymphadenitis. *Histopathology.* 1990;17:91–93.
50. Konstantinopoulos PA, Dezube BJ, March D, Pantanowitz L. HIV associated intramammary lymph adenopathy. *Breast J.* 2007;13:192–195.
51. Lindfors KK, Kopans DB, McCarthy KA, et al. Breast cancer metastasis to intramammary lymph nodes. *Am J Roentgenol.* 1986;146:133–136.
52. Kinoshita T, Yashiro N, Yoshigi J, et al. Inflammatory intramammary lymph node mimicking the malignant lesion in dynamic MRI. A case report. *J Clin Imaging.* 2002;26:258–262.
53. Gunhan-Bilgen I, Memis A, Ustun EE. Metastatic intramammary lymph nodes: mammographic and ultrasonographic features. *Eur J Radiol.* 2001;40:24–29.
54. Nassar A, Cohen C, Cotsonia G, Carlsong G. Significance of intramammary lymph nodes in the staging of breast cancer: correlation outcome. *Breast J.* 2008;14:147–152.
55. Rampaul RS, Dole OT, Mitchell M, et al. Incidence of intramammary nodes in completion mastectomy specimens after axillary node sampling: implications for conservation therapy. *Breast J.* 2008;17:195–198.
56. Shen J, Hunt KK, Mirza NQ, et al. Intramammary lymph node metastases are an independent predictor of poor outcome in patients with breast carcinoma. *Cancer.* 2004;101:1330–1337.
57. Biddle DA, Evans HL, Kemp BL, et al. Intraparenchymal nevus cell aggregates in lymph node. A possible diagnostic pitfall with malignant melanoma and carcinoma. *Am J Surg Pathol.* 2003;27:673–681.
58. Ridolfi RL, Rosen PP, Thaler H. Nevus cell aggregates associated with lymph nodes: estimated frequency and clinical significance. *Cancer.* 1977;39:164–171.

Metastases in the Breast from Nonmammary Malignant Neoplasms

25

It is important to consider metastatic tumor in the differential diagnosis when faced with a breast lesion that has unusual clinical, radiologic, gross, or microscopic features. The nonmammary primary lesion may be a new, occult neoplasm not evident to the patients' physicians. The preoperative clinical workup of an apparently healthy patient with a breast mass is often perfunctory and unlikely to exclude an occult malignant extramammary primary tumor. Even if a history of a previously treated nonmammary malignant tumor is known by the surgeon preoperatively, the information may not be communicated to the pathologist.

A lesion in the breast is the initial manifestation of a nonmammary malignant neoplasm in a minority of patients who have metastatic tumor in the breast. The occult primary tumor is usually a carcinoma, and one of the most common sites is the lung (1–4). The TTF1 immunostain is positive in pulmonary carcinoma but not in mammary carcinoma. A surprising number of the occult lung lesions have been small cell carcinomas (1,2,4). Other sites of occult, clinically inapparent neoplasms that have presented with metastases in the breast include the kidneys, stomach, ovaries (5,6), and intestinal carcinoid tumors (7–9). Previously diagnosed tumors that have given rise to metastases in the breast, sometimes rather late in the clinical course of the patient, include malignant melanoma (3,10), sarcomas (3), carcinoma of the lung (10,11), transitional cell carcinoma of the urinary bladder (12), and clear cell carcinoma of the kidney (13). Several types of malignant lymphoma have sometimes been included under the heading of metastases in the breast. However, in the breast these neoplasms are best regarded as primary tumors or as part of a systemic disease affecting the lymphoid system. A review of records for a 92-year period in one hospital revealed that about one-third of the nonmammary malignant tumors found in the breast originated from an occult tumor (4). Overall, the most common primary tumors that gave rise to mammary metastases were, in decreasing order of frequency, carcinoma of the lung, cutaneous malignant melanoma, carcinoma of the stomach, and clear cell carcinoma of the kidney.

On the one hand, adenocarcinomas of the gastrointestinal tract, especially the colon and rectum, are rarely the source of metastatic carcinoma in the breast, despite their relatively high frequency in the population at large (14). On the other hand, carcinoid tumors of the small bowel are a surprisingly frequent source of metastases in one or both breasts (7,9,15,16). Without knowledge of an extramammary primary, metastatic carcinoid tumor in the breast can be mistaken for a primary mammary carcinoma with endocrine differentiation (9,16) or for invasive lobular carcinoma.

Mammary metastases from medulloblastoma (17), rhabdomyosarcoma (18,19), and neuroblastoma have been reported in children and adults. Metastatic melanoma presenting clinically as a breast tumor may be difficult to recognize if the primary lesion is occult or if the pathologist is not informed that the patient received prior treatment for such a lesion (20). When a breast mass is discovered in a man known to have prostatic carcinoma, histochemical studies for mucin and immunohistochemical studies for prostate-specific antigen (PSA) and prostatic acid phosphatase should be performed (21,22). However, PSA has been detected by immunostains in breast carcinomas from men and women; therefore, a positive result is not by itself diagnostic of metastatic prostatic carcinoma (23,24). Examining the tissue for estrogen receptor is not likely to be helpful, because this protein can be found in mammary and prostatic carcinomas. Comparison of the histologic

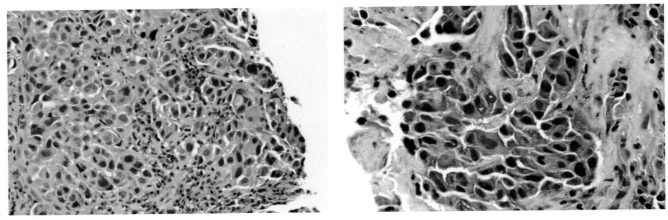

Figure 25.1 **Metastatic lung carcinoma. A:** Large cell adenocarcinoma in a needle core biopsy specimen of the breast. Without a history of pulmonary carcinoma, this tumor could be interpreted as mammary carcinoma. **B:** Intracytoplasmic mucin appears magenta with the mucicarmine stain. The patient had a histologically identical large cell carcinoma of the lung treated previously.

appearances of the prostatic and mammary tumors is essential. A collision tumor consisting of metastatic prostatic carcinoma in a solid papillary carcinoma of the male breast has been described (25).

Radiographically, metastatic lesions tend to be discrete, round shadows without spiculation (3). They are usually not distinguishable from circumscribed primary papillary, medullary, or colloid breast carcinomas. Microcalcifications are very uncommon but have been described in metastatic ovarian carcinoma (26,27). Metastatic foci in the breast are more often solitary than multiple initially, but they may become multiple and bilateral with progression of the patient's clinical course (3).

Some clinical features are helpful in recognizing that a neoplasm in the breast is a metastatic tumor. The average interval to the development of a mammary metastasis is approximately 2 years for patients with previously treated cancer. Usually, there have already been metastases at other sites, or they are detected coincidentally. Isolated metastases initially limited to the breast are uncommon.

Metastases have been described in ipsilateral axillary lymph nodes in a substantial proportion of patients with metastatic nonmammary tumor in the breast, generally as a manifestation of systemic spread.

An unusual histologic pattern and clinical information about a prior neoplasm are the best clues for identifying a metastatic tumor in the breast. It is important to be sensitive to morphologic patterns that are not typical for breast carcinoma, but some histologic appearances present especially difficult problems because histologically similar tumors arise in the breast as well as in other organs. Included in this group are pulmonary large cell carcinoma (Fig. 25.1), mucinous (colloid), mucoepidermoid, and clear cell carcinomas (Fig. 25.2) as well as malignant melanoma (Fig. 25.3). Metastatic ovarian carcinomas have generally been serous (26,27) rather than mucinous, and may be mistaken for papillary mammary carcinoma in the absence of a known ovarian primary (5), especially if there is also metastatic tumor in axillary lymph nodes (26,28) (Fig. 25.4). Metastatic endometrial carcinoma with a solid

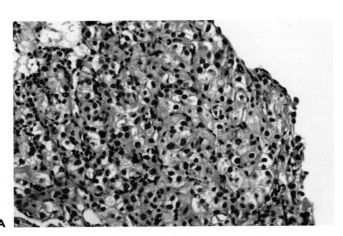

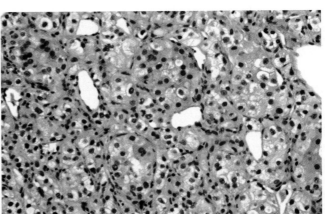

Figure 25.2 **Metastatic renal carcinoma. A:** A needle core biopsy specimen of the breast showing metastatic tumor with an alveolar structure and cytoplasmic clearing. **B:** The cells in this metastatic lesion from the kidney resemble apocrine carcinoma with clear cell change.

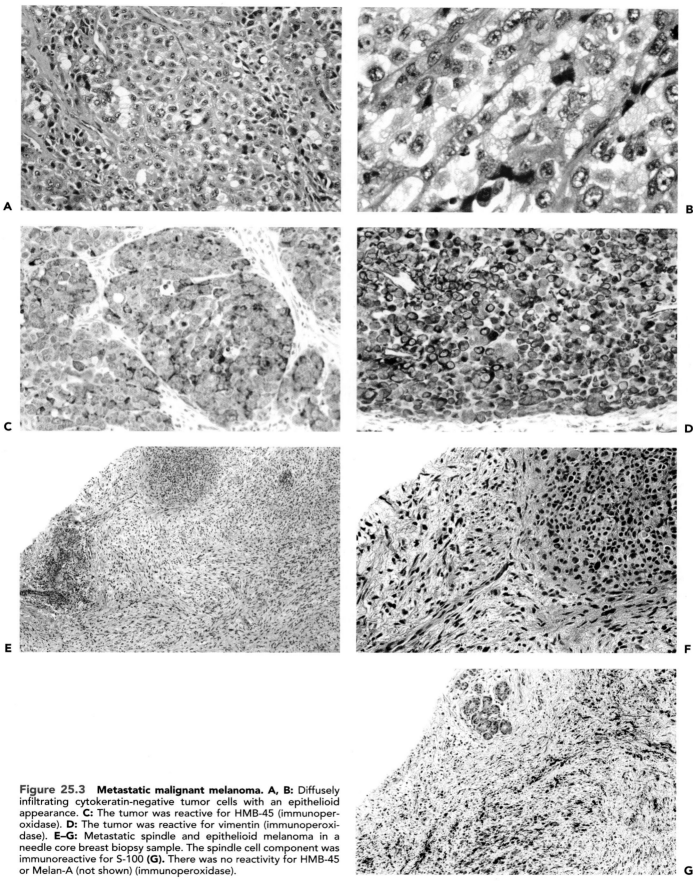

Figure 25.3   Metastatic malignant melanoma. A, B: Diffusely infiltrating cytokeratin-negative tumor cells with an epithelioid appearance. **C:** The tumor was reactive for HMB-45 (immunoperoxidase). **D:** The tumor was reactive for vimentin (immunoperoxidase). **E–G:** Metastatic spindle and epithelioid melanoma in a needle core breast biopsy sample. The spindle cell component was immunoreactive for S-100 **(G).** There was no reactivity for HMB-45 or Melan-A (not shown) (immunoperoxidase).

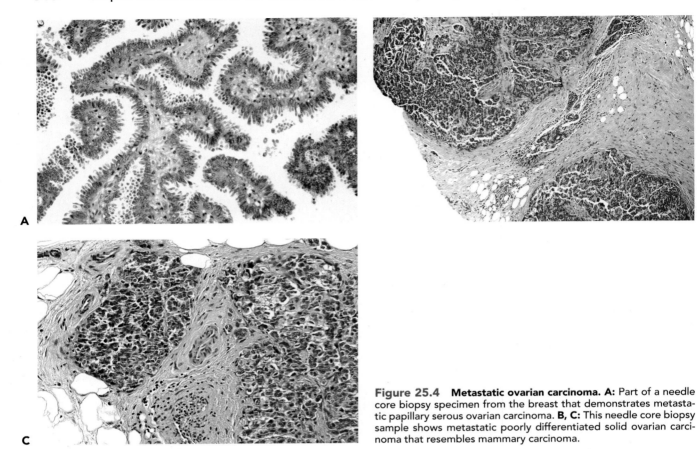

Figure 25.4 **Metastatic ovarian carcinoma. A:** Part of a needle core biopsy specimen from the breast that demonstrates metastatic papillary serous ovarian carcinoma. **B, C:** This needle core biopsy sample shows metastatic poorly differentiated solid ovarian carcinoma that resembles mammary carcinoma.

growth pattern may mimic poorly differentiated or solid papillary mammary carcinoma (29).

The immunostain for WT1, a nuclear marker associated with ovarian and peritoneal serous papillary carcinomas, has been reported to be nonreactive in mammary carcinomas (26,30,27), with the possible exception of rare instances of invasive micropapillary breast carcinoma (31,32) and mucinous mammary carcinomas (31,33). This is of interest because of the reported upregulation of the WT1 gene in breast carcinomas (34,35) and the observation that higher WT1 messenger ribonucleic acid (mRNA) levels were associated with a relatively poor prognosis in a series of 99 breast carcinoma patients with a median follow-up of 48 months (36). Focal cytoplasmic reactivity for WT1 in breast carcinomas noted in one report (34) is not considered a positive result. Because the majority of ovarian carcinomas are CA125 positive, and this marker is negative in almost all mammary carcinomas other than invasive micropapillary and mucinous carcinomas, nuclear reactivity for WT1 and cytoplasmic reactivity for CA 125 strongly favors metastatic ovarian carcinoma over primary mammary carcinoma (30,32).

Metastatic endometrial carcinoma with a solid growth pattern may mimic poorly differentiated mammary carcinoma (29) (Fig. 25.5). Among sarcomas metastatic to the breast, hemangiopericytoma (37), leiomyosarcoma (38), and malignant fibrous histiocytoma (38) may be difficult to distinguish from primary mammary sarcomas and some metaplastic mammary carcinomas (Fig. 25.6). Metastatic medullary carcinoma of the thyroid gland has been described growing in the breast with the pattern of infiltrating lobular carcinoma (39,40). Papillary and follicular carcinoma of the thyroid gland may rarely metastasize to the breast (41). Thyroid carcinoma will be immunoreactive for TTF1 and thyroglobulin, two markers not expressed in mammary carcinoma. Carcinoma of the lung has diverse histologic appearances some of which may resemble mammary carcinoma. Papillary carcinoma of the lung can produce cystic papillary metastases that mimic primary papillary carcinoma of the breast. Knowledge that carcinoma of the lung was previously diagnosed or is currently present and access to histologic sections of the lung tumor are vital aides in this circumstance. Most pulmonary carcinomas are immunoreactive for TTF1. An exceedingly rare source of metastatic tumor in the breast is mesothelioma, particularly the epithelioid variant. Immunoreactivity for D2-40, podoplanin, and calretinin strongly favors mesothelioma over carcinoma (42).

The limited sample of a needle core biopsy specimen is not likely to provide all of the information that would help to distinguish between a primary and a metastatic tumor. A search should be made for in situ carcinoma to confirm origin in the breast, but since this cannot be found in all primary mammary lesions the absence of in situ carcinoma

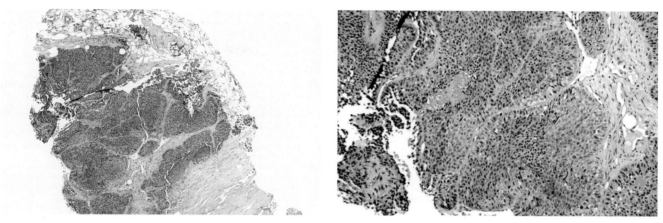

Figure 25.5 Metastatic endometrial carcinoma. A, B: The solid growth pattern subdivided into large alveolar nests in this needle core biopsy specimen of a metastatic endometrial carcinoma resembles the structure of solid papillary mammary carcinoma.

is not conclusive evidence that one is dealing with a metastasis. Metastatic tumor often surrounds and displaces normal appearing breast parenchyma that typically shows little or no hyperplasia. A peripheral lymphocytic infiltrate and stroma reaction are not unusual at the site of metastatic tumor in the breast as well as in primary breast carcinomas. The finding of more than two grossly evident tumor nodules should lead one to consider metastatic tumor, especially if the histologic pattern is unusual. Lymphatic

tumor emboli may result from metastases in the breast as well as from primary breast carcinomas. Diffuse lymphatic spread of metastatic tumor within the breast can occur, rarely producing the clinical appearance of inflammatory carcinoma.

The distinction between a primary breast tumor and a metastasis in the breast is critical for treatment. When an occult extramammary neoplasm presents with a breast metastasis, the workup of the patient will be influenced

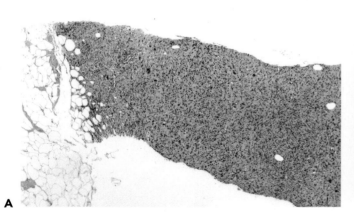

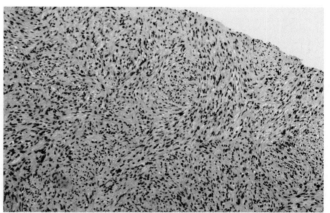

Figure 25.6 Metastatic leiomyosarcoma. A, B: This needle core biopsy specimen shows a dense tumor composed of interlacing spindle cells with eosinophilic cytoplasm. The tumor cells were immunoreactive for smooth muscle actin. **C:** The source of the metastasis shown here was a primary leiomyosarcoma of the groin resected 1-year earlier.

by morphologic features of the tumor that may suggest one of more particular primary sites. Mastectomy is not appropriate for metastatic tumor in the breast in most cases, but it may be performed to obtain local control of multifocal, bulky ulcerated, necrotic or otherwise symptomatic lesions. Wide excision can be supplemented by radiotherapy to the breast for radiosensitive neoplasms, and axillary dissection may be performed, especially if the lymph nodes seem grossly involved. Emphasis should necessarily be placed on systemic treatment appropriate to the primary lesion. Metastatic involvement of the breast is a manifestation of generalized metastases in virtually all cases. The prognosis depends on the clinical characteristics of the specific neoplasm.

REFERENCES

1. Kelly C, Henderson D, Corris P. Breast lumps: rare presentation of oat cell carcinoma of lung. *J Clin Pathol.* 1988;41:171–172.
2. McCrea ES, Johnston C, Haney PJ. Metastases to the breast. *Am J Roentgenol.* 1983;141:685–690.
3. Toombs BD, Kalisher L. Metastatic disease in the breast; clinical, pathologic and radiographic features. *Am J Roentgenol.* 1977;129:673–676.
4. Georgiannos SN, Aleong JC, Goode AW, Sheaff M. Secondary neoplasms of the breast. A survey of the 20th century. *Cancer.* 2001;92:2259–2266.
5. Elit LM, Cunnane MF. Breast metastasis from ovarian carcinoma: report of two cases and literature review. *J Surg Pathol.* 1995; 1:69–74.
6. Ron I-G, Inbar M, Halpern M, Chaitchik S. Endometrioid carcinoma of the ovary presenting as primary carcinoma of the breast. A case report and review of the literature. *Acta Obstet Gynecol Scand.* 1992;71:81–83.
7. Harrist TJ, Kalisher L. Breast metastasis; an unusual manifestation of a malignant carcinoid tumor. *Cancer.* 1977;40:3102–3106.
8. Kashlan RB, Powell RW, Nolting SF. Carcinoid and other tumors metastatic to the breast. *J Surg Oncol.* 1982;20:25–30.
9. Upalakolin JN, Collins LC, Tawa N, Parangis G. Carcinoid tumors in the breast. *Am J Surg.* 2006;191:799–805.
10. Sneige N, Zachariah S, Fanning TV, et al. Fine needle aspiration cytology of metastatic neoplasms in the breast. *Am J Clin Pathol.* 1989;92:27–35.
11. Domanski HA. Metastases to the breast from extramammary neoplasms. A report of six cases with diagnosis by fine needle aspiration cytology. *Acta Cytol.* 1996;40:1293–1300.
12. Belton AL, Stull MA, Grant T, Shepard MH. Mammographic and sonographic findings in metastatic transitional cell carcinoma of the breast. *Am J Roentgenol.* 1997;168:511–512.
13. Vassalli L, Ferrari VD, Simoncini E, et al. Solitary breast metastases from a renal cell carcinoma. *Breast Cancer Res. Treat.* 2001;68: 29–31.
14. Alexander HR, Turnbull AD, Rosen PP. Isolated breast metastases from gastrointestinal carcinomas. *J Surg Oncol.* 1989;42:264–266.
15. Landon G, Sneige N, Ordonez NG, Mackay B. Carcinoid metastatic to breast diagnosed by fine-needle aspiration biopsy. *Diagn Cytopathol.* 1987;3:230–233.
16. Mosunjac MB, Kochhar R, Mosunjac MI, Lau SK. Primary small bowel carcinoid tumor with bilateral breast metastases. Report of 2 cases with different clinical presentations. *Arch Pathol Lab Med.* 2004;128:292–297.
17. Kapila K, Sarkar C, Verma K. Detection of metastatic medulloblastoma in a fine needle breast aspirate. *Acta Cytol.* 1996;40: 384–385.
18. Hogge JP, Magnant CM, Lage JM, Zuurbier RA. Rhabdomyosarcoma metastatic to the breast. *Breast J.* 1996;2:270–274.
19. Kwan WH, Choi PHK, Li CK, et al. Breast metastasis in adolescents with alveolar rhabdomyosarcoma of the extremities: report of two cases. *Pediatr Hemat Oncol.* 1996;13:277–285.
20. Ravdel L, Robinson WA, Lewis K, Gonzalez R. Metastatic melanoma in the breast: a report of 27 cases. *J Surg Oncol.* 2006;94:101–104.
21. Choudhury M, DeRosas J, Papsidero L, et al. Metastatic prostatic carcinoma to the breast or primary breast carcinoma. *J Urol.* 1982;19:297–299.
22. Green LK, Klima M. The use of immunohistochemistry in metastatic prostatic adenocarcinoma to the breast. *Hum Pathol.* 1991;22:242–246.
23. Bodey B, Body B Jr., Kaiser HE. Immunocytochemical detection of prostate specific antigen expression in human breast carcinoma cells. *Anticancer Res.* 1997;17:2577–2581.
24. Yu H, Levesque MA, Clark GM, Diamandis EP. Enhanced prediction of breast cancer prognosis by evaluating expression of p53 and prostate-specific antigen in combination. *Br J Cancer.* 1999;81:490–495.
25. Sahoo S, Smith RE, Potz JL, Rosen PP. Metastatic prostatic adenocarcinoma within a primary solid papillary carcinoma of the male breast. Application of immunohistochemistry to a unique collision tumor. *Arch Pathol Lab Med.* 2001;125:1101–1103.
26. Recine MA, Deavers MT, Middleton LP, et al. Serous carcinoma of the ovary and peritoneum with metastases to the breast and axillary lymph nodes. *Am J Surg Pathol.* 2004;28:1646–1651.
27. Goldstein NS, Uzieblo A. WT1 Immunoreactivity in uterine papillary serous carcinomas is different from ovarian serous carcinomas. *Am J Clin Pathol.* 2002;117:541–545.
28. Duda RB, August CZ, Schink JC. Ovarian carcinoma metastatic to the breast and axillary node. *Surgery.* 1991;110:552–556.
29. Moore DH, Wilson DK, Hurtean JA, et al. Gynecologic cancers metastatic to the breast. *J Am Coll Surg.* 1998;187:178–181.
30. Tornos C, Soslow R, Chen S, et al. Expression of WT1, CA 125, and GCDF-15 as useful markers in the differential diagnosis of primary ovarian carcinomas versus metastatic breast cancer to the ovary. *Am J Surg Pathol.* 2005;29:1482–1489.
31. Domfeh AB, Carley AL, Striebel JM, et al. WT1 immunoreactivity in breast carcinoma: selective expression in pure and mixed mucinous subtypes. *Mod Pathol.* 2008;21:1217–1223.
32. Lee AHS, Paish EC, Marchio C, et al. The expression of Wilms' tumour-1 and Cal25 in invasive micropapillary carcinoma of the breast. *Histopathology.* 2007;51:824–828.
33. Rowsell C, Hanna WM, Kahn HJ. WT-1 expression in breast carcinomas with mucinous morphology. *Mod Pathol.* 2008;21(suppl l):52A.
34. Silberstein GB, Van Horn K, Strickland P, et al. Altered expression of the WT1 Wilms' tumor suppressor gene in human breast cancer. *Proc Natl Acad Sci U. S. A.* 1997;94:8132–8137.
35. Loeb DM, Evron E, Patel CB, et al. Wilms' tumor suppressor gene (WT1) is expressed in primary breast tumors despite tumor-specific promoter methylation. *Cancer Res.* 2001;61:921–925.
36. Miyoshi Y, Ando A, Egawa C, et al. High expression of Wilms' tumor suppressor gene predicts poor prognosis in breast cancer patients. *Clin Cancer Res.* 2002;8:1167–1171.
37. Breitbart AS, Harris MN, Vazquez M, Mitnick JR. Metastatic hemangiopericytoma of the breast. *N. Y. State J Med.* 1992;92: 158–160.
38. Shukla R, Pooja B, Radhika S, et al. Fine-needle aspiration cytology of extramammary neoplasms metastatic to the breast. *Cytopathology.* 2005;32:193–197.
39. Kiely N, Williams N, Wilson G, Williams RJ. Medullary carcinoma of the thyroid metastatic to breast. *Postgrad Med J.* 1995;72: 744–754.
40. Ali SD, Teichberg S, Attie JN, Susin M. Medullary thyroid carcinoma metastatic to breast masquerading as infiltrating lobular carcinoma. *Ann Clin Lab Sci.* 1994;24:441–447.
41. Loureiro MM, Leite VH, Boavida JM, et al. An unusual case of papillary carcinoma of the thyroid with cutaneous and breast metastases only. *Eur J Endocrinol.* 1997;137:267–269.
42. Ordoñez NG. Immunohistochemical diagnosis of epitheloid mesothelioma. An update. *Arch Pathol Lab Med.* 2005;129: 1407–1414.

Pathologic Effects of Therapy

26

RADIATION

The breasts may be exposed to radiation during diagnostic procedures such as mammography and fluoroscopy (1,2) or in the course of radiotherapy administered to another organ such as mediastinal radiotherapy for Hodgkin disease (3–6). The low-dose exposure in these situations has been associated with an increased risk for the subsequent development of breast carcinoma (1–3). Wendland et al. (7) reported that the standard incidence ratio (SIR) for breast carcinoma among Hodgkin disease patients who received radiotherapy was 3.17 with a 95% confidence interval (CI) of 2.66 to 3.79 when compared with the general population. The SIR for radiated female Hodgkin disease patients compared to nonradiated patients was 1.90. In the same study, the SIR for breast carcinoma in nonradiated Hodgkin disease patients when compared with the general population was also elevated (1.67;95% CI:1.24–2.20). Each of these differences was statistically significant, indicating that women who had been treated for Hodgkin disease had an elevated risk for breast carcinoma, which was enhanced in radiated women.

No structural changes attributable to low-dose, incidental radiation are evident when the mammary glandular tissue is examined histopathologically. Patients treated for Hodgkin disease have carcinomas that tend to be poorly differentiated but in other respects are not significantly different pathologically from tumors that arise in women without prior irradiation (5). Almost all of the postradiation carcinomas have been ductal with rare examples of infiltrating lobular and special types such as mucinous carcinoma (8). Approximately 15% of the carcinomas are intraductal. The carcinomas are more likely to be bilateral and to occur in the medial part of the breast (8,9).

Patients who have received supradiaphragmatic radiotherapy for the treatment of Hodgkin disease are candidates to be under surveillance for the early detection of breast carcinoma. In the absence of randomized, controlled clinical trials, the efficacy of various screening modalities has not been established in this circumstance. Mammography was reported to have high sensitivity for detecting carcinomas in the breast of women radiated for

Hodgkin disease, especially when calcifications were present (9–11). However, there is a risk for inducing cancer with frequently repeated mammography at an early age. Ultrasonography may be employed as an adjunct to mammography but cannot be relied on as a primary screening modality because of a relatively high frequency of false positive findings (12). Magnetic resonance imaging (MRI) has proven to be effective for detecting tumor-forming, largely invasive carcinomas in women with a genetic predisposition to breast carcinoma, but it has less sensitivity than mammography for intraductal carcinoma (13). On this basis, MRI would appear to be a useful adjunct for screening radiated Hodgkin disease patients.

Radiation of the breast for mammary carcinoma in the course of breast-conserving treatment involves levels of exposure that produce alterations in nonneoplastic as well as neoplastic breast tissues. Radiation-induced histologic changes must be distinguished from recurrent carcinoma in the interpretation of a posttreatment biopsy specimen. When the normal breast is compared with a preradiation specimen, the major changes in normal breast are apparent in terminal duct–lobular units (14) (Figs. 26.1–26.3). The most notable changes are (a) collagenization of intralobular stroma, (b) thickening of periacinar and periductular basement membranes, (c) atrophy of acinar and ductular epithelium, (d) cytologic atypia of residual epithelial and myoepithelial cells, and (e) relatively prominent acinar myoepithelial cells that tend to be preserved to a greater extent than the epithelial cells. Generally, the effects on the larger ducts are less pronounced than are those in lobules following primary radiotherapy. Apocrine epithelium is susceptible to developing severe cytologic atypia after therapeutic radiotherapy, especially in hyperplastic foci. When evaluating a posttreatment biopsy, it is useful to examine the pretreatment specimen for evidence of apocrine metaplasia. In a minority of specimens, one may also find atypical fibroblasts in the interlobular stroma.

Substantial variation in the severity of changes in the lobules can be observed from one patient to another, and on occasion, they may be virtually indistinguishable from physiologic atrophy. In a given patient, most of the lobular tissue responds in a uniform fashion if the entire breast has

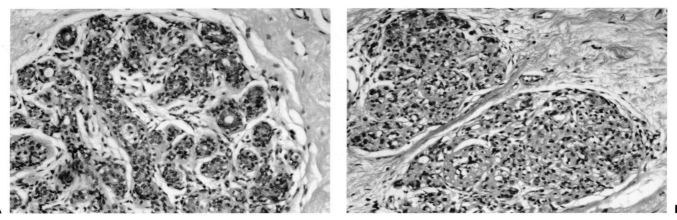

Figure 26.1 Radiation atrophy of lobules. A: A normal lobule in the breast of a 35-year-old woman after a lumpectomy for infiltrating duct carcinoma and before the start of radiotherapy. **B:** Lobules in the same breast 3 years after radiotherapy. This needle core biopsy procedure was performed for mammographically detected calcifications in recurrent carcinoma. The posttreatment lobules exhibit moderate radiation atrophy, including sclerosis of intralobular stroma, thickening of basement membranes around lobular glands, atrophy of epithelial cells, and cytoplasmic clearing in myoepithelial cells.

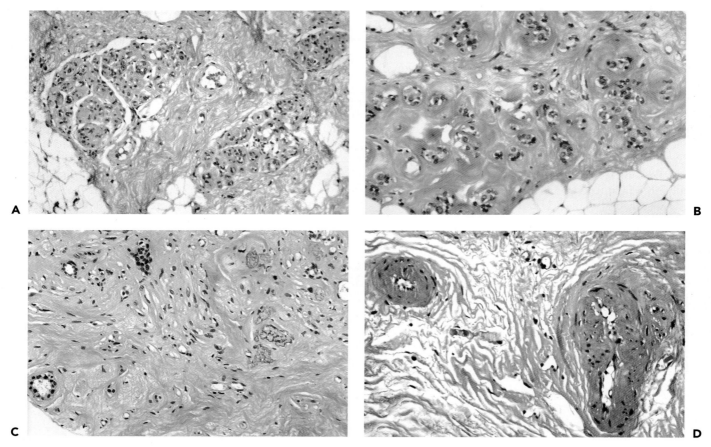

Figure 26.2 Radiation atrophy of lobules and vascular changes. A: Severe atrophy with persistent lobular structure. **B:** Nearly complete effacement of a lobule. Note thick periglandular basement membranes. **C:** Severe lobular atrophy with calcifications. **D:** Mild sclerosis of small arteries.

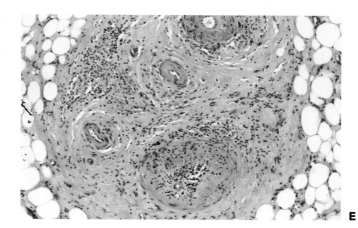

Figure 26.2 *(continued)* **E:** Arteritis following radiotherapy.

been radiated. Generally, the effects on the larger ducts are less pronounced following primary radiotherapy than are the effects on lobules. Differences in the severity of radiation changes between individual patients do not appear to be correlated with radiation dosage, patient age, posttreatment interval, or the use of adjuvant chemotherapy (14).

Moore et al. (15) studied 120 breast specimens obtained at various intervals (less than 1 year to more than 6 years) after radiotherapy. They observed statistically significant differences between pre- and posttreatment specimens with the latter showing the aforementioned alterations resulting from radiation. However, radiation-induced changes did not "show significant alterations over the various time intervals," indicating stable morphologic changes.

Fat necrosis and atypia of stromal fibroblasts are more common close to "boosted" or implanted areas (16). Radiation-induced vascular changes are not ordinarily seen after external beam radiotherapy, but they may occur where a boost dose has been delivered. Cytologic and architectural markers of radiation effect in larger blood vessels include fragmentation of elastica, endothelial atypia, and myointimal proliferation that leads to vascular sclerosis. Prominent, cytologically atypical endothelial cells are also apparent in capillaries. Epithelial atypia may occur

in the larger ducts of the breast where it is usually superimposed on preexisting hyperplasia or apocrine metaplasia (Figs. 26.4–26.6).

Cytologic atypia in nonneoplastic epithelium can create diagnostic problems if one is unaware of the typical appearance of radiation-induced atrophy of the breast (14,17,18). In situ lobular and intraductal carcinoma persisting after radiation therapy remain largely intact so that the affected lobules and ducts are filled and often expanded with a neoplastic cell population that differs little or not at all from the pretreatment appearance of the carcinoma (Figs. 26.7–26.8). In one study the grade of recurrent intraductal carcinoma after breast conservation with radiotherapy was the same as the pretreatment lesion in 95 of 113 cases (84%) (19). Therefore, it is essential to have slides of the pretreatment carcinoma available for comparison with a posttreatment biopsy to help in distinguishing between recurrent carcinoma and radiation atypia.

Apocrine metaplasia is sensitive to radiation effect and tends to exhibit cytologic atypia that can be striking after radiation treatment. Knowledge that apocrine metaplasia was present in the pretreatment specimen can be helpful in correctly interpreting the posttreatment biopsy with radiation atypia in apocrine metaplasia. Frequently, little or no

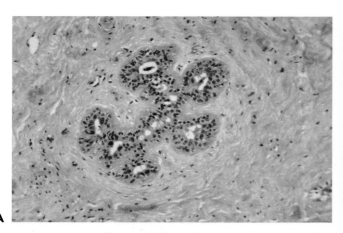

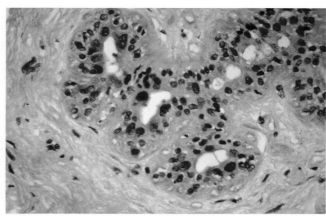

Figure 26.3 **Radiation atypia in a small duct. A, B:** Isolated epithelial cells bordering on the duct lumen have enlarged hyperchromatic nuclei. Thickening of the basement membrane is evident.

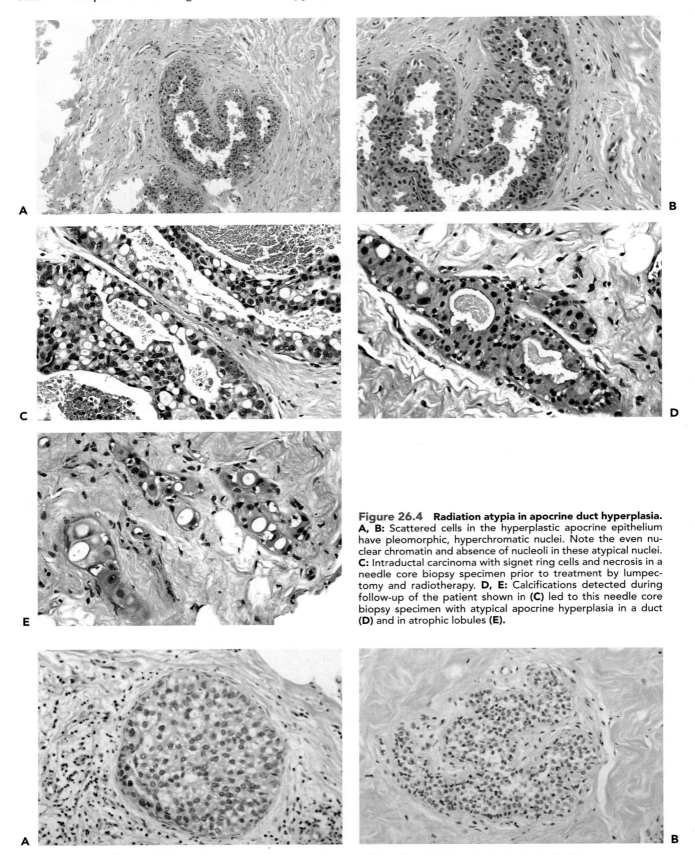

Figure 26.4   Radiation atypia in apocrine duct hyperplasia. A, B: Scattered cells in the hyperplastic apocrine epithelium have pleomorphic, hyperchromatic nuclei. Note the even nuclear chromatin and absence of nucleoli in these atypical nuclei. **C:** Intraductal carcinoma with signet ring cells and necrosis in a needle core biopsy specimen prior to treatment by lumpectomy and radiotherapy. **D, E:** Calcifications detected during follow-up of the patient shown in **(C)** led to this needle core biopsy specimen with atypical apocrine hyperplasia in a duct **(D)** and in atrophic lobules **(E)**.

Figure 26.5   Radiation atypia in terminal ducts with atypical lobular hyperplasia. A, B: After an initial excisional biopsy, the patient received radiotherapy. Intraductal carcinoma is shown in **(A)** and atypical lobular hyperplasia in **(B)**.

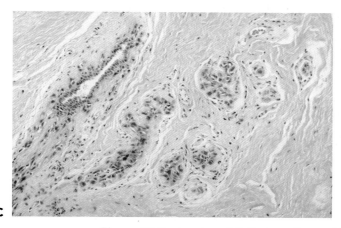

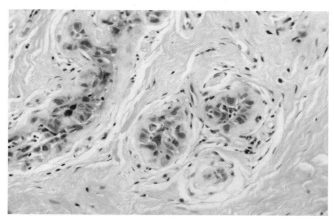

C

D

Figure 26.5   *(continued)* **C, D:** A needle core biopsy procedure performed 2 years later revealed marked cytologic atypia in these terminal ducts, probably in foci of atypical lobular hyperplasia shown in **(B)** that were present prior to treatment.

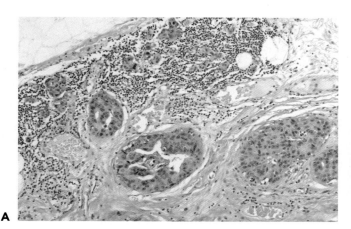

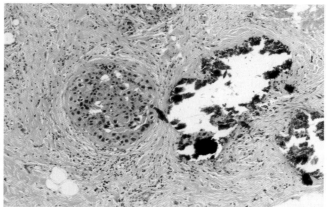

A

B

Figure 26.6   Recurrent intraductal carcinoma after radiotherapy. A: Intraductal carcinoma in a needle core biopsy specimen. The patient had a wide excision of the lesional area followed by radiotherapy. **B:** A follow-up mammogram 4 years later revealed calcifications, leading to another needle core biopsy procedure. The specimen illustrated here shows intraductal carcinoma similar to that in **(A)**. **C:** This section is from the excision performed after the diagnosis of recurrent intraductal carcinoma. A tissue defect caused by the needle core biopsy procedure is in the upper left corner. The current carcinoma is histologically very similar to the pretreatment lesion.

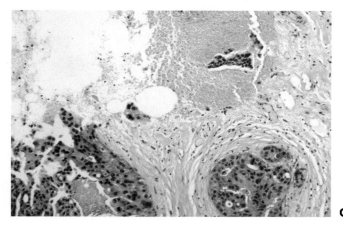

C

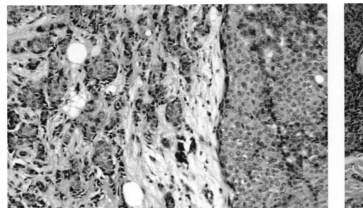

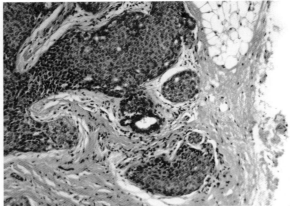

A

B

Figure 26.7 **Recurrent carcinoma after radiotherapy.** **A:** Intraductal and infiltrating poorly differentiated duct carcinoma before radiotherapy. **B:** This specimen from a needle core biopsy procedure performed 1 year after radiotherapy shows intraductal carcinoma identical to that on the right in **(A)**.

microscopic change attributable to treatment is evident when pre- and postradiation samples of in situ carcinoma are compared. From time to time radiated invasive tumor contains cells with multiple hyperchromatic nuclei or there is focal necrosis that was not seen in the pretreatment biopsy, and it may be suspected that these are radiation effects in residual tumor.

In a study of invasive breast recurrences after conservation therapy with radiotherapy in women 40 years or younger at diagnosis, Sigal-Zafrani et al. (20) found no significant differences in histologic type, grade, and hormone receptor expression between primary and recurrent tumors. New carcinomas that arose outside the index quadrant were more likely to differ from the initial primary tumor than were recurrences in the same quadrant.

Therapeutic radiotherapy for breast carcinoma has been associated with a significantly increased relative risk for carcinoma of the esophagus and lung and for myeloid leukemia (21–23). However, the overall incidence of such neoplasms appears to be low with about 160 cases observed in a cohort of 33,763 women with breast carcinoma who had radiotherapy (21).

CHEMOTHERAPY

Treatment-related histologic changes may be detected in mammary carcinoma and in nonneoplastic breast tissue examined after patients have received chemotherapy. Chemotherapy effect is most often encountered when patients with locally advanced or inflammatory carcinoma have been given high-dose systemic therapy preoperatively (24). The morphologic changes in this situation are often the result of the combined effect of multiple agents administered as neoadjuvant therapy, sometimes complicated by radiotherapy.

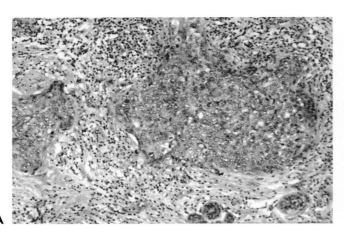

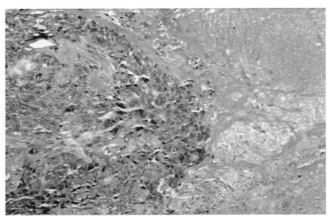

A

B

Figure 26.8 **Recurrent infiltrating carcinoma.** **A:** Infiltrating poorly differentiated duct carcinoma with a prominent lymphocytic reaction before treatment. **B:** One year after lumpectomy and radiotherapy, recurrent carcinoma was partially necrotic and devoid of lymphocytic reaction but otherwise similar to the pretreatment tumor.

In general, the histopathologic effects of systemic chemotherapy can be correlated with the extent of clinical response. The greatest histopathologic alterations are usually found in patients who appear clinically to have complete resolution of their neoplasm (25–27). However, it is not unusual to observe dissociation between the posttherapy clinical picture and the histologic findings, as when the patient seems to have had a complete clinical response but histologic examination of the breast reveals residual tumor. Pu et al. (28) investigated pathologic features in a pretreatment needle core biopsy specimen as a guide for predicting a complete pathologic response to neoadjuvant chemotherapy. Among complete responders, 80% had tumor necrosis in the core biopsy sample, whereas necrosis was found in 17% of nonresponders.

Mammography may suggest a response in patients treated with neoadjuvant chemotherapy, but this procedure is not reliable for predicting the pathologic status of the breast. There is not a consistent correlation between the pretreatment histologic grade of the tumor and pathologic evidence of response to therapy. When no residual tumor is detectable grossly in the breast, approximately 60% of patients are found to have persistent carcinoma histologically. Usually, similar chemotherapy effects are found in the primary tumor and in axillary nodal metastases.

The fundamental manifestation of chemotherapy effect is a decrease in tumor cellularity (Figs. 26.9–26.10). Rajan et al. (27) observed a decrease in median tumor cellularity from 40% in pretreatment core biopsies to 10% in tumors resected after neoadjuvant chemotherapy. There was considerable variation of changes in cellularity among clinical response categories. Many tumors appeared to have a pronounced decrease in tumor cellularity with minimal reduction in size.

In the most extreme situation, no residual carcinoma may be detectable, an occurrence reported in 6.7% to 10% of cases (26,29). If the breast of a patient who has a complete clinical response is examined histologically soon after treatment, residual degenerated and infarcted necrotic invasive carcinoma may be recognized by the loss of normal staining properties and decreased architectural detail. With the passage of time, the degenerated invasive carcinoma is absorbed. Healed sites of previous infiltrating carcinoma may be appreciated because of residual architectural distortion characterized by fibrosis, stromal edema, increased vascularity composed largely of thin-walled vessels, and a chronic inflammatory cell infiltrate (Fig. 26.10) (30). There is some evidence that intraductal carcinoma and lymphatic tumor emboli may be relatively more resistant to treatment than invasive carcinoma, so that these sites can serve as sanctuaries for persistent carcinoma. In a minority of

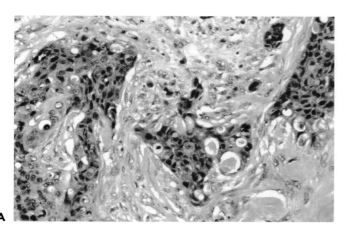

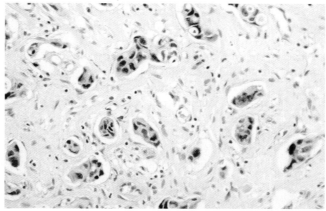

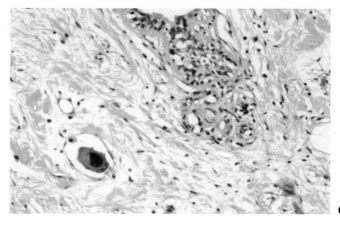

Figure 26.9 Chemotherapy effect. A: Poorly differentiated infiltrating duct carcinoma in a biopsy specimen from a patient who subsequently received doxorubicin (Adriamycin) and radiotherapy. **B:** This needle core biopsy sample was obtained from the breast after the patient had a partial clinical response. Small nests of carcinoma cells with pleomorphic hyperchromatic nuclei are present in the collagenous stroma. Peritumoral shrinkage simulates lymphatic invasion. **C:** A markedly enlarged hyperchromatic cell in a lymphatic space is shown near an atrophic lobule. The cytologic changes in the carcinoma are attributable largely to the chemotherapy.

A

B

C

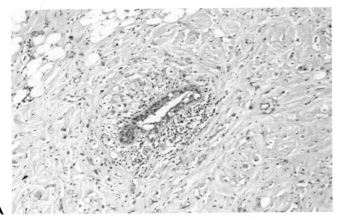
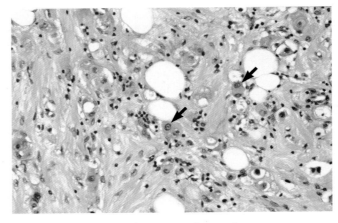

A **B**

Figure 26.10 Chemotherapy effect in the breast. A, B: This needle core biopsy sample was obtained after a partial clinical response to chemotherapy. Isolated residual carcinoma cells *(arrows)* are dispersed in the fibrotic mammary stroma, accompanied by a scattering of lymphocytes.

instances, the only residual carcinoma found after complete clinical response in the breast consists of lymphatic tumor emboli, intraductal carcinoma, or both (Fig. 26.11). Rabban et al. (31) reported finding intralymphatic carcinoma in the breasts of 11 of 146 (7.5%) patients treated with neoadjuvant chemotherapy, including 6 (4%) whose only residual carcinoma was intralymphatic.

Fibrosis and atrophy of lymphoid tissue are characteristic features of chemotherapy effect at sites of metastatic carcinoma in lymph nodes (32) (Fig. 26.12). Cytokeratin immunostaining is essential for detecting minimal residual carcinoma in lymph nodes or in the breast after neoadjuvant chemotherapy (33).

Residual in situ and invasive carcinoma cells may appear morphologically unaltered, but in most cases they exhibit histologic and cytologic changes that reflect chemotherapy treatment effect (25,29,30,34,35). The cells are enlarged due to increased cytoplasmic volume. The cytoplasm often contains vacuoles and eosinophilic granules (30,32,35). Cell borders are typically well defined, and the cells tend to shrink away from the stroma (35) (Fig. 26.9). Some carcinoma cells have enlarged,

pleomorphic, and hyperchromatic nuclei (24). The tumor cells retain immunohistochemical reactivity for cytokeratin and epithelial membrane antigen.

Nonneoplastic breast parenchyma is also altered following high-dose cytotoxic chemotherapy, but the changes are more subtle than those induced in the tumor (35). The glandular elements undergo diffuse atrophy causing a reduction in the number of lobules and the size of existing lobules (20,32,36). Cytologic atypia may be seen in duct and lobular epithelial cells, but in many cases these changes are not attributable specifically to treatment effect. Comparison with a pretreatment specimen is particularly helpful in this situation. Regressive changes may also be found in the lymphoid tissue of axillary lymph nodes (15).

ABLATION THERAPY

Several methods of in situ tumor ablation have been investigated. These include interstitial laser therapy, radiofrequency ablation, cryoablation, and microwave ablation

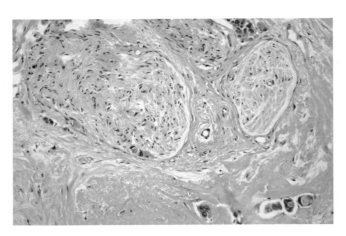

Figure 26.11 Chemotherapy effect in lymphatic tumor emboli. The clusters of carcinoma cells in a nerve and in lymphatic channels show cytologic changes related to chemotherapy. The patient had a complete clinical response to chemotherapy, and this was the extent of histologically detectable residual carcinoma.

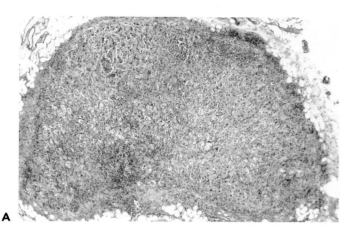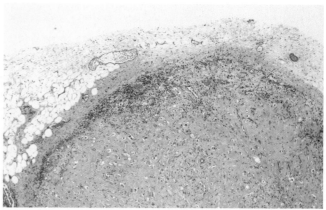

Figure 26.12 **Chemotherapy effect in a lymph node with metastatic carcinoma. A:** Carcinoma diffusely involves a lymph node before therapy. **B:** After chemotherapy, the tumor is largely necrotic in a background of fibrosis and lymphoid atrophy.

(37). All of these procedures use an image-guided technique to insert a probe into the lesion. Cryoablation destroys the tumor by freezing it. The other methods destroy the tumor with heat generated by various energy sources. At present, these techniques are considered to be investigational for the treatment of breast carcinoma. Histologic changes induced by these procedures appear to be limited to the lesion and the immediate surrounding tissue.

Interstitial laser therapy has been investigated as a method for causing the thermal destruction of small primary breast carcinomas (38,39). Thermal energy is generated with a laser probe inserted into the tumor. Bloom et al. (38) studied the pathologic changes associated with laser tumor ablation and observed a series of grossly identifiable concentric rings around the probe tract. Tissue in zone 1, immediately around the defect produced by the probe, appeared charred. Zone 2 surrounding the charred surface of the cavity exhibited coagulative necrosis and "wind swept" nuclei typically seen in surgical cautery effect. The third zone consisted of carcinoma that appeared to be histologically intact without necrosis or inflammation. A fourth zone consisted of necrotic tumor that appeared to be infarcted causing "conventional tinctorial affinities to be erased." The outermost zone 5 was composed of vascular proliferation with thrombosis, inflammation, and fat necrosis in parenchyma outside the tumor. The authors concluded that two mechanisms were involved in tumor destruction by interstitial laser therapy: direct thermal damage centrally and infarction at the periphery due to thrombosis of blood vessels at the perimeter. Zone 3 was found to decrease in size with the passage of time, whereas zone 4 enlarged over time. This observation was interpreted as evidence that the zone 3 carcinoma that appeared to be histologically intact had been rendered nonviable by the laser and that it underwent progressive degenerative change causing it to be incorporated into the necrotic zone 4.

In situ thermal destruction of breast carcinoma has also been achieved by applying radio frequency energy with

probes inserted into the tumor (40). Histologic examination reveals heat-induced tumor necrosis similar to that caused by the laser probe.

The histologic effects of cryoablation are well established 7 days after treatment at which time the affected tissue displays coagulative necrosis surrounded by a zone of fat necrosis and scar formation (41). Residual in situ or invasive carcinoma may be found beyond the perimeter of the necrotic tissue. Cyroprobe-assisted lumpectomy is a procedure in which freezing is used to convert a nonpalpable ultrasound-detected lesion into a palpable target that can be excised without the need for wire localization (42). The tissue is affected in much the same manner as occurs when cryoablation is performed, but excisional surgery is done promptly after procedure, while the tissue is still frozen. In a study of six specimens obtained by this method, Sahoo et al. (42) found that alterations in the tissue caused by freezing compromised grading of carcinomas and interfered with distinguishing between in situ and invasive components, assessing mitoses, and detecting vascular invasion. The histologic effects of freezing included retraction artifact, shrinkage of cells, nuclear smudging, and cytoplasmic eosinophilia. Ki67 expression was not appreciably altered by freezing when compared with samples obtained before treatment, but estrogen and progesterone receptor expression was substantially less after freezing. The authors concluded that "without the availability of prior needle core biopsy specimens, the quality of the cryoprobe-assisted lumpectomy specimens would not have been reliable for tumor typing and grading or for immunohistochemical studies."

REFERENCES

1. Boice JD, Manson RR, Rosenstein M. Breast cancer in women after repeated fluoroscopic examinations of the chest. *J Natl Cancer Inst.* 1977;159:823–832.
2. Hildreth NG, Shore RE, Dvoretsky PM. The risk of breast cancer after irradiation of the thymus in infancy. *N Engl J Med.* 1989;321:1281–1284.
3. Anderson N, Lokich J. Bilateral breast cancer after cured Hodgkin's disease. *Cancer.* 1990;65:221–223.
4. O'Brien PC, Barton MB, Fisher R, for Australian Radiation Oncology Lymphoma Group (AROLG). Breast cancer following treatment for Hodgkin's disease: the need for screening in a young population. *Austral Radiol.* 1995;39:271–276.

5. Yahalom J, Petrek JA, Biddinger PW, et al. Breast cancer in patients irradiated for Hodgkin's disease: a clinical and pathological study of 45 events in 37 patients. *J Clin Oncol.* 1992;10:1674–1681.
6. Bhatia S, Robison LL, Oberlin O, et al. Breast cancer and other second neoplasms after childhood Hodgkin's disease. *N Engl J Med.* 1996;334:745–751.
7. Wendland MMM, Tsodikov A, Glenn MJ, Gaffney DK. Time interval to the development of breast carcinoma after treatment for Hodgkin's disease. *Cancer.* 2004;101:1275–1282.
8. Cutuli B, Borel C, Dhermain F. Breast cancer occurring after treatment for Hodgkin's disease: analysis of 133 cases. *Radiother Oncol.* 2001;59:247–255.
9. Tarvidon AA, Garnier ML, Beaudre A, Grinsky T. Breast carcinoma in women previously treated for Hodgkin's disease: clinical and mammographic findings. *Eur Radiol.* 2003;9:1666–1671.
10. Dershaw DD, Yahalom J, Petrek JA. Breast carcinoma in women previously treated for Hodgkin disease: mammographic evaluation. *Radiology.* 1992;184:421–423.
11. Diller L, Nancarrow CM, Shaffer K, et al. Breast cancer screening in women previously treated for Hodgkin's disease: a prospective cohort study. *J Clin Oncol.* 2002;20:2085–2091.
12. Tehe W, Wilson ARM. The role of ultrasound in breast cancer screening. A consensus statement by the European Group for Breast Cancer Screening. *Eur J Cancer.* 1998;34:449–450.
13. Neubauer H, Li M, Kuehne-Heid R, et al. High grade and non-high grade ductal carcinoma in situ on dynamic MR mammography: characteristic findings for signal increase and morphological pattern of enhancement. *Br J Radiol.* 2003;76:3–12.
14. Schnitt SJ, Connolly JL, Harris JR, Cohen RB. Radiation-induced changes in the breast. *Hum Pathol.* 1984;15:545–550.
15. Moore GH, Schiller JE, Moore GK. Radiation-induced hisopathologic changes of the breast. The effects of time. *Am J Surg Pathol.* 2004;28:47–53.
16 Girling AC, Hanby AM, Millis RR. Radiation and other pathological changes in breast tissue after conservation treatment for carcinoma. *J Clin Pathol.* 1990;43:152–156.
17. Pedio G, Landolt V, Zobeli L. Irradiated benign cells of the breast: a potential diagnostic pitfall in fine needle aspiration cytology. *Acta Cytol.* 1989;32:127–128.
18. Peterse JL, Thunnissen FBJM, van Heerde P. Fine needle aspiration cytology or radiation-induced changes in non-neoplastic breast lesions. Possible pitfalls in cytodiagnosis. *Acta Cytol.* 1989;33:176–180.
19. Mills RR, Pinder SE, Ryder K, et al. Grade of recurrent *in situ* and invasive carcinoma following treatment of pure ductal carcinoma *in situ* of the breast. *Br J Cancer.* 2004;90:1538–1542.
20. Sigal-Zafrani B, Bollet MA, Antoni G, et al. Are ipsilateral invasive recurrences in young (<40 years) women more aggressive than their primary tumors? *Br J Cancer.* 2007;97:1046–1052.
21. Roychoudhuri R, Evans H, Robinson D, Moller H. Radiation-induced malignancies following radiotherapy for breast cancer. *Br J Cancer.* 2004;91:868–872.
22. Zablotska LB, Neugut AI. Lung carcinoma after radiotherapy in women treated with lumpectomy or mastectomy for primary breast carcinoma. *Cancer.* 2003;97:1404–1411.
23. Curtis RE, Boice JD Jr, Stoval M, et al. Risk of leukemia after chemotherapy and radiation treatment for breast cancer. *N Eng J Med.* 1992;326:1745–1751.

24. Rasbridge SA, Gillett CE, Seymour A-M, et al. The effects of chemotherapy on morphology, cellular proliferation, apoptosis and oncoprotein expression in primary breast carcinoma. *Br J Cancer.* 1994;70:335–341.
25. Brifford M, Spyratos F, Tubiana-Huhn M, et al. Sequential cytopunctures during pre-operative chemotherapy for primary breast cancer. *Cancer.* 1989;63:631–637.
26. Feldman LD, Hortobagyi GN, Buzdar AU, et al. Pathological assessment of response to induction chemotherapy in breast cancer. *Cancer Res.* 1986;46:2578–2581.
27. Rajan R, Poniecka A, Smith TL, et al. Changes in tumor cellularity of breast carcinoma after neoadjuvant chemotherapy as a variable in the pathologic assessment of response. *Cancer.* 2004;100:1365–1373.
28. Pu RT, Schott AF, Sturtz DE, et al. Pathologic features of breast cancer associated with complete response to neoadjuvant chemotherapy. Importance of tumor necrosis. *Am J Surg Pathol.* 2005;29:354–358.
29. Frierson HF Jr, Fechner RE. Histologic grade of locally advanced infiltrating ductal carcinoma after treatment with induction chemotherapy. *Am J Clin Pathol.* 1994;102:154–157.
30. Sharkey FE, Addington SL, Fowler LJ, et al. Effects of preoperative chemotherapy on the morphology of resectable breast carcinoma. *Mod Pathol.* 1996;9:893–900.
31. Rabban JT, Glidden D. Kwan ML, Chen Y-Y. Pure and predominantly pure intralymphatic breast carcinoma after neoadjuvant chemotherapy. An unusual and adverse pattern of residual disease. *Am J Surg Pathol.* 2009;33:256–263.
32. Aktepe F, Kapucuoglu N, Pak I. The effects of chemotherapy on breast cancer tissue in locally advanced breast cancer. *Histopathology.* 1996;29:63–67.
33. Pinder SA, Provenzano E, Earl H, Ellis IO. Laboratory handling and histology reporting of breast specimens from patients who received neoadjuvant chemotherapy. *Histopathology.* 2007;50:409–417.
34. McCready DR, Hortobagyi GN, Kau SW, et al. The prognostic significance of lymph node metastases after preoperative chemotherapy for locally advanced breast cancer. *Arch Surg.* 1989;124:21–25.
35. Sahoo, S, Lester SC. Pathology of breast carcinomas after neoadjuvant chemotherapy. An overview with recommendations on specimen processing and reporting. *Arch Pathol Lab Med.* 2009;133:633–642.
36. Kennedy S, Merino MJ, Swain SM, Lippman ME. The effects of hormonal and chemotherapy on tumoral and non-neoplastic breast tissue. *Hum Pathol.* 1990;21:192–198.
37. Simmons RM. Ablative techniques in the treatment of benign and malignant breast disease. *J Am Coll Surg.* 2003;197:334–338.
38. Bloom KJ, Dowlat K, Assad L. Pathologic changes after interstitial laser therapy of infiltrating breast carcinoma. *Am J Surg.* 2001;182:384–388.
39. Dowlatshahi K, Fan M, Gould VE, et al. Stereotactically guided laser therapy of occult breast tumors. *Arch Surg.* 2000;135:1345–1352.
40. Jeffrey SS, Birdwell RL, Ikeda DM, et al. Radiofrequency ablation of breast cancer. First report of an emerging technology. *Arch Surg.* 1999;134:1064–1068.
41. Roubidoux MA, Sabel MS, Bailey JE, et al. Small (<2.0 cm) breast cancers: mammographic and US findings at US-guided cryoablation-initial experience. *Radiology.* 2004;233:857–867.
42. Sahoo S, Talwalkar SS, Martin AW, Chagpar AB. Pathologic evaluation of cryoprobe-assisted lumpectomy for breast cancer. *Am J Clin Pathol.* 2007;128:238–244.

Breast Lesions in Men and Children

27

Needle core biopsy and fine needle aspiration of the male breast are uncommon procedures, and they are even less frequent in children. A review of fine needle aspirations of the breast performed in three large academic programs in the United States from 1990 to 2000 revealed that about 4% of 14,026 specimens were obtained from men (1). The most frequent diagnoses were gynecomastia and carcinoma. A pathology group servicing several community hospitals in the Netherlands received 26 core biopsy specimens of the male breast between 1993 and the end of 2002, or 2.6 specimens per year (2). The diagnoses were reported as gynecomastia, benign or carcinoma.

BENIGN PROLIFERATIVE LESIONS OF THE MALE BREAST

Gynecomastia is the most common clinical and pathologic abnormality of the male breast. Mammary enlargement may be due to a discrete, nodular increase in subareolar tissue, or a diffuse accumulation of tissue. Both breasts are affected in the majority of patients at all ages. Gynecomastia is a frequent adverse side effect of some medications used to treat prostatic hyperplasia (3) and may occur in men who receive antiretroviral treatment for HIV (4). The initial clinical signs of gynecomastia are breast enlargement and a palpable mass that may be accompanied by pain or tenderness. The palpable mass is located in the central subareolar region in most patients. Carcinoma arising in gynecomastia can usually be detected as a localized, asymmetric area of firmness.

Mammography is helpful for distinguishing between gynecomastia and carcinoma and may identify carcinoma developing in gynecomastia (5). Two mammographic patterns associated with gynecomastia are a dendritic, retroareolar density with prominent radial extensions into the breast and a triangular subareolar density lacking radiating extensions. Ultrasound has also proven to be useful in the diagnosis of gynecomastia.

The microscopic features of gynecomastia are similar regardless of etiologic factors (6,7). Three phases of proliferative change have been described. Florid gynecomastia, ordinarily seen soon after onset, is characterized by prominent epithelial proliferation in ducts, typically with flat and micropapillary structure (Fig. 27.1). Mitoses may be found in the epithelium. There is usually concomitant myoepithelial cell hyperplasia. The increased amount and cellularity of periductal stroma are accompanied by prominent vascularity, edema, and a round cell infiltrate. Intermediate gynecomastia has florid and fibrous components. It constitutes a transitional phase in maturation of the lesion (Fig. 27.2). Fibrous or inactive gynecomastia typically occurs after the lesion has been present for 12 months or longer. The epithelial proliferation tends to be less conspicuous than in the florid phase but prominent hyperplasia can persist (Fig. 27.3). The stroma is more collagenous, with less edema, and there is reduced vascularity. Pseudoangiomatous hyperplasia of the stroma may be found in any phase of gynecomastia, but it tends to be more pronounced in the florid and intermediate stages. (Fig. 27.4).

The cytologic features and growth pattern of the epithelial proliferation in ducts may be atypical. This occurs most often in the florid phase. Atypical features are the focal development of fenestrated and solid growth patterns, and papillary proliferation in which a cytologically atypical cell appears to overgrow the dimorphic population that characterizes florid gynecomastia (Fig. 27.5). Mitotic activity is variable but it may be pronounced in ducts exhibiting atypical hyperplasia. Nuclear estrogen receptor immunoreactivity is present in the epithelial cells in most examples of gynecomastia. Uncommon proliferative epithelial changes found in gynecomastia include lobule formation, pseudolactational hyperplasia, apocrine metaplasia, cysts, and squamous metaplasia (Fig. 27.6).

Gynecomastia-like hyperplasia of the female breast is composed of stromal and ductal proliferative elements that duplicate the appearance of true gynecomastia in men (8,9). The majority of the patients are premenopausal. The lesion is either palpable or it is detected as an asymmetric density on mammography (10). The radiologic findings are not specific, and in some instances, no lesions may be detected on the mammogram (8,10).

Intraductal papillomas can arise in the male breast (11). The usual presenting symptom is nipple discharge that is

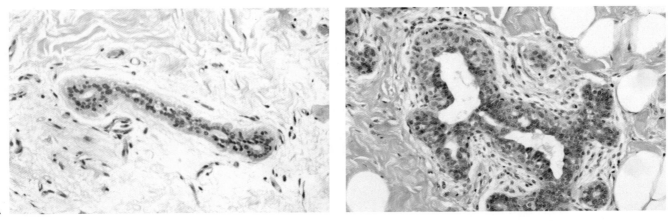

Figure 27.1 Gynecomastia, florid. A: A normal duct in the breast of a 75-year-old man. **B:** Gynecomastia with hyperplasia of myoepithelial cells and edema of the periductal stroma.

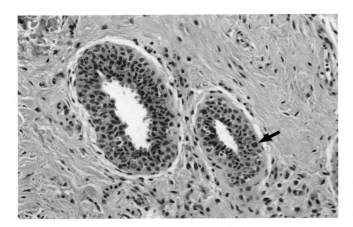

Figure 27.2 Gynecomastia, intermediate. An intermediate phase lesion with compact epithelial and myoepithelial hyperplasia. An epithelial mitotic figure is present *(arrow)*. Note the periductal edema and hypervascularity.

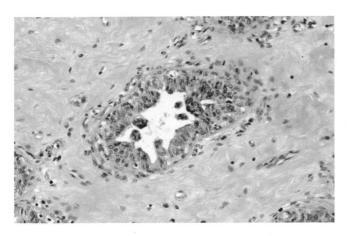

Figure 27.3 Gynecomastia, inactive. This focus features micropapillary epithelial hyperplasia and a mild increase in periductal vascularity. The periductal stroma is collagenized.

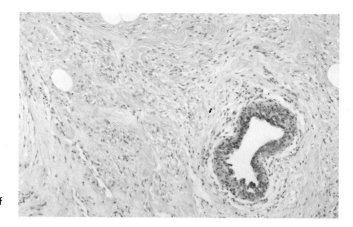

Figure 27.4   Gynecomastia. Pseudoangiomatous hyperplasia of the stroma surrounds a duct with myoepithelial hyperplasia.

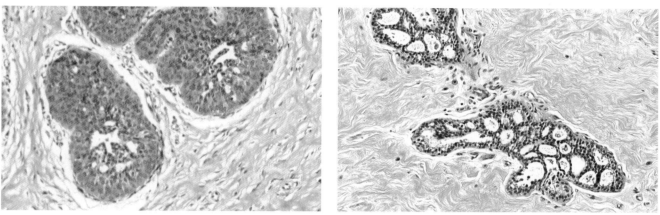

Figure 27.5   Gynecomastia with atypical duct hyperplasia. A: The proliferation is almost entirely epithelial with a minimal myoepithelial component. **B:** Atypical cribriform duct hyperplasia.

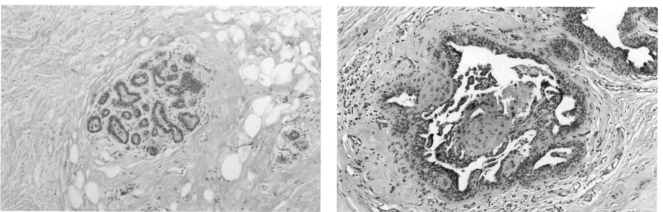

Figure 27.6   Gynecomastia. A: Lobule formation in a male breast. **B:** Florid gynecomastia with squamous metaplasia in hyperplastic duct epithelium.

bloody or blood tinged. Microscopic examination reveals an orderly papillary structure composed of cuboidal or columnar cells. Because of the relatively high proportion of papillary carcinomas of the male breast, all male papillary tumors should be carefully evaluated pathologically. Approximately 5% of the reported examples of *florid papillomatosis* of the nipple have been in men (12). Nearly half of these lesions have contained carcinoma.

Fibroepithelial tumors of the male breast usually arise in a background of gynecomastia. Some lesions classified as *fibroadenoma* or *phyllodes tumor* are probably nodular foci of gynecomastia (13,14). Most cystosarcomas in men have been histologically and clinically benign. Some of the male patients with fibroepithelial lesions had been treated with estrogens, resulting in concomitant gynecomastia with lobular differentiation (14). Digital fibroma-like inclusions were found in the stroma of a fibroadenoma from a man who had been treated with Lupron for prostatic carcinoma (15).

Other benign conditions in the male breast include *duct ectasia* (16) and *fibrocystic changes* (17), both often coexistent with gynecomastia. Myofibroblastoma is a relatively common benign mesenchymal tumor of the male breast (see Chapter 23).

CARCINOMA OF THE MALE BREAST

Breast carcinoma in men accounts for not more than 1% of all breast carcinomas (18). There is a straight-line relationship between incidence and age among men (19). This differs from female breast carcinoma, which has a less steep slope of incidence after age 50 (20). A study of male breast carcinoma cases in Florida revealed an increase from 56 in 1985 to 132 in 2000, representing a significant rise in incidence (21). The age-specific incidence was highest in men older than 85 years.

Between 1973 and 1998, the incidence of breast carcinoma in men reported to the National Cancer Institute rose from 0.86 to 1.08 per 100,000 men ($p < 0.001$) (22). The rise in incidence is probably a function of overall aging of the population.

The majority of male breast carcinomas are located centrally in a retroareolar position. The cumulative risk for bilaterality is 3% or less. Carcinoma is found in about 75% of male patients with a mass and bloody discharge. Serous discharge alone may indicate intraductal carcinoma (23). Age at diagnosis averages about 60 years, but breast carcinoma has been diagnosed in adult males at virtually all ages. Almost 90% of male breast carcinomas express estrogen receptor (24). HER2/*neu* expression is found in male breast carcinoma less frequently than in female breast carcinoma (25).

Mammograms of men with breast carcinoma typically reveal distinct lesions with invasive margins that contrast sharply with the surrounding fatty tissue (26,27), but carcinoma may be obscured by gynecomastia. Cystic papillary carcinoma produces a discrete round mass that may contain calcifications (28). Microcalcifications are found in 9% to 30% of male breast carcinomas studied mammographically (29,30).

Approximately 85% of male mammary carcinomas are of the ordinary infiltrating duct variety (31–33) (Fig. 27.7). An intraductal component is found in 35% to 50% of male and 75% of female infiltrating duct carcinomas (31). Extensive intraductal carcinoma constituting more than 25% of the tumor and involving surrounding breast, is uncommon in men. The majority of the invasive tumors are moderately or poorly differentiated (33) (Fig. 27.8), but low-grade and tubular carcinomas have been described (31–33) (Fig. 27.9). The structure of male infiltrating duct carcinoma duplicates carcinomas in the female breast, including cribriform, comedo, papillary, solid, or gland-forming patterns. Papillary carcinomas, often with a prominent cystic component, are relatively more common among men than women, constituting 3% to 5% of male carcinomas (31–33) but only 1% to 2% of carcinomas in women (Fig. 27.10). The majority of male papillary carcinomas are intracystic and noninvasive.

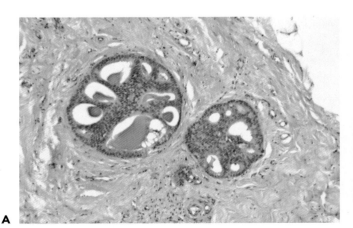
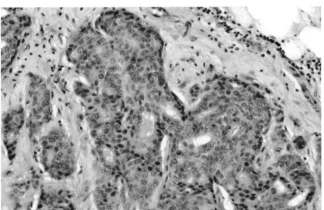

A   **B**

Figure 27.7   Male breast carcinoma. The patient was a 75-year-old man with a palpable tumor. **A, B:** The needle core biopsy specimen reveals cribriform intraductal carcinoma **(A)** and moderately differentiated infiltrating duct carcinoma that has cribriform features **(B).**

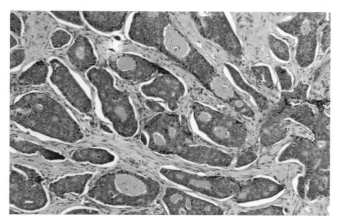

Figure 27.8   Male breast carcinoma. Infiltrating duct carcinoma with a cribriform structure and foci of necrosis.

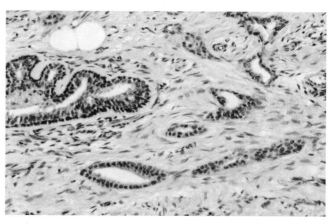

Figure 27.9   Male breast carcinoma. Tubular carcinoma composed of angular glands infiltrating around a duct.

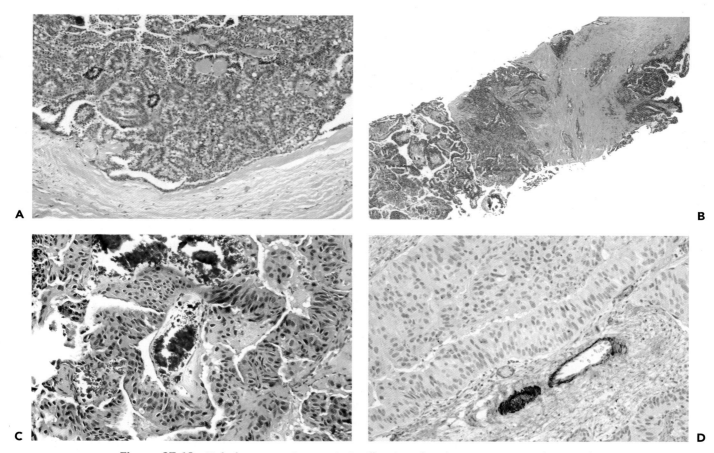

Figure 27.10   Male breast carcinoma. A: Papillary intraductal carcinoma protrudes into the lumen of a cystically dilated duct. **B:** Low magnification view of the needle core biopsy sample from a 67-year-old man. Cystic papillary intraductal carcinoma is shown at both ends of the sample with invasive carcinoma in the center. **C:** Part of the cystic papillary intraductal carcinoma in **(B)** with calcifications. **D:** Actin reactivity is absent from the papillary carcinoma. Vascular structures are actin-positive (immunoperoxidase).

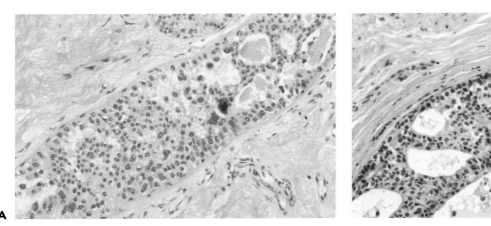

Figure 27.11   Male breast carcinoma, intraductal. Two views of cribriform intraductal carcinoma. **A:** The duct is cut longitudinally. Microcalcification is present. The patient was a 44-year-old man who presented with serous nipple discharge and a mass. **B:** Part of a duct with cribriform intraductal carcinoma cut transversely in a 70-year-old man.

Because lobular differentiation is so rarely seen in the male breast, the existence of lobular carcinoma has been questioned in this setting. Isolated examples of "small cell carcinoma" or lobular carcinoma have been described (34–36). The microscopic appearance of the lesions depicted in some papers is consistent with invasive lobular carcinoma. In situ lobular carcinoma has reportedly been found (34,35). E-cadherin negative invasive pleomorphic lobular carcinoma in a 44-year-old man was reported by Maly et al. (37). Absence of E-cadherin reactivity is now a requisite for making a diagnosis of lobular carcinoma in the male breast.

Other uncommon types of invasive carcinoma encountered in the male breast include medullary, mucinous and adenoid cystic tumors. Carcinoma with osteoclast-like giant cells has been reported in the male breast.

About 6% of male breast carcinoma patients also have metachronous prostatic carcinoma (38). These patients do not appear to have a more aggressive form of prostatic carcinoma than occurs in men without breast carcinoma, and it does not occur at an earlier age. On occasion, the distinction between a primary carcinoma of the breast and metastatic prostatic carcinoma may be difficult. Both types of carcinoma can express estrogen receptors. Patients with prostatic adenocarcinoma treated with estrogens invariably have gynecomastia, which may exhibit atypical papillary epithelial hyperplasia. In men with known prostatic carcinoma, the diagnosis of mammary carcinoma is relatively easy in the presence of convincing evidence of intraductal carcinoma, usually cribriform or comedo in type, or the finding of invasive growth patterns such as tubular, medullary, mucinous, or cystic papillary carcinoma. Greater difficulty is encountered with poorly differentiated carcinoma that lacks an intraductal component. The immunohistochemical demonstration of prostate-specific antigen (PSA) favors a diagnosis of metastatic prostatic carcinoma, whereas finding intracellular mucin supports a diagnosis of mammary carcinoma. However,

aberrant expression of PSA detected by immunohistochemistry has been reported in breast carcinomas from men (39) and women (40). Strong nuclear reactivity for androgen receptor is typically associated with prostatic carcinoma, but it also occurs in mammary carcinomas, especially the apocrine type.

A review of 282 cases of male breast carcinoma reported by 10 US population-based cancer registries revealed that 10.4% were intraductal (41). The histologic appearances of intraductal carcinoma in men include comedo, cribriform, solid, micropapillary, and papillary patterns (Fig. 27.11). When intraductal carcinoma arises in gynecomastia, it is sometimes possible to find transitions from atypical hyperplasia in gynecomastic ducts to intraductal carcinoma (42). Comedo necrosis and epithelial clear cell change are features more strongly associated with intraductal carcinoma than with hyperplasia in gynecomastia.

Staging of axillary nodal status in men can be effectively accomplished by sentinel lymph node (SLN) biopsy (43,44). Combined data from several reports included 23 men. SLNs were identified in 22 (95.7%). The SLN was positive in 9 (41%) of the 22 cases, with 3 positive at the time of frozen section. In a subset of 19 men with a T1 tumor, 8 (42%) had a positive SLN.

Prognosis is significantly related to stage at diagnosis as determined by tumor size and nodal status (31,45–47). The presence of lymphatic tumor emboli negatively influences prognosis (48). Many investigators have concluded that male and female patients with the same stage of disease have a similar prognosis (22,31,49,50).

BREAST TUMORS IN CHILDREN

Juvenile papillomatosis (JP) is a localized benign proliferative lesion that usually occurs in women younger than 30 years. Two-thirds of the patients are younger than 25. JP is uncommon prior to puberty and after the age of 40 years (51,52).

The typical clinical finding is a solitary, firm, discrete unilateral tumor that is palpably suggestive of a fibroadenoma. Bilateral JP, that may be synchronous or metachronous, is occasionally encountered. Very rare instances of multifocal tumors have been reported. Separate coexistent fibroadenomas are common.

Few descriptions of the mammographic findings in JP are available because mammography is usually not performed preoperatively in these young women. The films reveal a localized area of increased density with a border that is generally not as well defined as that of a fibroadenoma (52,53). The sonographic appearance of JP is that of an inhomogeneous, ill-defined mass with hypoechoic areas largely at the periphery (53,54).

At the time of diagnosis, patients with JP report a frequency of a positive family history for breast carcinoma that is similar to that of patients who have mammary carcinoma (55), and with further follow-up, the frequency of a positive family history exceeds 50% (56). The female relatives most likely to be affected by breast carcinoma are their mothers and maternal aunts of JP patients. Breast carcinoma has only rarely been seen in the sisters of JP patients.

Histologic examination reveals a spectrum of benign proliferative fibrocystic changes that are present in varying proportions in individual cases. Cysts and duct hyperplasia are constant features (Fig. 27.12). The epithelium of cysts and proliferative foci frequently exhibits apocrine metaplasia. Stasis of secretion in cysts and ducts is manifested by collections of lipid-laden histiocytes. Sclerosing adenosis, lobular hyperplasia, and fibroadenomatoid hyperplasia are variably present. In most cases, the ductal proliferative changes consist of usual hyperplasia. Sometimes, the ductal hyperplasia has a radial scar pattern. Atypical changes in the ductal hyperplasia include cribriform or micropapillary growth patterns and intraductal necrosis. In one series, significant atypia was detected in 40% of lesions and intraductal necrosis in 15% (56).

Ten percent to 15% of patients with JP also have breast carcinoma (52,56,57). Virtually all of these women have had a positive family history for breast carcinoma, usually affecting their mother or a maternal aunt (56,57). The types of breast carcinoma that have been encountered associated with JP include intraductal carcinoma, lobular carcinoma in situ, infiltrating duct carcinoma, and secretory (juvenile) carcinoma. Most of these patients have had carcinoma and JP diagnosed concurrently. With few exceptions, the carcinoma was within and appeared to arise from the JP. A review of 41 patients with at least 10 years of follow-up after the diagnosis of JP (median follow-up of 14 years) found that breast carcinoma subsequently developed in four patients (10%) after an interval of 5 to 15 years (56). These patients were 25 to 42 years old when JP was diagnosed, and thus all

A

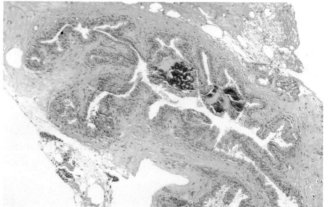

B

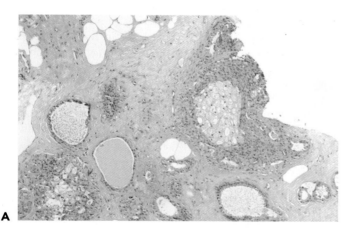

C

Figure 27.12 Juvenile papillomatosis. A–C: This needle core biopsy specimen is from a 2-cm breast tumor in an 18-year-old girl. The diagnostic features are cysts, cystic and papillary apocrine metaplasia, duct hyperplasia and stasis with accumulation of histiocytes. Calcifications are present in the papillary epithelium in **(B)**.

were past the mean age for JP. Three of the patients had multifocal or bilateral JP.

Excisional biopsy for JP is often performed for JP with little margin. Incomplete excision probably predisposes to local recurrence, but this may occur even when the margins appear to be adequate histologically. Reexcision of the biopsy site would be prudent if the lesion has not been grossly excised or if there is severe atypia. Unless carcinoma is found in the tumor, no treatment is necessary after complete excisional biopsy. Mammography should be employed judiciously, especially for patients younger than 35 years of age, during follow-up. Ultrasonography is a useful alternative to mammography. Female relatives of JP patients, especially on the maternal side, are advised to have regular breast surveillance.

Papillary duct hyperplasia and *papillomas* are infrequent breast lesions in patients younger than 30 years old (58). Most patients are female with a median age of 17 years (59). The majority (70%) are 15 to 25 years of age. The most frequent presenting symptom is a mass. Less than 20% of patients have nipple discharge, which may be bloody or clear. Any part of the breast may be affected, but periareolar or subareolar lesions are most common. Very few patients have been subjected to mammography, and the results are non-specific (59). Microcalcifications have been found in a few cases.

Three microscopic growth patterns have been described. *Sclerosing papilloma* has been found in nearly 50% of cases. This radial scar-like lesion is fundamentally a papilloma distorted and disrupted by a desmoplastic proliferation of myoepithelial and stromal cells (Fig. 27.13). Small clusters of epithelial cells incorporated into the stromal proliferation can be mistaken for invasive carcinoma. Lobules may be included in the sclerosing proliferation.

About one-third of the lesions are *papillomas* without sclerosis, limited to a single focus. Papillomas occur in one or more dilated ducts that contain papillary fronds of epithelial cells in single or multiple layers, supported by fibrovascular stroma. Infrequent mitoses may be encoun-

tered in the epithelium. Myoepithelial cell hyperplasia is variably present.

Papillary hyperplasia involving multiple ducts (papillomatosis) is encountered in about 25% of cases. Papillary fronds supported by fibrovascular stroma are seen in some foci, but the hyperplasia often has a solid or micropapillary pattern. In micropapillary areas, the nuclei of hyperplastic epithelial cells tend to become smaller and more hyperchromatic at the tips of individual papillae (Fig. 27.14). Myoepithelial cell hyperplasia may be present. Some lesions exhibit cytologic atypia.

Most patients with one of the types of papillary duct hyperplasia can be managed by excisional biopsy. In one series, recurrences in the breast were detected in 16% of patients after a median interval of 3 years (59). Information presently available supports the view that papillary duct hyperplasia does not predispose children and young women to develop breast carcinoma at an early age.

Juvenile atypical duct hyperplasia is a microscopic ductal proliferative lesion that has been described in female patients 18 to 26 years old, with a mean age of 21 years at diagnosis (60). The ductal hyperplasia has been found in biopsies of breast "thickening" or in specimens from patients who underwent reduction mammoplasty for "mammary hypertrophy." Histologic examination reveals widely separated, individual ducts with micropapillary or cribriform epithelial hyperplasia (Fig. 27.15). In the typical specimen, the area between the hyperplastic ducts is occupied by dense, collagenous stroma in which there are also widely spaced ducts without hyperplasia and lobules, an important diagnostic feature that is difficult to appreciate in the limited sample of a needle core biopsy specimen (Fig. 27.16). The hyperplastic changes tend to develop focally rather than diffusely in the epithelium of an affected duct. In some ducts, the hyperplastic epithelium forms a lace-like network in the lumen. Myoepithelial cells detected by immunostains are present in a continuous or discontinuous fashion. Juvenile atypical duct hyperplasia is exceedingly rare in young males (Fig. 27.17).

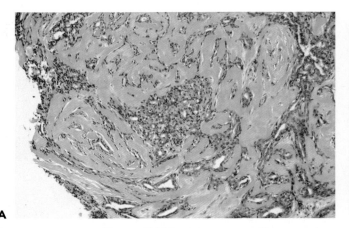
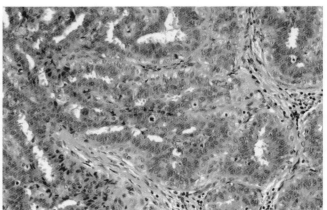

A

B

Figure 27.13   Sclerosing papilloma. A: This needle core biopsy specimen from a breast tumor in a 19-year-old girl shows areas of dense sclerosis with epithelium compressed into slender cords. **B:** A portion of the lesion with florid duct hyperplasia.

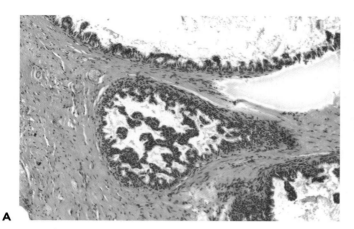

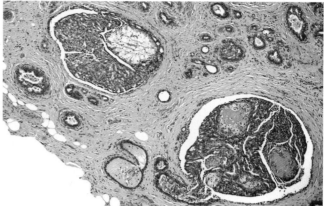

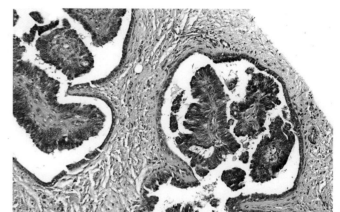

Figure 27.14 Papillomatosis. A: The patient was a 17-year-old girl with a breast mass. Multiple dilated ducts with micropapillary hyperplasia are present. **B, C:** This patient had multiple intraductal papillomas. Note the stromal histiocytes in the papillomas in **(B)**.

Fibroadenomas account for at least 75% of breast tumors in children (61). Most are similar histologically to comparable tumors in young adult women (62). Between 5% and 10% of fibroadenomas in adolescent girls attain a substantial size and have been termed "giant fibroadenoma." The dimensions that qualify for the adjective "giant" are not well documented and therefore these lesions are best simply referred to as fibroadenomas. Fibroadenomas are also discussed in Chapter 7.

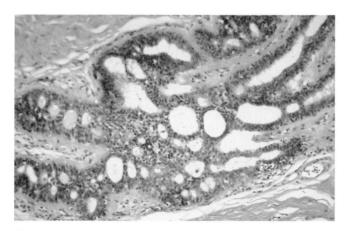

Figure 27.15 Juvenile atypical duct hyperplasia. Cribriform hyperplasia is present in this biopsy from an area of breast thickening in a 21-year-old woman.

Phyllodes tumors that occur in this age group have the same histologic characteristics as comparable tumors in adults (39) (Fig. 27.18). Important features that distinguish phyllodes tumor from fibroadenomas in children include areas of cellular stromal overgrowth relative to the epithelium, a tendency for cellularity to be greatest in the subepithelial stroma, the presence of stromal mitoses, especially in the subepithelial zone, and an invasive border in some cases. Although most phyllodes tumors in children follow a benign clinical course after excision, instances of local recurrence and systemic metastases have been reported (63,64).

Breast carcinoma is extremely unusual in children (65–67). A literature review published in 1977 listed 74 cases reported between 1888 and 1972 (65). Most of the patients have been girls, with an average age of about 13 years. With few exceptions, the presenting sign has been a mass. Histologically, a substantial number of the tumors have been of the secretory (juvenile) type (see Chapter 18), but other forms of carcinoma commonly found in adults have also been described in children. Small cell carcinoma of the breast in children is a highly malignant neoplasm that is difficult to distinguish from lymphoma and embryonal rhabdomyosarcoma in routine sections unless in situ carcinoma is found. Immunoreactivity for cytokeratin should be detectable, and the cells are not reactive with markers for lymphoma or myosarcoma.

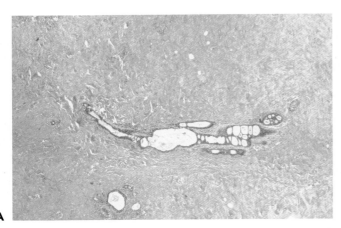

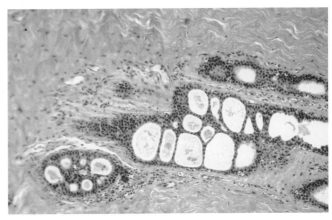

Figure 27.16 **Juvenile atypical duct hyperplasia. A, B:** This specimen was obtained from a reduction mammoplasty performed for juvenile hypertrophy in a 23-year-old woman. Cribriform hyperplasia is a focal abnormality in the duct. Note the broad expanse of collagenous stroma.

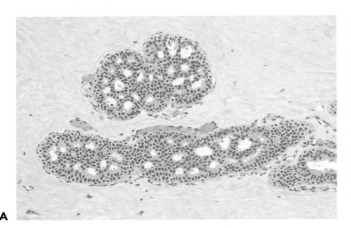

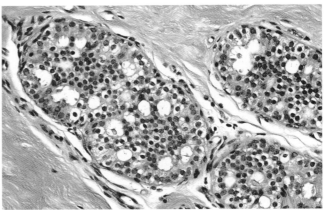

Figure 27.17 **Juvenile atypical duct hyperplasia, male. A:** This specimen is from a 14-year-old boy who presented with bilateral breast enlargement. The stroma lacks the cellularity of gynecomastia. **B:** Atypical cribriform duct hyperplasia in a 19-year-old boy with bilateral breast enlargement.

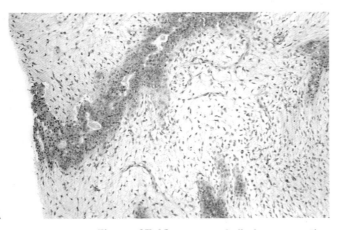

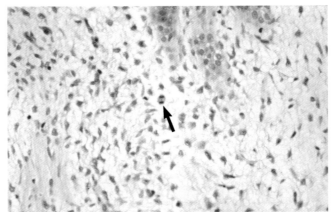

Figure 27.18 **Benign phyllodes tumor.** This needle core biopsy specimen was obtained from a breast mass in a 15-year-old female. **A:** Epithelial hyperplasia and variably cellular stroma are shown. **B:** Magnified view of **(A)** showing a mitotic figure in the stroma *(arrow)*.

REFERENCES

Benign Proliferative Lesions of the Male Breast

1. Siddiqui MT, Zakowski MF, Ashfaq R, Ali SZ. Breast masses in males: multi-institutional experience on fine needle aspiration. *Diagn Cytopathol.* 2002;26:87–91.
2. Westenend PJ. Core needle biopsy in male breast lesions. *J Clin Pathol.* 2003;56:863–865.
3. Green L, Wysowski DK, Fourcroy JL. Gynecomastia and breast cancer during finasteride therapy. *N Engl J Med.* 1996;335:823.
4. Schinina V, Rizzi WB, Zaccarelli M, et al. Gynecomastia in male HIV patients. MRI and US findings. *J Clin Imaging.* 2002;26:309–313.
5. Michels LG, Gold RH, Arndt RD. Radiography of gynecomastia and other disorders of the male breast. *Radiology.* 1977;122:117–122.
6. Bannayan GA, Hajdu SI. Gynecomastia: clinicopathologic study of 351 cases. *Am J Clin Pathol.* 1972;57:431–437.
7. Andersen JA, Gram JB. Gynecomasty. Histological aspects in a surgical material. *Acta Path Microbiol Immunol Scand.* 1982;90:185–190.
8. Kang Y, Wile M, Schinella R. Gynecomastia-like changes of the female breast. A clinicopathologic study of 4 cases. *Arch Pathol Lab Med.* 2001;125:506–509.
9. Umlas J. Gynecomastia-like lesions in the female breast. *Arch Pathol Lab Med.* 2000;124:844–847.
10. Seland DLG, Korbin CD, Lester SC, et al. Gynecomastiod hyperplasia: imaging findings in six patients. *Radiology.* 2000;214:553–555.
11. Navas MDM, Povedano JLR, Mendivil EA, et al. Intracystic papilloma in male breast: ultrasonography and pneumocystography diagnosis. *J Clin Ultrasound.* 1993;21:38–40.
12. Waldo ED, Sidhu GS, Hu AW. Florid papillomatosis of male nipple after diethylstilbesterol therapy. *Arch Pathol.* 1975;99:364–366.
13. Ansah-Boateng Y, Tavassoli FA. Fibroadenoma and cystosarcoma phyllodes of the male breast. *Mod Pathol.* 1992;5:114–116.
14. Bartoli C, Zurrida SM, Clemente C. Phyllodes tumor in a male patient with bilateral gynecomastia induced by oestrogen therapy for prostatic carcinoma. *Eur J Surg Oncol.* 1991;17:215–217.
15. Shin SJ, Rosen PP. Bilateral presentation of fibroadenoma with digital fibroma-like inclusions in the male breast. *Arch Pathol Lab Med.* 2007;131:1127–1129.
16. Tedeschi LG, McCarthy PE. Involutional mammary duct ectasia and periductal mastitis in a male. *Hum Pathol.* 1974;5:232–236.
17. Banik S, Hale R. Fibrocystic disease in the male breast. *Histopathology.* 1988;12:214–216.

Carcinoma of the Male Breast

18. Ewertz M, Holmberg L, Karjalainen S, et al. Incidence of male breast cancer in Scandinavia 1943–1982. *Int J Cancer.* 1989;43:27–31.
19. Hultborn R, Friberg S, Hultborn KA. Male breast carcinoma. I. A study of the total material reported to the Swedish Cancer Registry 1958–1967 with respect to clinical and histopathologic parameters. *Acta Oncol.* 1987;26:241–256.
20. Anderson WF, Althuis MD, Brinton LA, Devesa SS. Is male breast cancer similar or different than female breast cancer? *Breast Cancer Res Treat.* 2004;83:77–86.
21. Hodgson N, Button JH, Franceschi D, et al. Male breast cancer: is the incidence increasing? *Ann Surg Oncol.* 2004;11:751–755.
22. Giordano SH, Cohen DS, Buzdar AM, et al. Breast carcinoma in men. A population based study. *Cancer.* 2004;101:51–57.
23. Hittmair AP, Lininger RA, Tavassoli FA. Ductal carcinoma in situ (DCIS) in the male breast: a morphologic study of 84 cases of pure DCIS and 30 cases of DCIS associated with invasive carcinoma-a preliminary report. *Cancer.* 1998;83:2139–2149.
24. Rosen PP, Menendez-Botet CJ, Nisselbaum JS, et al. Estrogen receptor in lesions of the male breast. *Cancer.* 1976;37:1866–1868.
25. Rudlowski C, Friedrichs N, Faridi A, et al. HER-2/neu gene amplification and protein expression in primary male breast cancer. *Breast Cancer Res Treat.* 2004;84:215–223.
26. Dershaw DD. Male mammography. *Am J Roentgenol.* 1986;146:127–131.
27. Chantra PK, So GJ, Wollman JS, Bassett LW. Mammography of the male breast. *Am J Roentgenol.* 1995;164:853–858.
28. Sonksen CJ, Michell M, Sundaresan M. Case report: intracystic papillary carcinoma of the breast in a male patient. *Clin Radiol.* 1996;51:438–439.
29. Ouimet-Oliva D, Hebert G, Ladouceur J. Radiographic characteristics of male breast cancer. *Radiology.* 1978;129:37–40.
30. Dershaw DD, Borgen PI, Deutch BM, Liberman L. Mammographic findings in men with breast cancer. *Am J Roentgenol.* 1993;160:267–270.
31. Heller KS, Rosen PP, Schottenfeld D, et al. Male breast cancer. A clinicopathologic study of 97 cases. *Ann Surg.* 1978;188:60–65.
32. Burga AM, Fadare O, Lininger RA, Tavassoli FA. Invasive carcinomas of the male breast: a morphologic study of the distribution of histologic subtypes and metastatic patterns in 778 cases. *Virchows Arch.* 2006;449:507–512.
33. Visfeldt J, Sheike O. Male breast cancer. I. Histologic typing and grading of 187 Danish cases. *Cancer.* 1973;32:985–990.

34. Nance KVA, Reddick RL. In situ and infiltrating lobular carcinoma of the male breast. *Hum Pathol.* 1989;20:1220–1222.
35. Sanchez AG, Villanueva AG, Redondo C. Lobular carcinoma of the breast in a patient with Klinefelter's syndrome: a case with bilateral synchronous histologically different breast tumors. *Cancer.* 1986;57:1181–1183.
36. Yogore II, MG, Sahgal S. Small cell carcinoma of the male breast. Report of a case. *Cancer.* 1977;39:1748–1751.
37. Maly B, Maly A, Pappo I, et al. Pleomorphic variant of invasive lobular carcinoma of the male breast. *Virchows Arch.* 2005;446:344–345.
38. Leibowitz SB, Garber JE, Fox EA, et al. Male patients with diagnoses of both breast cancer and prostate cancer. *Breast J.* 2003;9:208–212.
39. Carder PJ, Speirs V, Ramsdale J, Lansdown MRJ. Expression of prostate specific antigen in male breast cancer. *J Clin Pathol.* 2005;58:69–71.
40. Bodey B, Bodey B Jr., Kaiser HE. Immunohistochemical detection of prostate specific antigen-expression in human breast cancer cells. *Anticancer Res.* 1997;17:2577–2581.
41. Stalsbert H. Thomas DB, Rosenblatt KA, et al. Histologic types and hormone receptors in breast cancer in men: a population-based study in 282 United States men. *Cancer Causes Control.* 1993;4:143–151.
42. Scheike O, Visfeldt J. Male breast cancer. 4. Gynecomastia in patients with breast cancer. *Acta Pathol Microbiol Scand A.* 1973;81:359–365.
43. Cimmino VM, Degnim AC, Sabel MS, et al. Efficacy of sentinel lymph node biopsy in male breast cancer. *J Surg Oncol.* 2994;76:74–77.
44. Albo D, Ames FC, Hunt KK, et al. Evaluation of lymph node status in male breast cancer patients; a role for sentinel lymph node biopsy. *Breast Cancer Res Treat.* 2003;77:9–14.
45. Adami H-O, Hakulinen T, Ewertz M, et al. The survival pattern in male breast cancer. An analysis of 1429 patients from the Nordic countries. *Cancer.* 1989;64:1177–1182.
46. Ciatto S, Iossa A, Bonardi R, Pacini P. Male breast carcinoma: review of a multicenter series of 150 cases. *Tumori.* 1990;76:555–558.
47. Hultborn R, Friberg S, Hultborn KA, et al. I. Male breast carcinoma. II. A study of the total material reported to the Swedish Cancer Registry 1958–1967 with respect to treatment prognostic factors and survival. *Acta Oncol.* 1987;26:327–341.
48. Joshi MG, Lee AKC, Loda M, et al. Male breast carcinoma: an evaluation of prognostic factors contributing to a poorer outcome. *Cancer.* 1996;77:490–498.
49. Borgen P, Senie RT, McKinnon WMP, et al. Carcinoma of the male breast. Analysis of prognosis compared with matched female patients. *Ann Surg Oncol.* 1997;4:385–388.
50. Anan K, Mitsuyama S, Nishihara K, et al. Breast cancer in Japanese men: does sex affect prognosis? *Breast Cancer.* 2004;11:180–186.

Breast Tumors in Children

51. Rosen PP, Cantrell B, Mullen DL, De Palo A. Juvenile papillomatosis (Swiss cheese disease) of the breast. *Am J Surg Pathol.* 1980;4:3–12.
52. Rosen PP, Holmes G, Lesser ML, et al. Juvenile papillomatosis and breast carcinoma. *Cancer.* 1985;55:1345–1352.
53. Kersschot EAJ, Hermans M-E, Pauwels C, et al. Juvenile papillomatosis of the breast: sonographic appearance. *Radiology.* 1988;169:631–633.
54. Hidalgo F, Llano JM, Marhuenda A. Juvenile papillomatosis of the breast (Swiss cheese disease). *Am J Roentgenol.* 1997;169:912.
55. Rosen PP, Lyngholm B, Kinne DW, Beattie Jr. EJ. Juvenile papillomatosis of the breast and family history of breast carcinoma. *Cancer.* 1982;49:2591–2595.
56. Rosen PP, Kimmel M. Juvenile papillomatosis of the breast: a follow-up study of 41 patients having biopsies before 1979. *Am J Clin Pathol.* 1990;93:599–603.
57. Bazzocchi F, Santini D, Martinelli G, et al. Juvenile papillomatosis (epitheliosis) of the breast. *Am J Clin Pathol.* 1986;86:745–748.
58. Rosen PP. Papillary duct hyperplasia of the breast in children and young adults. *Cancer.* 1985;56:1611–1617.
59. Wilson M, Cranor ML, Rosen PP. Papillary duct hyperplasia of the breast in children and young women. *Mod Pathol.* 1993;6:570–574.
60. Eliasen CA, Cranor ML, Rosen PP. Atypical duct hyperplasia of the breast in young females. *Am J Surg Pathol.* 1992;16:246–251.
61. Bower R, Bell ML, Ternbergh JL. Management of breast lesions in children and adolescents. *J Pediatr Surg.* 1976;11:337–346.
62. Ashikari R, Farrow JH, O'Hara J. Fibroadenomas in the breast of juveniles. *Surg Gynecol Obstet.* 1971;32:259–262.
63. Rajan PB, Cranor ML, Rosen PP. Cystosarcoma phyllodes in adolescent girls and young women: a study of 45 patients. *Am J Surg Pathol.* 1998;22:64–69.
64. Leveque J, Meunier B, Wattier E, et al. Malignant cystosarcoma phyllodes of the breast in adolescent females. *Eur J Obstet Gynecol Reprod Biol.* 1994;54:197–203.
65. Ashikari H, Jun MY, Farrow JH, et al. Breast carcinoma in children and adolescents. *Clin Bull.* 1977;7:55–62.
66. Roisman I, Barak V, Robinson E, et al. Breast malignancies in adolescents in Israel (1967–1989). *Breast Dis.* 1992;5:149–168.
67. Corpron CA, Block CT, Singletary SE, Andrass RJ. Breast cancer in adolescent females. *J Pediatr Surg.* 1995;30:322–324.

Pathologic Changes Associated with Needling Procedures

28

Direct penetration of the lesion is sought when a needle core biopsy is obtained. The core biopsy samples may remove some or all calcifications and/or a discrete tumor. The effects of the procedure on surrounding tissue are usually not apparent clinically in imaging studies. Follow-up mammography performed 6 months after stereotactic 14-gauge biopsy revealed no mammographically detectable architectural distortion attributable to the procedure in 24 patients studied by Kaye et al. (1). In two instances, there were fewer calcifications in postbiopsy mammograms and a 6-mm fibroadenoma contained a 2 × 3 mm defect. These and other observations suggest that the procedure usually does not cause long-standing structural changes in the breast outside the lesion that might interfere with later radiographic studies.

Nonetheless, traumatic changes do occur in and around the needle core biopsy site, and they can affect the interpretation of the subsequent excisional biopsy. Virtually all excisional biopsy specimens obtained after needle biopsy or localization procedures contain foci of hemorrhage in the breast stroma (2). Blood within the lumens of ducts and lobules not involved by the pathologic process as well as in epithelial structures in the lesional area is a frequent manifestation of a recent needling procedure (3) (Fig. 28.1). Fragments of epidermis may be dislodged into the breast by the needle if a small skin incision is not made before inserting the needle. Epidermoid inclusion cysts may be formed from displaced skin epithelium (Fig. 28.1) (4). The healing needle core biopsy site typically forms scar tissue. The maturity of the scar depends on the interval that has elapsed. Some of these reactive foci have stromal mitoses and myofibroblastic hyperplasia that should not be mistaken for a neoplastic process (5). Gel foam or similar material is often injected into the biopsy site after the tissue has been removed to improve hemostasis.

Disruption of the epithelium in the lesion may result in displacement of epithelial cells into the needle track and into stroma in the lesional area. This can produce a pattern that simulates invasive carcinoma (1,3,6,7) (Figs. 28.2 and 28.3). Displacement of benign or carcinomatous epithelium is suggested by finding scattered, isolated fragments of epithelium in artificial spaces within the breast stroma. At the needle biopsy site, the displaced epithelium is accompanied by hemorrhage, fat necrosis, inflammation, hemosiderin-laden macrophages, or granulation tissue and scar. Displaced epithelium that is not in the biopsy site may not be accompanied by a stromal reaction. This can lead to the mistaken diagnosis of invasive carcinoma in a benign lesion (Fig. 28.4). It is not unusual to find fragments of sloughed epithelium in the lumens of ducts and cysts that resemble displaced epithelium in the stroma. Rarely, intraductal carcinoma entirely dislodged in a duct lumen may simulate lymphatic invasion. Immunostains for p63 and D2-40 can be helpful in such situations. Displaced carcinomatous epithelium in vascular spaces is indistinguishable from intrinsic lymphatic or vascular invasion (3,6) (Figs. 28.5–28.7). The extent to which breast-needling procedures contribute to the hematogenous or lymphatic dispersal of tumor cells has not been determined.

The p63 immunostain for myoepithelial cells can be helpful for confirming the presence of epithelial displacement if p63-positive nuclei can be demonstrated around the extralesional epithelial cells (Fig. 28.8). Coincidentally, it must be possible to detect p63-positive myoepithelial cells in the lesion that was sampled by the core biopsy. Myoepithelial cells are more likely to be present if the primary lesion is benign, but they can also be found in in situ carcinomas. Failure to find p63-positive nuclei in association with the extralesional epithelium is not by itself diagnostic of invasive carcinoma, even if the lesion contains p63-positive myoepithelium, because only a minority of epithelial cells in a proliferative lesion are contiguous to myoepithelium that can accompany displaced epithelial fragments. When p63-positive cells can be demonstrated as evidence of epithelial displacement, they are usually associated with a minority of the displaced epithelium.

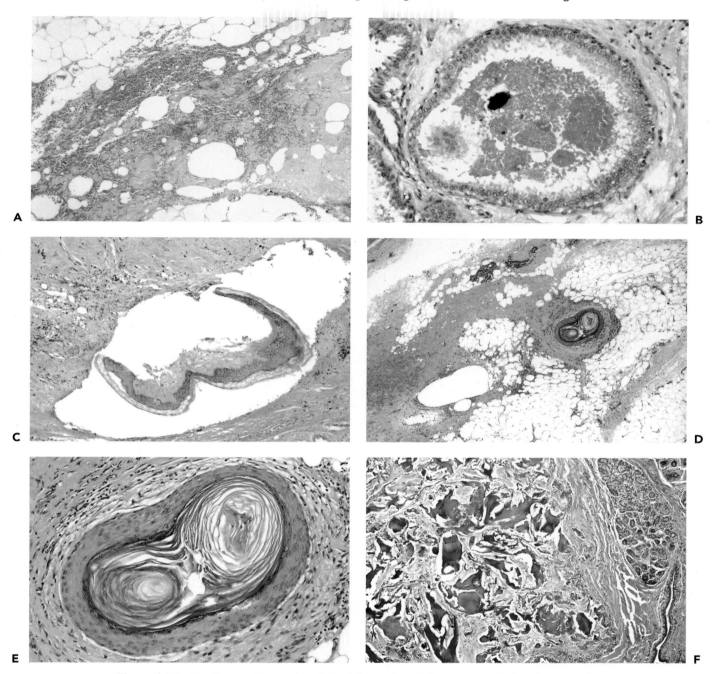

Figure 28.1 Needle core biopsy site. A: Fresh hemorrhage in breast stroma 5 days after a needle core biopsy procedure. **B:** Intraductal hemorrhage with a calcification near a needle core biopsy procedure performed for nonpalpable microcalcifications. The lesion proved to be tubular carcinoma. This duct exhibits columnar cell hyperplasia. **C:** A recently detached fragment of skin in a needle core biopsy track. **D, E:** This fragment of detached epidermis is adjacent to a needle core biopsy track in the lower left corner. The epidermis has formed a cyst and become encapsulated in granulation tissue. **F:** Gel foam in a healing needle core biopsy site.

Epithelial displacement into the stroma was found in three of five surgical biopsy specimens from patients with intraductal carcinoma and in three of seven papillary intraductal carcinomas studied by Boppana et al. (6). Lee et al. (7) drew attention to epithelial displacement in granulation tissue adjacent to a benign papillary tumor simulating invasive carcinoma and others have encountered the same

problem around papillary intraductal carcinomas that were excised after a needle core biopsy (8). Epithelial displacement can be difficult to distinguish from invasion when intraductal carcinoma is present (Figs. 28.5 and 28.9).

Youngson et al. (2) reported finding displaced epithelium in biopsies of papillary duct hyperplasia and papilloma, as well as in association with various types of

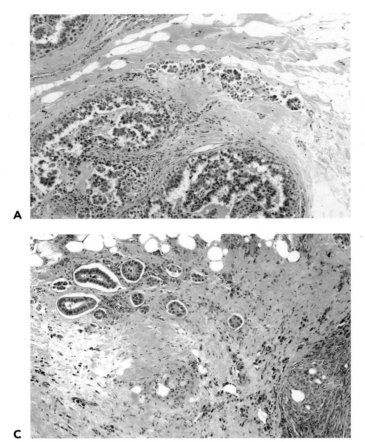

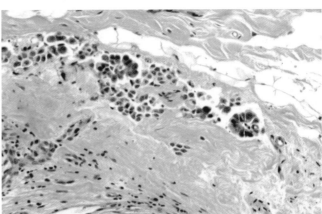

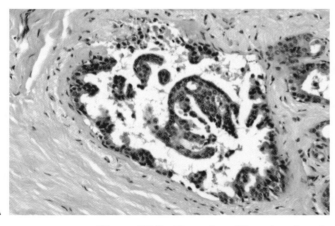

Figure 28.2 Epithelial displacement in postbiopsy excision. A, B: Displaced fragments of intraductal carcinoma are shown in the stroma near the site of a needle core biopsy procedure performed 7 days previously. Note the absence of reactive changes in the stroma and the well-preserved cytologic appearance of the displaced tumor cells. **C:** Displaced papillary intraductal carcinoma in granulation tissue next to a needle core biopsy site 16 days after the procedure. The carcinoma cells in lacunar retraction spaces resemble lymphatic tumor emboli.

intraductal carcinoma, invasive carcinoma, and phyllodes tumor. The average interval between the needling procedure and excisional biopsy was 10 days, with as long as 28 days having elapsed in one case. Intravascular or intralymphatic fragments of benign or malignant epithelium were present in seven cases, six of which also had stromal displacement. One of these women, who had extensive intraductal carcinoma associated with stromal displacement and lymphatic tumor emboli in the breast, also had clusters of carcinoma cells in the subcapsular sinuses of two axillary lymph nodes (Fig. 28.10).

Hoorntje et al. (9) reported finding displaced carcinoma cells in 11 of 22 (50%) needle tracts after 14 gauge needle biopsy procedures. Prospectively, these authors found displaced carcinoma in 7 or 11 (64%) of needle tracks examined 7 to 35 days (median interval, 25 days)

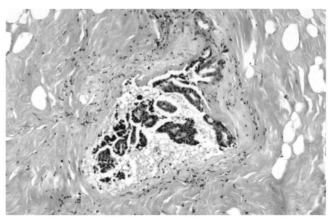

Figure 28.3 Disruption of intraductal carcinoma in postbiopsy excision. A: Portions of the intraductal carcinoma have been dislodged from the basement membrane and are displaced into the duct lumen after a needle core biopsy procedure. **B:** Another area in the specimen shown in **(A)** with severe disruption of intraductal carcinoma. The detached epithelial fragments have remained within the confines of the basement membrane.

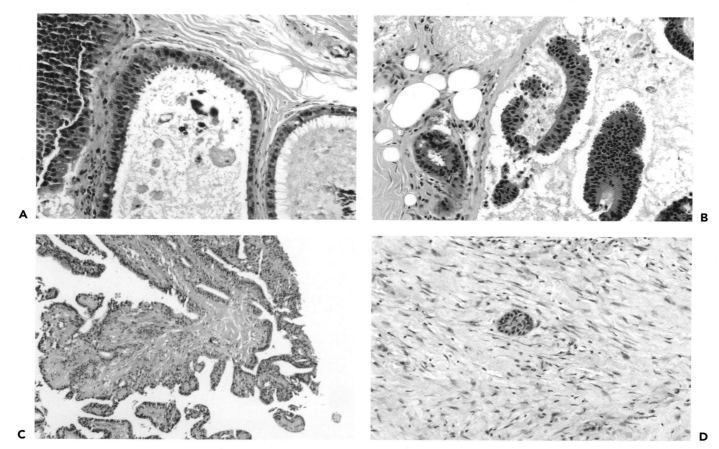

Figure 28.4   Displaced epithelium in benign lesions. A: This patient had a nonpalpable focus of microcalcifications detected by mammography. A needle core biopsy procedure revealed cystic apocrine metaplasia with calcifications and secretion. **B:** The needle core biopsy site in the subsequent excisional biopsy contained these detached fragments of epithelium surrounded by secretion, which led to an erroneous diagnosis of mucinous carcinoma. Note the apocrine "snouts" on the lumenal surface and smooth basal edge of the epithelium. The basement membrane is visible at the junction of the tissue on the left and the cyst lumen on the right. One small intact gland is shown on the left. **C:** This needle core biopsy specimen of a papilloma was obtained from an 8-mm nonpalpable mammographically detected tumor. **D:** The excisional biopsy specimen obtained 2 weeks after the core biopsy procedure produced the specimen shown in **(C)** contained residual papilloma and granulation tissue with displaced benign epithelial cell clusters, one of which is shown here.

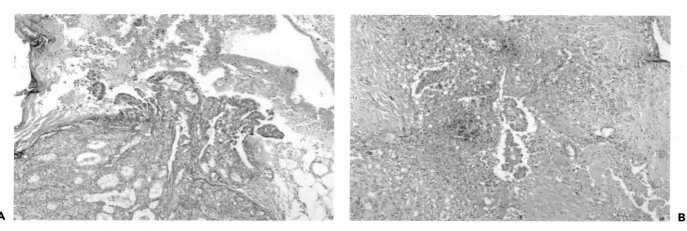

Figure 28.5   Epithelial displacement in intraductal carcinoma. The needle core biopsy specimen from a 1.3-cm palpable tumor revealed intraductal carcinoma. **A:** Solid papillary intraductal carcinoma is shown here in the subsequent excisional biopsy performed 12 days later. **B:** This is part of the needle core biopsy site adjacent to intraductal carcinoma. Displaced fragments of carcinoma are surrounded by hemorrhage and granulation tissue in the needle biopsy site.

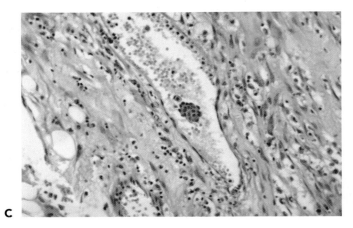

C

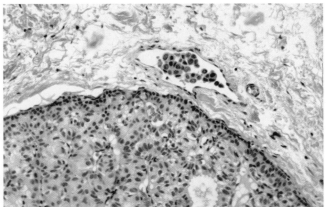

Figure 28.5 *(continued)* **C:** This cluster of carcinoma cells was found in a dilated vascular channel near the needle core biopsy site. No intrinsic invasive carcinoma was found in any of the specimens from this patient.

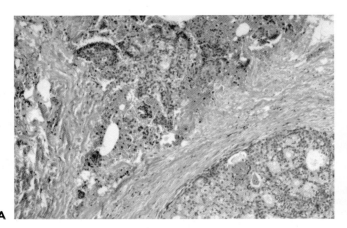

A

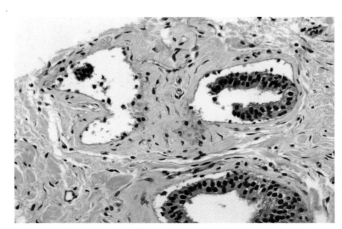

B

Figure 28.6 Epithelial displacement in intraductal carcinoma.   A: This excisional biopsy specimen was obtained after a needle core biopsy performed on a nonpalpable mammographically detected lesion revealed intraductal carcinoma. Shown here is the needle core biopsy site with displaced carcinoma next to cribriform intraductal carcinoma. **B:** A cluster of carcinoma cells is shown in a lymphatic space next to the intraductal carcinoma.

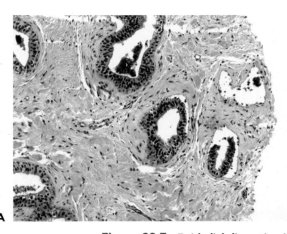

A

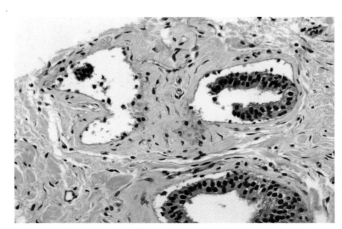

B

Figure 28.7 Epithelial disruption in a needle core biopsy specimen. A, B: Epithelium in these hyperplastic ducts has been partially dislodged from the basement membranes. The loose fragment in the duct lumen near the edge of the tissue simulates carcinoma in a lymphatic space. Nuclei of partially detached myoepithelial cells are visible at the perimeter of the ducts.

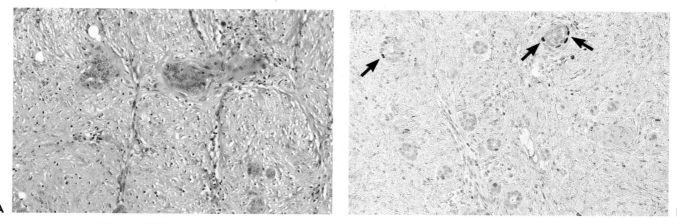

Figure 28.8   Displaced epithelium with p63-reactive myoepithelial cells in a postbiopsy scar. This patient underwent a needle core biopsy procedure that showed a sclerosing papilloma. These images are from the subsequent excisional biopsy specimen that contained residual papilloma. **A:** Displaced epithelial fragments in scar tissue at the needle core biopsy site. **B:** Myoepithelial cells display nuclear p63 reactivity *(arrows)* around some displaced epithelial cell fragments (immunoperoxidase).

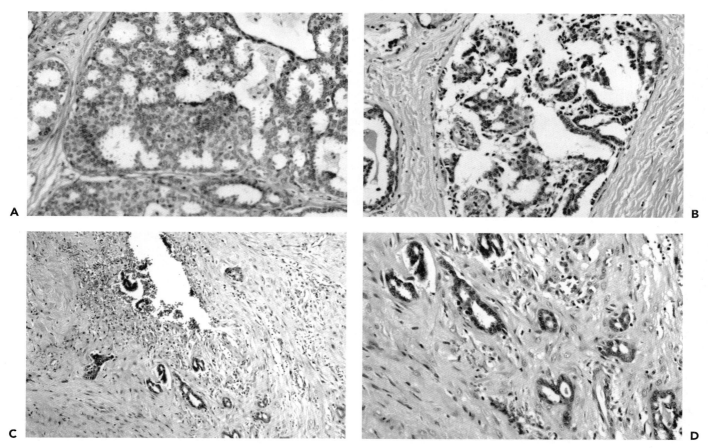

Figure 28.9   Epithelial displacement in intraductal carcinoma. A: Cribriform intraductal carcinoma as it appeared in an excisional biopsy specimen 8 days after a needle core biopsy procedure for a mammographically detected lesion. **B:** Disrupted intraductal carcinoma in the excisional biopsy specimen. **C, D:** Displaced epithelial fragments in the needle core biopsy site are indistinguishable from invasive tubular carcinoma.

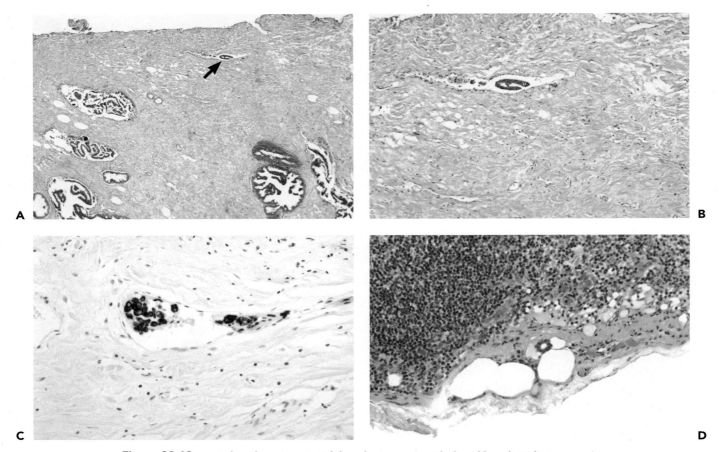

Figure 28.10 **Intraductal carcinoma with lymphatic tumor emboli and lymph node metastasis.**
A, B: This excisional biopsy specimen is from a procedure performed 8 days after a needle core biopsy sampling of mammographically detected calcifications revealed intraductal carcinoma. There is a U-shaped group of carcinoma cells in the lymphatic space near the upper border of the tissue *(arrow)*. **B:** Magnified view of the intralymphatic carcinoma. **C:** Other cells in lymphatic spaces are shown here to be immunoreactive for CAM 5.2 cytokeratin (immunoperoxidase). **D:** Metastatic carcinoma that formed a ring in the subcapsular sinus of a lymph node obtained in an axillary lymph node dissection performed because lymphatic tumor emboli were demonstrated in the excisional biopsy specimen shown in **(A–C).**

after 14-gauge needle biopsy. The frequency of epithelial displacement in the needle track has been substantially reduced since the introduction of vacuum-assisted stereotactic biopsy with an 11-gauge needle (10).

The long-term viability of displaced epithelium at the biopsy site in the breast, whether benign or malignant, is uncertain. Diaz et al. (11) found epithelial displacement in 32% of excisions performed after a needle core biopsy procedure. Displacement was less frequent after vacuum-assisted biopsy than when an automated gun device was used. The observation that the incidence of detectable epithelial displacement was inversely related to the post-core biopsy interval led these investigators to conclude that displaced epithelium underwent degenerative changes in some instances.

Nonetheless, the fate of displaced epithelium in all cases remains undetermined. Tumor seeding of the dermis of the skin was reported by Stolier et al. (12), leading to local recurrence at the biopsy site in one case. Chao et al. (13) described two patients who had subcutaneous recurrence of

carcinoma in a needle core biopsy track 12 and 17 months postbiopsy. A third patient was found to have microscopic carcinoma in the skin in a mastectomy specimen. The risk of cutaneous recurrence can be substantially reduced if the biopsy site in the skin can be included in the subsequent surgical excision.

The potential contribution of epithelial displacement induced by a core biopsy to local recurrence in the breast after breast conservation surgery and radiotherapy is also of concern. Thurfjell et al. (14) studied 303 consecutive women with nonpalpable carcinomas treated by excision. The majority had undergone a preoperative needle core biopsy procedure (71%) and postoperative radiotherapy (82%). Overall, 33 or 11% of the women developed a local recurrence after median follow-up of 5.4 years. On the basis of the location of the recurrence and the position of the needle track, it was considered likely that recurrences were attributable to epithelial displacement in three women who did not receive radiotherapy. Chen et al. (15) investigated the role of epithelial displacement in local recurrence by comparing women who underwent needle core biopsy before excision and those who had a needle localization biopsy as the diagnostic procedure. In a series of 551 consecutive patients treated with conservation surgery and radiotherapy, the frequency of local recurrence after a mean follow-up of 4.9 years in the core biopsy group (2.3%) was not significantly different from the needle localization group (5.4%).

As noted previously, the risk of local recurrence in the skin may be reduced by excising the skin puncture site at the time of breast conservation surgery. However, it is not always practical or cosmetically beneficial to excise the skin or the entire parenchymal biopsy track, and it has been suggested that postoperative radiotherapy can be relied on to eliminate displaced carcinoma cells in most cases (9).

Epithelial displacement presents the pathologist with a challenging diagnostic problem. Eliciting a history of a previous needling procedure may help prevent inappropriate interpretation of a specimen. A malignant diagnosis should not be based solely on the presence of epithelium within the stroma, since epithelial displacement has been observed following needling procedures in benign breast lesions, notably papillary duct hyperplasia and intraductal papilloma.

The significance of carcinomatous lymphovascular emboli in the setting of epithelial displacement remains uncertain. Until further clinical information becomes available, the finding of lymphatic tumor emboli is considered a risk factor for transport of carcinoma cells to axillary lymph nodes even when conventional stromal invasion cannot be identified. Carter et al. (16) introduced the term *benign transport* to describe instances that they concluded were iatrogenic displacement of carcinoma cells to axillary lymph nodes. It was suggested that benign transport could be recognized by the absence of reactive changes indicative of tumor growth at the site of carcinomatous nodal involvement and the presence of foamy histiocytes, presumably also displaced, associated with the carcinoma.

At present, there is no objective method for determining with certainty whether a micro deposit of epithelial cells arrived in a sentinel lymph node (SLN) as a result of intrinsic invasion at the primary site or because of iatrogenic mechanical displacement. Even if the phenomenon of mechanical transport were proved to occur, the clinical significance of displaced carcinoma cells in SLN or other axillary lymph nodes will remain uncertain. The indeterminate nature of these findings was highlighted by Carter and Page (17), who stated that they "look forward to the future development of laboratory assays that will correctly differentiate small lymph node deposits that are truly metastatic . . . from those minimal deposits that are unlikely to have any significant impact on the patient and those deposits that have been benignly transported to the lymph node as a cleanup-mechanism by the lymphatic system." Each case requires careful scrutiny that takes into consideration the histologic and immunohistochemical appearances of the primary tumor and epithelial microdeposits in the lymph node and the presence or absence of epithelial displacement at the primary site.

The presence of microdeposits of carcinoma cells in a lymph node capsule or subcapsular sinus is regarded as metastatic carcinoma, usually classified as "isolated tumor cells," in most instances even when no intrinsic invasion has been found in the breast. These patients often have carcinoma cells in lymphatic spaces in the breast parenchyma near the needling procedure. One unusual patient presented with a clinically enlarged axillary lymph node diffusely involved by metastatic carcinoma 7 years after a mastectomy for intraductal carcinoma that was diagnosed by needle biopsy. Lymph nodes removed from the axilla at the time of mastectomy had no carcinoma identified in routine sections. On review, the site of the needle core biopsy in the breast exhibited carcinoma cells in lymphatic channels. The viability of in situ carcinoma cells that may have been displaced into vascular channels and possibly deposited in sites outside the breast is unknown, but the case just described raises the possibility that these cells could persist for a substantial period of time and acquire invasive characteristics.

REFERENCES

1. Kaye MD, Vicinanza-Adami CA, Sullivan ML. Mammographic findings after stereotaxic biopsy of the breast performed with large-core needles. *Radiology.* 1994;192:149–151.
2. Youngson BJ, Cranor M, Rosen PP. Epithelial displacement in surgical breast specimens following needling procedures. *Am J Surg Pathol.* 1994;18:896–903.
3. Youngson BJ, Liberman L, Rosen PP. Displacement of carcinomatous epithelium in surgical breast specimens following stereotaxic core biopsy. *Am J Clin Pathol.* 1995;103:598–602.
4. Davies JD, Nonni A, Costa HFD. Mammary epidermoid inclusion cysts after wide-core needle biopsies. *Histopathology.* 1997;31:549–551.
5. Gobbi H, Tse G, Page DL, et al. Reactive spindle cell nodules of the breast after core biopsy or fine-needle aspiration. *Am J Clin Pathol.* 2000;113: 288–294.
6. Boppana S, May M, Hoda S. Does prior fine-needle-aspiration cause diagnostic difficulties in histologic evaluation of breast carcinomas? *Lab Invest.* 1994;70:13A.
7. Lee KC, Chan JKC, Ho LC. Histologic changes in the breast after fine-needle aspiration. *Am J Surg Pathol.* 1994;18:1039–1047.
8. Douglas-Jones AG, Verghese A. Diagnostic difficulty arising from displaced epithelium after core biopsy in intracystic papillary lesions of the breast. *J Clin Pathol.* 2002;55:780–783.
9. Hoorntje LE, Schipper MEI, Kaya A, et al. Tumour cell displacement after 14G breast biopsy. *Eur J Surg Oncol.* 2004;30:520–525.
10. Liberman L. Impact of image-guided core biopsy on the clinical management of breast disease. In: Rosen PP, Hoda SA, eds. *Breast Pathology: Diagnosis by Needle Core Biopsy.* 2nd ed. New York: Lippincott, Williams & Wilkins; 2006:314–324.
11. Diaz LK, Wiley EL, Venta LA. Are malignant cells displaced by large-gauge needle core biopsy of the breast? *Am J Roentgenol.* 1999;173:1303–1313.
12. Stolier A, Skinner J, Levine EA. A prospective study of seeding of the skin after core biopsy of the breast. *Am J Surg.* 2000;180:104–107.
13. Chao C, Torosian MH, Boraas MC, et al. Local recurrence of breast cancer in the stereotactic core needle biopsy site: case reports and review of the literature. *Breast J.* 2001;7:124–127.
14. Thurfjell MG, Jansson T, et al. Local breast cancer recurrence cause by mammographically guided punctures. *Acta Radiologica.* 2000;41:435–440.
15. Chen AM, Haffty BG, Lee CH. Local recurrence of breast cancer after breast conservation therapy in patients examined by means of stereotactic core-needle biopsy. *Radiology.* 2000;225:707–712.
16. Carter BA, Jensen RA, Simpson JF, et al. Benign transport of breast epithelium into axillary lymph nodes after biopsy. *Am J Clin Pathol.* 2000;113: 259–265.
17. Carter BA, Page DL. Sentinel lymph node histopathology in breast cancer: minimal disease versus artefact. *JCO.* 2006;24:1978–1979.

Specimen Processing, Pathologic Examination, and Reporting

29

SPECIMEN PROCUREMENT AND FIXATION

The performance of needle core biopsy (NCB) procedures for *palpable* breast lesions is currently considered the appropriate initial step in evaluating these abnormalities. NCB of *nonpalpable* radiographically detected breast lesions, under the guidance of various imaging techniques (i.e., ultrasound, stereotactic guidance or magnetic resonance imaging, MRI) is becoming increasingly common (1).

A variety of sampling instruments, employing either spring-loaded or vacuum-assisted mechanisms, are available. Instruments utilizing vacuum-assisted mechanisms safely yield specimens with minimum artifact that sample a relatively large area with a single needle insertion (2). By contrast, spring-loaded sampling devices yield artifact-prone, relatively smaller biopsy specimens, which necessitate multiple insertions if a larger volume of tissue is to be obtained.

Immediately after procurement, the NCB specimen should be placed in 10% formalin. Prompt formalin fixation preserves cytologic and architectural detail, and ensures optimal immunohistochemical (IHC) staining. Calcifications are detectable in surgical biopsy specimens after formalin fixation for periods of 2 or more weeks. Longer periods of fixation have been reported to result in radiographic disappearance of calcifications (3).

REQUISITION FORM

The requisition form submitted with the NCB specimen should include the following information: patient name, age and gender, laterality of the specimen, indication for the procedure, clinical diagnosis, sampled site, and any specific information regarding individual parts of the specimen (e.g., the presence or absence of calcifications). The name of the submitting physician and the date of the procedure must also be provided. As per the latest American Society of Clinical Oncology/College of American Pathologists (ASCO/CAP) guidelines, the time of specimen procurement *and* of its placement in fixative must be recorded in the requisition form (4).

The sampled site is generally indicated by a clock-face designation and distance from the nipple (e.g., right breast, 2 o'clock, N4) indicating that the specimen was taken from the upper-inner quadrant of right breast at the 2 o'clock position from a site 4 cm from the center of the nipple. Multiple palpable as well as impalpable lesions may be simultaneously sampled via NCB, safely and efficiently, and this practice favorably impacts patient management (5,6).

The pathologic findings in any previously performed breast biopsy procedure must be conveyed in the requisition form. Relevant history of prior treatment (e.g., surgery, radiation, hormone modulation therapy, or chemotherapy) that could affect the histology of the breast should be provided. Information regarding any known systemic disease that may also affect the breast (e.g., neoplasm at another site, diabetes mellitus, sarcoidosis, vasculitis, etc.) should be detailed. Family history of breast or ovarian carcinoma, or of *BRCA1* or *BRCA2* mutations, should be included. Ideally, the instrument utilized to procure NCB specimens should also be stated.

The specimen container must be labeled with patient and specimen identification information that must match identifying information on the accompanying specimen requisition form.

GROSS DESCRIPTION

A gross description should be recorded for each specimen with documentation of the number of samples, the range (and aggregate extent) of their lengths, and any other notable feature (e.g., color). The entire specimen including any apparent blood clot must be processed for

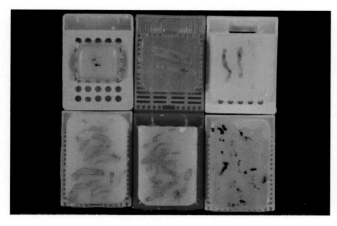

Figure 29.1 Demonstration of the wide array of dimensions of needle core biopsy specimens in a random set of tissue blocks. Note the minuscule dimension of the NCB specimen in the pink tissue block on the top-left, and the numerous tightly packed NCB specimens in the green tissue block on the bottom-right. The bottom row demonstrates haphazard placement of needle core biopsy samples in three tissue blocks rather than the orderly arrays of NCB in the top row.

histologic evaluation. The bottom surface of the lid of the specimen container should be routinely examined for tissue that may be stuck to it. If the material in a sample is too abundant to be placed in one tissue cassette (i.e., >10.0 cm in aggregate length), the cores should be separated into groups of approximately equal number and size (Fig. 29.1). Formalin fixation causes minimal shrinking of tissue. The shrinkage effect has been estimated to be 7% for 16-gauge tru-cut biopsy samples from the liver (7). The number of cassettes corresponding to each sample should be recorded, and each cassette should be labeled with a unique identifier.

Dipping of NCB specimens in dyes that are routinely available in a surgical pathology laboratory, such as methylene blue or eosin, increases the visibility of the embedded tissue in the paraffin block (Fig. 29.2). Inking of breast NCB specimens at the time of gross examination

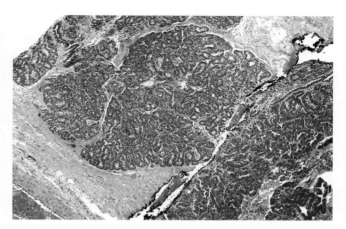

Figure 29.3 Inked needle core biopsy specimens. The samples were inked with blue ink at the time of gross examination. The ink is visible in the resultant histologic sections shown here (H&E).

has been proposed as a relatively simple, inexpensive, and effective way to reduce the possibility of specimen mix-up during the processing of the tissue in the pathology laboratory (Fig. 29.3). All NCB specimens from a patient are inked with a single color. The next set of NCB specimens from another patient is inked with a different color, and so on. The color of the ink used for a case should be noted in the gross description. Three discrepancies were discovered in a study of 1,000 core biopsies that were inked sequentially with 6 different colors. In one instance, the error was related to switching of a tissue block. In another case, the error was related to incorrect labeling, and in a third, the error was typographic (8). Of course, no laboratory procedure can guard against the misidentification of specimens in the radiology office where NCB samples are usually obtained.

SPECIMEN PROCESSING

Routine methods of paraffin embedding, sectioning, and staining with hematoxylin and eosin (H&E) can be used for NCB specimens from the breast. A "fast-track" method for rapid processing of NCB specimens has been described (9). However, compliance with regulatory processing standards and achievement of optimal histologic and IHC staining should be ensured before the routine adoption of this technique (10).

The NCB samples must be embedded in a manner that positions them at approximately the same plane in the paraffin block. Histological sections should be 4 to 5 μm thick. Microscopic examination of at least three "levels" (interval sections) is recommended. These levels are generally taken approximately 50 μm apart, but could be closer depending on quantity of material available. Evaluation of three-step sections reportedly maximizes the chances of visualizing microcalcifications in NCB samples (11). Examination of a minimum of five levels has been recommended to ensure maximum sensitivity for detecting "atypical foci" (12) and of six levels to ensure "accurate" diagnosis (13).

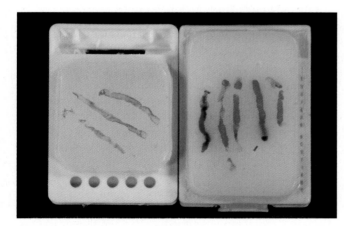

Figure 29.2 Visibility of needle core biopsy in tissue blocks. Dipping the needle core biopsies in methylene blue **(left)** or eosin **(right)** render the samples more readily visible in the tissue block. This is helpful to the histotechnologist when cutting histologic sections.

It is important not to exhaust the NCB tissue in the preparation of initial histologic sections to preserve material for IHC studies that may be necessary to establish or refine a diagnosis. If laboratory resources allow, intervening sections cut between the various stained levels can be mounted unstained on labeled slides and saved for possible IHC studies. Such a protocol saves tissue, time, and effort that may be subsequently spent in the retrieval and processing of tissue blocks. If recuts are made at a second sitting for immunostains, one new recut slide should always be submitted for H&E staining (14).

CORRELATION WITH RADIOLOGIC FINDINGS

Because radiologic findings are often stated in the requisition forms and NCBs of the breast are usually performed under some form of radiographic guidance, pathologists should be acquainted with the fundamentals of breast imaging and reporting. Radiographic techniques commonly employed to study the breast include ultrasound (US), mammography (including digital mammography), MRI, and positron emission tomography (PET).

NCB can be performed under stereotactic image guidance (i.e., mammographic guidance). Mammography using low-dose ionizing radiation can detect masses, architectural distortion, or calcifications. For a mammographically detected *mass* (or lesion causing architectural distortion), the radiology report usually states its density, shape, and borders. On mammography, a mass suspicious for malignancy may be dense and irregular with spiculated edges. For mammographically detected abnormal *calcifications*, the radiology report usually describes their morphology and distribution. Calcifications suspicious for malignancy may be linear ("casting-type"), branching, and/or pleomorphic. Digital breast tomosynthesis is an evolving enhanced mammographic technique that increases lesional visibility and localization by reducing "noise."

US-imaging utilizes high-frequency sound waves to study breast diseases. The echogenicity of a lesion vis-à-vis that of subcutaneous adipose tissue and the orientation of the lesion in relation to the skin of the breast are usually reported in US reports. A lesion may be "isoechoic" (having the same echogenicity as adipose tissue, e.g., a lipoma), "anechoic" (e.g., a cyst), "hyperechoic" (normal fibrofatty breast tissue), or "hypoechoic" (most clinically significant lesions). On US, a lesion suspicious for malignancy may be hypoechoic with a "taller than wide" orientation. An US-guided biopsy procedure is relatively simple and quick to perform if the target lesion can be visualized.

MRI of the breast is based on the premise that neoplasms incite neovascularity, which results in locally increased blood flow and permeability. Injection of contrast (intravenous gadolinium) leads to enhanced and accelerated deposition of contrast in the region of the tumor ("wash-in") and accelerated dissipation of contrast ("wash-out"). MRI can evaluate lesional morphology (shape and border) and the kinetics of contrast enhancement (initial and delayed). On MRI, a lesion suspicious for malignancy may be irregular in outline with rim enhancement and exhibit characteristic kinetics. MRI of the breast has diagnostic and screening applications (e.g., evaluation of occult tumor, extent of tumor, multifocality, multicentricity, response to neoadjuvant chemotherapy, recurrence, and in the screening of high-risk women).

PET screening of the breast assesses the level of glycolysis in tissues after injecting a patient with a radiotracer with an unstable nucleus. PET scans of the breast have been used in a limited fashion with mixed results for screening in high-risk patients, for evaluating recurrences, and for evaluating response to chemotherapy or hormonal therapy.

The ACR BI-RADS (American College of Radiology's Breast Imaging-Reporting and Data System) is used in reporting findings on mammography and has also been applied to the reporting of findings on US and MRI. BI-RADS category 1 indicates a negative study, category 2 a benign abnormality, category 3 an abnormality that is probably benign (requiring short interval, typically 4- to 6-month, follow-up), category 4 a "suspicious" abnormality (requiring biopsy), and category 5 a lesion that is highly suggestive of malignancy (requiring appropriate action). Category 0 is used for an incomplete evaluation (requiring additional imaging) and category 6 for a biopsy-confirmed malignancy. Routine interval screening is recommended for categories 1 and 2. NCB or excisional biopsy (if appropriate) is usually performed for category 4 and 5 cases.

The concordance of the clinical impression, imaging results, and pathologic findings is often referred to as the "triple-test." It is important to ensure that the clinical and radiographic findings are consistent with the pathologic findings on NCB. Re-biopsy with NCB or an excisional biopsy is usually recommended for discordant cases (i.e., cases that fail the "triple-test").

The histopathologic diagnosis ought to be based entirely on the microscopic appearance of the sampled tissue in the NCB specimen. The results of a pathologic interpretation that is not consistent with the clinical impression should be discussed with the submitting radiologist or responsible clinician to ensure that the sample is representative of the lesion. A written note of this discussion should be kept with the pathology records of the case. The repeated procurement of minuscule or otherwise inadequate samples (e.g., blood only) should be discussed with the appropriate clinician.

NCB specimens derived from a target with calcifications, as demonstrated by mammography, should undergo specimen radiography immediately after the procedure, and the presence of calcification in the sampling should be confirmed (Fig. 29.4). This process makes it possible to

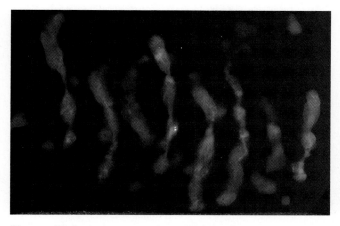

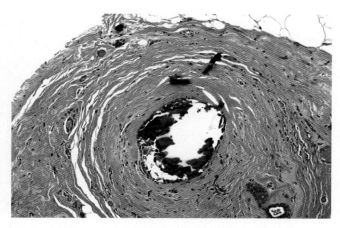

Figure 29.4 Specimen radiograph of a breast needle core biopsy specimen. This NCB specimen radiograph shows a solitary focus of calcification in one **(center)** of several samples. Optimally, the radiologist should select the samples with calcifications and submit them separately from those without calcifications.

Figure 29.5 Calcifications in a duct showing shattering (fracturing) effect. A few fragments of displaced calcified debris are present above the duct. Occasionally the entire focus of calcification may shatter and become dislodged (H&E).

identify and segregate the NCB samples containing calcifications from those without visible calcifications before submission to the pathology laboratory. The cores with and without calcifications from each biopsy site can then be immersed in fixative in separately labeled containers. Alternatively, the two sets of cores can be placed into separate tissue cassettes, differentiated by color and/or label, and submitted in a single container. The method chosen to separate specimens before submission to the pathology laboratory should be standardized within a given institution. The practice of separating the specimens with and without calcifications is useful for correlation with the mammogram. The diagnostic yield has been reported to be higher in the segregated cores containing calcifications (15), although equally careful attention must be paid to samples with and without calcifications.

Calcifications can be visualized in x-ray images of paraffin blocks and they remain detectable in this condition for an indefinite period. Radiographic study of paraffin blocks is helpful to determine the location of calcifications. Calcifications that are less than 100 μm (0.1 mm) in maximum dimension are unlikely to be radiographically visible (16). Consequently, histologically detected calcifications of minuscule proportions cannot be assumed to represent the calcifications seen in a clinical mammogram.

One possible explanation for the occasional lack of histologic visualization of calcification in NCB material obtained for mammographically detected microcalcification is their loss during histologic sectioning. This may occur either due to discarding of shavings containing calcifications in the microtome or "fracturing" of the calcifications when they are hit by the microtome blade, resulting in ejection of shattered calcific debris, in the course of preparation of levels (Fig. 29.5). Indeed, radiography of histologic shavings has provided evidence for both eventualities (17). It is also important to be aware of the possibility that calcifications from vacuum-assisted core biopsy procedures may be

aspirated into the debris canister of the instrument (18). Other explanations for "missing" calcification are inadequate sampling, mislabeling of samples, and failure to recognize calcium deposits in histologic sections. This is more likely to occur with calcium oxalate than with calcium phosphate calcifications.

Whenever a biopsy procedure is performed for calcifications, the pathology report should specify whether calcific deposits are microscopically evident, and the type of breast tissue in which they are located (Fig. 29.6). If calcifications are described in the radiograph of the NCB specimens and none are initially evident histologically, the slides should be examined for calcium oxalate (weddelite) crystals. These crystals do not stain with the H&E stain but are birefringent with polarized light (19). Calcium oxalate crystals are usually located in cysts lined by apocrine epithelium (Fig. 29.7) and may rarely elicit a foreign body-type giant cell reaction in the cyst or in periductal stroma.

Correlation with imaging findings is crucial to the reporting of NCB specimens, as exemplified even by the seemingly innocuous finding of histologically unremarkable adipose tissue—an instance that may represent either fatty breast parenchyma, a lipoma, or a missed target.

FROZEN SECTION EXAMINATION

In general, frozen section examination (FSE) should not be performed on NCB samples regardless of whether these are obtained from radiographically detected nonpalpable breast lesions or from palpable tumors. This recommendation is based on the following observations: (a) interpretation of diagnostically difficult lesions is compromised by frozen section artifact, increasing the risk of misdiagnosis, and (b) part of the diagnostic tissue may be exhausted in the process of preparing the frozen section slide. Notwithstanding the foregoing, a recent study of FSE of 59 cases of

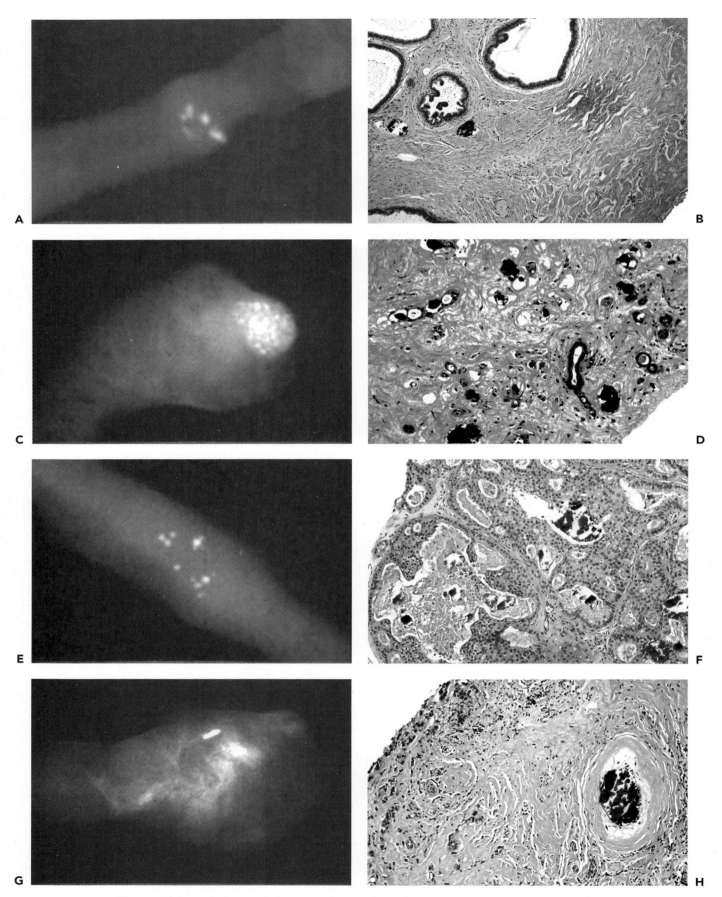

Figure 29.6 **Radiology-pathology correlation of needle core biopsy samples. A, B:** Stromal calcifications. **C, D:** Sclerosing adenosis. **E, F:** Intraductal carcinoma. **G, H:** Invasive duct carcinoma with a sclerotic and calcified duct.

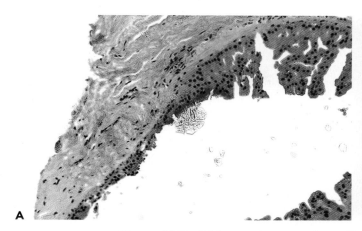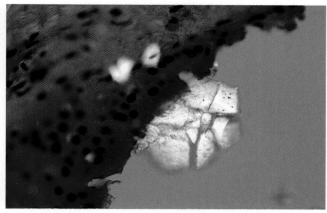

Figure 29.7 Calcium oxalate crystals. A: The crystals are barely visible in a focus of cystic-papillary apocrine hyperplasia on routine light microscopy (H&E). **B:** Birefringent calcium oxalate crystals are readily demonstrated by polarizing microscopy (**B**, H&E).

ultrasound-guided NCB of breast found no false-positive and two false-negative results; with the sensitivity, specificity, positive predictive value (PPV), and negative predictive value (NPV) of this technique being 95%, 100%, 100%, and 90%, respectively, in this series (20).

In practice, FSE of an NCB specimen from a nonpalpable breast tumor is clinically warranted only in exceptionally rare and emergency situations. Optimally, a request for a FSE on an NCB specimen should be discussed with the responsible pathologist pre-operatively. FSE is a particularly inappropriate method for rendering a diagnosis if nonsurgical ablation of a tumor or neoadjuvant chemotherapy is being considered. It is imperative to reach a diagnosis with "permanent," H&E-stained paraffin sections before these treatments, which could radically alter the histology of target lesion, are initiated.

TOUCH IMPRINT CYTOLOGY

Touch imprint cytology (TIC) of an NCB specimen is a technique that provides a cytologic diagnosis without the risks of tissue loss attendant on preparing a frozen section (21,22). However, this procedure substitutes the limitations of cytologic preparation for those of frozen sections. Imprints are subject to drying artifacts and other distortions that may present substantial pitfalls for inexperienced, and even some experienced, pathologists.

The TIC is prepared by either "touching" (i.e., gently compressing) or "rolling" the NCB specimen on glass slides. Air-dried slides are suitable for the Diff–Quik stain. Alcohol-fixed slides may be used for either H&E or Papanicolaou stains. TIC has the potential of improving patient management in "one-stop" breast clinics by providing a prompt diagnosis. Kulkarni et al. reported a 95% adequacy rate and 55% malignant rate in 819 cases in a recent series from such a setting (23). This method of evaluating NCB may also be of value in the immediate assessment of specimen adequacy, thus reducing the number of insufficient

specimens. The interpretation of low-grade carcinoma and fibroadenoma in a TIC preparation may be particularly challenging. Consequently, it is recommended that TIC of breast NCB specimens be undertaken only by pathologists or cytologists who examine this type of material with sufficient frequency to maintain a high level of proficiency and work in close collaboration with radiologists and surgeons who routinely perform the NCB procedure.

"Core wash cytology" examination utilizes cells taken from the fixative fluid in which the NCB is placed. The "core wash" is subjected to liquid-based preparation and then stained by the routine Papanicolaou method. This technique has been successfully employed for the immediate diagnosis of NCB of the breast, and in a series of 30 cases was found to have better morphology and fewer insufficient diagnoses than TIC (6.6% vs. 13.3%) (24). Core wash cytology entails diagnostic risks that are similar to those of TIC.

PATHOLOGIC REPORTING

The pathology report of a NCB specimen should render the diagnosis in a concise and clinically meaningful manner. A detailed microscopic description of the histologic findings is not necessary if the specific diagnosis is clearly stated. For example, it is sufficient to report "fibroadenoma" without listing the microscopic characteristics. On occasion, microscopic details may be added to the diagnosis to convey additional clinically significant information, as for example in the diagnosis: "fibroadenoma with cellular stroma; recommend excision to rule-out phyllodes tumor."

When a carcinoma is diagnosed, the presence or absence of invasion must be stated if this can be ascertained. For in situ carcinoma, the diagnosis should state the type (ductal or lobular), nuclear grade, and presence of luminal necrosis and calcification. In cases of ductal carcinoma in situ (DCIS), the architectural pattern, such as solid cribriform and micropapillary should be mentioned. A high degree of concordance in the classification of intraductal carcinoma has been found between NCB and excisional biopsy specimens in the same patient. Jackman et al. found comedo-type of intraductal carcinoma in 91% of excisions after a diagnosis of histologically similar intraductal carcinoma in an NCB specimen and in 15% of excisions following the diagnosis of noncomedo intraductal carcinoma in NCB samples (25).

The diagnosis of invasive carcinoma should describe the subtype of tumor (ductal, lobular, or special type—tubular or mucinous), associated in situ carcinoma, presence of lymphovascular invasion and any significant benign proliferative lesions. Information may be limited for microinvasive carcinoma. If possible, the nuclear grade of microinvasive tumor cells should be reported. Studies of the classification of invasive breast carcinoma diagnosed in NCB and subsequent excised specimens show a concordance rate of 72% to 82% (26). The presence of in situ carcinoma supports the primary mammary origin of invasive carcinoma, and this information may be clinically relevant. However, the determination of extensive intraductal component (>25% of tumor mass composed of DCIS and extension of DCIS beyond the invasive component) is not possible in an NCB specimen.

The nuclear and histologic grade (both on a three-tier scale) can be reported for an NCB specimen of invasive carcinoma of the breast. Evaluation of the mitotic count is unreliable in NCB samples as it is usually underestimated, especially if fewer than four samples are available for examination (27). Comparison of the grading of invasive ductal carcinomas in NCB and excisional biopsy specimens from the same tumor reveals a tendency by pathologists to assign a lower grade on the NCB specimen, but an agreement rate of up to 84% has been reported for poorly differentiated breast carcinomas (grade 3), the type of carcinoma most likely to benefit from neoadjuvant chemotherapy (28).

The most important histologic factors that determine the prognosis of breast carcinoma are lymph node involvement, tumor size, and histologic grade. Only one of these three factors, histologic grade, can be assessed in NCB material.

The determination of tumor size on NCB material is unreliable because the samples are taken randomly and may not represent the maximum tumor extent. In one study, NCB specimens underestimated tumor size in 79% of cases (29), and in another report tumor size determined from an NCB specimen was "upstaged" in 72% of cases upon assessment of size in the excised tissue (30). However, it may be useful to routinely include the largest single histologically contiguous size of invasive carcinoma in a single needle core sample in an NCB specimen. This information is particularly significant in the event that little or no residual invasive carcinoma is detected in the subsequent excisional biopsy specimen.

Stereotactic vacuum-assisted NCB procedures remove a "substantial quantity of tissue" and complete extirpation

of the tumor may occur in 20% of nonpalpable invasive carcinomas (31). If the size of invasive carcinoma is not routinely provided prospectively, then it is important to document it retrospectively in the event that no residual invasive carcinoma is identified upon excision (i.e., include the invasive size in an addendum to the NCB specimen report and also include the size information from the NCB material in the excisional biopsy report).

E-cadherin immunostaining should be employed in those circumstances when there is difficulty in distinguishing ductal from lobular carcinoma. This applies to in situ or invasive lesions (32). The cytoplasmic membranes of tumor cells are immunoreactive for E-cadherin in virtually all ductal lesions, and display fragmented, weak, or absent reactivity in lobular carcinomas. p120 catenin immunostaining may also be helpful in distinguishing ductal and lobular carcinomas (including its pleomorphic variant) (33,34). The p120 catenin immunostain is localized on the cytoplasmic membrane in ductal-type of neoplastic cells and appears within the cytoplasm in lobular carcinoma cells.

The assessment of lymphovascular involvement (LVI) by tumor cells in NCB specimens is not reliable due to the limited samples obtained and the potential for retraction artifact. A sensitivity of only 8% and PPV of 87% for LVI was reported in one study (28). Adherence to established histologic criteria for LVI (i.e., location of LVI away from tumor, presence of endothelial cells around tumor, difference between the shape of tumor embolus and space within which it lies) and confirmatory immunostains for endothelial cells such as CD31, D2-40, or WT1 may be helpful in confirming the presence of lymphovascular channel invasion (35).

Some pathologists routinely resist the reporting of benign inactive breast tissue as "normal" even if it is the only histopathologic finding and yield to the temptation of using the all-encompassing rubric: "fibrocystic changes." The use of the latter term as a diagnosis without specifying the specific elements of those changes is clinically unhelpful. In the absence of fibrocystic changes, a diagnosis of breast tissue with physiologic changes can be offered (e.g., atrophy) depending on the findings that are present.

STANDARDIZED REPORTING

Standardized forms listing the majority of potential diagnoses are a useful method for reporting breast pathology findings in routine cases. Such a checklist is an efficient way to record the diagnosis in a comprehensive manner, and for the development of a database.

The major drawback to the use of formatted diagnoses is the rigidity of the report, which tends to give equal weight to all components and presents the histologic findings in an inflexible sequence. In a particular case, certain diagnoses may require emphasis by being given priority in the report as well as by additional commentary. If the preformatted report does not offer sufficient latitude to rearrange the diagnostic components when necessary, the pathologist should have the option to issue a nonstructured diagnosis. This is especially important if critical information cannot be conveyed by amplifying the formatted text with comments.

In the United Kingdom, a scoring system (category classification) has been adopted for reporting NCB specimens (36). All NCB samples of the breast are classified as B1 to B5, with the assigned designation appearing prominently in each report. B1 is normal or inadequate (e.g., fibrosis), B2 is benign (e.g., sclerosing adenosis), B3 is benign with uncertain malignant potential (e.g., atypical hyperplasia), B4 is suspicious (e.g., minimal diagnostic tissue or crushed/distorted tissue), and B5 is positive (e.g., in situ or invasive carcinoma). In general, an excisional biopsy procedure might be performed if clinically indicated for categories B1 and B2 and local excision would follow for categories B3–B5. Although the system may appear "restrictive," it helps "concentrate the mind of the pathologist when writing a report" (31). A microscopic description or comments may be added at the pathologists' discretion. In a recent study, the B4 category was shown to have a high PPV: 74.2% (range: 62.5%–90.6%), the PPV of B5 category was more than 99%, and the PPV of the B3 category was reported to be 19.1% (37).

ROLE OF THE NCB SPECIMEN PATHOLOGY REPORT IN PATIENT CARE

The NCB procedure is highly accurate for the diagnosis of most breast lesions with a PPV for the diagnosis of invasive carcinoma of 98% to 99.8% (38). The pathologic diagnosis made on NCB samples can be, and often is, a key determinant in planning optimal management. Nonetheless, it cannot be relied upon to provide comprehensive data equal to that which can be obtained from an excisional biopsy specimen. In a series of 1,168 NCB specimens, there was complete histologic agreement with the diagnosis rendered on the subsequently excised specimens in 83% of cases (39). Consideration must be given to the potential limitations of NCB specimen diagnosis in the formulation of treatment plans. In a series of 952 consecutive cases, the overall false-negative rate of NCB specimens was 9.1%, based on the results of a standard radiology follow-up protocol for all patients (40). The pathologic report for an NCB specimen from the breast must be integrated with the clinical history, physical examination, and radiographic findings to plan the management of an individual patient.

The diagnosis rendered for an NCB specimen obviously applies only to information available from that sample. Final characterization of the lesion must be based on pathologic data from the NCB and excised specimens. It is

therefore essential that the pathologist entrusted with the responsibility of diagnosing the subsequent surgical specimen have slides available from the NCB sample. It is substandard practice for a patient to undergo an excision for a lesion diagnosed in another institution on an NCB specimen without prior review of NCB slides at the hospital where the surgical procedure is to be performed (41).

Some diagnoses of NCB specimens could qualify for the designation of "critical." An example of this would be the unexpected diagnosis of carcinoma in an NCB specimen from a mass in a young woman that was clinically expected to be a fibroadenoma. It has been proposed that a list of such "critical" diagnoses for various organ systems and types of biopsies should be customized for each institution (42).

ANCILLARY STUDIES ON NEEDLE CORE BIOPSY SPECIMENS

Hormone Receptors

An NCB specimen is suitable in most cases for the assessment of prognostic markers. The IHC detection of estrogen receptors (ER) in the NCB specimen correlated with the receptor status of a subsequent surgical excision specimen in 73% of cases in one study (43). Agreement between the NCB and excised specimens of breast carcinoma was observed in 69% of cases for progesterone receptors (PR), a substantial discrepancy that the authors attributed to greater heterogeneity of receptor expression. A trend toward higher expression of ER in NCB specimens than in excision samples may be attributable to more rapid specimen fixation of the former (44). According to ASCO/CAP recommendations, the optimal fixation time for ancillary IHC testing is 24 to 48 hours, but less than 6-hour fixation is considered sufficient for NCB specimens (45). Underfixation is more deleterious to ER and HER2/*neu* testing by immunostaining or fluorescent in situ hybridization (FISH) testing than is overfixation (46).

The "H-score" (histochemical score) system can be used for reporting IHC hormone receptor results (47). The H-score is derived from *multiplying* the percentage of immunostained tumor cells by the staining intensity factor (Table 29.1).

The "Allred Score" is another method of quantifying immunostaining for ER and PR (48). This method yields the *sum* of the estimated proportion and intensity of positive tumor cells (Table 29.2).

Scoring of hormone receptor results remains nonstandardized at this time (49). In most cases, the percentage of tumor cells staining and the strength of immunoreactivity (on a four-tier scale: negative, weak, intermediate, and strong) should be reported, for example, 75% of invasive carcinoma cells show moderate staining for ER. In this regard, four practical caveats deserve iteration. First, positive and negative internal "controls" must not be overlooked.

TABLE 29.1
THE H (HISTOCHEMICAL)-SCORE SYSTEM FOR QUANTIFYING IMMUNOHISTOCHEMICAL STAINING OF ER AND PR

Obtaining the H-score

1. Record percentage of cells staining	0–100
2. Record staining intensity factor	0–4
0: negative, 1: weak, 2: moderate, 3: strong	
3. *Multiply* percentage of cells staining by the staining intensity factor to obtain the H (histochemical)-score	

Interpreting the H-score

0–50	Negative
51–100	Weak–positive (1+ positive)
101–200	Moderate–positive (2+ positive)
201–300	Strong–positive (3+ positive)

Adapted from Snead DR, Bell JA, Dixon AR, et al. Methodology of immunohistological detection of oestrogen receptor in human breast carcinoma in formalin-fixed, paraffin-embedded tissue: a comparison with frozen section methodology. *Histopathology.* 1993;23:233–238.

Ideally, hormone receptor immunoreactivity in normal breast glandular tissue, if available, should be confirmed. Second, the status of receptors cannot be reliably calculated if only a minute amount of tumor is present in an NCB specimen. Third, the complete absence of immunoreactivity in tissue for ER and PR (in all neoplastic and nonneoplastic breast tissue, and in control tissue) is most likely due to technical failure, such as absence of primary antibody or error in technique. This finding may also be the result of loss of immunogenicity of tissue being tested due to underfixation. In such situations, the use of vimentin or another ubiquitous antibody is helpful to assess the immunocompetence of the tissue. Fourth, optimal testing for prognostic markers depends on an NCB sample that is representative of a particular tumor. In tumors that show heterogeneity of grade, multifocality or multicentricity, retesting on appropriately selected tumor tissue from excised specimens may be indicated.

TABLE 29.2
THE ALLRED SCORING SYSTEM FOR QUANTIFYING IMMUNOHISTOCHEMICAL STAINING OF ER AND PR

This method yields the *sum* of the estimated proportion and intensity of positive tumor cells

Obtaining the Allred score

1. Score proportion of "positive" cells from 0 to 5
   0: total negativity in tumor cells, 1: 1% positive cells, 2: 10% positive cells, 3: 33% positive cells, 4: 66% positive cells, 5: 100% positive cells
2. Score intensity of staining from 0 to 3
   0: no staining in tumor cells, 1: weak staining, 2: intense staining, 3: strong staining
3. Add proportion score and intensity score to obtain the Allred score. Total score could range from 0 to 8

Interpreting the Allred score

A score of >2 (i.e., ≥"3") has been adjudged the minimum score for defining ER-positive breast carcinoma

Adapted from Ellredge RM, Allred DC. Clinical aspects of estrogen and progesterone receptors. In Harris JR, Lippman ME, Morrow M, Osborne CK, eds. *Diseases of the Breast.* Philadelphia: Lippincott Williams Wilkins; 2004:603–617.

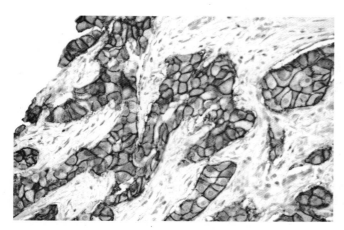

Figure 29.8 3+ Immunoreactivity of HER2/*neu* in carcinoma. Uniform 3+ intense membrane staining of >30% of tumor cells in an invasive carcinoma (Herceptest).

HER2/*neu*

The use of trastuzumab, lapatinib, and related medications in patients with metastatic breast carcinoma relies on the reliable determination of HER2/*neu* status on tumor tissue. A variety of technologies exist to assess HER2/*neu* status (50), either through the detection of protein expression or through gene amplification. The former is detectable by immunohistochemistry (Fig. 29.8) and the latter by various in situ hybridization techniques.

The IHC detection of HER2/*neu* is the most commonly used technique. The scoring system for HER2/*neu* immunoreactivity in breast cancer in the 2007 ASCO/CAP guidelines is outlined in Table 29.3.

ASCO/CAP guidelines recommend FISH confirmation for all cases judged to be 2+ by immunohistochemistry. The assessment of HER2/*neu* in NCB material and correlation with the excision biopsy material had a 92% concordance rate in one study, with 100% of patients being selected for appropriate therapy (51).

HER2/*neu* protein expression levels observed by IHC are directly, if not always consistently, related to HER2/*neu* gene amplification detected by FISH or related techniques. Variations in accuracy, reproducibility, and precision of IHC testing techniques, interobserver variation in IHC interpretation, and most importantly inconsistent IHC expression of HER2/*neu* protein in variably fixed tumor tissues have cast doubt on the reliability and efficiency of IHC even for primary "screening."

For the aforementioned reasons, it is more accurate to determine HER2/*neu* status via techniques that detect gene amplification. These techniques include FISH, currently considered the "gold standard" for determining HER2/*neu* status, chromogenic in situ hybridization (CISH), and silver in situ hybridization (SISH). The latter two techniques are reportedly comparable to FISH and offer the advantage of being permanent, and thus available for retrospective review (52–54). FISH, CISH, and SISH techniques can all be performed on NCB material.

In the Department of Pathology at New York Presbyterian Hospital-Weill Cornell Medical Center, ER, PR, and HER2/*neu* immunostains are routinely performed for all invasive carcinomas on NCB specimens. FISH confirmation is obtained for immunohistochemically equivocal (2+) cases. Immunostains for ER and PR are routinely performed on intraductal carcinomas.

Other Ancillary Tests

Washings from NCB specimens have been demonstrated to yield sufficient numbers of epithelial cells to allow sorting by *flow cytometry*. This methodology facilitates a variety of molecular and genetic analyses (55).

Preliminary studies indicate that it is possible to obtain sufficient ribonucleic acid (RNA) for transcriptional profiling by complementary deoxyribonucleic acid (cDNA) microarray from samples of breast carcinoma derived from appropriately processed NCB samples of breast carcinoma

TABLE 29.3
THE ASCO/CAP SCORING SYSTEM FOR QUANTIFYING IMMUNOHISTOCHEMICAL STAINING OF HER2/*neu*
0: No overexpression of HER/*neu*: No staining is observed in invasive tumor cells
1: No overexpression of HER/*neu*: Weak, incomplete membrane staining in any proportion of invasive tumor cells, or weak, complete membrane staining in less than 10% of cells
2: Equivocal of HER/*neu*: Complete membrane staining that is nonuniform or weak but with obvious circumferential distribution in at least 10% of cells, or intense complete membrane staining in ≤30% of tumor cells
3: Overexpression of HER/*neu*: Uniform intense membrane staining of >30% of invasive tumor cells

Adapted from Wolff AC, Hammond ME, Schwartz JN, et al. American Society of Clinical Oncology/College of American Pathologists guideline recommendations for human epidermal growth factor receptor 2 testing in breast cancer. *J Clin Oncol.* 2007;25:118–145.

(56). Tissue sections taken from NCB material have been suitable for Oncotype DX 21 gene recurrence score testing if sufficient material is available. Akashi-Tanaka et al. (57) found that half of cases of NCBs submitted for such testing yielded insufficient RNA for testing. However, the remaining specimens were "highly predictive" of response to neoadjuvant endocrine therapy. Patients with low, rather than intermediate or high, Oncotype DX 21 gene recurrence scores responded better and tended to have a better relapse-free survival.

Numerous other cancer "biomarkers" are available for testing on NCB material, including the ASCO-recommended cancer biomarker: urokinase-type plasminogen activator (uPA) and its inhibitor: plasminogen activator inhibitor (PAI-1) (58). Extraordinary ancillary tests on NCB material may be performed for clinically valid indications at the request of the treating physician, but these will generally be part of a research protocol.

Current CAP regulatory guidelines dictate that when ancillary IHC testing is performed, the pathology report should specify the antibody clone, the general form of detection used, and the scoring system used. Deviations from standard processing or antigen retrieval techniques should be included. Appropriate negative and positive controls should be used and documented (59).

REFERENCES

1. Iwase T, Takahashi K, Gomi N, et al. Present state of and problems with needle core biopsy for non-palpable breast lesions. *Breast Cancer.* 2006;13:32–37.
2. Nakano S, Sakamoto H, Ohtsuka M, et al. Evaluation and indications of ultrasound-guided vacuum assisted core needle breast biopsy. *Breast Cancer.* 2007;14:292–296.
3. Moritz JD, Luftner-Nagel S, Westerhof JP, et al. Microcalcifications in breast core biopsy specimens: disappearance at radiography after storage in formaldehyde. *Radiology.* 1996;200:361–363.
4. Wolff AC, Hammond ME, Schwartz JN, et al. American Society of Clinical Oncology/College of American Pathologists guideline recommendations for human epidermal growth factor receptor 2 testing in breast cancer. *J Clin Oncol.* 2007;25:118–145.
5. Liberman L, Dershaw DD, Rosen PP, et al. Core needle biopsy of synchronous ipsilateral breast lesions: impact on treatment. *Am J Roentgenol.* 1996;166:1429–1432.
6. Senn Bahls E, Dupont Lampert V, Oelschlegel C, et al. Multitarget stereotactic core-needle breast biopsy (MSBB)—an effective and safe diagnostic intervention for non-palpable breast lesions: a large prospective single institution study. *Breast.* 2006;15:339–346.
7. Riley TR III, Ruggiero FM. The effect of processing on liver biopsy core size. *Dig Dis Sci.* 2008;53:2775–2777.
8. Renshaw AA, Kish R, Gould EW. The value of inking breast cores to reduce specimen mix-up. *Am J Clin Pathol.* 2007;127:271–272.
9. Ragazzini T, Magrini E, Cucci MC, et al. The fast-track biopsy: description of a rapid histology and immunohistochemistry method for evaluation of preoperative breast core biopsies. *Int J Surg Pathol.* 2005;13:247–252.
10. Yaziji H, Taylor CR. Begin at the beginning, with the tissue! The key message underlying the ASCO/CAP Task-force Guideline Recommendations for HER2 testing. *Appl Immunohistochem Mol Morphol.* 2007;15:239–241.
11. Grimes MM, Karageorge LS, Hogge JP. Does exhaustive search for microcalcifications improve diagnostic yield in stereotactic core needle breast biopsies? *Mod Pathol.* 2001;14:350–353.
12. Renshaw A. Adequate histologic sampling of breast core needle biopsies. *Arch Pathol Lab Med.* 2001;125:1055–1057.
13. Kumaraswamy V, Carder PJ. Examination of breast needle core biopsy specimens performed for screen-detected microcalcification. *J Clin Pathol.* 2007;60:681–684.
14. Hoda SA, Rosen PP. Contemporaneous H&E sections should be standard practice in diagnostic immunopathology. *Am J Surg Pathol.* 2007;31:1627.
15. Margolin FR, Kaufman L, Jacobs RP, et al. Stereotactic core biopsy of malignant calcifications: diagnostic yield of cores with and without calcifications on specimen radiographs. *Radiology.* 2004;233:251–254.
16. Dahlstrom JE, Sutton S, Jain S. Histologic–radiologic correlation of mammographically detected microcalcification in stereotactic core biopsies. *Am J Surg Pathol.* 1998;22:256–259.
17. Winston JS, Geradts J, Liu DF, et al. Microtome shaving radiography: demonstration of loss of mammographic microcalcifications during histologic sectioning. *Breast J.* 2004;10:200–203.
18. Friedman PD, Sanders LM, Menendez C, et al. Retrieval of lost microcalcifications during stereotactic vacuum-assisted core biopsy. *Am J Roentgenol.* 2003;180:275–284.
19. Tornos C, Silva E, el-Naggar A, et al. Calcium oxalate crystals in breast biopsies. The missing microcalcifications. *Am J Surg Pathol.* 1990;14:961–968.
20. Brunner AH, Sagmeister T, Kremer J, et al. The accuracy of frozen section analysis in ultrasound-guided core needle biopsy of breast lesion. *BMC Cancer.* 2009;9:341.
21. Carmichael AR, Berresford A, Sami A, et al. Imprint cytology of needle core-biopsy specimens of breast lesion: is it best of both worlds? *Breast.* 2004;13:232–234.
22. Kass R, Henry-Tillman RS, Nurko J, et al. Touch preparation of breast core needle specimens is a new method for same-day diagnosis. *Am J Surg.* 2003;186:737–742.
23. Kulkarni D, Irvine T, Reves RJ. The use of core biopsy imprint cytology in the 'one-stop' breast clinic. *Eur J Surg Oncol.* 2009;35:1037–1040.
24. Wauters CA, Sanders-Eras CT, Kooistra BW, et al. Modified core wash cytology procedure for the immediate diagnosis of core needle biopsies of breast lesions. *Cancer Cytopathol.* 2009;117:333–337.
25. Jackman RJ, Nowels KW, Shepard MJ, et al. Stereotaxic large-core needle biopsy of 450 nonpalpable breast lesions with surgical correlation in lesions with cancer and atypical hyperplasia. *Radiology.* 1994;193:91–95.
26. Hoda SA, Harigopal M, Harris GC, et al. Expert opinion: what should be included in reports of needle core biopsies of breast? *Histopathology.* 2003;43:87–90.
27. McIlhenny C, Doughty JC, George WD, et al. Optimum number of core biopsies for accurate assessment of histologic grade in breast cancer. *Br J Surg.* 2002;89:84–85.
28. Harris GC, Denley HE, Pinder SE, et al. Correlation of histologic prognostic factors in core biopsies and therapeutic excisions of invasive breast carcinoma. *Am J Surg Pathol.* 2003;27:11–15.
29. Sharifi S, Peterson M, Baum J. Assessment of pathologic prognostic factors in breast core needle biopsies. *Mod Pathol.* 1999;12:941–945.
30. Lara JF, Abellar RG, Singh NV. Benefits and pitfalls of tumor size and/or volume determination on core needle biopsy in invasive breast cancer: a year of experience from a community hospital. *Mod Pathol.* 2005;18(suppl 1):39A.
31. Shousha S. Issues in the interpretation of breast core biopsies. *Int J Surg Pathol* 2003;11:167–176.
32. Goldstein NS, Bassi D, Watts JC, et al. E-cadherin reactivity of 95 noninvasive ductal and lobular lesions of the breast. Implications for the interpretation of problematic lesions. *Am J Clin Pathol.* 2001;115:534–542.
33. Dabbs DJ, Bhargava R, Chivukula M. Lobular versus ductal breast neoplasms: the diagnostic utility of p120 catenin. *Am J Surg Pathol.* 2007;31:427–437.
34. Chivukula M, Haynik DM, Brufsky A, et al. Pleomorphic lobular carcinoma in situ (PLCIS) on breast core needle biopsies: clinical significance and immunoprofile. *Am J Surg Pathol.* 2008;32:1721–1726.
35. Hoda SA, Hoda RS, Merlin S, et al. Issues relating to lymphovascular invasion in breast carcinoma. *Adv Anat Pathol.* 2006;13:308–315.
36. Ellis IO, Humphrey S, Mitchell M, et al. Guidelines for breast needle core biopsy handling and reporting in breast screening assessment. Best practice No. 179. *J Clin Pathol.* 2004;57:897–902.
37. El-Sayed ME, Rakha EA, Reed J, et al. Predictive value of needle core biopsy diagnoses of lesions of uncertain malignant potential (B3) in abnormalities detected by mammographic screening. *Histopathology.* 2008;53:650–657.
38. Liberman L, Dershaw D, Rosen PP. Stereotaxic core biopsy of breast carcinoma: accuracy at predicting invasion. *Radiology.* 1995;194:379–381.
39. Crowe JP, Rim A, Patrick RJ, et al. Does core needle breast biopsy accurately reflect breast pathology? *Surgery.* 2003;134:523–528.
40. Shah VL, Raju U, Chitale D, et al. False-negative core needle biopsies of the breast. An analysis of clinical, radiologic, and pathologic findings in 27 consecutive cases of missed breast cancer. *Cancer.* 2003;97:1824–1831.
41. Rosen PP. Review of 'outside' pathology before treatment should be mandatory. *Am J Surg Pathol.* 2002;26:1235–1236.
42. Huang EC, Kuo FC, Fletcher CD, et al. Critical diagnoses in surgical pathology: a retrospective single-institution study to monitor guidelines for communication of urgent results. *Am J Surg Pathol.* 2009;33:1098–1102.
43. Zidan A, Christie Brown JS, Peston D, et al. Oestrogen and progesterone receptor assessment in core biopsy specimens of breast carcinoma. *J Clin Pathol.* 1997;50:27–29.
44. Douglas-Jones A, Coletti N, Morgan J, et al. Comparison of core oestrogen receptor (ER) assay with excised tumor: intratumoral distribution of ER in breast carcinoma. *J Clin Pathol.* 2001;54:951–955.
45. Hanna W, O'Malley FP, Barnes P, et al. Updated recommendations from the Canadian National Consensus Meeting on Her2/neu testing in breast cancer. *Curr Oncol.* 2007;14:149–153.
46. Goldstein NS, Ferkowicz M, Odish E, et al. Minimum formalin fixation time for consistent estrogen receptor immunohistochemical staining of invasive breast carcinoma. *Am J Clin Pathol.* 2003;120:86–92.

47. Snead DR, Bell JA, Dixon AR, et al. Methodology of immunohistological detection of oestrogen receptor in human breast carcinoma in formalin-fixed, paraffin-embedded tissue: a comparison with frozen section methodology. *Histopathology*. 1993;23:233–238.

48. Ellredge RM, Allred DC. Clinical aspects of estrogen and progesterone receptors. In Harris JR, Lippman ME, Morrow M, Osborne CK, eds. *Diseases of the Breast*. Philadelphia, PA: Lippincott Williams Wilkins; 2004: 603–617.

49. Fisher ER, Anderson S, Dean S, et al. Solving the dilemma of the immunohistochemical and other methods used for scoring estrogen receptor and progesterone receptor in patients with invasive breast carcinoma. *Cancer*. 2005;103:164–173.

50. Penault-Llorca F, Bilous M, Dowsett M, et al. Emerging technologies for assessing HER2 amplification. *Am J Clin Pathol*. 2009;132:539–548.

51. Mueller-Holzner E, Fink V, Frede T, et al. Immunohistochemical determination of HER2 expression in breast cancer from core biopsy specimen: a reliable predictor of HER2 status of the whole tumour. *Breast Cancer Res Treat*. 2001;69:13–19.

52. Van de Vijver M, Bilous M, Hanna W, et al. Chromogenic in situ hybridization (CISH) for the assessment of HER2 status in breast cancer: an international validation ring study. *Breast Cancer Res*. 2007;9:R68.

53. Shousha S, Peston D, Amo-Takyi B, et al. Evaluation of automated silver-enhanced in situ hybridization (SISH) for detection of HER2 gene amplification in breast carcinoma excision and core biopsy specimens. *Histopathology*. 2009;54:248–253.

54. Sauter G, Lee J, Bartlett JM, et al. Guidelines for human epidermal growth factor receptor 2 testing: biologic and methodologic considerations. *J Clin Oncol*. 2009;27:1323–1333.

55. Stoler DL, Stewart CC, Stomper PC. Breast epithelium procurement from stereotactic core biopsy washings: flow cytometry-sorted cell count analysis. *Clin Cancer Res*. 2002;8:428–432.

56. Symmans WF, Ayers M, Clark EA, et al. Total RNA yield and microarray gene expression profiles from fine needle aspiration biopsy and core-needle biopsy samples of breast carcinoma. *Cancer*. 2003;97:2960–2971.

57. Akashi-Tanaka S, Shimizu C, Ando M, et al. 21-gene expression profile assay on core needle biopsies predicts responses to neoadjuvant endocrine therapy in breast cancer patients. *Breast*. 2009;18:171–174.

58. Thomssen C, Harbeck N, Dittmer J, et al. Feasibility of measuring the prognostic factors uPA and PAI-1 in core needle biopsy breast cancer specimens. *JNCI*. 2009;101:1028–1029.

59. Commission on Laboratory Accreditation. *AP Checklist*. Northfield, IL. CAP. Available at: http://www.cap.org/apps/cap.

Index

Page numbers followed by f indicate figures; by t indicate tables.

A

Ablation therapy, pathologic effects of, 326–327
Abscess, bacteria-caused, 26
Acantholytic metaplastic carcinoma, 198f
Acid-fast bacteria, 25
Acinic cell carcinoma, 73
ACR BI-RADS. *See* American College of Radiology's
    Breast Imaging-Reporting and Data System
    (ACR BI-RADS)
Actinomycotic infection, 26
Adenoid cystic carcinoma
    with basaloid features, 223–224, 227f
    grades, 223, 224
    growth patterns of, 223, 224f
    with perineural invasion, 223, 226f
    radiation therapy and, 226
    size of, 223
    staining of, 226
Adenolipoma, 284f
Adenomatous polyposis, familial, 274
Adenomyoepithelioma, 52–59
    in adenosis, 54f
    with infarction, 56f
    mistaken for carcinoma, 55f
    myoepithelial carcinoma in, 57f–58f
    with myoepithelial cell hyperplasia, 57f
    with myoid differentiation, 56f
    with sebaceous and squamous differentiation,
        55f–56f
Adenosis
    adenomyoepithelioma in, 54f
    apocrine, 66, 68f–69f
    florid, 61, 63f, 64f
    florid papillomatosis with, 49
    intraductal carcinoma, 69–70
    microglandular, 72–76
    papilloma with, 30f
    sclerosing, 61, 64f–66f, 71f, 72f, 73f
    tubular, 67, 70f, 71f
    tumor, 61, 62f–63f
Adenosquamous carcinoma, low-grade, 194–195,
    196f–197f
Adolescent giant fibroadenomas, 77
Age distribution
    columnar cell hyperplasia, 111
    ductal hyperplasia, 97
    fibroadenoma, 77
    intraductal carcinoma, 119, 120
    LCIS, 246
    PASH, 275, 276
    phyllodes tumor, 86
    secretory carcinoma, 229, 231
AJCC. *See* American Joint Committee on Cancer
    Staging Manual (AJCC)
ALH. *See* Atypical lobular hyperplasia (ALH)
Alveolar invasive lobular carcinoma, 266, 267f
American College of Radiology's Breast Imaging-
    Reporting and Data System (ACR BI-RADS),
    350
American Joint Committee on Cancer Staging
    Manual (AJCC) guidelines, 147
American Society of Clinical Oncology/College of
    American Pathologists (ASCO/CAP)
    guidelines, 348, 357
Amylase, 73
Amyloidosis, 21, 21f
Amyloid tumor, 21
ANA. *See* Antinuclear antibody (ANA)
Anaplastic large cell lymphoma, 303

Anatomy of breast, 1–3
Ancillary studies of NCB specimens, 355–358
    HER2/*neu*, 357, 357f
    hormone receptors, 355–356
Angiogenesis
    associated with breast carcinomas, 154–155
    invasive duct carcinoma with, 155f
Angiolipoma, nonparenchymal, 292f, 293f
Angiomatosis, 291, 291f
Angiosarcoma
    growth patterns, 294
    intermediate and high-grade, 294, 296f
    MRI and, 293
    parenchymal, 294
    peripheral vascular component, 295
    tumor grade, 295
Antinuclear antibody (ANA), 19
Apocrine adenosis, 66, 68f–69f
Apocrine carcinoma, 284
    atypical, 213
    cytologic features, 213, 216
    diagnosis on basis of size, 213, 215
    with histiocytoid features, 221f
    infiltrating, 218–219
    invasive, 217f, 219f
    in papillary lesions, 218
    prognosis of, 222
    with signet ring cells, 219
Apocrine differentiation in pleomorphic invasive
    lobular carcinoma, 266, 270f
Apocrine intraductal carcinoma, 124f, 213, 214f
    apocrine metaplasia with, 214f
    arising in apocrine adenosis, 215f
    clear cell type, 217f
    with lobular extension, 218f
Apocrine metaplasia
    with atypia and apocrine intraductal carcinoma,
        214f
    atypical ductal hyperplasia with, 109f
    cystic and papillary, 45–48
    cystic micropapillary, 215f
    in papilloma, 218f
    papilloma with, 31f
    RSL with, 39–40
    in sclerosing adenosis, 68f
Argyrophilic granules, in mucinous carcinoma,
    206
Arteritis, giant cell, 18–19, 18f
ASCO/CAP guidelines. *See* American Society of
    Clinical Oncology/College of American
    Pathologists (ASCO/CAP) guidelines
Aspergillus infection, 21
Asteroid bodies, 16
Atrophy
    lobular, 246–247, 248f
        radiation-induced, 320f
    menopausal epithelial, 3–4, 5f
    sclerosing adenosis with, 64f
Atypical ductal hyperplasia
    with apocrine metaplasia, 107, 109f
    borderline, 107–108, 110f
    breast carcinoma risk and, 118–119
    with calcification, 106f
    columnar cell, 108–117, 109f
    with cytologic atypia, 107, 109f–110f
    gynecomastia with, 331f
    juvenile, 336, 337f, 338f
    with lobular extension, 105–107, 107f
    micropapillary, 106f–107f, 109f

mucocele-like lesions, 209
needle core biopsy, diagnosis by, 117–118
pathology of, 104–108
Atypical hemangioma, 290, 290f
Atypical hyperplasia
    papilloma with, 36f
    pregnancy-like, 6, 7f
    in sclerosing adenosis, 68, 70f
Atypical lobular hyperplasia (ALH), 111–117, 115f,
    247, 257–260, 322f–323f
    diagnosis of, 257–258
        needle core biopsy, 259–260
        surgical biopsy, 259–258
    risk for carcinoma in, 258–259
Atypical papillomas, defined, 37
Axillary dissection, 141

B

Bartonella infection, 26
Basal-like carcinomas
    clinical studies, 159
    neoadjuvant therapy for, 159
    risk for local recurrence, 159
Basal-like phenotype
    defined, 157
    histologic features associated with, 158–159
    Invasive duct carcinoma with, 158f
Benign mesenchymal tumors
    angiomatosis, 291, 291f
    fibromatosis, 274, 275f, 276f, 282
    fibrous tumor, 274, 276f
    granular cell tumors, 283–284, 283f
    hamartoma, 284
    hemangioma, 286–287, 289, 290, 291
    hibernoma, 286, 286f
    leiomyoma, 285, 285f
    lipoma, 285, 286
    myofibroblastoma, 276, 277, 278, 279–280,
        279f–282f, 282–283
    PASH, 275–276
    tumors of nerve and nerve sheath origin, 284
Benign papillary tumors
    collagenous spherulosis, 37–39
    cystic and papillary apocrine metaplasia,
        45–48
    florid papillomatosis of nipple, 48–49
    intraductal papilloma, 27–37
    radial sclerosing lesions, 39–44
    subareolar sclerosing duct hyperplasia, 44–45
    syringomatous adenoma of nipple, 49–50
Benign phyllodes tumor, 86, 87f, 89f–91f, 93f–94f,
    95, 338f
Bilaterality in invasive lobular carcinoma,
    263–264
Blastomyces infection, 21
Blood vessel invasion, 154
Bloody nipple discharge, 9
Borderline atypical ductal hyperplasia, 107–108,
    110f
Breast Cancer Surveillance Consortium, 144
Breast carcinoma
    angiogenesis associated with, 154–155
    in children, 337
    in males, 332–334. *See also* Male breast lesions
    radiotherapy for Hodgkin disease and, 319
        supradiaphragmatic, 319
    risk for, atypical ductal hyperplasia, 118–119
    RR increased, 118, 119
    standard incidence ratio (SIR) for, 319

Breast conserving surgery
    for atypical hyperplasia, 141
    for medullary carcinoma, 189
Breast-conserving treatment, 319
Breast development, infantile, 1
Burkitt lymphoma, 303

C

Calcifications
    associated with intraductal carcinoma, 8f
    atypical ductal hyperplasia with, 106f
    columnar cell change with, 111, 112f
    in columnar cell lesions, 116
    cystic and papillary apocrine metaplasia with, 47f
    in ductal hyperplasia, 97
    in fibroadenoma, 77, 79f
    granular, in mucocele-like lesions, 208f
    intraductal carcinoma, associated with, 119–120
    in necrotic core of intraductal comedo carcinoma, 130–132
    ossifying, 114f, 116, 116f
    papillary carcinoma with, 176f
    pregnancy-like changes with, 6f
    pseudolactational changes with, 6f
    in tubular carcinoma, 162f
Calcium oxalate crystals, 15f
California Cancer Registry, 183
Capillary hemangioma, 287, 289, 289f
Carcinoembryonic antigen (CEA), 284
Cat-scratch disease, mammary lesions from, 26
Cavernous hemangioma, 287, 288f
CCH. *See* Columnar cell hyperplasia (CCH)
CCL. *See* Columnar cell lesions (CCL)
CDNA. *See* Complementary deoxyribonucleic acid (cDNA)
CEA. *See* Carcinoembryonic antigen (CEA)
CGH. *See* Comparative genomic hybridization (CGH)
CHC. *See* Cystic hypersecretory carcinoma (CHC)
Chemotherapy pathologic effect
    in breast, 325f, 326f
    histopathologic, 325, 326
    in lymphatic tumor emboli, 326f
    in lymph node with metastatic carcinoma, 327f
CHH. *See* Cystic hypersecretory hyperplasia (CHH)
Children: breast tumors
    breast carcinoma, 337
    fibroadenomas, 337
        vs. phyllodes tumors, 337
    juvenile atypical duct hyperplasia, 336, 337f, 338f
    juvenile papillomatosis (JP), 334–336
    papillary duct hyperplasia, 336
    phyllodes tumors, 337, 338f
        vs. fibroadenomas, 337
Chloroma, 308
Chondrolipoma, 284, 285f
Chondromyxoid metaplasia, 73
Chondrosarcoma, 298
Chromogenic in situ hybridization (CISH), 357
CISH. *See* Chromogenic in situ hybridization (CISH)
C-kit expression, in phyllodes tumor, 92
CK5/6 stains, in papillary carcinoma, 178
CK14 stains, in papillary carcinoma, 178
Classic invasive lobular carcinoma, 264f, 266, 272
Clear cell cytology, 6, 8, 8f
Clear cell type, intraductal carcinoma, 122–124, 123f
Clinging carcinoma. *See* Flat micropapillary intraductal carcinoma
Coccidioides infection, 21
Collagenized myofibroblastoma, 280, 280f
Collagenous spherulosis, 37–39, 226
    cribriform intraductal carcinoma in, 129
    with degenerative changes, 38f
    ductal hyperplasia with, 103–104, 104f
    LCIS in, 252, 255f
    in papilloma, 37f, 38f
    with in situ carcinoma, 38f
Columnar cell change (CCC), 108, 111, 111f–112f, 116
    tubular carcinoma and, 167

Columnar cell duct hyperplasia, coexistence with LCIS, 246
Columnar cell hyperplasia (CCH), 108, 109f, 111–117, 112f, 167–168
    with cytologic atypia, 111, 114f
    intraductal carcinoma and, 111, 114f–115f
    Ki67 indices of, 116
    LCIS and, 111, 115f
    with mild atypia, 111, 113f
    with moderate atypia, 111, 113f
Columnar cell lesions (CCL)
    calcifications in, 112f, 113f, 114f, 116, 116f
    carcinoma risk and, 117
    cytologic features of, 111
    by excisional biopsy, 117
    Ki67 index, 116
Comedo carcinoma
    calcifications, 130–132
    grading of, 136
    intraductal, 129–133
Comparative genomic hybridization (CGH), 56
Complementary deoxyribonucleic acid (cDNA), 357
Complex fibroadenoma, 68
Complex hemangioma, 289, 290f
Congo red–stain, 21
Connecticut Tumor Registry, 119
Cordylobia anthropophaga infection, 24
Core wash cytology, 353
Coumadin anticoagulant treatment, 9
Cribriform atypical ductal hyperplasia, 107, 108f–109f
Cribriform carcinoma, 237, 238, 239, 240
    invasive, 239f
Cribriform hyperplasia, 98, 99f, 101f–102f, 103f
Cribriform intraductal carcinoma, 129, 130f
Cryoablation, 85
    histologic effects of, 327
Cryptococcus infection, 21
Crystalline calcification, 112f, 113f, 114f, 116
Cutaneous myiasis, 23–24
Cyclosporin A, 77
Cylindroma, 223
Cyroprobe-assisted lumpectomy, 327
Cystic apocrine metaplasia, 45–48
Cysticercosis, 23, 24f
Cystic hypersecretory carcinoma (CHC)
    growth pattern of, 236
    hyperchromatic nuclei in, 234f
    intraductal, 235f, 236
    in lobules, 235f
Cystic hypersecretory hyperplasia (CHH), 6, 233
Cystic papilloma, 27, 28f
    with florid adenosis, 30f
Cytokeratin, 11
    immunostaining, 326
    markers in lymphoma, 307
Cytokeratin stains
    BE12, 178
    CK5/6, 178
    CK14, 178
    invasive duct carcinoma with, 157f
    invasive lobular carcinoma detection and, 268f
Cytologic atypia, 319, 321, 323f, 326
    atypical ductal hyperplasia with, 107, 109f–110f
    columnar cell hyperplasia with, 111, 114f
Cytologic pleomorphism in LCIS, 250–251

D

D2-40 antibody, lymphatic tumor emboli by, 150, 154
DCIS. *See* Ductal carcinoma in situ (DCIS)
Degeneration, in collagenous spherulosis, 38f
Dermatobia hominis infection, 23
Dermatomyositis, 19
Diabetic mastopathy, 19–21, 20f
Dimorphic papillary carcinoma, 177f
Dislodged fragment of carcinoma, 132, 132f–133f
Ductal carcinoma in situ (DCIS), 353
    coexistence with LCIS, 253, 255f
Ductal hyperplasia
    age distribution, 97
    atypical, pathology of, 104–108
    calcifications in, 97

    with collagenous spherulosis, 103–104, 104f
    florid. *See* Florid ductal hyperplasia
    vs. intraductal carcinoma, quantitative criteria, 104
    micropapillary, 98–99, 99f–100f
    with myoepithelial cells, 102, 103f
    with necrosis, 100, 102f
    papilloma with, 29f
    radiation atypia in, 322f
    squamous carcinoma in, 203f
    subareolar sclerosing, 44–45
    usual, patholgy of, 98–104
Ductal involvement
    of atypical lobular hyperplasia, 260f
    of LCIS, 252, 253f–254f
Duct carcinoma, invasive, 6f
Duct ectasia, 16f, 332
    mammary, 13–15, 14f
    and mastitis, 15f
    and stasis, 16f

E

E-cadherin
    defined, 267
    expression in invasive duct carcinoma *vs.* invasive lobular carcinoma, 267, 269
    immunoreactivity, 269
    intraductal carcinoma by, 135
    in invasive lobular carcinoma, 267, 269–270
    in LCIS, 247, 252
    mutations, 250
    small cell intraductal carcinoma, 125–126
    stain, 37
    in tubulolobular carcinoma, 166
    usage of, 354
Echinococcus granulosus, 23
Ectasia, mammary duct, 13–15
EGFR. *See* Epidermal growth factor receptor (EGFR)
Elastin, 39
Elastosis
    in stroma of invasive duct carcinoma, 156
    tubular carcinoma with, 166f
EMA. *See* Epithelial membrane antigen (EMA)
Embryology, 1
EMH. *See* Extramedullary hematopoiesis (EMH)
Encapsulated papillary carcinoma, 177–178
Endometrial carcinoma, metastatic, 314, 316, 317f
Endothelial hyaluronan receptor-1 (LYVE-1) antibody
    lymphatic tumor emboli by, 153
Epidermal growth factor receptor (EGFR), 73
Epidermoid inclusion cysts, 340
Epithelial cells
    displacement of, 340–341, 342f, 346–347
    in papillary carcinoma, 171, 175f
Epithelial changes in gynecomastia, 329, 331f
Epithelial hyperplasia
    in fibroadenoma, 81, 83
    in phyllodes tumor, 90, 93f–94f
Epithelial membrane antigen (EMA), 73, 284
Epithelioid myofibroblastoma, 280, 281f
Epstein–Barr virus (EBV)
    in medullary carcinoma, 187
Erdheim–Chester disease, 9, 17
Estrogen receptors, 229, 355
    Allred score system for, 355, 356t
    H-score system for, 355, 356t
    invasive lobular carcinoma, 271f
Excisional biopsy, 340, 342, 343f–346f
Extracellular mucin, papillary carcinoma with, 176f
Extralobular ducts, 2
Extramedullary hematopoeisis (EMH), 286–287
Extranodal sinus histiocytosis with massive lymphadenopathy, 309

F

Familial adenomatous polyposis (FAP), 274
FAP. *See* Familial adenomatous polyposis (FAP)
Fat, invasive lobular carcinoma obscured by, 265f
Fat necrosis, 9, 10f–11f
FEA. *See* Flat epithelial atypia (FEA)
Fibroadenoma
    age distribution of, 77

Fibroadenoma (*continued*)
  complex, 78
    with fibrocystic changes and pregnancy-like
      hyperplasia, 81*f*
    with sclerosing adenosis, 82*f*
  diagnosis and management, 83
  epithelial hyperplasia in, 81, 83
  growth patterns, 78, 79*f*
  juvenile, 81, 83*f*
  with sclerosis and calcification, 77, 79*f*
  stroma in, 78
  treatment, 85
  vs. phyllodes tumor, 83, 84*f*
  in young and elderly women, 78, 79*f*
Fibroadenomatoid mastopathy, 77, 78*f*
Fibrocystic changes, 332
Fibroepithelial neoplasms
  fibroadenoma, 77–86
  fibroadenomatoid mastopathy, 77
  phyllodes tumor, 86–95
Fibromatosis, 274, 275*f*, 276*f*, 282
Fibrosarcoma, 298
Fibrosis
  invasive lobular carcinoma obscured by, 265*f*
  periductal, in mammary duct ectasia, 14
Fibrous gynecomastia. *See* Inactive gynecomastia
Fibrous sclerosis, 29
Fibrous tumor, 274, 276*f*
"Filaria dance sign," 23
Filariasis, 23, 24*f*
FISH. *See* Fluorescent in situ hybridization (FISH)
Flat epithelial atypia (FEA), 108, 117
Flat micropapillary intraductal carcinoma, 111,
  115*f*, 128–129
Florid adenosis, 61, 63*f*
  cystic papilloma with, 30*f*
  in pregnancy, 64*f*
Florid ductal hyperplasia, 102*f*, 103*f*
  with histiocytes, 100–101, 102*f*
  vs. moderate ductal hyperplasia, 100
  with necrosis, 100, 100*f*–102*f*
  with streaming, 99, 101*f*
Florid gynecomastia, 329, 330*f*, 331*f*
Florid papillomatosis, 332
  of nipple, 48–49
Florid sclerosing adenosis, 9
Fluorescent in situ hybridization (FISH), 355
Focal fibrous disease, 274
Follicular phase, 3
Frozen section diagnosis
  of intraductal carcinoma, 120–121, 120*f*
  of invasive duct carcinoma, 144, 146*f*
Frozen section examination (FSE), of NCB
  specimens, 351, 353
FSE, of NCB specimens. *See* Frozen section
  examination (FSE), of NCB specimens
Fungal infections, 23

G
Gadolinium uptake, 263
Galactocele, 12–13
GCDFP-15. *See* Gross cystic disease fluid protein-
  15 (GCDFP-15)
Gel foam in needle core biopsy, 340, 341*f*
Giant cell arteritis, 18–19, 18*f*
Giant cells, 78
  in medullary carcinoma, 189
  osteoclast-like, mammary carcinoma with, 237,
    238*f*, 239*f*
  in phyllodes tumor, 90*f*
Glands, under tubular carcinoma, 162–163
Glycogen-rich carcinoma, 242–243, 242*f*
Grading
  adenoid cystic carcinoma, 223, 224
  of comedo carcinoma, 136
  of intraductal carcinoma, 127*t*, 135–137
  of invasive duct carcinomas, 148
  Scarff–Bloom–Richardson system, 150*t*
Granular calcifications, 111, 112*f*, 119–120
Granular cell tumors, 283–284, 283*f*
Granulation tissue
  epithelial displacement in, 341, 341*f*, 343*f*
  intraductal carcinoma in, 342*f*
Granulocytic leukemia, 308–309, 309*f*
Granulocytic sarcoma, 308–309

Granulomatous lobular mastitis, 15–16
Granulomatous lobulitis, 16, 17*f*
Granulomatous mastitis, 15–16
Gross cystic disease fluid protein-15 (GCDFP-15),
  14, 73
Growth patterns
  of adenoid cystic carcinoma, 223, 224*f*
  angiosarcoma, 294
  cribriform carcinoma, 239
  of cystic hypersecretory carcinoma, 236
  fibroadenoma, 78, 79*f*
  fibromatosis, 274
  invasive lobular carcinoma, 264, 265*f*, 266*f*
  juvenile papillomatosis, 336
  of leukemic infiltration, 309
  mammary carcinoma with osteoclast-like giant
    cells, 237
  medullary carcinoma, 188, 189
  metaplastic carcinoma, 191–192
  mucinous carcinoma, 205–206, 207*f*
  of non-Hodgkin lymphoma, 306
  papillary carcinoma, 172*f*
  prognosis of, 226
  secretory carcinoma, 229
Gynecomastia, 1
  with atypical ductal hyperplasia, 331*f*
  clinical signs of, 329
  diagnosis of, 329
    mammography, 329
  intermediate, 329, 330*f*
  phases of, 329
  pseudoangiomatous hyperplasia and, 329, 331*f*
Gynecomastia-like hyperplasia, 329

H
Hamartoma, 284
Hellenzellen, 6
Hemangioma
  atypical, 290, 290*f*
  capillary, 287, 289, 289*f*
  cavernous, 287, 288*f*
  complex, 289, 290*f*
  diagnosis of, 291
  nonparenchymal mammary, 292
  perilobular, 286, 287*f*
  venous, 291, 291*f*
Hemangiopericytoma, 298, 299, 300*f*
Hemorrhage
  after needle core biopsy, 340, 341*f*
  in breast infarct, 9
  invasive duct carcinoma with, 145*f*
Hemosiderin, 340
HER2/*neu* expression, 357
  secretory carcinoma and, 229
Heterologous metaplasia carcinoma, 199
Hibernoma, 286, 286*f*
Histiocytes, 335
  in fat necrosis, 9
  florid ductal hyperplasia with, 100–101, 102*f*
  in mammary duct ectasia, 13, 14*f*
Histiocytic lymphoma, 303
Histiocytoid lobular carcinoma, 266, 269*f*
Histiocytoma, malignant fibrous, 298, 299*f*
Histochemical score system, 355, 356*t*
Histologic grade, invasive duct carcinoma with,
  149*f*
Histologic grading, of invasive duct carcinoma, 148
Histology of breast, 1–3
Histoplasma capsulatum infection, 21
Hodgkin disease, 307–308
Hormone receptors, 355–356
HPV. *See* Human papilloma virus (HPV)
H-score system, 355, 356*t*
Human papilloma virus (HPV)
  in medullary carcinoma, 187
Hyperelastosis, 14
Hyperplasia
  atypical
    ductal. *See* Atypical ductal hyperplasia
    lobular, 111, 116, 257–260, 322*f*, 323*f*
    papilloma with, 36*f*
    pregnancy-like, 6, 7*f*
    in sclerosing adenosis, 68, 70*f*
  columnar cell, 108–117, 109*f*
  cribriform, 98, 99*f*, 101*f*–102*f*, 103*f*

ductal. *See* Ductal hyperplasia
epithelial
  in fibroadenoma, 81, 83
  in phyllodes tumor, 90, 93*f*–94*f*
florid. *See* Florid ductal hyperplasia
lactational, 3*f*–4*f*
micropapillary, 98–99, 99*f*–100*f*
mild, 98, 98*f*, 100*f*
moderate, 98–101, 99*f*, 100*f*
myoepithelial cell, 54*f*, 57*f*
pseudolactational, 5–6

I
Immature breast, 1, 2*f*
Immunohistochemistry
  metaplastic carcinoma, 200–201
  papillary carcinoma by, 177
  tubular carcinoma by, 165*f*
Immunoreactivity
  invasive micropapillary carcinoma, 244
  in medullary carcinoma, 189
  phyllodes tumor, 92
  tubulolobular carcinoma, 166–167
Immunostain markers, 59
Immunostains, 11, 29, 39, 49, 52, 307
  34BE12, 166–167, 177, 178, 200
  CK5/6, 157–158, 177, 178
  CK14, 157–158, 177, 178
  E-cadherin, 247, 251, 252, 253, 268*f*
  Ki67, 287, 294, 295
  p63, 31, 102, 134, 139, 163, 174, 181, 340, 345*f*
Implant-associated mastitis, 19*f*
Inactive gynecomastia, 329, 330*f*
Infarct
  with atypical cells, 12*f*
  breast, 9, 11
  of papillary carcinoma, 183*f*
Infarction
  adenomyoepithelioma with, 56*f*
  in hemangiomas, 289
  in papillary carcinoma, 181
  papillomas with, 31, 34, 34*f*
Infections
  bacterial, 6
  fungal, 23
  mycobacterial, 24–26
  nontuberculous bacterial, 26
  parasitic, 23–24
Infiltrating, myofibroblastoma, 280, 282*f*
Infiltrating carcinoma. recurrence after
  radiotherapy, 324*f*
Infiltrating duct carcinoma in males, 332*f*, 333*f*
Inflammatory and reactive tumors
  amyloid tumor, 21
  breast infarct, 9, 11
  diabetic mastopathy, 19–21
  fat necrosis, 9
  galactocele, 12–13
  granulomatous mastitis, 15–16
  inflammatory pseudotumor, 17
  mammary duct ectasia, 13–15
  plasma cell mastitis, 13
  silicone mastitis, 19
  vasculitis, 17–19
Inflammatory pseudotumor, 17, 18*f*
Interstitial laser therapy, 327
Intracytoplasmic mucin
  intraductal carcinoma, 123*f*
  papillary carcinoma with, 175*f*, 180–181
  tubular carcinoma with, 164*f*
Intracytoplasmic mucin vacuoles in LCIS, 251
Intraductal carcinoma, 332, 334
  in adenosis, 66, 69–70
  arising in sclerosing adenosis, 134–135
  associated with
    mucinous carcinoma, 205, 206*f*
    mucocele-like lesions with, 207
    small cell carcinoma, 240
  and atypical columnar cell hyperplasia, 111, 114*f*
  calcifications, 8*f*
  CCH and, 111, 114*f*–115*f*
  clinical diagnosis of, 119–120
  coexistence with LCIS, 253, 255*f*
  epithelial displacement in, 341, 342, 342*f*–345*f*
  frequency of, 119

frozen-section diagnosis of, 120–121
grading of, 127t, 135–137
histologic appearances of, 334
with invasion, 139, 140f
in invasive micropapillary carcinoma, 243
with lobular extension in medullary carcinoma, 189
with lymphatic tumor emboli and lymph node metastasis, 346f
and microinvasion, 137–139
micropapillary, 127–129
and myoepithelial cells, 122f
with obliterative sclerosis, 133
pathology of, 121–135
in radial sclerosing lesions, 135
recurrent, after radiotherapy, 323f
reporting necrosis in, 127t
signet ring cells in, 122, 123f
size of, 137
tubular carcinoma with, 167f
Intraductal papilloma, 27–37
in the male breast, 329, 332
Intraductal squamous carcinoma, 202, 203f
Intramammary lymph nodes, 309, 310f–311f, 311
Invasion
blood vessel, 154
intraductal carcinoma with, 139, 140f
in solid papillary carcinoma, 177–178, 181, 182f–185f
Invasive carcinoma
diagnosis of, 340, 343f, 347
LCIS and, 261
Invasive duct carcinoma
with angiogenesis, 155f
elastosis in stroma of, 156
frozen section diagnosis of, 144, 146f
with hemorrhage, 145f
histologic and nuclear grading of, 148
histologic grade, 149f
lacking myoepithelium, 156
and lobular carcinoma, 145f
with lymphatic tumor emboli, 150, 152f
lymphoplasmacytic infiltration in, 151f
with myoepithelial markers, 156
with necrosis, 153f–154f
nuclear grade, 151f
with perineural invasion, 155
risk for local recurrence, 154
with shrinkage artefact, 152f–153f
size, 144, 146
MRI and, 148
and multifocal tumor, 147–148
and needle core biopsy specimen, 147
and prognosis, 147
special types of, 237–244
tumors subset of, 144
Invasive lobular carcinoma
in benign phyllodes tumor, 268f
cytologic features of, 264, 266
diagnostic sonography for, 263
E-cadherin expression, 267, 269–270
frequency of bilaterality in, 263–264
growth patterns, 264, 265f, 266f
histology of, 264
lobular carcinoma in situ in, 266, 267f, 268f
with lymphocytic reaction, 266f
mammographic manifestation of, 263
metastatic, 270–272
minimal lesion, 267f, 268f
obscured by fat and by fibrosis, 265f
pleomorphic and histiocytoid types, 266, 269f
prevalence in older women, 263
prognosis, 272
with signet ring cells, 269f
symptoms of, 263
trabecular variant, 267f
variant forms of, 264, 266
Invasive lobular carcinoma vs. ductal carcinoma
age factors in, 263
contralateral carcinoma in, 263
E-cadherin expression in, 267, 270f
neoadjuvant therapy for, 272
Invasive micropapillary carcinoma, 243–244, 243f
Invasive squamous carcinoma, 202, 203f
Isolated tumor cells, 347

J
JP. See Juvenile papillomatosis (JP)
Juvenile fibroadenoma, 81, 83f
Juvenile papillomatosis (JP), 334–336
excisional biopsy for, 336
histologic examination of, 335
mammographic findings in, 335
sonographic appearance of, 335

K
Keloidal, fibromatosis, 274, 275f
Ki67 immunostain, 287, 294, 295
Ki67 index, 116

L
Lactating adenoma, 81, 83f
Lactating glands, 4f
Lactational hyperplasia, 3f–4f
Lactiferous ducts, 1–2
Lactiferous sinus, 2
Lamprocytosis, 6
Lapatinib, 357
LCIS. See Lobular carcinoma in situ (LCIS); Lobular carcinoma in situ (LCIS)
Leiomyoma, 285, 285f
Leiomyomatous hamartoma, 285, 286f
Leiomyosarcoma, 295, 297, 298f
metastatic, 317f
Leukemic infiltration, 308, 309
growth pattern of, 309
Linear calcifications, 119–120
Lipid rich carcinoma, 241–242, 242f
Lipofuscin pigment, 2
Lipomas, 285, 286
diagnosis of, 286
spindle cell, 279, 280, 282, 286
Lipomatous myofibroblastoma, 279
Liposarcoma, 298, 298f
Loa loa infection, 23
Lobular cancerization, 121
Lobular carcinoma
invasive, 263–273
invasive duct carcinoma and, 145f
in males, 334
Lobular carcinoma in situ (LCIS), 69, 246–257, 261
in adenosis, 69
in collagenous spherulosis, 252, 255f
with columnar cell change, 111, 115f
columnar cell duct hyperplasia and, 246
cytologic features, 251–252
cytologic pleomorphism in, 250–251
diagnosis of, 247, 251, 253
differential, 253
ductal involvement, 253f–254f
E-cadherin immunostain in, 247, 251, 252, 253
histopathologic appearance of, 246
intracytoplasmic mucin vacuoles in, 251
intraductal carcinoma and, 135
invasion and, 255–256
in invasive lobular carcinoma, 261, 266, 267f, 268f
marker lesion, 261
precursor to, 261
loss of cohesion of neoplastic cells in, 247
glandular lumina and, 247
mosaic pattern, 252f
in postmenopausal women, 246, 251, 252
retrospective studies, 257
sclerosing adenosis and, 71f, 246, 252f, 256
tubular adenosis with, 71f
tubular carcinoma and, 169f
Lobular extension
atypical ductal hyperplasia with, 105–107, 107f
intraductal carcinoma with, 121f
Lobules
altered by pregnancy-like change, 3–5
anatomy, 2
atrophy, 246–247, 248f
radiation-induced, 320f
cystic hypersecretory carcinoma into, 235f
in fibrocollagenous stroma, 2f
in mammary adipose tissue, 2f
progressive recruitment of, 3

Lobulitis
granulomatous, 16, 17f
lymphocytic, 21f
Low-grade adenosquamous carcinoma, 194–195, 196f–197f
Low-grade papillary carcinoma, 173f–174f
Lumpectomy
for intraductal carcinoma, 141, 157
for papillary carcinoma, 181
for tubular carcinoma, 170
Lupron, 332
Lupus erythematosus, 19
Lupus mastitis, 19
Luteal phase, 3
LVI. See Lymphovascular involvement (LVI)
Lymphatic tumor emboli
chemotherapy effect in, 326f
by D2-40 antibody, 150, 154
intraductal carcinoma with, 346f
invasive duct carcinoma with, 150, 152f, 153–154
in invasive lobular carcinoma, 267
by LYVE-1 antibody, 153
Lymphocytic leukemia, 309, 309f
Lymphocytic lobulitis, 21f
Lymphocytic reaction
invasive lobular carcinoma with, 264, 266f. See also Lymphoepithelioma-like carcinoma
Lymphoepithelioma-like carcinoma, 264
Lymphoid and hematopoietic tumors, 303–311
extranodal sinus histiocytosis with massive lymphadenopathy, 309
Hodgkin disease, 307–308
intramammary lymph nodes, 309–311
leukemic infiltration, 308, 309
non-hodgkin lymphoma, 303, 306, 307
plasmacytic tumors, 308
Lymphomas
anaplastic large cell, 303
appearance of, 306
Burkitt, 303
histiocytic, 303
malignant, 304f–306f
MALT, 303
non-hodgkin, 303, 306, 307
signet ring cell, 306
T-cell, 303
Lymphoplasmacytic infiltration, in invasive duct carcinoma, 151f
Lymphoplasmacytic reaction, of medullary carcinoma, 187, 188f
Lymphovascular involvement (LVI), assessment of, 354
Lysozyme, 73
LYVE-1. See Endothelial hyaluronan receptor-1 (LYVE-1)

M
Magnetic resonance imaging (MRI), 1, 16, 319, 350
angiosarcomas and, 293
for atypical ductal hyperplasia, 97
for intraductal carcinomas, 120
for invasive lobular carcinoma, 263
vs. mammography, for intraductal carcinoma, 120
size and, 148
Male breast lesions
benign proliferative, 329, 331–332
fibroepithelial tumors, 332
gynecomastia, 329
intraductal papillomas, 329, 332
carcinoma, 332–334
age factors in, 332
estrogen receptor expression, 332, 334
intraductal, 332, 334
prognosis of, 334
prostatic carcinoma and, 334
vs. female breast carcinoma, 332
Malignant fibrous histiocytoma, 298, 299f
Malignant lymphoma, 304f–306f
in PASH, 306f
Malignant neoplasms, nonmammary, metastases in breast from, 313–318
Malignant phyllodes tumor, 89, 92f–93f
MALT. See Mucosa-associated lymphoid tissue (MALT)

Mammary carcinoma with osteoclast-like giant cells, 237, 238f, 239f
Mammary duct ectasia, 13–15
Mammograms, 332
Mammography, 1, 309, 319, 325, 340, 343f, 350
  of fat necrosis, 9
  for invasive lobular carcinoma, 263
  vs. MRI for invasive lobular carcinoma, 263
  vs. ultrasonography for invasive lobular carcinoma, 263
Markers
  cytokeratin, 307
  endothelial
    lymphatic tumor emboli by, 153
  for intraductal carcinoma, 136
  for metaplastic carcinoma, 191, 200
  myoepithelial, 102–103
    invasive duct carcinoma with, 156
    for tubular carcinoma, 163–164
  for papillary carcinoma, 174
  spindle cell intraductal carcinomas, 124–125
  of stromal proliferative activity, 83, 95
Mast cells, in invasive duct carcinoma, 150
Mastectomy, 346, 347
  for intraductal carcinoma, 141
  for lymphatic tumor emboli, 154
  for medullary carcinoma, 189
  for tubular carcinoma, 169
Mastitis
  AIDS-related, 26
  granulomatous, 15–16
  implant-associated, 19f
  lupus, 19
  plasma cell, 13
  silicone, 19
  tuberculous, 24–26, 25f
Mastopathy, diabetic, 19–21, 20f
Matrix-producing carcinoma, 200
Medullary carcinoma
  EBV in, 187
  giant cells in, 189
  histopathologic features of, 187
  HPV in, 187
  intraductal carcinoma with lobular extension, 189
  lymphoplasmacytic reaction of, 187
  metastatic, 316
  microscopic circumscription of, 188
  prognosis of, 189
  syncytial growth pattern of, 188, 189f
Melanoma, metastatic malignant, 313, 315f
Menopause
  hormonal alterations during and after, 3
  postmenopausal LCIS, 252f
Menstrual phase, 3
Mesenchymal neoplasms
  benign mesenchymal tumors, 274–292
  sarcomas, 292–300
Messenger ribonucleic acid (mRNA), 316
Metaplastic carcinoma
  acantholytic type, 198f
  distinction from sarcoma, 199
  growth patterns in, 191–192
  heterologous, 199
  immunohistochemical studies, 200–201
  low-grade adenosquamous carcinoma, 194–195, 196f–197f
  matrix-producing variant, 200
  osteocartilaginous metaplasia, 199f
  with osteosarcomatous differentiation, 199f
  prognosis of, 201
  spindle cell type, 193f–195f
  squamous metaplasia, 192f
Metastases in breast, from nonmammary malignant neoplasms, 313–318
Metastatic carcinoma
  in intramammary lymph node, 309, 311
  lobular, 270–272
  lymph node with, chemotherapy effect in, 327f
Metastatic squamous carcinoma, 202, 204
MGA. *See* Microglandular adenosis (MGA)
MIB-1, 83
Microcalcification, 332, 334f, 336
Microglandular adenosis (MGA), 72–76, 74f
  carcinoma arising in, 73–74, 76
  immunoreactivity of, 73

Microinvasion, intraductal carcinoma and, 137–139
Micropapillary atypical ductal hyperplasia, 106f–107f, 109f
Micropapillary carcinoma, invasive, 243–244, 243f
Micropapillary ductal hyperplasia, 98–99, 99f–100f
Micropapillary intraductal carcinoma, 127–129
Microscopic circumscription, of medullary carcinoma, 188
Mild hyperplasia, 98, 98f, 100f
Moderate ductal hyperplasia, 98–101, 99f, 100f
Morphologic changes, radiation-induced, 321
Mosaic pattern of LCIS, 252f
MRI. *See* Magnetic resonance imaging (MRI)
MRNA. *See* Messenger ribonucleic acid (mRNA)
Mucin
  extracellular
    papillary carcinoma with, 176f
  intracytoplasmic
    intraductal carcinoma, 123f
    papillary carcinoma with, 175f, 180–181
    tubular carcinoma with, 164f
Mucinous carcinoma, 319
  argyrophilic granules in, 206
  benign and malignant, 209
  granular calcification in, 208f
  mucocele-like lesions in, 207–208, 208f
  pure, 205, 210–211
Mucocele-like lesions
  with atypical ductal hyperplasia, 209
  benign, 207, 208f
  intraductal carcinoma, 207
  in mucinous carcinoma, 207–208, 208f
Mucosa-associated lymphoid tissue (MALT), 303
Multiple papillomas, 27
Mycobacterial infections, 24–26
Mycobacterium abscesses, 26
Mycobacterium fortuitum, 26
Mycobacterium tuberculosis infection, 24–26
Myeloperoxidase, 308
Myiasis, cutaneous, 23–24
Myoepithelial carcinoma, in adenomyoepithelioma, 57f–58f
Myoepithelial cell hyperplasia, 54f
  adenomyoepithelioma with, 57f
Myoepithelial cells
  anatomy and histology, 2
  ductal hyperplasia with, 102, 103f
  intraductal carcinoma and, 122f
  markers, 102–103
  papillomas with, 33f
  p63 immunostain for, 340, 345f
Myoepithelial markers, 11
Myoepithelial neoplasms
  adenomyoepithelioma, 52–59
  myoepithelioma, 59–60
Myoepithelioma, 52, 59–60
Myoepithelium
  invasive duct carcinoma lacking, 156
  papillary carcinoma lacking, 177
  in solid papillary carcinoma, 177
Myofibroblastic hyperplasia, 340
Myofibroblastoma, 276, 277, 278, 279–280, 279f–282f, 282–283, 332
  epithelioid variant of, 280, 281f
  infiltrative variant of, 280, 282f
Myofibroblasts, in PASH, 276
Myoid cells, plump, 280
Myoid differentiation, adenomyoepithelioma with, 56f
Myoid hamartoma, 285, 286f
Myoid metaplasia
  around atrophic duct, 5f
  of myoepithelial cells, 5f
  sclerosing adenosis with, 67f
Myxoid myofibroblastoma, 280, 282f
Myxoid stroma, fibroadenomas with, 80f

N

National Cancer Institute, 332
NCB specimens. *See* Needle core biopsy (NCB) specimens
Necrosis. *See also* Fat necrosis
  ductal hyperplasia with, 100, 102f
  invasive duct carcinoma with, 153f–154f
  reporting in intraductal carcinoma, 127t

Needle core biopsy, 3
  atypical ductal hyperplasia, diagnosis of, 117–118
  epithelial displacement in, 340–342, 342f–345f, 346–347
  gel foam in, 340, 341f
Needle core biopsy (NCB) specimens, 348–358
  ancillary studies, 355–358
  fixation of, 348
  frozen section examination, 351, 353
  gross description, 348–349
  inked, 349f
  pathology report of, 353–354
  processing of, 349–350
  procurement, 348
  radiologic findings, correlation with, 350–351
  requisition form, 348
  role of, pathology report in patient care, 355
  size and, 147
  standardized reporting, 354–355
  touch imprint cytology, 353
Needling procedures, pathological changes associated with, 340–347, 345f
Negative predictive value (NPV), 353
Neoadjuvant chemotherapy, 325, 326
  effect in tumor cellularity, 325, 326f
Neoplastic cells, loss of cohesion in LCIS, 247
Nerves and nerve sheath, tumors originating in, 284
Neuroendocrine intraductal carcinoma, 124–125
Neuron-specific enolase (NSE), 240
Neutrophils, 25
Nipple, 1–2
  florid papillomatosis of, 48–49
  syringomatous adenoma of, 49–50
Non-Hodgkin lymphoma, 303, 306, 307
  growth patterns of, 306
Non-Langerhans cell histiocytosis, 9
Nonmammary malignant neoplasms, metastases in breast from, 313–318
Nonparenchymal angiolipoma, 292f, 293f
Nonparenchymal mammary hemangioma, 292
Nontuberculous bacterial infections, 26
NPV. *See* Negative predictive value (NPV)
NSE. *See* Neuron-specific enolase (NSE)
Nuclear estrogen receptor immunoreactivity in gynecomastia, 329
Nuclear grade, invasive duct carcinoma with, 151f
Nuclear grading, of invasive duct carcinoma, 148

O

Oat cell carcinoma. *See* Small cell carcinoma
Obliterative sclerosis, intraductal carcinoma with, 133
Ochrocytes, 2, 13, 14f
Oncoprotein expression in apocrine adenosis, 66
Ossifying calcifications, 114f, 116, 116f, 169
Osteocartilaginous metaplasia, metaplastic carcinoma, 199f
Osteochrondrosarcoma, 299f
Osteoclast-like giant cells, mammary carcinoma with, 237, 238f, 239f
Osteogenic sarcoma, 298
Osteosarcomatous differentiation, metaplastic carcinoma with, 199f
Ovarian carcinoma, metastatic, 314, 316f

P

Paget disease
  of nipple epidermis, 49
  and tubular carcinoma: differential diagnosis, 161
Pagetoid spread of LCIS, 252, 253, 253f
Papillary apocrine metaplasia, 45–48
Papillary carcinoma
  arising in papilloma, 176f
  with calcification, 176f
  diagnosis of, 178, 180
  with dimorphic differentiation, 177f
  encapsulated, 177
  epithelial cells in, 171, 175f
  with extracellular mucin, 176f
  fibrovascular stroma in, 171
  growth patterns of, 172f
  by immunohistochemistry, 177

infarction in, 181
with intracytoplasmic mucin, 175f, 180–181
invasion in, 181
lacking myoepithelium, 177
low-grade, 173f–174f
in males, 332, 333f
prognosis, 183
risk of local recurrence, 181
snouts in, 175f
solid, 171, 177, 178f–185f
treatment, 181
Papillary hyperplasia involving multiple ducts, 336, 337f
Papillary intraductal carcinoma, 134
tubular carcinoma with, 169f
Papilloma, 336
collagenous spherulosis in, 37f, 38f
with ductal hyperplasia, 29f
infarcted, 9, 11, 12f
infarction in, 9
intraductal, 27–37
papillary carcinoma arising in, 176f
Papillomatosis, 27, 336, 337f
florid, of nipple, 48–49
juvenile, 334–336
Parasitic infections, 23–24
Parenchyma, 347
Parenchymal angiosarcoma, 294
PAS. See Periodic acid-Schiff (PAS) stain
PASH. See Pseudoangiomatous stromal hyperplasia (PASH)
Patient care, role of NCB specimens pathology report in, 355
Periductal fibrosis, 14
in mammary duct ectasia, 14
Periductal stroma, histology, 2
Periductal stromal tumors, 86
Perilobular hemangioma, 286, 287f
Perineural invasion
adenosis with, 69f
invasive duct carcinoma with, 155
Periodic acid-Schiff (PAS) stain, 5, 14, 229, 251
PET. See Positron emission tomography (PET)
Phyllodes tumor (PT)
age distribution of, 86
benign, 86, 87f, 89f–91f, 93f–94f, 95
diagnosis, 86
epithelial hyperplasia in, 90, 93f–94f
fibroadenoma vs., 83, 84f
malignant, 89, 92f–93f
papillary, 88f
stroma in, 86, 89–90, 92
Physiologic morphology of breast, 3–8
P63 immunostain, 31, 340, 345f
Plasma cell mastitis, 13
Plasmacytic tumors, 308
Plasmacytoma, 308f
Pleomorphic adenomas, 52
Pleomorphic invasive lobular carcinoma
estrogen and progesterone receptors and, 266
P63 markers, 102
for metaplastic carcinoma, 191, 193
for papillary carcinomas, 174, 177, 181
Polyarteritis, 19
Polyposis, familial adenomatous, 274
Positive predictive value (PPV), 27, 353
Positron emission tomography (PET), 350
Postbiopsy scar, 340, 345f
PPV. See Positive predictive value (PPV)
Precocious puberty, 1
Pregnancy
florid adenosis in, 64f
secretory changes associated with, 3
Pregnancy-like change. See Pseudolactational hyperplasia
Premature thelarche, 1
Primary amyloid tumors, 21
Processing of NCB specimens, 349–350
Procurement of NCB specimens, 348
Progesterone receptors, 3, 229, 355
Allred score system for, 355, 356t
H-score system for, 355, 356t
Prognosis
of angiosarcoma, 295
invasive duct carcinoma, 147

invasive micropapillary carcinoma, 244
of medullary carcinoma, 189
of metaplastic carcinoma, 201
papillary carcinoma, 183
small cell carcinoma, 240
squamous carcinoma, 204
tubular carcinoma, 169–170
Proliferative phase, 3
Prostate-specific antigen (PSA), 334
Prostatic carcinoma, 313, 314
PSA. See Prostate-specific antigen (PSA)
Pseudoangiomatous hyperplasia, 329, 331f
Pseudoangiomatous stromal hyperplasia (PASH), 86
age distribution of, 275, 276
bilateral involvement, 276
fascicular, 278f, 279f
malignant lymphoma in, 306f
mistaken for angiosarcoma, 287
myofibroblasts in, 276
phyllodes tumor with, 91f
Pseudolactational hyperplasia
atypical, 6, 7f
with calcification, 5, 6f
physiologic morphology of, 5
Pseudolymphoma, 307, 307f
Pseudomonas aeruginosa infection, 26
Pseudotumor, inflammatory, 17, 18f
PT. See Phyllodes tumor (PT)
Puberty, 1, 2f
Pulmonary carcinoma, metastatic, 313, 314f
Pulmonary small cell carcinoma, 241

Q

Quantitative criteria, in diagnosis of atypical ductal hyperplasia, 104–105

R

Radial scar, 39
tubular carcinoma arising in, 163f
Radial sclerosing lesions (RSL), 39–44
intraductal carcinoma in, 135
and tubular carcinoma: differential diagnosis, 164–165
Radiation, pathologic effects
arteritis, 321f
atrophy of lobules, 320f
ductal atypia, 321f–323f
histologic changes, 319
recurrent intraductal carcinoma after radiotherapy, 323f
Radiation therapy
adenoid cystic carcinoma and, 226
role of, in secretory carcinoma, 232
Radiologic findings, correlation with NCB specimens, 350–351
Radiotherapy, for intraductal carcinoma, 141
Recurrence
after radiotherapy
carcinoma, 324f
intraductal carcinoma, 323f
hemangiopericytoma, 299
invasive duct carcinoma, 157
medullary carcinoma, 189
role of core biopsy-induced epithelial displacement in, 346–347
Reed-Sternberg cells, 307
Renal carcinoma, metastatic, 314f
Reports on NCB specimens
pathology report, 353–354
in patient care, 355
standardized reports, 354–355
Requisition form, NCB specimens, 348
Reticulin stain, 11
Retraction artefact. See Shrinkage artefact
Retrospective study, of LCIS, 257
Ribonucleic acid (RNA), 357
RNA. See Ribonucleic acid (RNA)
Rosai–Dorfman disease, 309
RSL. See Radial sclerosing lesions (RSL)

S

S-100, 5, 59
Salmonella infection, 26
Sarcoidosis, 16, 17f

Sarcoma
angiosarcoma, 293–295
distinction from metaplastic carcinoma, 197, 199
fibrosarcoma, 298
granulocytic, 308–309
hemangiopericytoma, 298, 299, 300f
leiomyosarcoma, 295, 297, 298f
liposarcoma, 298, 298f
malignant fibrous histiocytoma, 298, 299f
osteogenic and chondrosarcomas, 298
Scar
radial, 39
tubular carcinoma arising in, 163f
tissue, 340, 345f
Scarff–Bloom–Richardson grading system, 150t
Schaumann bodies, 16
Schistosomiasis, 23, 25f
Schwannoma, 284, 284f
Scleroderma, 19
Sclerosing adenosis, 61, 64f–66f
with apocrine intraductal carcinoma, 72f
atypical hyperplasia in, 68, 70f
complex fibroadenoma with, 82f
with intraductal carcinoma, 72f
intraductal carcinoma arising in, 134–135
with lobular carcinoma in situ, 71f
with microinvasive lobular carcinoma, 73f
and tubular carcinoma: differential diagnosis, 163–164
Sclerosing lobular hyperplasia, 77
Sclerosing papilloma, 336
Sclerosis
fibroadenoma with, 79f
papilloma with, 32f
Scoring system for VNPI, 127, 129t
Secretory carcinoma
with apocrine cytology, 230f
ETV6-NTRK3 gene fusion in, 229
growth patterns, 229
HER2/neu expression and, 229
radiation therapy in, role of, 232
STAT5a and, 229
Secretory hyperplasia in fibroadenoma, 81
Secretory phase, 3
SEER. See Surveillance, Epidemiology, and End Results (SEER)
Sentinel lymph node (SLN), 347
biopsy, 334
mapping, 190
for tubular carcinoma, 170
Shrinkage artefact, invasive duct carcinoma with, 152f–153f
Signet ring cell
in intraductal carcinomas, 122, 123f
invasive lobular carcinoma with, 269f
in lobular carcinoma in situ, 71f
lymphoma, 306
Silicone mastitis, 19
Silver in situ hybridization (SISH), 357
SISH. See Silver in situ hybridization (SISH)
Size
adenoid cystic carcinoma, 223
of intraductal carcinoma, 137
of invasive duct carcinomas, 144, 146–147
SLN. See Sentinel lymph node (SLN)
Small cell carcinoma, 240–241, 241f, 334
intraductal, 125–126
Solid intraductal carcinoma, 129, 131f
Solid invasive lobular carcinoma, 266f
Solid papillary carcinoma, 171, 177, 178f–185f
with mucinous differentiation, 182f
Solid papilloma, 31f
Solitary papilloma, 27
Sonography
in diagnosis of invasive lobular carcinoma, 263
for nonparenchymal mammary hemangiomas, 292
Spindle cell carcinoma
of breast, 192, 193f
intraductal, 124, 125f
metaplastic, 193f–195f
Spindle cell lipomas, 279, 280, 282, 286
Spindle cell neoplasms, 60
Spirometra, 23
Squamocolumnar junction, 1–2

Squamous carcinoma
  in duct hyperplasia, 203f
  intraductal, 202, 203f
  invasive, 202, 203f
  metaplastic, 202, 204
  prognosis of, 204
Squamous metaplasia, 2, 11
  metaplastic carcinoma, 192f
  papilloma with, 34, 35f
Stroma
  alterations, in tubular carcinoma, 167
  collagenization in intraductal papilloma, 78
  epithelial displacement, 340
  in fibroadenoma, 78
  fibrofatty, 5f
  intralobular, 2f
  of invasive duct carcinoma, elastosis in, 156
  in phyllodes tumor, 86, 89–90, 92
  pseudoangiomatous hyperplasia of, 329, 331f
Stromal inflammatory cell infiltrates, 148, 150
Stromal mitoses, 340
Stromal reaction, 340
Subareolar sclerosing duct hyperplasia, 44–45
Surveillance, Epidemiology, and End Results
  (SEER), 95, 119
Syncytial growth pattern, of medullary carcinoma,
  188, 189f
Syringomatous adenoma of nipple, 49–50

T
Taenia solium infection, 23
Tamoxifen treatment, 141

T-cell lymphoma, 303
Therapy: pathologic effect
  ablation therapy, 326–327
  chemotherapy, 324–326
  pretreatment *vs.* posttreatment specimen, 319,
    321, 324, 325, 326
  radiation, 319–324
TIC. *See* Touch imprint cytology (TIC)
Touch imprint cytology (TIC), 353
Trabecular invasive lobular carcinoma, 267f
Trastuzumab, 357
Trichinella infection, 23
Triple-negative carcinoma
  defined, 157
  invasive duct carcinoma with, 158f
Tuberculosis, 24–26, 25f
Tuberculous mastitis, 24–26, 25f
Tubular adenomyoepithelioma, 52
Tubular adenosis, 67, 70f
  LCIS in, 256f
  with lobular carcinoma, 71f
Tubular carcinoma
  calcifications in, 162f
  carcinomatous ductules in, 162f
  diagnosis of, 165
  differential diagnosis of, 163–165
  with elastosis, 166f
  glands of, 162–163, 164f
  histological sections of, 161–162
  immunohistochemistry, 165f
  with intracytoplasmic mucin, 164f
  with intraductal carcinoma, 167f

and LCIS, 169f
  in male, 333f
  with papillary intraductal carcinoma, 169f
  prognosis, 169–170
  in radial scar, 163f
  and RSL: differential diagnosis, 40, 43, 164–165
  and sclerosing adenosis: differential diagnosis,
    163–164
  size, 161
  stromal alterations in, 163, 165f, 167
Tubulolobular carcinoma
  defined, 165, 166f
  immunoreactivity in, 166–167
  size, 166

U
Usual ductal hyperplasia, 98–104

V
Van Nuys Prognostic Index (VNPI), 127, 129t
Vascular endothelial growth factor (VEGF), 237
Vascular spaces, carcinoma cells in, 340, 344f, 347
Vasculitis, 17–19
VEGF. *See* Vascular endothelial growth factor
  (VEGF)
Venous hemangioma, 291, 291f
VNPI. *See* Van Nuys Prognostic Index (VNPI)

W
Wegener granulomatosis, 19
Wuchereria bancrofti infection, 23